CLINICAL TEXTBOOK OF ADDICTIVE DISORDERS

Clinical Textbook
of Addictive Disorders

THIRD EDITION

Edited by
RICHARD J. FRANCES
SHELDON I. MILLER
AVRAM H. MACK

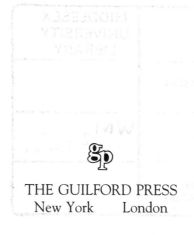

THE GUILFORD PRESS
New York   London

© 2005 The Guilford Press
A Division of Guilford Publications, Inc.
72 Spring Street, New York, NY 10012
www.guilford.com

Printed in the United States of America

This book is printed on acid-free paper.

Last digit is print number: 9   8   7   6   5   4   3   2   1

Library of Congress Cataloging-in-Publication Data

Clinical textbook of addictive disorders / edited by Richard J. Frances, Sheldon I.
Miller, Avram H. Mack.—3rd ed.
    p. cm.
  Includes bibliographical references and index.
  ISBN 1-59385-174-X (hardcover)
  1. Substance abuse.   2. Alcoholism.   I. Frances, Richard J.   II. Miller, Sheldon I.
III. Mack, Avram H.
  RC564.C55 2005
  616.86—dc22
                                                                        2004026092

About the Editors

Richard J. Frances, MD, is Clinical Professor in the Department of Psychiatry at New York University School of Medicine and Director of Public and Professional Education at Silver Hill Hospital in New Canaan, Connecticut. He is also in private practice in New York City. Dr. Frances was former President and Medical Director at Silver Hill Hospital; was founding president of the American Academy of Addiction Psychiatry; and helped found and chaired the Council of Addiction Psychiatry for the American Psychiatric Association. He is the author of several hundred articles and several books, and is on numerous editorial boards of journals. Dr. Frances frequently lectures on addiction psychiatry and has appeared numerous times as a guest on *Court TV*.

Sheldon I. Miller, MD, is the Lizzie Gilman Professor of Psychiatry and former Chairman of the Department of Psychiatry and Behavioral Sciences at Northwestern University. During his career, he has served on many boards and committees of many national and local organizations. Dr. Miller has authored or coauthored over 60 scientific articles, chapters, and books. He is Editor-in-Chief of the *American Journal on Addictions* and was a founder of the American Academy of Addiction Psychiatry. Dr. Miller is on the Board of Directors of the Accreditation Council for Graduate Medical Education and the American Board of Emergency Medicine. He also currently serves as Vice Chair of the American Psychiatric Association's Council on Medical Education and Lifelong Learning.

Avram H. Mack, MD, is Assistant Professor of Psychiatry at the Institute of Psychiatry of the Medical University of South Carolina in Charleston. He is a graduate of the University of Michigan–Ann Arbor and of Cornell University

Medical College. Dr. Mack has extensive experience in organized medicine and psychiatry. His other areas of interest in psychiatry have included development, the psychiatric presentation of medical disorders, and the history of psychiatric classification. As a child and forensic psychiatrist, he has treated or evaluated individuals with addictions in many different settings, including general inpatient, outpatient, correctional, juvenile justice, and community. Dr. Mack has lectured to medical groups, bar associations, patient groups, and other mental health professionals as well.

Contributors

Michelle C. Acosta, PhD, Department of Psychiatry, St. Luke's–Roosevelt Hospital Center, New York, New York

D. Andrew Baron, PhD, Department of Psychiatry and Behavioral Medicine, Temple University, Philadelphia, Pennsylvania

David A. Baron, DO, MSEd, Department of Psychiatry and Behavioral Medicine, Temple University, Philadelphia, Pennsylvania

Steven H. Baron, PhD, Department of Social Sciences, Montgomery County Community College, Blue Bell, Pennsylvania

Judith S. Beck, PhD, Beck Institute for Cognitive Therapy, Bala Cynwyd, Pennsylvania

Sheila B. Blume, MD, Department of Psychiatry, State University of New York at Stony Brook School of Medicine, Stony Brook, New York

Oscar G. Bukstein, MD, MPH, Department of Psychiatry, Western Psychiatric Institute and Clinic, Pittsburgh, Pennsylvania

Alisa B. Busch, MD, Department of Psychiatry, Harvard Medical School, Cambridge, Massachusetts; Alcohol and Drug Abuse Treatment Program, McLean Hospital, Belmont, Massachusetts

Kathleen M. Carroll, PhD, Department of Psychiatry, Yale University School of Medicine, New Haven, Connecticut; Department of Psychiatry, VA Connecticut Healthcare System, West Haven, Connecticut

Ricardo Castañeda, MD, Department of Psychiatry, New York University School of Medicine, New York, New York

Stephen L. Dilts, Jr., MD, MBA, Department of Psychiatry, Penn State College of Medicine, University Park, Pennsylvania; Department of Behavioral Health, WellSpan Health, York, Pennsylvania

Stephen L. Dilts, MD, PhD, Department of Psychiatry, University of Colorado Health Sciences Center, Denver, Colorado

Lance M. Dodes, MD, Department of Psychiatry, Harvard Medical School, Cambridge, Massachusetts

Caroline M. DuPont, MD, DuPont Clinical Research, Rockville, Maryland; Department of Psychiatry, Johns Hopkins University, Baltimore, Maryland

Robert L. DuPont, MD, Institute for Behavior and Health, Rockville, Maryland; Department of Psychiatry, Georgetown University, Washington, DC

Richard J. Frances, MD, Silver Hill Hospital, New Canaan, Connecticut; Department of Psychiatry, New York University School of Medicine, New York, New York; private practice, New York, New York

Hugo Franco, MD, Dual Diagnosis Unit, New York University Hospital, New York, New York; private practice, Eatontown, New Jersey

John Franklin, MD, Department of Psychiatry and Behavioral Sciences, Feinberg School of Medicine, Northwestern University, Chicago, Illinois

Marc Galanter, MD, Department of Psychiatry, New York University School of Medicine, New York, New York

Tony P. George, MD, Department of Psychiatry, Yale University School of Medicine, New Haven, Connecticut

Jon E. Grant, JD, MD, Department of Psychiatry and Human Behavior, Brown University, Providence, Rhode Island

Deborah L. Haller, PhD, Department of Psychiatry, St. Luke's–Roosevelt Hospital Center, New York, New York

Francis Hayden, MD, Department of Psychiatry, New York University School of Medicine, New York, New York

Anthony W. Heath, PhD, United Behavioral Health, Schaumburg, Illinois

James M. Hill, PhD, Department of Psychiatry, University of Medicine and Dentistry of New Jersey, Newark, New Jersey

Norman Hymowitz, MD, Department of Psychiatry, University of Medicine and Dentistry of New Jersey, Newark, New Jersey

Jeffrey P. Kahn, MD, Department of Psychiatry, Weill Medical College of Cornell University, New York, New York

Yifrah Kaminer, MD, Department of Psychiatry, University of Connecticut Health Center, Farmington, Connecticut

Cheryl Ann Kennedy, MD, Department of Psychiatry, University of Medicine and Dentistry of New Jersey, Newark, New Jersey

Edward J. Khantzian, MD, Department of Psychiatry, Harvard Medical School, Cambridge, Massachusetts

Kenneth L. Kirsh, PhD, Symptom Management and Palliative Care Program, Markey Cancer Center, University of Kentucky, Lexington, Kentucky

Herbert D. Kleber, MD, Department of Psychiatry, College of Physicians and Surgeons, Columbia University, New York, New York

Thomas R. Kosten, MD, Department of Psychiatry, Yale University School of Medicine, New Haven, Connecticut; Department of Psychiatry, VA Connecticut Healthcare System, West Haven, Connecticut

Petros Levounis, MD, The Addiction Institute of New York, St. Luke's–Roosevelt Hospital Center, and Department of Psychiatry, College of Physicians and Surgeons, Columbia University, New York, NY

Bruce S. Liese, PhD, Department of Family Medicine, University of Kansas Medical Center, Kansas City, Kansas

Marsha M. Linehan, PhD, Department of Psychology, University of Washington, Seattle, Washington

David Lussier, MD, Division of Geriatric Medicine, Montreal General Hospital, McGill University, Montreal, Quebec, Canada

Thomas R. Lynch, PhD, Department of Psychiatry and Behavioral Sciences, Duke University Medical Center, and Department of Psychology, Duke University, Durham, North Carolina

Avram H. Mack, MD, Institute of Psychiatry, Medical University of South Carolina, Charleston, South Carolina

Marylinn Markarian, MD, FEGS Continuing Day Program, Brooklyn, New York

Elinore F. McCance-Katz, MD, Department of Psychiatry, Virginia Commonwealth University, Richmond, Virginia

David McDowell, MD, Department of Psychiatry, Columbia University, New York, New York

Sheldon I. Miller, MD, Department of Psychiatry and Behavioral Sciences, Feinberg School of Medicine, Northwestern University, Chicago, Illinois

Edgar P. Nace, MD, Department of Psychiatry, University of Texas Southwestern Medical School, Dallas, Texas

Lisa M. Najavits, PhD, Department of Psychiatry, Harvard Medical School, Cambridge, Massachusetts; Trauma Research Program, McLean Hospital, Belmont, Massachusetts

Steven D. Passik, PhD, Symptom Management and Palliative Care Program, Markey Cancer Center, University of Kentucky, Lexington, Kentucky

Russell K. Portenoy, MD, Department of Pain Medicine and Palliative Care, Beth Israel Medical Center, New York, New York

Marc N. Potenza, MD, Department of Psychiatry, Yale University, New Haven, Connecticut

M. Zachary Rosenthal, PhD, Department of Psychiatry and Behavioral Sciences, Duke University Medical Center, Durham, North Carolina

Richard N. Rosenthal, MD, Department of Psychiatry, St. Luke's–Roosevelt Hospital Center, and Department of Psychiatry, College of Physicians and Surgeons, Columbia University, New York, New York

Steven J. Schleifer, MD, Department of Psychiatry, University of Medicine and Dentistry of New Jersey, Newark, New Jersey

Sidney H. Schnoll, MD, Purdue Pharma LP, Stamford, Connecticut

M. Duncan Stanton, PhD, School of Professional Psychology, Spalding University, Louisville, Kentucky; The Morton Center, Louisville, Kentucky

Ralph E. Tarter, PhD, School of Pharmacy, University of Pittsburgh, Pittsburgh, Pennsylvania

Roger D. Weiss, MD, Department of Psychiatry, Harvard Medical School, Cambridge, Massachusetts; Alcohol and Drug Abuse Treatment Program, McLean Hospital, Belmont, Massachusetts

Joseph Westermeyer, MD, Department of Psychiatry, Minneapolis VA Hospital, University of Minnesota, Minneapolis, Minnesota

Monica L. Zilberman, MD, PhD, Institute of Psychiatry, University of São Paulo, São Paulo, Brazil

Sheldon Zimberg, MD, Department of Psychiatry, College of Physicians and Surgeons, Columbia University, New York, New York

Preface

This third edition of the *Clinical Textbook of Addictive Disorders* appears 20 years after the founding of the American Academy of Addiction Psychiatry (AAAP). During this period, major progress has occurred in both general psychiatry and addiction psychiatry. There has been movement ranging from description of the phenomenology of psychiatric disorders, including substance use disorders (SUDs), to the beginnings of understanding neurobiological mechanisms, pathophysiology, genetic and family influences, and etiology. Addiction treatment research, including that for comorbid conditions, has advanced and the development of evidence-based guidelines for addiction treatment has been launched. While treatment methods are still very much tied to the craft and art of psychotherapy (including self-help and spirituality), dissemination of research findings and evidence-based treatment approaches will add to the quality of care of patients.

Unfortunately, our advances in the understanding of addiction psychiatry are not necessarily associated with reductions in the incidence of substance use. The magnitude of use seems to be subject to fads and fluctuations in perceptions of risk of use. Over the past 30 years there have been important variations in the use of substances by age, gender, ethnic, and racial groups. The most recent estimate on the cost of substance use is for 1998, with the cost of drug abuse directly estimated at $143.4 billion (Office of National Drug Control Policy, 2001) and the costs of alcohol abuse projected to be $185 billion (Harwood, 2000). This figure (estimated in 1992) reflects the estimated 8.3% of the population ages 12 or older who were current illicit drug users in 2002 and perhaps also includes the 2.6% of the population ages 12 or older who were current users of psychotherapeutic drugs taken nonmedically in 2002. The rate of current drug use among adolescents in 2002 was 11.6%, but that rate was surpassed by young adults (ages 18–25 years) at 20.2%. As for alcohol, an estimated 120 million Americans ages 12 or older reported being current drinkers of alcohol in the 2002 survey (51%). In terms of diagnosis, an estimated 22 million Americans in 2002 were classified with substance dependence or abuse (9.4% of the total population ages 12 or older). Of these, 3.2 million were classified with dependence on or abuse of both alcohol and illicit drugs, 3.9 million were dependent on or abused illicit drugs but not alcohol, and 14.9 million were dependent on or abused alcohol but not illicit drugs (Office of Applied Studies, 2003). As for children, according to the Monitoring the Future study, Ecstasy use among 12th graders finally began to lessen after increases since 1998 and use of illicit substances other than marijuana continued to decline among both 10th and 12th graders. Yet inhalant use increased and cocaine use remained steady among eighth graders (Johnston, O'Malley, Bachman, & Schulenberg, 2004). These numbers suggest that treatment and prevention efforts need to be tailored to particular diagnoses and to members of particular groups, as the magnitude of substance use remains large.

In order to address this great and costly social and medical problem, this textbook, written previously by the founders and many of the leaders of AAAP, again includes many of the prestigious, internationally renowned clinicians, educators, and researchers from the original pool of talent, with extensive revision and updating of their work. We have also added new chapters on the neuroscientific basis of addiction, gambling and other "behavioral" addictions, occupational issues and addiction, and dialectical behavior therapy of addicted borderline patients. Many excellent authors were added, and a third editor, Avram H. Mack, provides a fresh perspective. This new volume presents historical background, scientific basis, diagnostic tools, substance-specific information, and a full range of treatment approaches, including individual, group, self-help, family, cognitive-behavioral, psychodynamic, psychopharmacological, and integrated treatment for comorbid conditions. Competency in tailoring addiction treatment to specific concerns that relate to culture, ethnicity, spirituality, gender, age, legal and occupational problems, and medical and psychiatric comorbidity are all vital clinical skills covered throughout the book. Integrating the right combination of treatments for the addicted patient is at this point as much art as science.

Greater attention has been given to integrating treatment for co-occurring psychiatric disorders; medical conditions such as HIV/AIDS, hepatitis, and tuberculosis; and the psychosocial problems that complicate addictive illness. Clinicians need skills to tailor addiction treatment to women, different sociocultural groups, age-specific groups, the medically ill, and those with legal problems. Some of the newer treatment approaches are being formatted as manuals and advocate pure application of their methods. What is the reader of a volume like this to do with the disparate kinds of practices authors describe, when we still are at the infancy of scientifically based differential therapeutics? While controversy surrounds this area, we recommend integration and blending of many of these tools with the personality and style of the informed clinician and with respect for the particular and salient needs of each case. Slavish adherence to one method or school of thought, hammering every nail with the same hammer, is not what most experienced, skillful therapists do. Addiction treatment, especially psychotherapy and psychopharmacology, is still very much an art. However, even the experienced clinician must stay abreast of treatment outcome research, evidence-based approaches, and technical and pharmacological advances in the field. Knowledge of how to address comorbid problems is vital, and integration of treatment is the best approach. Patients will seek therapists with wisdom, compassion, modesty, honesty, knowledge, skill, and good judgment, and will want their therapists to be available, practical, affordable, and active. Increasingly, patients and their families come to treatment well armed with scientific knowledge and with high expectations that their health care expenditure is a value proposition, and they reasonably expect to see positive results from their efforts.

Addiction is a disease of denial, stigma, and hopelessness, and patients with severe mental illness and addictions more often than not suffer their darkest days without the compassionate, evidence-based care advocated in this volume, which can provide a path to a more productive and happier life that is frequently the product of recovery. Addiction is a disease of the brain and of the spirit. Helping patients and their families progress to acceptance of their illness, acceptance of a need for help, and making healthier choices to take action restores hope and is half the battle. Maintaining progress, developing a treatment alliance that leads to continued engagement in help, rebuilding of self-esteem and self-care, and development of coping skills that help prevent relapse are essential ingredients of successful treatment programs.

The mutual help that patients provide each other in self-help programs, groups, organized rehabilitation programs, network and family treatment, and through organized religion and in their daily encounters with others is a force that needs to be tapped by the skillful therapist. Some individuals with addictive disorders are particularly gifted at helping others or providing models of hope by communicating how they moved past their darkest days, accepted their illness, reached out for help, developed coping skills, and restored balance in their lives.

Exciting research is under way studying the familial patterns of genetic transmission, localization and sequencing of multiple genes and alleles for addiction and interaction with other illnesses, and how gene expression occurs. Effects on membrane chemistry, receptor sites, neurotransmission, neuroplasticity, apoptosis, and regeneration of nerve and glial cells, and localization of brain effects through imaging, are other areas of basic science that can lead to better targeted future treatments. Development of new agents that can provide neurotropic healing of damage caused by alcohol and other drugs and possibly other psychiatric illnesses such as manic–depression or schizophrenia is a distinct possibility.

Research (1) on health systems; (2) on effects of public health, advertising, and educational campaigns on decisions to use drugs, on prevention, and on early diagnosis; and (3) on cost effectiveness of treatment is also important. Integrating treatment for psychiatric and addictive disorders needs to be a higher priority, and barriers within systems of funding, treatment agencies, and training programs for staff need to be removed. Substance abuse clinicians must learn about other mental illnesses, and no one who works with mentally ill persons should be without addiction treatment training.

Two of us (R. J. F. and S. I. M.) were the founders of AAAP and have spent our careers in fostering training, education, and addiction psychiatry rotations for medical students, psychiatrists, addiction psychiatry fellows, other primary care physicians, nurses, social workers, psychologists, addiction counselors, and rehabilitation therapists. In addition to students and clinicians in these fields, this book will be of great interest to teachers, to those who work in the criminal justice system, and to others interested in learning more about addiction treatment. Practitioners, from beginners to the more experienced, will enhance their skills by reading this well-referenced textbook. At this point, psychiatry is the only medical specialty with a board-certified subspecialty in addictions. At present, approximately 2,000 board-certified addiction psychiatrists are able to provide consultation, education, and research, to spearhead the much larger number of clinicians engaged in treating the nation's number one public health problem.

A small but growing percentage of those with alcohol or other substance problems are properly screened, diagnosed, and treated, and lapses and relapses are a regular experience. The denial exhibited by addicted individuals—often present in their families and enabling workplaces—mirrored by society's lack of adequate funding for prevention and treatment, the absence of universal health care, and the criminal justice system's neglect of addiction and mental illness treatment are reasons most people do not get the help they need. The countertransference and attitudinal problems of staff can be an important barrier to treatment, and these can be reduced significantly when the clinician has a good knowledge of addictions and effective treatment tools at hand. While many clinicians may fear or dread working with addicts, those armed with the proper skills, attitude, and knowledge have wonderful opportunities to benefit their patients. We hope readers enjoy this volume and find the tools in it as useful as we do in helping addicted patients. Few people suffer more than addicts, few patients will gain more from the efforts they put into treatment, and we find no population more interesting, challenging, and rewarding to treat.

We wish to thank the many contributors to this volume; they have worked hard to provide comprehensive reviews in a timely manner so that readers receive the most up-to-date perspectives. Most importantly, we want to especially thank our respective wives, Marsha Frances, Sarah Miller, and Hallie Lightdale, MD, for their tireless support and care as we worked with pride on this project.

RICHARD J. FRANCES, MD
SHELDON I. MILLER, MD
AVRAM H. MACK, MD

REFERENCES

Harwood, H. (2000). *Updating estimates of the economic costs of alcohol abuse in the United States: Estimates, updated methods and data.* Available at www.drugabuse.gov/Infofax/costs.html

Johnston, L. D., O'Malley, P. M., Bachman J. G., & Schulenberg J. E. (2004). *Monitoring the future: National results on adolescent drug use.* Bethesda, MD: U.S. Department of Health and Human Services.

Office of Applied Studies. (2003). *Overview of findings from the 2002 National Survey on Drug Use and Health* (NHSDA Series H-21, DHHS Publication No. SMA 03–3774). Rockville, MD: Author.

Office of National Drug Control Policy. (2001). *The economic costs of drug abuse in the United States, 1992–1998* (Publication No. NCJ-190636). Washington, DC: Executive Office of the President.

Contents

PART IV. SPECIAL POPULATIONS

PART V. TREATMENTS FOR ADDICTIONS

PART I

FOUNDATIONS OF ADDICTION

CHAPTER 1

The Neurobiology
of Substance Dependence
Implications for Treatment

THOMAS R. KOSTEN
TONY P. GEORGE
HERBERT D. KLEBER

Tolerance, dependence, and addiction are all manifestations of brain changes resulting from chronic substance abuse and involve different brain pathways than those subserving acute drug reinforcement. Acute drug reinforcement appears to share a final common dopaminergic pathway from the ventral tegmental area of the brain to the nucleus accumbens. These acute processes are relatively unimportant for pharmacotherapy of dependence and addiction; instead, the neurobiology of changes associated with chronic use forms the basis for rational pharmacotherapy. This translation of neurobiology into effective treatments has been most successful for opioids, with more limited success for alcohol, nicotine, and stimulant dependence. Opioid treatments such as methadone, levo-alpha-acetyl methadol (LAAM), buprenorphine, and naltrexone act on the same brain structures and processes as addictive opioids, but with protective or normalizing effects. This concept of normalization is critical for effective treatments and is illustrated in this chapter, with opioids as the primary example. As we understand the molecular biology of dependence more fully, normalization appears to be a process very similar to learning and may involve similar changes in gene activation and neuronal long-term potentiation (LTP) and long-term depression (LTD) that appear to underlie learned behaviors and emotional states.

While the individual patient, rather than his or her disease, is the appropriate focus of treatment for substance abuse, an understanding of the neurobiology of dependence and addiction can clarify the rationales for treatment methods and goals. Patients who are informed about the brain origins of addiction also can benefit from understanding that their addiction has a biological basis and does not mean that they are "bad" people.

Brain abnormalities resulting from chronic use of nicotine, stimulants, opioids, alcohol, hallucinogens, inhalants, cannabis, and many other abused substances are underlying causes of dependence (the need to keep taking drugs to avoid a withdrawal syndrome) and addiction (intense drug craving and compulsive use). Most of the abnormalities associated with dependence resolve after detoxification, within days or weeks after the substance use stops. The abnormalities that produce addiction, however, are more wide-ranging, complex, and long-lasting. They may involve an interaction of environmental effects—for example, stress, the social context of initial opiate use, and psychological conditioning—and a genetic predisposition in the form of brain pathways that were abnormal even before the first dose of opioid was taken. Such abnormalities can produce craving that leads to relapse months or years after the individual is no longer opioid-dependent.

In this chapter we describe how drugs affect brain processes to produce drug liking, tolerance, dependence, and addiction. Although these processes are highly complex, like everything that happens in the brain, we try to explain them in terms that can be understood by patients. We also discuss the treatment implications of these concepts. Pharmacological therapy directly offsets or reverses some of the brain changes associated with dependence and addiction, greatly enhancing the effectiveness of behavioral therapies. Although researchers do not yet have a comprehensive understanding about how these medications work, it is clear that they often renormalize brain abnormalities that have been induced by chronic, high-dose abuse of various substances.

ORIGINS OF DRUG LIKING

Many factors, both individual and environmental, influence whether a particular person who experiments with drugs will continue taking them long enough to become dependent or addicted. For individuals who do continue, the drug's ability to provide intense feelings of pleasure is a critical reason.

When abused drugs travel through the bloodstream to the brain, they attach to specialized proteins on the surface of neurons that may be receptors, transporters, or even structural elements of the neurons. For example, opiates such as heroin bind to mu opioid receptors, which are on the surfaces of opiate-sensitive neurons, and have their effects by inhibiting the cyclic adenosine monophosphate (cyclic AMP) second messenger system. Inhibition occurs through a guanine nucleotide-binding (G)-protein-mediated coupling leading to a series of changes in phosphorylation for a wide range of intraneuronal proteins (Nestler, 2002). The linkage of heroin with the receptors imitates the linkage of endogenous opioids such as beta-endorphin with these same receptors and triggers the same biochemical brain processes that reward people with feelings of pleasure when they engage in activities that promote basic life functions, such as eating and sex. Opioids such as oxycodone or methadone are prescribed therapeutically to relieve pain, but when these exogenous opioids activate the reward processes in the absence of significant pain, they can motivate repeated use of the drug simply for pleasure.

One of the brain circuits activated by opioids and most, if not all, abused drugs is the mesolimbic (midbrain) reward system. This system generates signals in a part of the brain called the ventral tegmental area (VTA) that result in the release of the chemical dopamine (DA) in another part of the brain, the nucleus accumbens (N-Ac) (Figure 1.1). This release of DA into the N-Ac causes feelings of pleasure. Other areas of the brain create a lasting record or memory that associates these good feelings with the circumstances and environment in which they occur. These memories, called "conditioned associations," often lead to the craving for drugs when the abuser reencounters those persons, places, or things, and they drive abusers to seek out more drugs in spite of many obstacles.

Other abused drugs activate this same brain pathway, but via different mechanisms and by stimulating or inhibiting different neurons in this pathway.

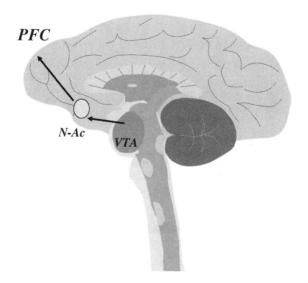

FIGURE 1.1. Mesolimbic dopamine ("reward") pathways. PFC, prefrontal cortex; N-Ac, nucleus accumbens; VTA, ventral tegmental area.

For example, opioids and cannabinoids can inhibit activity in N-Ac directly, whereas stimulants such as cocaine and amphetamine act indirectly by binding to various DA transporters and either inhibiting the reuptake of DA into the VTA neurons (cocaine) or actively pumping DA out of the VTA (amphetamine) at its synapse with the N-Ac neurons (Kosten, 2002; Stahl, 1998). Since stimulation of the DA D_2 receptor inhibits the cyclic AMP system, this increase in DA in the synapse leads to relative inhibition of the N-Ac neuron. The mechanism is more complex than this, however, since the D_1 receptor has the opposite effect on the cyclic AMP system (e.g., it increases the amount of cyclic AMP) and both D_1 and D_2 receptors are present on the N-Ac neurons. The presumption is that the D_2 receptor effects predominate perhaps simply due to more D_2 receptors, or due to a higher affinity of the D_2 than the D_1 receptors for DA. Other substances may be even more indirect in their stimulation. For example, nicotine and benzodiazepines stimulate ion channels for calcium/sodium and chloride, respectively (Stahl, 2002). The calcium/sodium channel is a nicotinic receptor that normally binds acetylcholine, while the chloride channel is associated with a gamma-aminobutyric acid (GABA) receptor. The stimulation of these ion channels can lead to depolarization of the VTA neuron and release of DA into the synapse between the VTA and N-Ac. The entry of calcium into the VTA neuron can also directly facilitate the merging of the synaptic vesicles in the VTA with the cell membrane, leading to release of DA from these vesicles (Kosten, 2002). For some substances, we do not yet have a clear idea of their biochemical mechanisms of reinforcement. For example, alcohol may act through the mu opioid receptor like heroin, or the GABA receptor like benzodiazepines. Inhalants have direct toxic effects on the structural proteins of neuronal membranes and may act directly to increase neurotransmission through the VTA to the N-Ac by damaging these structural proteins in neuronal membranes and allowing calcium entry into the VTA, thereby releasing DA vesicles into the synapse connecting the VTA with the N-Ac.

Particularly in the early stages of abuse, the drug's stimulation of the brain's reward system is a primary reason that some people take drugs repeatedly. However, the compulsion to use drugs builds over time to extend beyond a simple drive for pleasure. This increased compulsion is related to tolerance and dependence.

DRUG TOLERANCE, DEPENDENCE, AND WITHDRAWAL

From a clinical standpoint, withdrawal can be one of the most powerful factors driving dependence and addictive behaviors. This seems particularly true for opioids, alcohol, benzodiazepines, nicotine, and to a lesser extent stimulants such as cocaine. For hallucinogens, cannabinoids, or inhalants, withdrawal symptoms seem of more limited importance. Treatment of the patient's withdrawal symptoms is based on understanding how withdrawal is related to the brain's adjustment to these drugs after chronic repeated high doses.

Repeated exposure to escalating dosages of most drugs alters the brain, so that it functions more or less normally when the drugs are present and abnormally when they are not. Two clinically important results of this alteration are drug tolerance (the need to take higher and higher dosages of drugs to achieve the same effect) and drug dependence (susceptibility to withdrawal symptoms). Withdrawal symptoms occur only in patients who have developed tolerance.

Tolerance occurs because the brain cells that have receptors or transporters on them gradually become less responsive to the stimulation by the exogenous substances. For example, more opioid is needed to inhibit the cyclic AMP system in the N-Ac neurons, as well as to stimulate the VTA brain cells of the mesolimbic reward system to release the same amount of DA in the N-Ac. Therefore, more opioid is needed to produce pleasure comparable to that provided in previous drug-taking episodes. The mechanism for this reduction in response is related to the cyclic AMP coupling for opioids, but direct reductions in the number of receptors or increases in the number of transporters can occur. For example, it appears that after chronic cocaine inhibition of the DA transporter, the number of DA receptors decreases, while the number of transporters may increase to compensate for this chronic overstimulation of the N-Ac DA receptors and chronic inhibition of the transporter (Kosten, 2002). These changes associated with tolerance might be considered an attempt by the brain to attain relative homeostasis in the face of the disruption induced by these abused drugs. Tolerance to alcohol may be due to a more complex series of neurobiological changes at the neuronal and molecular levels, and involve GABA, opioid, DA, and other neurochemical systems, including the excitatory amino acid neurotransmitters such as glutamate and its multiplicity of receptor subtypes (Fadda & Rossetti, 1998). Tolerance to cannabinoids probably has a similar mechanism to opioids, since the cannabinoid CB_1 receptor is also a G-protein-coupled, cyclic AMP type receptor (Kosten, 2000; Stahl, 1998). Tolerance to hallucinogens such as lysergic acid (LSD) probably involves changes in the serotonergic $5HT_2$ receptors, which involve the phosphoinositol phosphate (PIP) second messenger system, but this system's relationship to chronic LSD use has not been as extensively studied as the cyclic AMP system for the opioids and cannabinoids (Kosten, 2000).

Opioids provide an outstanding example to illustrate how the neurobiological changes associated with tolerance are related to dependence and withdrawal symptoms. Opioid dependence and some of the most distressing opioid withdrawal symptoms stem from changes in the locus coeruleus (LC), another important brain system at the base of the brain (Figure 1.2). Neurons in the LC produce noradrenaline (NA) and widely distribute it to other parts of the brain including the cerebral cortex, brainstem, and various subcortical regions, where

A. Baseline

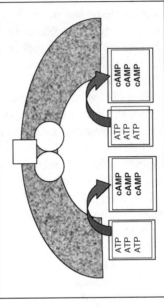

B. Acute opioid inhibition of converting enzyme

C. Chronic opioid leads to increased converting enzyme activity

D. Discontinuing opioid leads to increased cyclic AMP due to loss of inhibition by opioid

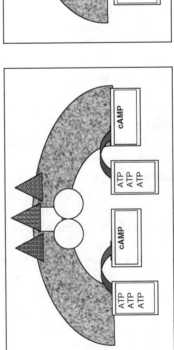

FIGURE 1.2. Neuronal coupling of receptor to G protein and adenyl cyclase (converting enzyme) at baseline (Panel A), changes during acute opiate effects (Panel B), changes after chronic opiate use (Panel C), and changes during acute opiate withdrawal (Panel D). After "resetting" of opiate receptors with naltrexone, the number of receptors appears to increase to match the increased converting enzyme activity (see text).

it stimulates wakefulness, breathing, blood pressure, and general alertness, among other functions. When opioid molecules link to mu receptors on brain cells in the LC, they suppress the neurons' release of NA, resulting in drowsiness, slowed respiration, and low blood pressure—familiar effects of opioid intoxication. With repeated exposure to opioids, however, LC neurons adjust by increasing their level of activity. Now, when opioids are present, their suppressive impact is offset by this heightened activity, with the result that roughly normal amounts of NA are released and the patient feels more or less normal. When opioids are not present to suppress the LC brain cells' enhanced activity, however, the neurons release excessive amounts of NA, triggering jitters, anxiety, muscle cramps, and diarrhea. Figure 1.2 illustrates this development of opiate tolerance and withdrawal.

Other brain areas in addition to the LC also contribute to the production of opiate withdrawal symptoms, including the mesolimbic reward system. For example, opioid tolerance that reduces the VTA's release of DA into the N-Ac may prevent the patient from obtaining pleasure from normally rewarding activities such as eating. These changes in the VTA and the DA reward systems, though not fully understood, form an important brain system underlying craving and compulsive drug use.

TRANSITION TO ADDICTION

As we have seen, the pleasure derived from various drugs' activation of the brain's natural reward system promotes continued drug use during the initial stages of opioid addiction. Subsequently, repeated exposure to these drugs induces the brain mechanism of dependence, which leads to daily drug use to avert the unpleasant symptoms of drug withdrawal for many substances, although for some drugs, withdrawal symptoms are minimal and may contribute minimally to dependence features and relapse after discontinuation. Further prolonged use of drugs that produce dependence lead to more long-lasting changes in the brain that may underlie the compulsive drug-seeking behavior and related adverse consequences that are the hallmarks of addiction. Recent research has generated several models to explain how habitual drug use produces changes in the brain that may lead to drug addiction. In reality, the process of addiction probably involves components from each of these models, as well as other features.

The "Changed Set Point" Model

The "changed set point" model of drug addiction has several variants based on the altered neurobiology of the DA neurons in the VTA and of the NA neurons of the LC during the early phases of withdrawal and abstinence. The basic idea is that drug abuse alters a biological or physiological setting or baseline. One variant, by Koob and LeMoal (2001), is based on the idea that neurons of the mesolimbic reward pathways are naturally "set" to release enough DA in the N-Ac to produce a normal level of pleasure. Koob and LeMoal suggest that abused drugs cause addiction by initiating a vicious cycle of changing this set point, such that the release of DA is reduced when normally pleasurable activities occur and these abused drugs are not present. Similarly, a change in set point occurs in the LC, but in the opposite direction, such that NA release is increased during withdrawal, as described earlier, thus accounting for both the positive (drug liking) and negative (drug withdrawal) aspects of drug addiction.

A specific way that the DA neurons can become dysfunctional relates to an alteration in their baseline ("resting") levels of electrical activity and DA release (Grace, 2000). In this second variant of the changed set point model, this resting level is the result of two factors that influence the amount of resting DA release in the N-Ac: cortical excitatory (glutamate) neurons that drive the VTA DA neurons to release DA, and autoreceptors ("brakes") that shut down further release when DA concentrations become excessive. Activation of various types of receptors by abused substances, such as mu opiate receptors by heroin, initially bypasses these brakes and leads to a large release of DA in the N-Ac. However, with repeated drug use, the brain responds to these successive large DA releases by increasing the number and strength of the brakes on the VTA DA neurons. Eventually, these enhanced "braking" autoreceptors inhibit the neurons' resting DA release. When this happens, the dependent addict will take even more of the abused drug, such as heroin, to offset the reduction of normal resting DA release. When he or she stops the drug use, a state of DA deprivation will result, manifesting in dysphoria (pain, agitation, and malaise) and other withdrawal symptoms, which can lead to a cycle of relapse to drug use.

A third variation on the set point change emphasizes the sensitivity to environmental cues that leads to drug wanting or craving rather than just reinforcement and withdrawal (Breiter et al., 1997; Robinson & Berridge, 2000). During periods when the drug is not available to addicts, their brains can remember the drug, and desire or craving for the drug can be a major factor leading to drug use relapse. This craving may represent increased activity of the cortical excitatory (glutamate) neurotransmitters, which drive the resting activity of the DA-containing VTA neurons, as mentioned, and also drive the LC NA neurons. As the glutamate activity increases, DA will be released from the VTA, leading to drug wanting or craving, and NA will be released from the LC, leading to increased withdrawal symptoms, particularly with opiates such as heroin. This theory suggests that these cortical excitatory brain pathways are overactive in addiction, and reducing their activity would be therapeutic. Basic scientists and clinicians are currently researching compounds called "excitatory amino acid antagonists" to see whether this potential treatment strategy really can work.

Thus, several mechanisms in the LC and VTA–N-Ac brain pathways may be operating during addiction and relapse. The excitatory cortical pathways may produce little response in the VTA during the resting state, leading to reductions in DA. However, when the addict is exposed to cues that produce craving, the glutamate pathways may get sufficiently active to raise DA and stimulate desire for a greater high. This same increase in glutamate activity will raise NA release from the LC to produce a dysphoric state predisposing to relapse and continued addiction.

The Cognitive Deficits Model

The cognitive deficits model of drug addiction proposes that individuals who develop addictive disorders have abnormalities in an area of the brain called the prefrontal cortex (PFC). The PFC is important for regulation of judgment, planning, and other executive functions. To help us overcome some of our impulses for immediate gratification in favor of more important or ultimately more rewarding long-term goals, the PFC sends inhibitory signals to the VTA DA neurons of the mesolimbic reward system.

The cognitive deficits model proposes that PFC signaling to the meso-limbic reward system is compromised in individuals with addictive disorders; as a result, they have reduced ability to use judgment to restrain their impulses and are predisposed to compulsive drug-taking behaviors. Consistent with this model, stimulant drugs such as methamphetamine appear to damage the specific brain circuit—the frontostriatal loop—that carries inhibitory signals from the PFC to the mesolimbic reward system. In addition, a recent study using magnetic resonance spectroscopy showed that chronic alcohol abusers have abnormally low levels of GABA, the neurochemical that the PFC uses to signal the reward system to release less DA (Behar et al., 1999). As well, the cognitive deficits model of drug addiction could explain the clinical observation that heroin addiction is more severe in individuals with antisocial personality disorder—a condition that is independently associated with PFC deficits (Raine, Lencz, Bihrle, LaCasse, & Colletti, 2000).

In contrast to stimulants and perhaps alcohol, heroin apparently damages the PFC but not the frontostriatal loop. Therefore, individuals who become heroin addicts may have some PFC damage that is independent of their opioid abuse, either inherited genetically or caused by some other factor or event in their lives. This preexisting PFC damage, which predisposes individuals to impulsivity and lack of control, may be important for most individuals who become addicted to drugs, and the additional PFC damage from chronic repeated drug abuse, particularly abuse of stimulants, increases the severity of these problems (Kosten, 1998).

THE IMPORTANT ROLE OF STRESS

That drug abuse patients are more vulnerable to stress than the general population is a clinical truism. Numerous preclinical studies have documented that physical stressors (e.g., foot shock or restraint stress) and psychological stressors can cause animals to reinstate drug use (e.g., Shaham, Erb, & Stewart, 2000). Furthermore, stressors can trigger drug craving in addicted humans (Sinha, Catapano, & O'Malley, 1999). One potential explanation for these observations is that abused drugs, including opiates and stimulants, raise levels of cortisol, a hormone that plays a primary role in stress responses; cortisol, in turn, raises the level of activity in the mesolimbic reward system (Kreek & Koob, 1998). By these mechanisms, stress may contribute to the abuser's desire to take drugs in the first place, as well as to his or her subsequent compulsion to keep taking them.

PHARMACOLOGICAL INTERVENTIONS AND TREATMENT IMPLICATIONS

In summary, the various biological models of drug addiction are complementary and broadly applicable to chemical addictions. We next illustrate how long-term pharmacotherapies for opioid dependence, such as methadone, naltrexone, and buprenorphine, can counteract or reverse the abnormalities underlying dependence and addiction. These agents are particularly informative, because they are an agonist, antagonist, and partial agonist, respectively. We do not review short-term treatments for relieving withdrawal symptoms and increasing abstinence but refer readers elsewhere for detailed neurobiological explanations for various abstinence initiation approaches (see Kosten & O'Connor, 2003).

Methadone, a long-acting opioid medication with effects that last for days, causes dependence, but because of its sustained stimulation of the mu receptors, it alleviates craving and compulsive drug use. In addition, methadone therapy tends to normalize many aspects of the hormonal disruptions found in addicted individuals (Kling et al., 2000; Kreek, 2000; Schluger, Borg, Ho, & Kreek, 2001). For example, it moderates the exaggerated cortisol stress response (discussed earlier) that increases the danger of relapse in stressful situations.

Naltrexone is used to help patients avoid relapse after they have been detoxified from opioid dependence. Its main therapeutic action is to occupy mu opioid receptors in the brain with a 100-fold higher affinity than agonists such as methadone or heroin, so that addictive opioids cannot link up with them and stimulate the brain's reward system. Naltrexone does not activate the G-protein-coupled cyclic AMP system and does not increase or decrease levels of cyclic AMP inside the neuron, and it does not promote these brain processes that produce feelings of pleasure (Kosten & Kleber, 1984). An individual who is adequately dosed with naltrexone does not obtain any pleasure from addictive opioids and is less motivated to use them. An interesting neurobiological effect of naltrexone is that it appears to increase the number of available mu opiate receptors, which may help to renormalize the imbalance between the receptors and G-protein coupling to cyclic AMP (Kosten, 1990). Naltrexone is also sometimes used to detoxify patients rapidly from opioid dependence. In this situation, while naltrexone keeps the addictive opioid molecules away from the mu receptors, clonidine may help to suppress the opioid-induced excessive NA output that is a primary cause of withdrawal (Kosten, 1990). Clonidine is capable of this withdrawal relief because alpha-adrenergic autoreceptors are co-localized with mu opiate receptors on the neurons of the LC, and both receptor types inhibit cyclic AMP synthesis through similar inhibitory G proteins.

Buprenorphine's action on the mu opioid receptors elicits two different therapeutic responses within the brain cells, depending on the dose. At low doses, buprenorphine has effects like methadone, but at high doses, it behaves like naltrexone, blocking the receptors so strongly that it can precipitate withdrawal in highly dependent patients (i.e., those maintained on more than 40 mg methadone daily). Several clinical trials have shown that buprenorphine is as effective as methadone, when used in sufficient doses (Kosten, Schottenfeld, Ziedonis, & Falcioni, 1993; Oliveto, Feingold, Schottenfeld, Jatlow, & Kosten, 1999; Schottenfeld, Pakes, Oliveto, Ziedonis, & Kosten, 1997). Buprenorphine has a safety advantage over methadone, since high doses precipitate withdrawal rather than the suppression of consciousness and respiration seen in overdoses of methadone and heroin. Thus, buprenorphine has less overdose potential than methadone, since it blocks other opioids and even itself as the dosage increases. Finally, buprenorphine can be given three times per week, simplifying observed ingestion during the early weeks of treatment.

SUMMARY

Dependence and addiction are most appropriately understood as chronic medical disorders, with frequent recurrences to be expected. The neurobiology of these disorders is becoming well understood, but much remains unknown about the genomic mechanisms that predispose to addictions and that are activated, perhaps irreversibly, by long-term drug use. The mesolimbic reward system appears to be central to the development of the direct clinical consequences of chronic abuse, including tolerance, dependence, and addiction. Other brain areas and neurochemicals, including cortisol, also are relevant to dependence and relapse. Pharmacological interventions for addiction are highly effective for opiates, and we have illustrated three different approaches using an agonist, an antagonist, or a partial agonist. However, given the complex biological, psychological, and social aspects of these diseases, they must be accompanied by appropriate psychosocial treatments. Clinician awareness of the neurobiological basis of drug dependence, and information sharing with patients, can provide insight into patient behaviors and problems, and clarify the rationale for treatment methods and goals.

ACKNOWLEDGMENT

This work was supported by Grant Nos. P50-DA-12762, K05-DA-00454, K12-DA-00167, R01-DA-13672, and R01-DA-14039 from the National Institute on Drug Abuse.

REFERENCES

Behar, K. L., Rothman, D. L., Petersen, K. F., Hooten, M., Delaney, R., Petroff, O. A., et al. (1999). Preliminary evidence of low cortical GABA levels in localized 1H-MR spectra of alcohol-dependent and hepatic encephalopathy patients. Am J Psychiatry, 156, 952–954.

Breiter, H. C., Gollub, R. L., Weisskoff, R. M., Kennedy, D. N., Makris, N., Berke, J. D., et al. (1997). Acute effects of cocaine on human brain activity and emotion. Neuron, 19, 591–611.

Fadda, F., & Rossetti, Z. L. (1998). Chronic ethanol consumption: From neuroadaptation to neurodegeneration. Prog Neurobiol, 56, 385–431.

Grace, A. A. (2000). The tonic/phasic model of dopamine system regulation and its implications for understanding alcohol and stimulant craving. Addiction, 95(Suppl 2), S119–S128.

Kling, M. A., Carson, R. E., Borg, L., Zametkin, A., Matochik, J. A., Schluger, J., et al. (2000). Opioid receptor imaging with PET and [18F]cyclofoxy in long-term, methadone-treated former heroin addicts. J Pharmacol Exp Ther, 295, 1070–1076.

Koob, G. F., & LeMoal, M. (2001). Drug addiction, dysregulation of reward, and allostasis. Neuropsychopharmacology, 24, 97–129.

Kosten, T. R. (1990). Neurobiology of abused drugs: Opioids and stimulants. J Nerv Ment Dis, 178, 217–227.

Kosten, T. R. (1998). Pharmacotherapy of cerebral ischemia in cocaine dependence. Drug Alcohol Depend, 49, 133–144.

Kosten, T. R. (2000). Drugs of abuse (Chapter 32 revision). In G. B. Katzung (Ed.), Basic and clinical pharmacology (8th ed., pp. 532–547). Stamford, CT: Appleton & Lange.

Kosten, T. R. (2002). Pathophysiology and treatment of cocaine dependence. In K. L. Davis, D. Charney, J. T. Coyle, & C. Nemeroff (Eds.), Neuropsychopharmacology: The fifth generation of progress (pp. 1461–1473). Baltimore: Lippincott/Williams & Wilkins.

Kosten, T. R., & Kleber, H. D. (1984). Strategies to improve compliance with narcotic antagonists. Am J Drug Alcohol Abuse, 10, 249–266.

Kosten, T. R., & O'Connor, P. G. (2003). Current concepts—management of drug withdrawal. *N Engl J Med, 348,* 1786–1795.

Kosten, T. R., Schottenfeld, R. S., Ziedonis, D., & Falcioni, J. (1993). Buprenorphine versus methadone maintenance for opioid dependence. *J Nerv Ment Dis, 181,* 358–364.

Kreek, M. J. (2000). Methadone-related opioid agonist pharmacotherapy for heroin addiction: History, recent molecular and neurochemical research and the future in mainstream medicine. *Ann NY Acad Sci, 909,* 186–216.

Kreek, M. J., & Koob, G. F. (1998). Drug dependence: Stress and dysregulation of brain reward pathways. *Drug Alcohol Depend, 51*(1–2), 23–47.

Nestler, E. J. (2002). From neurobiology to treatment: Progress against addiction. *Nat Neurosci, 5*(Suppl), 1076–1079.

Oliveto, A. H., Feingold, A., Schottenfeld, R., Jatlow, P., & Kosten, T. R. (1999). Desipramine in opioid-dependent cocaine abusers maintained on buprenorphine vs methadone. *Arch Gen Psychiatry, 56,* 812–820.

Raine, A., Lencz, T., Bihrle, S., LaCasse, L., & Colletti, P. (2000). Reduced prefrontal gray matter volume and reduced autonomic activity in antisocial personality disorder. *Arch Gen Psychiatry, 57*(2), 119–127.

Robinson, T. E., & Berridge, K. C. (2000). The psychology and neurobiology of addiction: An incentive-sensitization view. *Addiction, 95*(Suppl 2), S91–S117.

Schluger, J. H., Borg, L., Ho, A., & Kreek, M. J. (2001). Altered HPA axis responsivity to metyrapone testing in methadone maintained former heroin addicts with ongoing cocaine addiction. *Neuropsychopharmacology, 24*(5), 568–575.

Schottenfeld, R. S., Pakes, J. R., Oliveto, A., Ziedonis, D., & Kosten, T. R. (1997). Buprenorphine versus methadone maintenance treatment for concurrent opioid dependence and cocaine abuse. *Arch Gen Psychiatry, 54*(8), 713–720.

Shaham, Y., Erb, S., & Stewart, J. (2000). Stress-induced relapse to heroin and cocaine seeking in rats: A review. *Brain Res Brain Res Rev, 33,* 13–33.

Sinha, R., Catapano, D., & O'Malley, S. (1999). Stress-induced craving and stress response in cocaine dependent individuals. *Psychopharmacology, 142,* 343–351.

Stahl, S. M. (1998). Getting stoned without inhaling: Anandamide is the brain's natural marijuana. *J Clin Psychiatry, 59,* 566–567.

Stahl, S. M. (2002). Selective actions on sleep or anxiety by exploiting GABA-A/benzodiazepine receptor subtypes. *J Clin Psychiatry, 63,* 179–180.

CHAPTER 2

Historical and Social Context of Psychoactive Substance Use Disorders

JOSEPH WESTERMEYER

Historical and social factors are key to the understanding of addictive disorders. These factors affect the rates of addictive disorders in the community, the types of substances abused, the characteristics of abusive users, the course of these disorders, and the efficacy of treatment. Knowledge of these background features helps in understanding the genesis of these disorders, their treatment outcome, and preventive approaches.

Psychoactive substances subserve several human functions that can enhance both individual and social existence. On the individual level, desirable ends include the following: relief of adverse mental and emotional states (e.g., anticipatory anxiety before battle and social phobia at a party), relief of physical symptoms (e.g., pain and diarrhea), stimulation to function despite fatigue or boredom, and "time-out" from day-to-day existence through altered states of consciousness. Socially, alcohol and drugs are used in numerous rituals and ceremonies, from alcohol in Jewish Passover rites and the Roman Catholic Mass, to peyote in the Native American Church and the serving of opium at certain Hindu marriages. To a certain extent, the history of human civilization parallels the development of psychoactive substances (Westermeyer, 1999).

Paradoxically, these substances that bless and benefit our existence can also torment and decivilize us. Individuals, societies, and cultures began learning this disturbing truth millennia ago. We continue to rediscover this harsh reality today and will do so in the future, as though each new generation must learn afresh for itself. As our societies become more complex, so too do our psychoactive substances, our means of consuming them, and the problems associated with them. Preventive and treatment efforts, also age-old and wrought at great cost, are our forebears' gifts to us for dealing with psychoactive substance use gone astray (Anawalt & Berdan, 1992).

HISTORY AND ORIGINS

Prehistory

Methods for the study of psychoactive substance use disorders through time and space include the archaeological record, anthropological studies of preliterate societies, and the historical record. Archaeological data document the importance of alcohol commerce in late prehistorical and early historical times, both in the Mediterranean (where wine vessels have been discovered in numerous shipwrecks) and in China (where wine vessels have been found in burial sites). Poppy seed caches have been recorded in a prehistoric site in northern Turkey. Incised poppy capsules have been noted in the prehistoric headdresses of Cretan goddesses or priestesses, indicating an early awareness of opium harvest methods. Availability of carbohydrate in excess of dietary needs, fostered by neolithic farming technology and animal husbandry, permitted sporadic cases of alcohol abuse (Westermeyer, 1999).

Anthropological studies of preliterate societies have shown the almost universal use of psychoactive substances. Tribal and peasant societies of North and South America focused on the development of stimulant drugs (e.g., coca leaf, tobacco leaf, and coffee bean) and numerous hallucinogenic drugs (e.g., peyote). They used hallucinogens for ritual purposes and stimulant drugs for secular purposes, such as hard labor or long hunts. New World peoples discovered diverse modes of administration, such as chewing, nasal insufflation or "snuffing," pulmonary inhalation or "smoking," and rectal clysis (DuToit, 1977). African and Middle Eastern ethnic groups produced a smaller number of stimulants, such as qat, and hallucinogens, such as cannabis (Kennedy, Teague, & Fairbanks, 1980). Groups across Africa and the Eurasian land mass obtained alcohol from numerous sources, such as honey, grains, tubers, fruits, and mammalian milk. Certain drugs were also used across vast distances, such as opium across Asia and the stimulant betel nut from South Asia to Oceania. Old World peoples primarily consumed drugs by ingestion prior to Columbus's travel to the New World.

Early History

Historical records of alcohol, opium, and other psychoactive substances appear with the earliest Egyptian and Chinese writings. Opium was described as an ingested medication in these first documents, especially for medicinal purposes. Mayan, Aztec, and Incan statues and glyphs indicated drug use for ritual reasons (Furst, 1972). Medieval accounts recorded traditional alcohol and drug use. Travelers of that era often viewed use patterns in other areas as unusual, aberrant, or problematic; examples include reports of Scandinavian "beserker" drinkers by the English and reports by Crusaders of Islamic military units or "assassins" intoxicated on cannabis. Along with animal sacrifice and the serving of meat, the provision of alcohol, betel, opium, tobacco, or other psychoactive substances came to have cultural, ritual, or religious symbolism, including hospitality toward guests (Smith, 1965). Affiliation with specific ethnic groups, social classes, sects, and castes was associated with consumption of specific psychoactive substances. For example, one group in India consumed alcohol but not cannabis, whereas an adjacent group consumed cannabis but not alcohol (Carstairs, 1954). Altered patterns of psychoactive use have signaled other, more fundamental cultural changes (Caetano, 1987). Religious identity could be tied to alcohol or drug consumption. For example, wine has been a traditional aspect of Jewish, Catholic, and certain other Christian rituals and ceremonies, whereas some Islamic, Hindu, Buddhist, and fundamentalist Christian sects prohibit alcohol drinking. In addition to distinguishing people from one another, substance use may serve to maintain cooperation and communication across ethnic groups and social classes, from Africa (Wolcott, 1974) to Bolivia (Heath, 1971).

Cultural and Social Change

In recent centuries, political, commercial, and technical advances have influenced the types, supply, cost, and availability of psychoactive substances, along with modes of administration (Westermeyer, 1987). International commerce, built on cheaper and more efficient transportation, and increasing income have fostered drug production and distribution. Increasing disposable income has resulted in greater recreational intoxication (Caetano, Suzman, Rosen, & Voorhees-Rosen, 1983). Development of parenteral injection for medical purposes was readily adapted to recreational drug self-administration in the mid-1800s, within several years of its invention. Purification and modification of plant compounds (e.g., cocaine from the coca leaf, morphine and heroin from opium, and hashish oil from the cannabis plant) produced substances that were both more potent and more easily smuggled and sold illicitly. Laboratory synthesis has produced drugs that closely mimic naturally occurring substances (e.g., the stimulant amphetamines, the sedative barbiturates and benzodiazepines, the opioid fentanyl, and the hallucinogen lysergic acid) that are more potent and often cheaper than purified plant compounds.

Historical and cultural factors may theoretically affect the pharmacokinetics and pharmacodynamics of psychoactive substance, just as the pharmacology of these substances may affect their historical and traditional use. A case in point is the flushing reaction observed among a greater-than-expected number of Asians and Native Americans (but neither universal in these peoples, nor limited to them). Absence of alcohol use among the northern Asian peoples who subsequently peopled much of East Asia and the Americas is a likely explanation, but the exact reason is unknown. The flushing reaction associated with alcohol (Johnson & Nagoshi, 1990) has been offered as a reason for two opposite phenomena:

1. The low rates of alcoholism among Asian peoples, who presumably find the reaction aversive and hence drink little—although rates are increasing across much of Asia (Ohmori, Koyama, et al., 1986).
2. The high rates of alcoholism among certain Native American groups, who presumably must "drink through" their flushing reaction to experience other alcohol effects.

Flushing may be more or less desirable, depending upon how the culture values this biological effect. Among many East and Southeast Asian peoples influenced by Buddhist precepts, flushing is viewed as the emergence of cupidity or rage, with implied loss of emotional control. Modal differences in alcohol metabolism have also been observed among ethnic groups, and these differences support arguments in favor of biological causation. However, the intraethnic differences in alcohol metabolism greatly exceed the interethnic differences (Fenna, Mix, Schaeffer, & Gilbert, 1971). Despite some minimal pharmacokinetic differences among people of different races, the observed differences appear to be more due to pharmacodynamics; that is, the influence of people vis-à-vis the drug (i.e., their traditions, taboos, expectations, and patterns of use) appears to exert greater influence than the drug vis-à-vis the people (e.g., rates of absorption and catabolism and flushing reactions). Pharmacodynamic factors related to culture and pharmacokinetic factors related to biological inheritance and environmental influences probably both play roles in the individual's experience with psychoactive substances.

As psychoactive substance use developed into substance abuse in many advanced civilizations, social and cultural means evolved to control usage. One method was law and law enforcement. Aztecs utilized this method in pre-Columbian times to limit the frequency and amount of drinking (Anawalt & Berdan, 1992). Later, in the post-Columbian period, England countered its "gin plague" with a tax on imported alcohol-containing beverages (Thurn, 1978), and its later "opium epidemic" with prescribing laws (Kramer, 1979). Another method has been religious stricture. Perhaps the first organized religion to prescribe abstinence from alcohol was Hinduism. Early Buddhist leaders counseled abstinence from alcohol as a means of quitting earthly bondage to achieve contentment in this life and eternal nirvana after death. Islam became the third great religion to adopt abstinence from alcohol, reportedly when a town was sacked as a result of a drunken nighttime guard. The gin plague in England spawned several abstinence-oriented Christian sects, despite the earlier status of wine as a Christian sacramental substance (Johnson & Westermeyer, 2000). The Church of Jesus Christ of Latter-Day Saints (the group popularly known as the Mormons) forbids any use of psychoactive substances, including caffeine and nicotine.

In addition to religion as a preventive measure, religion has also served as a therapy for psychoactive substance abuse. Native Americans and Latin Americans, plagued with high rates of alcoholism, have joined fundamentalist Christian sects as a means of garnering social support while resisting peer pressures to drink (Mariz, 1991). Many Native Americans have joined the Native American Church, in which peyote is a sacramental substance but alcohol is proscribed (Albaugh & Anderson, 1974).

Patterns of Psychoactive Substance Use

Traditional patterns of psychoactive substance use in most societies were episodic, coming at times of personal celebrations (e.g., birth and marriage), rituals (e.g., arrivals, departures, and changes in status), and seasonal celebrations (e.g., harvest and New Year). Exceptions to this pattern were daily or at least occasional use of alcohol as a foodstuff and use of various stimulants (e.g., betel-areca, tea and coffee, and coca leaf) in association with long, hard labor (e.g., paddy rice or taro farming and silver mining). Daily beer or wine drinking was limited to Europe, especially the para-Mediterranean wine countries and central grain-beer countries. Such daily or "titer" use is not without its problems, even when socially sanctioned. Hepatic cirrhosis and other organ damage (e.g., to brain, bone marrow, neuromuscular system, and pancreas) may result from long-term, daily use of more than 2–4 ounces of alcohol, depending on body weight (Baldwin, 1977). Daily use of stimulants, especially if heavy or addictive, can lead to biomedical or psychosocial problems, such as oral cancers in the case of betel-areca chewing (Ahluwalia & Ponnampalam, 1968) or psychobehavioral changes in the case of coca leaf chewing (Negrete, 1978).

Socially sanctioned, episodic psychoactive substance use may involve heavy use, with marked intoxication or drunkenness (Bunzel, 1940). In a low-technology environment, this pattern may cause few problems, although psychotomimetic drugs such as cannabis can cause toxic psychosis (Chopra & Smith, 1974). In a high-technology environment, with modern methods of transportation and industrial machinery, intoxication even at mild traditional levels may be life threatening (Stull, 1972). Binge-type alcohol problems include delirium tremens, fights, sexually transmitted disease, and falls.

Among other consequence of technology and advanced civilization are widespread substance abuse epidemics, or long-lasting endemics. In the pre-

Columbian era, sporadic cases of acute and chronic substance abuse problems had been known for at least a millennium, and probably longer. However, relatively sudden, massive substance abuse increases appeared early in the post-Columbian era. One of these was the English gin epidemic or gin plague (Thurn, 1978), which began in the late 1600s and continued for several decades. Transatlantic intercontinental trade and the beginnings of the Industrial Revolution were the immediate causes. At about the same time, opium epidemics broke out in several Asian countries. The origins of these epidemics were somewhat different. The post-Columbian spread of tobacco smoking to Asia introduced the inhabitants to inhalation as a new mode of drug administration. This new route of administration applied to an old drug, opium, produced a combination more addictive than the old opium-eating tradition. Governmental pressures against tobacco smoking (which was viewed as wasteful and associated with seditious elements) probably accelerated the popularity of opium smoking. Subsequently, European colonialism and international trade contributed to the import of Indian opium to several East Asian countries. Opium epidemics also occurred somewhat later in Europe and North America (Kramer, 1979). Although East Asian countries have largely controlled their opium problems, opiate endemics continue in Southeast and South Asia, the Middle East, parts of Europe, and North America.

HISTORICAL MODELS OF SUBSTANCE USE

Although ceremonial alcohol use is widely appreciated, the ceremonial use of drugs is not so well known. Peyote buttons are a sacramental substance in the Native American Church (Bergman, 1971). Hallucinogen use for religious purposes still occurs among many South American ethnic groups (DuToit, 1977). Supernatural sanctions, both prescribing use within certain bounds and proscribing use outside these bounds, inveigh against abuse of these substances by devotees. Thus, ceremonial or religious use tends to be relatively safe. Examples of abuse do occur, however, such as the occasional Catholic priest who becomes alcoholic, beginning with abuse of sacramental wine.

Secular but social use of alcohol and drugs occurs in numerous quasi-ritual contexts. Drinking may occur at annual events, such as New Year or harvest ceremonies (e.g., Thanksgiving in the United States). Weddings, births, funerals, and other family rituals are occasions for alcohol or drug use in many cultures. Marking of friendships, business arrangements, or intergroup competitions can virtually require substance use in some groups. For example, the *dutsen* in German-speaking Central Europe is a brief ritual in which friends or associates agree to address each other by the informal *du* ("thou") rather than by the formal *Sie* ("you"). Participants, holding an alcoholic beverage in their right hands, link their right arms, toast each other, and drink with arms linked.

The use of betel-areca, pulque or cactus beer, coca leaf, and other intoxicants has accompanied group work tasks, such as harvests or community *corvée* obligations (e.g., maintaining roads, bridges, and irrigation ditches). Although substance use may be heavy at ceremonial events, even involving intoxication, the social control of the group over dosage and the brief duration of use augurs against chronic abuse (although problems related to acute abuse may occur). Problems can develop if the group's central rationale for existence rests on substance use (e.g., habitués of opium dens, taverns, and cocktail lounges). In these latter instances, group norms for alcohol or drug use may foster substance abuse rather than prevent it (Dumont, 1967).

Medicinal reasons for substance use have prevailed in one place or another with virtually all psychoactive substances, including alcohol, opium, cannabis, tobacco, the stimulants, and the hallucinogens (Hill, 1990). Insofar as substances are prescribed or administered solely by healers or physicians, abuse is rare or absent. For example, the prescribing of oral opium by Chinese physicians over many centuries had few or no adverse social consequences. On the other hand, self-prescribing for medicinal purposes carries risks. For example, certain Northern Europeans, Southeast Asians, and others use alcohol for insomnia, colds, pain, and other maladies—a practice that can and does lead to chronic alcohol abuse. Self-prescribing of opium by poppy farmers similarly antedates opium addiction in a majority of cases (Westermeyer, 1982). Thus, professional control over medicinal use has been relatively benign, whereas individual control over medicinal use of psychoactive compounds has often been problematic.

Dietary use of substances falls into two general categories: (1) the use of alcohol as a source of calories and (2) the use of cannabis and other herbal intoxicants to enhance taste. Fermentation of grains, tubers, and fruits into alcohol has been a convenient way of storing calories that would otherwise deteriorate. Unique tastes and eating experiences associated with beverage alcohol (e.g., various wines) have further fostered their use, especially at ritual, ceremonial, or social meals. Cannabis has also been used from the Middle East to the Malay Archipelago as a means of enhancing soups, teas, pastries, and other sweets. Opium and other substances have been served at South Asian ceremonies (e.g., weddings) as a postprandial "dessert."

Recreational use can presumably occur in either social or individual settings. Much substance use today occurs in recreational or "party" settings that have some psychosocial rationales (e.g., social "time-out" and meeting friends) but minimal or no ritual or ceremonial aspects. So-called recreational substance use in these social contexts may in fact be quasi-medicinal (i.e., to reduce symptoms associated with social phobia, low self-esteem, boredom, or chronic dysphoria). Even solitary psychoactive substance use can be recreational (i.e., to enhance an enjoyable event) or medicinal (i.e., to relieve loneliness, insomnia, or pain).

Other purposes exist but are not as widespread as those described earlier. In the 19th century, young European women took belladonna before social events in order to give themselves a ruddy, blushing complexion. A particular substance or pattern of use can represent a social or ethnic identity (Carstairs, 1954). Children may inhale household or industrial solvents as a means of mimicking adult intoxication (Kaufman, 1973). Intoxication may simply serve as a means for continuing social behaviors, such as fights or homicide, that existed previously without intoxication (Levy & Kunitz, 1969). Particular patterns of alcohol–drug production or use may represent rebellion by disenfranchised groups (Connell, 1961; Lurie, 1970).

HISTORY OF SUBSTANCE ABUSE TREATMENT

Historical and literary accounts have long documented individual attempts to draw back from the abyss of alcohol and drug abuse. At various times autobiographical, biographical, journalistic, and anecdotal, these descriptions list centuries-old recovery methods still employed today in lay and professional settings. Modalities include gradual decrease in dosage; symptomatic use of nonaddicting medications; isolation from the substance; relocation away from fellow users; religious conversion; group support; asylum in a supportive and nondemanding environment; and treatment with a variety of shamanistic, spiritual, dietary, herbal, and medicinal methods (Westermeyer, 1998).

Beginning with Galenic medicine, a key strategy has been to identify certain syndromes as having their etiology in alcohol and drug abuse. Once the etiology is determined, the specific treatment (i.e., cessation of substance abuse) can be prescribed. Examples of such substance-associated disorders include delirium tremens (i.e., alcohol and sedative withdrawal), withdrawal seizures, morphinism (i.e., opioid withdrawal), cannabis-induced acute psychosis, stimulant psychosis, and various fetal effects, such as fetal alcohol syndrome. Thus, description of pathophysiological and psychopathological processes, together with diagnostic labeling, has been a crucial historical step in the development of modern assessment and treatment for substance use disorders (Rodin, 1981).

Modern treatment approaches have their origins in methods developed by Benjamin Rush, a physician from the Revolutionary War era, who is often credited as the father of American psychiatry. Rush developed a categorization of drinkers and alcoholics. He further prescribed treatment that consisted of a period of "asylum" from responsibilities and from access to alcohol, to take place in a family-like setting, in a milieu of respect, consideration, and social support. As Rush's concepts were extrapolated to the growing American society, large state-supported institutions were developed—although some smaller, private asylums or sanitoria for alcoholics have persisted up to the current time (Johnson & Westermeyer, 2000).

Medical treatments can interact constructively with cultural factors. For example, taking disulfiram can serve as an excuse for Native American alcoholics to resist peer pressures to drink (Savard, 1968). Ethnic similarity between patients and staff appears to be more critical to the treatment process than in other medical or psychiatric conditions (Shore & Von Fumetti, 1972). Strong ethnic affiliation may be associated with more optimal treatment outcomes, although ethnic affiliation may change as a result of treatment (Westermeyer & Lang, 1975).

On a federal level, treatment for drug abuse (largely opiate dependence) began with the Harrison Act of 1914, which outlawed nonmedical use of opiate drugs. For a time, heroin maintenance was prescribed and dispensed in several clinics around the country. Although research studies were not conducted, case reports from these clinics indicated that many patients were able to resume stable lives while receiving maintenance doses of heroin. These clinics were phased out, largely because of political opposition. Two long-term, prison-like hospitals for opiate addicts were established (one in Kentucky and the other in Texas). Research in these institutions contributed greatly to our understanding of opiate addiction (and alcoholism, which was also studied), but the demonstrated inefficacy of prison treatment led to their demise as treatment facilities. These legal and medical approaches, beginning in 1914, were effective in reducing opiate dependence in the societal mainstream. However, certain occupational, geographical, and ethnic groups continued to use drugs that were made illicit by the Harrison Act. These included seamen, musicians, certain minority groups, and inhabitants of coastal–border areas involved in smuggling (e.g., San Antonio, Texas; Louisiana seaports; San Francisco, California; and New York City).

Following World War II, medical and social leaders were more aware of widespread mental disabilities in the country because of the high rate of psychiatric disorders among inductees and veterans. This led to the establishment of the National Institute of Mental Health (NIMH), which had divisions of alcoholism and drug abuse. By the 1970s, it became apparent that substance use disorders were widely prevalent. Numerous indices of alcohol abuse and alcoholism had been increasing since World War II, including hepatic cirrhosis and violence-related mortality. Endemic abuse of cocaine and opiates exploded into an epidemic in the late 1960s, followed by the appearance of stimulant and hallucinogen abuse. It was evident that the NIMH was not adequately addressing either the alcohol epidemic or the drug epidemic. This led to the formation of the National Institute on Alcohol Abuse and Alcoholism (NIAAA) and the National Institute on Drug Abuse (NIDA), both of which have equal status with the NIMH under the Alcohol, Drug Abuse, and Mental Health Administration (ADAMHA). Located within the Department of Health and Human

Services, ADAMHA has fostered the development of substance abuse research, training, clinical services, and prevention. Governmental support for these efforts has come largely from elected officials who have personally experienced psychoactive substance use disorders, either in themselves or in their families. For example, most of the last several American presidents have had a spouse, parent, sibling, offspring, or personal experience with a substance abuse disorder.

SOCIAL AND SELF-HELP MOVEMENTS

Abstinence-oriented social movements first appeared among organized religions (Johnson & Westermeyer, 2000). Certain South Asian sects, arising from early Persian religions and Hinduism, abstained from alcohol over two millennia ago. Buddhist clergy were forbidden to drink alcoholic beverages, and pious Buddhist laity were urged to refrain from drinking, or at least to drink moderately. Early on, Moslems were urged not to drink; tradition has it that Mohammed himself established abstinence for his followers. Abstinence-oriented Christian sects evolved in England and then in Central Europe at about the time of the gin epidemic.

Religiomania has long served as a cure for dipsomania and narcotomania. Opium addicts in Asia have gone to Buddhist monasteries in the hope that worship, meditation, or clerical asceticism would cure them, which it sometimes did (Westermeyer, 1982). Many Latin Americans and Native Americans with high rates of alcoholism have abandoned Catholicism and Anglicanism in favor of abstinence-prescribing fundamentalist Christian sects and the Native American Church (Albaugh & Anderson, 1974; Hippler, 1973). Children raised in these sects are taught the importance of lifelong abstinence from alcohol and other drugs of abuse. Despite this childhood socialization, those leaving these sects as adults can develop substance use disorders. Thus, the effects of various religions in preventing substance abuse disorders appear to persist only as long as one is actively affiliated with the group.

Abstinent societies not tied to specific religions began to appear in the 18th and 19th centuries. Examples include the Anti-Opium Society in China and the Women's Christian Temperance Union in the United States. These groups engaged in political action, public education, social pressure against addiction or alcoholism, and support for abstinence. These led eventually to prohibition movements that sought legal strictures against the production, sale, and/or consumption of psychoactive substances outside religious or medical contexts. In Asia, these movements began against tobacco (which was viewed in the 1600s and 1700s as a slothful habit associated with political sedition) and then later changed to oppose primarily opium. In Northern Europe and the United States, prohibition laws first involved opiates and cannabis but later expanded to include alcohol. As Moslem peoples emerged from colonial regimes, their nations passed anti-alcohol legislation that ranged from mild strictures for Moslems alone, to harsh measures against all inhabitants of the country.

Numerous self-help groups in the United States were founded during the Depression era. Many more were begun after World War II. These groups involved individuals who banded together to meet their common financial, social, or personal needs (Lieberman & Borman, 1976). Movements of the era differed in several important aspects from earlier abstinence-oriented groups as follows:

- Individuals could remain in their homes, families, and jobs rather than joining a separate sect or going off to an asylum or special group.
- Considerable structure was involved, with specific meetings and phased "step" recovery activities.
- The concept of a recovery process over time was introduced, as distinct from a sudden cure or conversion; this had biological, psychological, social, and spiritual dimensions.
- Organization was kept predominantly atomistic (i.e., autonomous small groups) rather than hierarchical.
- Membership required self-identity as an alcoholic or addict (i.e., supportive or concerned persons were excluded).

Like earlier movements, these self-help groups emphasized the importance of abstinence from psychoactive substance abuse (although tobacco and coffee are notably present at some Alcoholics Anonymous [AA] meetings today), reliance on a superior spiritual force (the "Higher Power"), and social affiliation or "fellowship" for mutual support. AA, perhaps the best known of these groups today, was first established in the United States. It has spread to many other parts of the world over the last 50 years and has served as a model for similar groups whose identity centers on other drugs and even other problems (i.e., Narcotics Anonymous, Cocaine Anonymous, Overeaters Anonymous, Gamblers Anonymous, and Emotions Anonymous [formerly Neurotics Anonymous]). Groups for those personally affected by alcoholism have also appeared, such as Alateen for the teenage offspring of alcoholic parents and Al-Anon for the spouses, parents, and other concerned associates of alcoholic persons. Over the last several years, the Adult Children of Alcoholics and Addicts (ACOAA) movement has also evolved to meet the needs of those distressed or maladaptive adults raised by alcoholic parents. Mothers Against Drunk Drivers (MADD) was originally formed to meet the support needs of parents whose children were killed by drunken auto drivers. MADD has since expanded its activities as a "watchdog" group that follows the records of legislators and judges in regard to alcohol-related legal offenses. The social and cultural composition of the self-help group appears to be an important factor in attracting clients and effecting therapeutic outcomes (Jilek-Aal, 1978).

FACTORS AFFECTING ALCOHOL–DRUG EPIDEMICS

Numerous factors contributed to the development of substance abuse "epidemics" or "plagues." One of the first of these, the gin epidemic (which involved other alcohol-containing beverages besides gin) in late 17th- and 18th-century England, was fostered by the following factors:

- English merchant ships returning empty from trips to its colonies loaded on gin, rum, and other alcohol-containing beverages as ballast before returning to England.
- Rum was derived from sugar cane grown with slave labor, and gin was from grains grown with indentured labor. With no import tax, calories of these alcohol-containing beverages were literally cheaper than calories of bread in London.
- The beginnings of the Industrial Revolution gave rise to repressive social conditions and a loss of traditional rural values, fostering widespread drunkenness with inexpensive beverage alcohol.
- Although traditions and social controls existed for the drinking of mead and ale, these traditions and controls did not extend to gin and rum drinking, with the result that daily excessive drinking appeared.

During this period, numerous sequelae of alcoholism were first recognized, including the description of the fetal alcohol syndrome (Rodin, 1981). The gin epidemic raged for several decades, perhaps as long as a century. It eventually receded under such pressures as an import tax on imported alcohol-containing beverages, anti-alcohol propaganda in the literature and art of the day, and evolution of abstinence-oriented Protestant sects for the working classes.

The opium epidemic in many countries of East and Southeast Asia began about the same time as the European alcohol epidemic. Several factors, some similar to the European situation but others different, contributed to the opium epidemic:

- Tobacco smoking was introduced to Asia from the New World; it became a popular pastime in smoking houses that were frequented by the artisans, artists, adventurists, and literati of the day.
- As European and New World concepts and artifacts flooded into Asia, tobacco-smoking houses were viewed as places of cultural change and even political sedition; they were gradually outlawed.

• Opium eating, primarily a medicinal activity that had never been a significant social problem, was combined with this new technology (i.e., drug consumption by volatilization and inhalation); recreational opium smoking subsequently became widespread.

• Political corruption, government inefficiency, and absence of statecraft skills to deal with widespread drug abuse, abetted by the political and economic imperialism of Western colonial powers, led to centuries of widespread opium addiction among various Asian nations. Some countries have reversed the problem in this century (e.g., Japan, Korea, China, and Manchuria); others have not (e.g., Thailand, Laos, Burma, Pakistan, Afghanistan, Iran, and India).

TRENDS IN PROBLEMS ACROSS TIME AND SPACE

The appearance of new drugs (or reappearance of old ones in new forms) exposed social groups to agents against which they had no sociocultural protection or "immunity"; that is, the community or nation had no tradition for problem-free, or at least controlled, use of the substance. Users themselves may not have perceived the actual risks associated with the new psychoactive substance. This situation also occurred when the group was familiar with the substance but in a different form. For example, traditions may exist for wine but not beer or distilled alcohol; pipe smoking may be subject to customs that do not extend to cigarette smoking.

Symbolic aspects of certain drugs or modes of drug administration may displace the issue from psychoactive substance use per se to associated issues of ethnic identity, cultural change, political upheaval, class struggle, or intergenerational conflict (Robbins, 1973). Examples include the following:

• Cannabis and hallucinogen use as antiauthority symbols in the late 1960s and 1970s.
• Alcohol abuse among indigenous peoples (Thompson, 1992).
• Illicit raising of poppy as a cash crop and opium smuggling by ethnic minorities in Asia (Westermeyer, 1982).

As drug use has spread in the last few centuries, drug production and commerce have become important economic resources in many areas. Early examples in the 1800s were the British trading companies in large areas of India, which depended for their wealth on opium sales to China. Numerous backward areas in the world today maintain their participation in national and world markets through their participation in illicit drug production and sales: Afghanistan, Burma, Laos, Mexico, Pakistan, and Thailand in opium and heroin; the Caribbean nations and Mexico in cannabis production and cocaine commerce; and several South and Central American countries in cocaine production and commerce. During the 1980s, several states in the United States counted cannabis as a major, albeit illicit, cash crop: North Carolina, Tennessee, Kentucky, Kansas, Nebraska, New Mexico, California, and Hawaii (Culhane, 1989).

Government instability, corruption, or inefficiency can cause or result from drug production, export, and/or smuggling today. Unstable countries in South Asia, the Middle East, Africa, and Latin America have become producers, transshippers, or importers of illicit drugs. Societal breakdown has led to substance abuse in some Moslem countries, contributing to a backlash of Islamic fundamentalism. Likewise, in the United States and Latin America, widespread alcoholism predates the shift to Christian fundamentalism.

Industrialization and technological advances have fostered a redefinition of substance abuse (Stull, 1972). An intoxicated or "hungover" (withdrawing) oxcart driver can effect limited damage, other than to cart, ox, and self. The alcohol- or drug-affected driver of a modern high-speed bus, the captain of a ferry boat, or the pilot of a jet transport can kill scores of people and destroy equipment and material worth millions of dollars. Handicraft artisans under the influence of drugs or alcohol can do little damage, whereas workers in a factory can harm themselves or others, as well as destroying expensive machinery and bringing production to a halt.

Since World War II, and especially since the 1960s, adolescent-onset substance abuse has escalated from rare sporadic cases to a high prevalence in many communities (Cameron, 1968). Several factors appear to have fostered it: widespread parental substance abuse, societal neglect of adolescents, poverty, rapid social changes, family breakdown, and political upheaval. Whatever the cause, the consequences are remarkably similar: undermining of normal adolescent psychosocial development, poor socialization of children to assume adult roles, lack of job skills, emotional immaturity, increased rates of adolescent psychiatric morbidity, and increased adolescent mortality from suicide, accidents, and homicide.

TRENDS IN TREATMENT AND PREVENTION

From the time of Benjamin Rush, two central treatment methods were established, based on the psychiatric treatment methods of the late 1700s: (1) "asylum" in a supportive environment away from drink and companion drinkers and (2) "moral treatment," consisting of a civil, respectful consideration for the recovering person (Johnson & Westermeyer, 2000). Both methods persist today and remain as two standard treatment strategies. They were not and are not inevitably successful. Consequently, other methods have been tried.

One of these methods was the substitution of one drug for another. For example, laudanum (combined alcohol and opiates) was once prescribed for alcoholism. Morphine, and later heroin, was recommended for opium addiction during the mid-1800s. This approach is not extinct, as exemplified by the frequent recommendation in the 1970s that alcoholics substitute cannabis smoking for alcohol. Currently, methadone is used for chronic opiate addicts who have failed attempts at drug-free treatment. Despite aversive selection factors, methadone maintenance patients tend to do well as long as they comply with treatment.

Detoxification became prevalent in the mid-1900s. Public detoxification facilities, established first in Eastern Europe, spread throughout the world. For many patients, this resource offers an entree into recovery. For others, "revolving door" detoxification may actually produce lifelong institutionalization on the installment plan (Gallant et al., 1973). The problem of the treatment-resistant public inebriate exists today in all parts of the United States.

The so-called Minnesota Model of treatment developed from several sources: a state hospital program (at Wilmar) and a later private program (at Hazelden), supplemented by the first day program for alcoholism (at the Minneapolis Veterans Administration Hospital). The characteristics of this "model" have varied over time as treatment has evolved and changed, and definitions still differ from one person to the next. However, characteristics often ascribed to the model include the following:

1. A period of residential or inpatient care, ranging from a few weeks to several months.
2. A focus on the psychoactive substance use disorder, with little or no consideration of associated psychiatric conditions or individual psychosocial factors.
3. Heavy emphasis on AA self-help concepts, resources, and precepts, such as the "12 steps" of recovery.
4. Referral to AA or another self-help group on discharge from residential or inpatient care, with minimal or no ongoing professional treatment.
5. Minimal or no family therapy or counseling (although family orientation to AA principles and Al-Anon may take place).
6. Negative attitudes toward ongoing psychotherapies and pharmacotherapies for substance use disorder or associated psychiatric disorder.

At the time of its evolution in the 1950s and 1960s, this model served to bridge the formerly separate hospital programs and self-help groups—a laudable achievement. However, if it is applied rigidly in light of current knowledge, some patients (who might otherwise be helped) will fail in or drop out of treatment. Nowadays, many treatment programs employ aspects of the old "Minnesota Model," integrating them flexibly with newer methods in a more individualized and patient-centered manner.

The workplace has been a locus of prevention, early recognition, referral for treatment, and rehabilitation. Following World War II, Hudolin and coworkers in Yugoslavia established factory- and farm–commune-based recovery groups, with ties to treatment facilities. Over the last two decades, alcoholism counselors have worked in similar "employee assistance programs" in the United States.

More sophisticated methods of pharmacotherapy have appeared recently, although these remain few in comparison with other areas of medicine. Safe detoxification is possible through increased basic and clinical appreciation of withdrawal syndromes. Disulfiram, naltrexone, buprenorphine, and methadone may be selectively prescribed as maintenance drugs in the early difficult months and years of recovery. Other medications are currently being investigated for use in special circumstances.

Recognition of comorbid conditions accompanying substance abuse has led to concurrent treatment for affective disorders, anxiety disorders, eating disorders, and pathological gambling. For certain chronic conditions (e.g., mild mental retardation, borderline intelligence, organic brain syndrome, or chronic schizophrenia), substance abuse treatment, rehabilitation, and self-help procedures need to be modified. Intensive outpatient programs, conducted during the day, evening, or weekend, assist certain patients to recover when other measures fail. These intensive outpatient programs are modeled after similar psychiatric programs. Much of the treatment time is spent in groups of various sizes, although individual and family sessions may occur as well. Staffing is typically multidisciplinary, with counselors, nurses, occupational and recreational therapists, psychologists, psychiatrists, and social workers. Monitoring of recovery in several contexts and by several sources (e.g., at work, by licensing agencies or unions, in the family, and with medical resources) appears to enhance outcome (Westermeyer, 1989).

Preventive techniques first applied to the gin epidemic are still useful today: control over hours and location of sales, taxes or duties to increase cost, changing of public attitudes via the mass media, education, and abstinence-oriented religion (Smart, 1982). The prolonged Asian opium epidemic demonstrated that laws alone are ineffective unless accompanied by socially integrated treatment; recovery programs; compulsory abstinence in identified cases; police pressure against drug production, commerce, and consumption; and follow-up monitoring. Experience with anti-alcohol prohibition laws in Europe and North America demonstrated the futility of outlawing substance use that was supported by many citizens. Adverse results from the Prohibition era in the United States included increased criminality associated with bootlegging alcohol, lack of quality control (e.g., methanol and lead contaminants), and development of unhealthy drinking patterns (e.g., surreptitious, rapid, without food, and in a deviant setting). Public interest groups such as MADD may aid in reducing certain alcohol- and drug-related problems. The United States has expended several 10's of billions of dollars since 1970 to reduce the supply of and demand for drugs. But mortality from hepatic cirrhosis, alcohol-related accidents, and suicide continue at an unprecedented level, especially among young American males. Work still remaining includes our learning from history (our own as well as that of others) to honing that aspect of statecraft aimed at eliminating our endemic substance abuse.

REFERENCES

Ahluwalia, H. S., & Ponnampalam, J. T. (1968). The socioeconomic aspects of betel-nut chewing. *J Trop Med Hyg, 71*, 48–50.

Albaugh, B., & Anderson, P. (1974). Peyote in the treatment of alcoholism among American Indians. *Am J Psychiatry, 131*, 1247–1256.

Anawalt, P. R., & Berdan, F. F. (1992). The Codex Mendoza. *Sci Am, 266*, 70–79.

Baldwin, A. D. (1977). Anstie's alcohol limit: Francis Edmund Anstie 1833–1874. *Am J Public Health, 67*, 679–681.

Bergman, R. L. (1971). Navaho peyote use: Its apparent safety. *Am J Psychiatry, 128*, 695–699.

Bunzel, R. (1940). The role of alcoholism in two Central American cultures. *Psychiatry, 3*, 361–387.

Caetano, R. (1987). Acculturation and drinking patterns among U.S. Hispanics. *Br J Addict, 82*, 789–799.

Caetano, R., Suzman, R. M., Rosen, D. H., & Voorhees-Rosen, D. J. (1983). The Shetland Islands: Longitudinal changes in alcohol consumption in a changing environment. *Br J Addict, 78*, 21–36.

Cameron, D. C. (1968). Youth and drugs: A world view. *JAMA, 206*, 1267–1271.

Carstairs, G. M. (1954). Daru and bhang: Cultural factors in the choice of intoxicant. *Q J Stud Alcohol, 15*, 220–237.

Chopra, G. S., & Smith, J. W. (1974). Psychotic reactions following cannabis use in East Indians. *Arch Gen Psychiatry, 30*, 24–27.

Connell, K. H. (1961). Illicit distillation: An Irish peasant industry. *Hist Stud Ireland, 3*, 58–91.

Culhane, C. (1989). Pot harvest gains across country. *USJ, 13*, 14.

Dumont, M. (1967). Tavern culture: The sustenance of homeless men. *Am J Orthopsychiatry, 37*, 938–945.

DuToit, B. M. (1977). *Drugs, rituals and altered states of consciousness.* Rotterdam, Netherlands: Balkema.

Fenna, D. L., Mix, O., Schaeffer, J., & Gilbert, A. L. (1971). Ethanol metabolism in various racial groups. *Can Med Assoc J, 105*, 472–475.

Furst, P. T. (1972). *Flesh of the gods: The ritual use of hallucinogens.* New York: Praeger.

Gallant, D. M., Bishop, M. P., Mouledoux, A., Faulkner, M. A., Brisolara, A., & Swanson, W. A. (1973). The revolving door alcoholic. *Arch Gen Psychiatry, 28*, 633–635.

Heath, D. (1971). Peasants, revolution, and drinking: Interethnic drinking patterns in two Bolivian communities. *Hum Organ, 30*, 179–186.

Hill, T. W. (1990). Peyotism and the control of heavy drinking: The Nebraska Winnebago in the early 1900s. *Hum Organ, 49*, 255–265.

Hippler, A. E. (1973). Fundamentalist Christianity: An Alaskan Athabascan technique for overcoming alcohol abuse. *Transcult Psychiatric Res Rev, 10,* 173–179.

Jilek-Aal, L. (1978). Alcohol and the Indian-White relationship: A study of the function of Alcoholics Anonymous among coast Salish Indians. *Confinia Psychiatr, 21,* 195–233.

Johnson, D. R., & Westermeyer, J. (2000). Psychiatric therapies influenced by religious movements. In J. Boehnlein (Ed.), *Psychiatry and religion: The convergence of mind and Spirit* (pp. 87–108). Washington, DC: American Psychiatric Press.

Johnson, R., & Nagoshi, C. (1990). Asians, Asian-Americans and alcohol. *J Psychoactive Drugs, 22,* 45–52.

Kaufman, A. (1973). Gasoline sniffing among children in a Pueblo Indian village. *Pediatrics, 51,* 1060–1065.

Kennedy, J. G., Teague, J., & Fairbanks, L. (1980). Quat use in North Yemen and the problem of addiction: A study in medical anthropology. *Cult Med Psychiatry, 4,* 311–344.

Kramer, J. C. (1979). Opium rampant: Medical use, misuse and abuse in Britain and the west in the 17th and 18th centuries. *Br J Addict, 74,* 377–389.

Levy, J. E., & Kunitz, S. J. (1969). Notes on some White Mountain Apache social pathologies. *Plateau, 42,* 11–19.

Lieberman, M. A., & Borman, L. D. (1976). Self-help groups. *J Appl Behav Sci, 12,* 261–303.

Lurie, N. O. (1970). The world's oldest on-going protest demonstration: North American Indian drinking patterns. *Pacific Hist Rev, 40,* 311–332.

Mariz, C. L. (1991). Pentecostalism and alcoholism among the Brazilian poor. *Alcoholism Treatment Q, 8,* 75–82.

Negrete, J. C. (1978). Coca leaf chewing: A public health assessment. *Br J Addict, 73,* 283–290.

Ohmori, T., Koyama, T., Chen, C. C., Yeh, E. K., Reyes, B. V., Jr., & Yamashita, I. (1986). The role of aldehyde dehydrogenase isozyme variance in alcohol sensitivity, drinking habits formation and the development of alcoholism in Japan, Taiwan and the Philippines. *Prog Neuropsychopharmacol Biol Psychiatry, 10,* 229–235.

Robbins, R. H. (1973). Alcohol and the identity struggle: Some effects of economic change on interpersonal relations." *Am Anthropol, 75,* 99–122.

Rodin, A. E. (1981). Infants and gin mania in 18th century London. *JAMA, 245,* 1237–1239.

Savard, R. J. (1968). Effects of disulfiram therapy in relationships within the Navaho drinking group. *Q J Stud Alcohol, 29,* 909–916.

Shore, J. H., & Von Fumetti, B. (1972). Three alcohol programs for American Indians. *Am J Psychiatry, 128,* 1450–1454.

Smart, R. G. (1982). The impact of prevention measures: An examination of research findings. In A. K. Kaplan (Ed.), *Legislative approaches to prevention of alcohol-related problems* (pp. 224–246). Washington, DC: Institute of Medicine.

Smith, W. R. (1965). Sacrifice among the Semites. In W. A. Lessa & E. Z. Vogt (Eds.), *Reader in comparative religion* (pp. 39–48). New York: Harper & Row.

Stull, D. D. (1972). Victims of modernization: Accident rates and Papago Indian adjustment. *Hum Organ, 31,* 227–240.

Thompson, J. W. (1992). Alcohol policy considerations for Indian people. *Am Indian Alsk Native Ment Health Res, 4,* 112–119.

Thurn, R. J. (1978). The gin plague. *Minn Med, 61,* 241–243.

Westermeyer, J. (1982). *Poppies, pipes and people: Opium and its use in Laos.* Berkeley: University of California Press.

Westermeyer, J. (1987). Cultural patterns of drug and alcohol use: An analysis of host and agent in the cultural environment. *UN Bull Narc, 39,* 11–27.

Westermeyer, J. (1989). Monitoring recovery from substance abuse: Rationales, methods and challenges. *Adv Alcohol Subst Abuse, 8,* 93–106.

Westermeyer, J. (1998). Historical–social context of psychoactive substance disorders. In R. J. Frances & S. I. Miller (Eds.), *Clinical textbook of addictive disorders* (2nd ed., pp. 14–32). New York: Guilford Press.

Westermeyer, J. (1999). The role of cultural and social factors in the cause of addictive disorders. *Psychiatr Clin North Am, 22,* 253–273.

Westermeyer, J., & Lang, G. (1975). Ethnic differences in use of alcoholism facilities. *Int J Addict, 10,* 513–520.

Wolcott, H. F. (1974). *African Beer Garden of Bulawayo: Integrated drinking in a segregated society.* New Brunswick, NJ: Rutgers Center of Alcoholism Studies.

PART II

ASSESSMENT OF ADDICTION

CHAPTER 3

Psychological Evaluation
of Substance Use Disorder
in Adolescents and Adults

RALPH E. TARTER

Psychological evaluation is directed at characterizing cognitive, emotional, and behavioral processes. The evaluation of substance use disorders thus focuses on multiple domains of psychological functioning. The instruments selectively reviewed in this chapter satisfy the following criteria: (1) the psychometric properties have been empirically established, (2) the measures have practical utility, and, (3) they are applicable to diverse populations.

It has been previously argued that the assessment of substance abuse should use comparable measures in clinical and research settings (Rounsaville, 1993). The ultimate usefulness of psychological measurement is to delineate the unique factors within the individual that predispose to substance use onset, sustain habitual consumption, and impede psychosocial adjustment. Moreover, a comprehensive evaluation should directly guide the selection of prevention and treatment strategies that are most likely to be successful. In the managed care environment, where there is an emphasis on cost containment and empirical documentation, it is invaluable to obtain as much information as possible that could expedite effective treatment.

Psychological evaluation must also accommodate contemporary understanding of the disorder. Hence, evaluation must encompass an approach that aligns with an appreciation of the multifactorial etiology of substance use disorder. A multivariate assessment protocol is therefore necessary to characterize the individual fully. Finally, it needs to be recognized that manifold psychological disturbances presage, are concomitant to, and emerge as consequences of chronic substance use. A comprehensive psychological evaluation must therefore encompass the natural history of the disorder.

This chapter is divided into three sections. First, I discuss the scope and requirements of a psychological assessment. Next, the methods for conducting a psychological assessment are described. A presentation of a decision-tree format that links the results of psychometric evaluation to specific modes of treatment concludes the chapter.

SCOPE AND ATTRIBUTES OF COMPREHENSIVE ASSESSMENT

Three broad categories of processes require psychological evaluation in cases of known or suspected substance abuse: cognition, emotion, and behavior. A disturbance in one domain may or may not involve a disturbance in another. For instance, among individuals with a substance use disorder, some are disturbed emotionally, whereas others primarily have a cognitive disorder. Hence, within a given diagnostic category, there is substantial heterogeneity in the population with respect to the profile of psychological disturbance. A major task is therefore to ascertain what processes are disturbed, the severity of disturbance, and the relationships among the various components of psychological functioning.

Importantly, the pattern of psychological disturbance is related to the type of facility in which the individual is obtaining treatment. For example, patients with alcohol use disorder in a gastroenterology service typically manifest less severe emotional disorder and present with better social adjustment than individuals treated in psychiatric facilities (Ewusi-Mensah, Saunders, & Williams, 1984). In contrast, patients with chronic liver disease are more likely to suffer acute and chronic hepatic encephalopathy compared to persons admitted to psychiatric facilities. Clinicians must therefore be cognizant of the general characteristics of the population from which their clients are drawn in order to design the most informative examination.

PSYCHOMETRIC STANDARDS

The information acquired from the psychological assessment must satisfy two basic requirements: validity and reliability.

Validity

Employed for either research or clinical purposes, a psychological test must have empirically documented validity. This ensures that the test results are factual; that is, the score is an accurate description of the individual. *Validity* has several facets. *Construct validity* means that the psychological processes claimed to be measured are, in fact, what are being assessed. For instance, it is essential to be confident that a poor score on a neuropsychological test of memory capacity is due to a central nervous system (CNS) disorder and is not spurious. Hence, utility of a particular instrument depends on its capacity to evaluate accurately the process intended to be measured.

In addition, psychological measures should have *predictive validity*; that is, the processes evaluated by the test should yield scores that predict the individual's behavior. For example, low scores on tests of educational aptitude should portend academic underachievement. High scores on tests of anxiety should predict avoidant social behavior. These predictions should be oriented to meaningful and specific domains of functioning, such as the person's potential to respond to a particular type of treatment or hold a certain type of job. Predictive validity is therefore an essential aspect of a comprehensive assessment, because it yields information that guides selection of the particular type of rehabilitation program that in turn impacts on long-term prognosis.

Finally, it should be noted that psychological testing is warranted only when the obtained data have *incremental validity*; that is, the test should yield information beyond what can be acquired from informal interviewing or casual observation. It is pointless to measure depression if the patient readily provides a self-report of symptoms. Psychometric procedures are most prudently utilized in situations where the objectivity of measurement yields information that is either too complex or too subtle to be obtained from observation or ordinary interaction with the client. Because it is both expensive and labor-intensive, clinicians should not request a psychological evaluation to merely confirm a clinical impression.

Reliability

Of the various types of reliability, two need to be considered here: test–retest and interrater reliability. *Test–retest reliability* refers to the temporal stability of the score. The clinical meaningfulness of test results is contingent upon its repeatability. Thus, any changes observed in the individual over time should reflect a true change in the person's status and not be due to random fluctuations of unknowable origin. A psychological test that has established test–retest reliability can be thus used repeatedly to monitor changes in status that occur during the course of treatment and aftercare.

The second type of reliability is *interrater reliability*. A test score obtained by one clinician should ideally be the same as the test administered by another, equally skilled clinician. In this fashion, confidence can be placed in the results. In effect, the results should not reflect the idiosyncratic interaction between the clinician and the client.

PSYCHOLOGICAL PROCESSES INTEGRAL
TO SUBSTANCE ABUSE

Cognitive processes encompass both cognitive style and cognitive capacity. Both aspects are relevant to understanding substance abuse. *Cognitive style* refers to the general strategy an individual uses to process information. For example, substantial evidence indicates that substance abusers are more inclined than the general population to analyze perceptual stimuli in a global, inarticulate manner (Sugerman & Schneider, 1976). This stable trait is referred to as *perceptual field dependence*. Significantly, field-dependence cognitive style appears to be related to treatment prognosis (Karp, Kissin, & Hustmeyer, 1970).

Another facet of cognitive style commonly found among substance abusers is *stimulus augmentation*—the propensity to magnify sensory input (Buchsbaum & Ludwig, 1980). Stimulus augmentation is overtly featured by impulsivity, behavioral disinhibition and sensation, or novelty seeking. Interestingly, this cognitive style correlates with low platelet monoamine oxidase (MAO) activity (Schooler, Zahn, Murphy, & Buchsbaum, 1978). Low platelet MAO activity is particularly associated with alcoholism in cases in which there is a comorbid antisocial disorder (Von Knorring, Bohman, Von Knorring, & Oreland, 1985).

Understanding the person's cognitive style may thus assist in treatment planning and in formulating a differential diagnosis. Unfortunately, the techniques for assessing this aspect of cognition have not been inculcated into general psychometric assessment practice, although it is possible to make inferences about perceptual field dependence by using a simple test measuring flexibility of perceptual closure (Jacobson, Pisani, & Berenbaum, 1970) and stimulus augmenting by measuring sensation-seeking behavior (Zuckerman, Bone, Neary, Mangelsdorff, & Brastman, 1972).

Another important aspect of cognition pertains to *attributional style*. In effect, individuals at high risk for substance abuse and currently active users are inclined mistakenly to harbor beliefs about the putative benefits of alcohol and other drugs (Finn, Sharkansky, Brandt, & Turcotte, 2000; Vernon, Lee, Harris, & Jang, 1996). Because these types of cognitions portend how an individual will behave, it is important also to assess attributional style.

Cognitive capacities are commonly impaired in people with alcohol use disorders as a result of CNS injury either directly caused by alcohol neurotoxicity or indirectly mediated by organ–system damage (e.g., hepatic encephalopathy, obstructive pulmonary disease, hypertension). Multiple factors typically compromise CNS functioning. Besides the direct effects of drugs or alcohol on the brain, these factors include trauma (e.g., head injuries from accidents and fights), poor nutrition, and exposure to toxic substances in the environment. The psychological evaluation must therefore not only be aimed at detecting and describing the pattern of CNS disturbances by means of validated neuropsychological tests but should also attempt to determine from other psychometric instruments (as well as from biomedical or laboratory tests) the possible etiological basis for the manifest disturbances.

Approximately 75% of individuals with alcohol dependence demonstrate some form of CNS disturbance, as measured by neuropsychological tests (Tarter & Edwards, 1985). Emerging findings also suggest that other forms of substance abuse are frequently associated with deficits on neuropsychological tests. Generally speaking, chronic alcohol abuse can cause both cognitive and physical damage to the brain that is typically expressed as visuomotor deficits, while verbal ability remains essentially intact. Impairments have also been frequently observed on tasks measuring abstract thinking and memory capacity, as well as on tests measuring visuospatial processes (Tarter & Ryan, 1983). These deficits appear to be most pronounced in individuals who are in less than optimal health, or who have experienced the cumulative effects of multiple CNS insults (Grant, Adams, & Reed, 1979). With respect to biomedical factors, a low-grade chronic hepatic encephalopathy may contribute substantially to the cognitive deficits found in cirrhotic alcoholics. This neuropsychiatric disturbance has a complex etiology. For example, the encephalopathy, revealed as poor performance on cognitive tests, is caused to large degree by the liver's failure to catabolize circulating neurotoxins (Tarter, Edwards, & Van Thiel, 1986). Furthermore, it should be noted that a hepatic encephalopathy may have a variety of other etiological determinants (Tarter et al., 1986). In effect, the manifest cognitive deficits have a multifactorial etiology.

Neuropsychological deficits associated with alcoholism are well documented. Indeed, two syndromes of cognitive disorder have been described. A dementia has been observed that is distinguishable according to both neuroanatomical and cognitive manifestations from the more florid amnestic or Korsakoff's syndrome (Wilkinson & Carlen, 1980). A number of other neurological conditions have also been described, although their neuropsychological manifestations have not yet been studied.

Less is known regarding neuropsychological sequelae following other types of substance abuse. Evidence has been presented indicating that the chronic use of phencyclidine (PCP), inhalants, benzodiazepines, heroin, cocaine, and amphetamines may be associated with neuropsychological impairments in some individuals (Parsons & Farr, 1981). One major methodological problem in this area of study is that it is not possible to ascertain the specific effects of a certain drug on CNS functioning, because polydrug abuse is the typical pattern of consumption. Also, the frequency and quantity of drug use are extremely variable; hence, determining a dose–effect relationship is difficult, if not impossible. These qualifications notwithstanding, the available evidence indicates that, as a group, substance abusers perform deficiently on certain neuropsychological tests indexing CNS integrity. As is the case among individuals with alcohol dependence, poor neuropsychological test performance has a multifactorial etiology. For instance, poor performance may be reflective of multiple minor brain injuries, poor overall health, and premorbid neurodevelopmental disorder.

Neuropsychological tests are very sensitive indicators of cerebral integrity (Lezak, Howieson, & Loring, 2004). In the early stages of a demential disease, these psychometric procedures complement neuroradiological procedures, where gross morphological injury may not be detectable upon visual inspection. Neuropsychological tests are especially informative for rehabilitation purposes, because the data describe functional cerebral integrity and, as such, characterize the person according to the cognitive processes (e.g., attention, memory, language, learning, and concentration) that are generally understood to be important for educational, vocational, and social adjustment. Indeed, it is the relationship between neurological status and these latter processes, rather than the test scores per se, that underscores the importance of the neuropsychological assessment.

Documenting cognitive capacity and efficiency via neuropsychological assessment is important for several reasons. During the drug withdrawal phase at the onset of rehabilitation, cognitive capacity may be too impaired for the person to achieve meaningful gains from didactic therapy or counseling. Assessment of the subjective effects of intoxication or withdrawal status from various substances of abuse has been developed by the Addiction Research Center (Haertzen, 1974). Handelsman and colleagues (1987) have also developed assessment instruments to evaluate severity of withdrawal.

A brief cognitive screening used on repeated occasions is an efficient method to determine the client's readiness for rehabilitation. Individuals with substantial cognitive limitations may not be able to solve daily problems, develop strategic plans to organize their lives, acquire insight into their problems, or benefit from vocational rehabilitation. A neuropsychological assessment can thus assist in formulation of a treatment plan and aftercare program. For instance, most persons respond to didactic psychotherapy, whereas those whose thinking is concrete benefit most from structured interventions that do require problem solving (Kissin, Platz, & Su, 1970). Furthermore, it is important to note that everyday activities such as driving a car, using power machinery, or performing tasks in which there are safety risks may be impaired because of CNS damage consequent to chronic heavy substance use. Neuropsychological testing, particularly in the area of psychomotor capacities, may therefore assist in the determination of injury risk to self and others.

Neuropsychological assessment has also been increasingly utilized as part of forensic evaluation. In criminal cases, objective quantitative assessment of cognitive capacities contributes to a better understanding the underlying causes of behavior disturbance. In this regard, expertise of the neuropsychologist who understands brain–behavior relationships that may be disrupted following alcohol or substance use can inform about the mechanisms underlying cognitive disturbances such as blackouts and anterograde amnesia.

In summary, systematic delineation of cognitive strengths and weaknesses, particularly as they relate to the onset and pattern of substance use behavior, is important for several reasons. For example, an attentional disorder or learning disability often precedes the onset of substance abuse (Tarter, Alterman, & Edwards, 1985). This has treatment implications, because it may be possible to prevent or treat the substance use behavior in some individuals by ameliorating the problem that initially motivated drug use. In addition, the assessment of cognitive deficits is important for understanding the person's everyday abilities, such as remembering appointments, following directions, and learning new information and skills. Demonstrating the presence of a cognitive deficit also informs about implementing a treatment plan that encompasses a cognitive rehabilitation component. For example, cognitive retraining by teaching the person compensatory strategies when there is an irreversible deficit, or by reestablishing a capacity that was not permanently impaired, affords the opportunity to maximize social and vocational adjustment within the framework of comprehensive rehabilitation.

Emotion

The intensity of emotional experience and appropriate expression of emotion are strongly associated with the quality of psychological adjustment. Conflicts over anger and guilt, and the display of intense emotional reactions commonly accompany substance use. These disruptive emotions may either presage substance use or emerge following drug use onset. Not uncommonly, consumption of psychoactive substances is motivated by a need to ameliorate negative affective states such as anger, depression, and fear. The inability to express emotions effectively in the social context, particularly negative feelings, is also frequently associated with drug abuse.

Emotional disturbance is often encompassed within psychopathology. From the psychometric perspective, clinically significant psychopathology is present when severity exceeds two standard deviations from the population mean. In effect, the severity score ranks in excess of the 95th percentile in the population on a trait (e.g., anxiety). Whether the magnitude of severity of psychopathological disturbance points to the need for treatment can only be determined by integrating the findings obtained from a diagnostic psychiatric interview and psychometric assessments. For example, anxiety or depression may foster substance abuse in an individual even if the severity is subthreshold for diagnosis. Notably, subthreshold negative affective states predispose to drug seeking (Khantzian, 1985). As pointed out by Dodes (1990), psychoactive drugs modulate affect in part by ameliorating negative feelings concomitant to helplessness and powerlessness.

It is important to be cognizant of the possibility that a psychiatric disorder may remit following effective treatment of substance abuse. It is not uncommon for psychopathological symptoms to dissipate in conjunction with abstinence from alcohol and drugs following the initial period of detoxification and withdrawal. Furthermore, it is essential to recognize that emotional distress can both precipitate and sustain a psychopathological disorder. Characterizing the client's emotional status therefore enables the clinician to determine the relation of psychopathology to substance abuse either as a predisposing condition, a correlate of the disorder, or a consequence of the disorder.

In contrast to diagnostic psychiatric assessment, psychological tests measure traits. The evaluation is thus concerned with quantifying the person on particular dimensions, whereas the psychiatric evaluation categorizes the person according to presence or absence of a disorder. Hence, commonly used psychiatric interviews such as the Schedule for Affective Disorders and Schizophrenia, Diagnostic Interview Schedule, and Structured Clinical Interview for DSM-III-R are concerned primarily with dichotomous classification. Whether a categorical or dimensional approach is utilized, the most frequently observed psychopathological disturbances comorbid to alcohol or drug abuse are anxiety and depression. However, virtually every Axis I and Axis II disturbance has been observed concomitant to substance use disorder (Dackis, Gold, Pottash, & Sweeney, 1985; Daley, Moss, & Campbell, 1987; Helzer & Pryzbeck, 1988; Peace & Mellsop, 1987; Weissman, 1988).

Behavior

The third component of a comprehensive psychological assessment pertains to determining the degree to which the individual's behavioral characteristics are related to substance abuse. Behavioral adjustment can be characterized in both microenvironment (e.g., family and friends) and macroenvironment (e.g., work, community, and school). Importantly, behavioral disposition, such as antisocial personality disorder, mitigates optimal functioning in a variety of social contexts. The point to be emphasized is that behavioral adjustment is the product of the interaction between the individual and the particular context. A behavioral characteristic (e.g., aggressiveness) can be adaptive in one context and maladaptive in another context.

Many behavioral characteristics have been shown to augment the risk for substance abuse, as well as to covary with substance abuse severity. The most commonly reported features include impulsivity, aggressivity, thrill seeking, poor goal persistence, hyperactivity, and social nonconformity (Spear, 2000; Tarter et al., 1999).

Cognition, emotion, and behavior comprise the major domains of psychological functioning. Notably, the facets of these three processes pertaining to self-regulation are indicators of a unidimensional trait termed *neurobehavioral disinhibition* (Tarter et al., 2003). The score on this trait is highly predictive of substance use disorder between childhood and young adulthood (Tarter et al., 2003). These findings indicate that a core disorder of psychological self-regulation underlies the risk for substance abuse (Tarter, Kirisci, Habeych, Reynolds, & Vanyukov, 2004). It should be emphasized, however, that there is substantial population heterogeneity with respect to the expression of these three domains of psychological functioning. At the individual level, therefore, a disturbance may be confined to only one area of functioning, may pervade all psychological domains, or (theoretically, at least) may not be present to a significant degree in any of the three areas.

METHODS OF PSYCHOLOGICAL ASSESSMENT

The overarching purpose of a psychological evaluation is to identify and quantify severity of problems integral to substance abuse that are amenable to modification. Based on evaluation results, interventions can thus be directed at changing the individual, the environment, or the quality of person–environment interaction to assist the client in terminating substance consumption from the person's behavioral repertoire.

In addition to promoting an intervention strategy, psychological assessment offers the opportunity to monitor quantitatively changes occurring during the course of treatment. The use of brief standardized self-report checklists or rating scales, for example, facilitates objective and quantitative documentation of therapeutic progress. One multivariate instrument designed for this purpose is the revised Drug Use Screening Inventory (Tarter, 1990). The obtained information not only provides ongoing feedback to the clinician but also serves the purpose of goal setting for the client. Furthermore, demonstrating to the client via objective and quantitative indices that he or she is benefiting from treatment serves the important purpose of sustaining motivation for continued investment in the rehabilitation. The following discussion reviews the most commonly used instruments for drug and alcohol assessment.

Alcohol and Drug Use

Consumption of alcohol and other drugs is closely linked to developmental processes. Not surprisingly, therefore, it unfolds in a more or less regular order. Typically, consumption begins with licit compounds (alcohol, tobacco) and progresses, if at all, to the use of illicit drugs. Although much has been written about the gateway hypothesis, in which drug use staging is presumably influenced by prior history of drug use (Kandel, 1975), the evidence to support this speculation is at best equivocal (Morral, McCaffrey, & Paddock, 2002). Rather, the progression across stages of substance use is most parsimoniously explained by severity of the predisposing liability (Vanyukov et al., 2003). In effect, the factors contributing to the risk for one type of drug abuse largely apply to all other abusable drugs.

The onset of use of each type of substance needs to be documented to describe fully the natural history of consumption. As each type of substance emerges in the person's history, it is essential to ascertain whether it has reached problematic severity to warrant a diagnosis of abuse or dependence. In addition, the occurrence of remission and number of lifetime episodes should be described. Moreover, polydrug use should be investigated because of the substantial lethal risk posed by the combined use of psychoactive drugs. For example, conjointly using alcohol and benzodiazepines is especially dangerous because of the risk of respiratory arrest.

To date, no single assessment measure evaluates all aspects of consumption behavior and its psychological manifestations. Certain instruments measure quantity and frequency, others measure severity, and yet others measure patterns of current and lifetime abuse. Several rating scales quantifying severity of alcohol problems in adults are, however, routinely used. The Michigan Alcoholism Screening Test (MAST; Selzer, 1971) is best known for this purpose. The MAST is easy to administer, because it consists of only 25 true–false statements. Paralleling the MAST, the Drug Abuse Screening Test (DAST; Skinner, 1982) is a self-report measure that is brief (20 items) and easy to score.

Alcohol problems can also be evaluated within a multivariate perspective employing the Alcohol Use Inventory (AUI; Wanberg & Horn, 1985). This instrument captures primarily the motivational aspects of alcohol use. The AUI, consisting of 228 items in a self-report format, can be administered to individuals or groups. A limiting characteristic of the AUI is that the questions are not phrased to inform about a specific time frame.

A frequently used instrument to assess problem severity is the Addiction Severity Index (McLellan, Luborsky, Woody, & O'Brien, 1980). This interview was designed to assist treatment planning. A homologous version has also been developed for adolescents. Referred to as the Teem Addiction Severity Index (T-ASI; Kaminer, Bukstein, & Tarter 1991), this semistructured interview informs about problem severity in multiple spheres of health and psychosocial functioning.

A subscale of the Minnesota Multiphasic Personality Inventory (MMPI)— the MacAndrew Alcoholism Scale (MAC)—consists of 49 items that differentiate persons with psychiatric disorders from those with substance use disorders. Another important feature of the MAC is that it assists in the assessment of particular characteristics associated with addiction, such as impulsivity, poor judgment, and sensation-seeking behavior. Also, when analyzed within the context of the MMPI validity scales, the MAC can identify persons who might be minimizing their substance abuse by endorsing socially desirable responses. It is important to note that individuals with substance abuse disorders who are court-ordered to receive a drug and alcohol evaluation are often motivated to hide or minimize their substance abuse (Shaffer, 1992).

Psychometric tests designed specifically for adolescent drug users have also been validated. The Personal Experience Inventory (PEI; Henly & Winters, 1988) and the Chemical Dependency Assessment Survey (Oetting, Beauvais, Edwards, & Waters, 1984) are two examples. The PEI, suitable for a clinical population, assesses multiple psychosocial domains that may be adversely affected by substance abuse.

The Drug Use Screening Inventory (DUSI; Tarter, 1990) is the most recently developed self-report that is in widespread use. This inventory has homologous forms for adolescents and adults. It profiles frequency of substance use behavior in conjunction with severity of disturbance in 10 spheres of functioning that are integral to both the etiology and sequelae of substance abuse. Each scale quantifies problem severity from 0 to 100%. The measurement domains are (1) substance use consequences, (2) psychiatric disorder, (3) health status, (4) behavior disorder, (5) school performance, (6) work adjustment, (7) social competence, (8) peer relationships, (9) family adjustment, and (10) leisure and recreation. The revised DUSI-R also contains a Lie scale as a validity check. The reliability and validity of the DUSI-R, as well as cutoff scores for diagnosis, are documented (Kirisci, Hsu, & Tarter, 1994; Tarter & Kirisci, 1997). Importantly, the overall problem density score in early adolescence is predictive of substance use disorder by young adulthood (Tarter & Kirisci, 2001).

It is readily apparent that psychological inventories that measure the multifaceted topology of alcohol and drug use have not been developed. The previously described procedures only clarify current use patterns and problem severity. Other information that can most easily be gathered in the course of an interview is also important to obtain. Questioning should therefore be directed at determining the following: (1) patterns of substance use (e.g., episodic vs. continuous), (2) context of substance use (solitary vs. social consumption), (3) availability of drugs and opportunity to access drugs in the social environment, (4) perceived importance of drugs, (5) expected and experienced effects of drugs on mood and behavior, and (6) family history of drug and alcohol abuse.

Health Status

There is no standardized instrument to assess health status in individuals with substance use disorders. This lack of instrumentation in a critical area of health care is the result of current health policy, which has shifted emphasis from health status to health care delivery and quality of life. Some general health surveys that are not specific to substance abuse but can be applied to this population are the Nottingham Health Profile (Hunt, McEwen, & McKenna, 1985), the Duke–University of North Carolina Health Profile (Parkerson et al., 1981), and the General Health Survey (Stewart, Hays, & Ware, 1988).

Psychiatric Disturbance

Substance abuse can occur conjointly with virtually any Axis I or Axis II psychiatric disorder. This has important treatment implications, the most obvious of which is that for some individuals, alcohol or drug consumption may constitute an attempt at self-medication. Hence, treatment of the primary disorder may in some circumstances be sufficient to ameliorate the substance use disorder. Alternatively, prolonged drug abuse may precipitate a psychiatric disturbance, either directly by inducing neurochemical changes or indirectly through stress or maladjustment concomitant to a substance abusing lifestyle. A major task is therefore to delineate the type and severity of psychiatric morbidity that may be present and to determine whether it preceded or developed after the substance use disorder.

Structured diagnostic interviews have been increasingly utilized in the objective formulation of substance use disorder diagnoses, as well as other psychiatric diagnoses. Several instruments, all with good psychometric properties, are currently available. The Structured Clinical Interview for DSM-III-R (SCID; Spitzer, Williams, & Gibbon, 1987) is presently the most frequently used instrument. Other structured interviews are the Diagnostic Interview Schedule (DIS; Robins, Helzer, Croughan, & Ratcliff, 1981) and the Schedule for Affective Disorders and Schizophrenia (SADS; Spitzer, Endicott, & Robins, 1975). There are some important differences among the SCID, DIS, and SADS. In contrast to the SCID and SADS, which are semistructured interviews requiring a high level of clinical skill to administer and interpret, the DIS is fully structured, so that it can be administered by paraprofessionals.

Three diagnostic interviews are available for adolescents. These include the Diagnostic Interview Schedule—Revised for Children (Costello, Edelbrock, & Costello, 1984), the Kiddie Schedule for Affective Disorders and Schizophrenia (Orvaschel, Puig-Antich, Chambers, Tabrizi, & Johnson, 1982), and the Diagnostic Interview for Children and Adolescents (Wellner, Reich, Herianic, Jung, & Amado, 1987). Each of these interviews also has a version that can be administered to a parent, so as to ensure accuracy of the evaluation.

By employing a structured psychiatric interview, it is possible to relate substance use involvement with psychiatric status. Myriad configurations of comorbidity are possible. The pattern of comorbidity has important ramifications for treatment. For example, if an affective disorder preceded the substance use disorder and is still present at the time of the assessment, it would suggest the need to treat this disorder as the primary condition.

Self-report questionnaires can also yield important information by quantifying the presence and severity of psychiatric disorder that is not severe enough to warrant a diagnosis but may nonetheless be a contributor to, or a consequence of, substance abuse. Thus, self-rating scales may provide a more valid picture of the severity of psychopathology than that afforded by only an interview. For example, the MMPI (Hathaway & McKinley, 1951) contains three validity scales that measure the person's test-taking attitude; hence, truthfulness and a response bias toward either over- or underreporting symptoms are documented. A disadvantage is that the MMPI profile does not yield a diagnosis. However, the configuration of scores in the 10 basic scales, in conjunction with the many specialized scales, makes it possible to identify personality disorders, family problems, health disturbances, and social maladjustment comprehensively.

Other self-report rating scales can be employed when either time or expertise is not available to conduct a structured interview or obtain an MMPI profile. The most commonly used test in this regard is the Symptom Checklist 90—Revised (Derogatis, 1983). This self-rating scale is brief and easy to score. Severity of psychopathology is quantified across nine dimensions of psychopathology.

The importance of evaluating psychopathology in the substance use disorders cannot be overemphasized. Treatment of the underlying psychiatric disorder may itself, in many cases, be sufficient to ameliorate a substance use disorder. For this reason, it is essential to document the type, onset, and presentation of psychopathology as it relates to alcohol or drug use behavior. In addition, documentation of psychiatric illness in other family members, using instruments such as the Family History Chart (Mann, Sobell, Sobell, & Pavan, 1985) and the Family Informant Schedule and Criteria (Manuzza, Fryer, Endicott, & Klein, 1985), can assist in obtaining a clear picture of the primary psychiatric disorder.

Personality

Certain personality characteristics are commonly associated with the etiology and maintenance of alcohol and drug abuse. The extent to which the particular feature presages the onset of substance use or is shaped by the long-term consequence of consumption needs to be ascertained on a case-by-case basis. Traits such as low self-esteem, impulsivity, aggressiveness, and behavioral undercontrol are highly prevalent in the drug-abusing population.

No single instrument currently assesses all dimensions of personality that may be relevant to understanding drug use behavior. The MMPI, described previously, is very useful for profiling psychopathology and facilitating the formulation and testing of hypotheses about specific personality characteristics. However, other inventories are also informative for elucidating the role of particular traits on the risk for and maintenance of drug abuse. Notably, the Multidimensional Personality Questionnaire (MPQ) quantifies traits that have frequently been found to be characteristic of alcoholics and drug abusers. Significantly, the traits comprising the MPQ scales have a strong heritable basis (Tellegen, 1982, 1985; Tellegen et al., 1988). Numerous other personality questionnaires have been developed; however, none measures traits that are so integrally linked to substance abuse as the MPQ.

Self-esteem disturbances are also present in substance-using individuals. Low self-esteem can occur in a number of areas of daily living and may be secondary to psychopathology. The Self-Esteem Inventory (Epstein, 1976) is a multidimensional scale with good breadth of coverage and superior psychometric properties. It taps aspects of psychological well-being that are not ordinarily covered by personality tests.

Cognition

A neuropsychological evaluation is important for a variety of reasons. It provides information regarding the person's amenability to treatment. For example, individuals who have a mental deficiency, have suffered neurological injury, or have dementia as the result of alcoholism or habitual drug use are unlikely to profit from insight-oriented treatment. In addition, in the early stages of substance withdrawal, cognitive assessment can determine whether mental confusion is present, in which case the benefit of participation in individual or group therapy is likely to be minimal. Importantly, emotional and behavioral changes associated with neurological impairment may impede rehabilitation. Hence, clarifying cognitive impairment due to CNS injury and dysfunction has important ramifications for treatment planning and aftercare, including long-term rehabilitation.

Tarter and Edwards (1987) proposed a three-stage assessment procedure for documenting neuropsychological functioning. At the outset, neuropsychological screening provides the opportunity to determine whether there is evidence of a CNS disturbance. If a neurocognitive impairment is not observed, the evaluation is terminated, thereby saving substantial time and cost. The second stage of evaluation involves delineation of cognitive abilities and limitations. In standardized batteries, complemented when necessary by specialized tests, cognitive capacity is quantified across multiple domains. Typically, this includes speech and language, attention, psychomotor efficiency, learning and memory, and abstract reasoning. The results at this stage can inform about lesion localization and lateralization. Several standardized neuropsychological batteries are currently in wide use. The Halstead–Reitan Battery (Reitan, 1955), Luria–Nebraska Neuropsychological Test Battery (Golden, 1981), and the Pittsburgh Initial Neuropsychological Test System (Goldstein, Tarter, Shelly, & Hegedus, 1983) are examples of multidomain assessment batteries. Based on the profile of results describing cognitive strengths and weaknesses, a decision is made regarding the need for focused comprehensive testing. This is the third and last stage of assessment. In-depth information is obtained regarding a particular cognitive domain. The results inform about "real-life" prospects of success. Moreover, the results inform about potential risks to the person. For example, it is important to describe psychomotor impairments fully if the client works with power machinery. Visuoperceptual disturbances must be comprehensively documented if the person drives a car. Similarly, if the clinician identifies a learning or memory deficit, it has direct ramifications for educational and vocational rehabilitation. The reader is referred to Nixon (1999) for a discussion of instrument selection for neuropsychological evaluation.

In interpreting the results of a neuropsychological evaluation, it is important to be cognizant of the multifactorial etiology of any identified impairment. Not only do alcohol and other drugs act directly on the brain but their habitual consumption may also induce organ–system injury, which in turn disrupts integrity of the brain. For example, cirrhosis, independent of alcoholism, causes hepatic encephalopathy, Thus, neuropsychological deficits commonly found in alcoholics may be, in large part, the result of advanced liver disease (Tarter, Van Thiel, & Moss, 1988). This fact is not inconsequential, because treatment of low-grade hepatic encephalopathy caused by alcoholic liver disease has been tentatively shown to improve cognitive capacities (McClain, Potter, Krombout, & Zieve, 1984). Thus, medically significant problems that potentially disrupt brain functioning should be recorded and incorporated into the treatment plan.

Family Adjustment

Family organization and quality of interaction among its members impact on the risk for and maintenance of substance abuse. Indeed, the transmission of alcoholism across generations is to some degree influenced by attitudes and rituals of the family pertaining to consumption (Steinglass, Bennett, Wolin, & Reiss, 1987). Inasmuch as the family is the primary influence shaping the values and behavioral patterns of children, parenting style and family environment exercise a profound influence on the child's development until at least adolescence, when psychoactive substance use may first become problematic.

From the standpoint of psychological evaluation, a number of issues must be addressed. First, it is essential to characterize the contribution of psychiatric disorder, including substance abuse, in the family. The greater the family density of substance use disorder and pervasiveness of psychiatric disorder in family members of the client undergoing evaluation, the more severe the psychological problems. Among young substance-abusing clients, it is especially important to record the presence and history of physical and sexual abuse as an etiological factor on any manifest psychological disturbances. Second, the causal relationship between family dysfunction and drug use behavior needs to be ascertained.

How substance abuse precipitated the family problems or, conversely, how family problems triggered substance abuse needs to be investigated in the course of the evaluation. Third, the reinforcement contingencies, if any, exercised by the family on the member with the substance abuse problem need to be analyzed. It thus needs to be determined whether substance abuse is ignored, punished, or positively reinforced. Fourth, the roles and status of each family member must be understood to the extent that individual maladjustment, conflict, and instability contribute to overall family dysfunction that in turn propels one member to consume alcohol or other psychoactive drugs.

Five self-report instruments are commonly used to quantify family functioning. The Family Environment Scale (FES; Moos, 1974; Moos & Moos, 1981) was the first instrument developed to evaluate family system functioning. The FES evaluates three major dimensions: (1) Relationships, (2) Personal Growth, and (3) Systems Maintenance. Each major dimension consists of several scales. The Relationship dimension encompasses scales that measure family conflict, cohesion, and expressiveness. The Personal Growth dimension includes scales that evaluate the family's emphasis on independence and achievement, as well as intellectual, religious, and recreational pursuits. The Systems Maintenance dimension contains scales that measure the family's success at organization and control. The Self-Report Family Inventory (SFI) is based on the theoretical orientation of the Beavers Systems Model of Family Functioning (Beavers & Hampson, 1990). It measures health/competence, level and type of conflict, communication patterns, cohesiveness, leadership, and emotional expression.

Epstein, Baldwin, and Bishop (1983) developed the Family Assessment Device (FAD) to evaluate current level of family functioning. The FAD can be administered to children as young as 12 years of age. In addition to providing a general functioning score, the FAD provides useful information pertaining to affective involvement, behavior control, family roles, problem solving, communication patterns, and affective responsiveness.

The Family Assessment Measure (FAM) focuses on the individual perceptions of each family member (Skinner, Steinhauer, & Santa Barbara, 1983; Steinhauer, Santa Barbara, & Skinner, 1984). The family system characteristics assessed by the FAM include affective involvement, control, role performance, task accomplishment, communication patterns, affective expression, and values and norms.

The Family Adaptability and Cohesion Evaluation Scales (FACES), developed by Olson, Russell, and Sprenkle (1980, 1983) and Olson and colleagues (1989) for both research and clinical applications, is another frequently used measure of family functioning. It takes only 10–15 minutes to administer and is appropriate for children (ages 10–12). It assesses three dimensions of family functioning: cohesion (degree of emotional bonding), adaptability (family power/roles/rules), and communication (dyadic patterns/styles).

Social Adjustment

Social adjustment is defined as the individual's success at fulfilling age-appropriate roles according to expectations (Barrabee, Barrabee, & Finesinger, 1955). The measurement domains encompass social support, social roles, social skills, peer affiliations, school and vocational adjustment, and recreation and leisure activities.

Social Functioning/Social Support

As previously discussed, the Addiction Severity Index (McLellan et al., 1980) profiles the individual's problems, including social support, along with psychological, legal, family, and vocational status. The Substance Abuse Problem Checklist (SAPC; Carroll, 1983) assesses social functioning in relation to treatment planning. An especially useful feature of the SAPC is its capacity to determine the client's readiness to initiate substance abuse treatment. The SAPC evaluates health status, personality, social relationships, vocational status, use of leisure time, religious orientation, and legal status. The Social Relationship Scale (SRS; McFarlane, Neale, Norman, Roy, & Steiner, 1981) is one of only a few instruments developed with the specific intention to measure social support. It assesses three facets of social support: (1) total number of individuals who make up the social support network, (2) type of relationships, and (3) quality of relationships. These facets of social adjustment are integral to prognosis following treatment for substance use disorders (see McLellan, 1986; Woody et al., 1983).

Peer Affiliations

A social network in which drug use is commonplace increases the likelihood that the individual will adopt this behavior. Ameliorating a substance abuse problem may thus require abandoning long-standing peer affiliations. Whether the quality of peer relationships is embedded in an antisocial behavior disposition needs to be evaluated. Antisociality impedes work, school, and family adjustment. One self-report measure, the revised Drug Use Screening Inventory (Tarter, 1990), described earlier, quantifies deviancy in both the individual and friendships.

Because the social environment is a major source of reinforcement, it is essential to identify the reward contingencies, role models, and contextual factors associated with alcohol or drug use. It should be recognized that the individual not only responds to the particular social environment but also seeks out an environment that has reinforcing value. Hence, during the course of the psychological assessment, an attempt should be made to learn why the substance abusing client seeks out social interactions that have maladaptive consequences.

Social Skills

Social skills deficits are common among substance abusers (Van Hasselt, Hersen, & Milliones, 1978). Deficiencies in assertiveness skills, refusal skills, and compliment-giving skills have all been documented. Poor ability to manage conflict in interpersonal situations may also be linked to a propensity for substance abuse. Moreover, the exacerbation of poor social skills by stress or anxiety potentiates the risk for substance use as a coping strategy. Consequently, describing the person's coping style also needs to be an integral component of the social skills assessment.

There are currently no standardized instruments for evaluating social skills. Various self-rating scales, although lacking in normative scores, have been employed for identifying the presence and severity of deficits and for targeting behaviorally focused interventions. The same limitations exist with respect to coping style; however, two measures that have been found to be informative are the Ways of Coping Scale (Folkman & Lazarus, 1980) and the Constructive Thinking Inventory (Epstein, 1987).

In conjunction with a social skills evaluation, it is important to document the individual's capacity to exercise the competencies required for everyday living. As society becomes more technologically complex, it is valuable to learn whether the individual is capable of performing the everyday tasks that are required for successful adjustment. For example, it is important to determine whether the individual can manage a bank account, use bankcard machines, access the Internet, obtain services information, utilize public transportation, and attend to personal needs with respect to food and clothing. Deficiencies in any of these areas exacerbate stress that in turn promotes the risk for substance use.

School Adjustment

The school is the primary social environment during adolescence. It is important to document school adjustment and academic performance of adolescent substance abusers. Drug accessibility and the adolescent's peer affiliation network are especially influential determinants of drug use initiation. Conduct problems and social deviance are also commonly associated with both poor school adjustment and substance abuse. The teacher version of the Child Behavior Checklist (CBCL; Achenbach & Edelbrock, 1983) affords the opportunity to identify and quantify severity of behavioral problems in the school environment. Also, comparing the findings to the parallel parent version enables the clinician to ascertain whether adjustment problems are confined to the school or are also present in the home.

Assessing the teacher's perceptions of a child's behavior in the classroom is a highly desired component of a comprehensive evaluation. The Disruptive

Behavior Rating Scale (Pelham & Murphy, 1987), based on DSM-III-R criteria (American Psychiatric Association, 1987), quantifies severity of conduct, and attention-deficit/hyperactivity and oppositional defiant disturbance. Another brief symptom rating scale that can be completed by the teacher is the Iowa Conners Teachers Rating Scale (Loney & Milich, 1982).

One important aspect of school adjustment pertains to the extent to which the child participates in athletics and other extracurricular activities. These activities indicate how well the person is socially integrated and accepted by peers. In addition, it is essential to evaluate academic achievement and learning aptitude in the basic skill areas. For example, learning disability compounded by low self-esteem may be a major factor propelling a youngster toward drug use, as well as other non-normative behaviors. Standardized learning and achievement tests can readily document whether a learning deficit is present.

Vocational Adjustment

Stress in the workplace fosters substance use as a coping strategy. Inability to meet work performance standards, conflicts with other employees or supervisors, an inconsistent work schedule, and low job satisfaction exemplify the common proximal causes of substance use. The impact of unemployment and underemployment as a source of stress also needs to be evaluated. In addition, extensive travel and associated social obligations may frequently place the individual in situations where alcohol consumption is expected. Over the long term, social drinking may lead to problems controlling intake.

Besides evaluating the job demands and workplace environment, it is essential to evaluate the client's behavioral disposition. For example, premorbid personality disorders contribute to job failure, which in turn predisposes the individual to substance abuse. Furthermore, it is important to evaluate substance abuse in the context of specific circumstances of the job. Access to addictive substances places the person at heightened risk simply by virtue of facile availability. Not surprisingly, bartenders have a high rate of alcohol abuse. The vocational evaluation must therefore identify the specific job-related characteristics that predispose the individual to substance abuse.

Recreation/Leisure Activities

Substance use is commonly circumscribed to recreational activities. Furthermore, an individual who does not have socially satisfying leisure activities may use alcohol or drugs to cope with the stress of boredom. This may be particularly problematic among members of the elderly population who have not developed a rewarding goal directed lifestyle following retirement. A somewhat similar problem may confront adolescents who have substantial unstructured time. Presently, there are no standardized procedures to evaluate recreation and leisure activities. As noted above, however, the DUSI-R (Tarter, 1990) screens for severity of problems related to leisure and recreation.

LINKING ASSESSMENT AND TREATMENT: THE DECISION-TREE PROCEDURE

A three-stage evaluation procedure provides a systematic framework for connecting assessment and treatment. The first stage involves brief screening using the DUSI-R (Tarter, 1990). At this stage, the areas of disturbance that point to the need for comprehensive evaluation are identified. In the second stage, a diagnostic evaluation is performed in the identified problem areas. This information in turn is applied to a focused, in-depth evaluation to formulate a multidisciplinary treatment plan.

Using a decision-tree multistage evaluation procedure has several advantages:

- The areas of disturbance can be quickly identified at minimal cost.
- Labor-intensive, comprehensive diagnostic evaluation is guided by the results obtained in initial screening.
- The client's rehabilitation needs are clearly delineated, based on aggregate findings from the initial screening and the comprehensive diagnostic evaluation.
- Once the required treatment interventions are specified, a coordinated intervention program can be developed. In this fashion, evaluation and treatment are integrally linked in an ongoing reciprocal and interactive manner.

Matching assessment results with treatment is rapidly becoming standard clinical practice. For example, Annis and Graham (1995) link treatment planning, including relapse prevention counseling, to particular client profiles on the Inventory of Drinking Situations (IDS; Annis, 1982). The IDS categorizes heavy alcohol abusers into four types: (1) the negative profile—individuals whose alcohol abuse is a consequence of negative emotions (e.g., boredom, anxiety, and depression); (2) the positive profile—individuals who drink heavily due to social pressure, wanting to have a good time, or wanting to relax; (3) low-testing personal control—individuals whose abuse of alcohol is undifferentiated, possibly due to lack of motivation to change and lack of awareness of the antecedents of abuse; and (4) low physical discomfort—individuals who also presents with an undifferentiated profile characterized by limited use of alcohol. Substance abuse treatment is thus individualized according to the four IDS client profiles. For example, in the case of the negative and positive profilers, the focus of intervention is on teaching alternate ways of coping with social pressures and interpersonal conflicts, teaching alternate forms of relaxation, providing assertiveness training, and resolving interpersonal stress. The point to be made is that psychological assessment is not an intellectual exercise. Rather, the information should be applied to improving treatment outcome. Toward that goal, psychological evaluation is pertinent to determining the client's readiness for treatment, designing the most appropriate treatment, monitoring change during the course of treatment, documentation of individual outcome, and determining effectiveness of the treatment program.

REFERENCES

Achenbach, T., & Edelbrock, C. (1983). *Manual for the Child Behavior Checklist and Revised Child Behavior Profile.* Burlington: University of Vermont, Department of Psychiatry.

American Psychiatric Association. (1987). *Diagnostic and statistical manual of mental disorders* (3rd ed., rev.). Washington, DC: Author.

Annis, H. M. (1982). *Inventory of Drinking Situations (IDS-100).* Toronto: Addiction Research Foundation of Ontario.

Annis, H. M., & Graham, J. M. (1995). Profile types on the Inventory of Drinking Situations: Implications for relapse prevention counseling. *Psychol Addict Behav, 9,* 176–182.

Barrabee, R., Barrabee, E. L., & Finesinger, J. E. (1955). A normative social adjustment scale. *Am J Psychiatry, 112,* 252–259.

Beavers, W. R., & Hampson, R. B. (1990). *Successful families: Assessment and intervention.* New York: Norton.

Buchsbaum, M., & Ludwig, A. (1980). Effects of sensory input and alcohol administration on visual evoked potentials in normal subjects and alcoholics. In H. Begleiter (Ed.), *Biological effects of alcohol.* New York: Plenum Press.

Carroll, J. F. (1983). *Substance Abuse Problem Checklist manual.* Eagleville, PA: Eagleville Hospital.

Costello, J., Edelbrock, C., & Costello, A. (1984). *The reliability of the NIMH Diagnostic Interview Schedule for Children: A comparison between pediatric and psychiatric referrals.* Pittsburgh, PA: Western Psychiatric Institute and Clinic.

Dackis, C. A., Gold, M. S., Pottash, A. L. C., & Sweeney, D. R. (1985). Evaluating depression in alcoholics. *Psychiatry Res, 17,* 105–109.

Daley, D., Moss, H. B., & Campbell, F. (1987). *Dual disorders: Counseling clients with chemical dependency and mental illness.* Center City, MN: Hazelden.

Derogatis, L. R. (1983). *SCL-90-R: Administration, scoring and procedures manual II* (rev.). Towson, MD: Clinical Psychometric Research.

Dodes, L. M. (1990). Addiction, helplessness, and narcissistic rage. *Psychoanal Q, 59,* 398–419.

Epstein, N. B., Baldwin, L., & Bishop, D. (1983). The McMaster Family Assessment Device. *J Marital Fam Ther, 9,* 213–228.

Epstein, S. (1976). Anxiety, arousal and the self-concept. In I. G. Sarason & C. D. Spielberger (Eds.), *Stress and anxiety.* Washington, DC: Hemisphere.

Epstein, S. (1987). *The constructive thinking inventory*. Amherst: University of Massachusetts, Department of Psychology.

Ewusi-Mensah, I., Saunders, J., & Williams, R. (1984). The clinical nature and detection of psychiatric disorders in patients with alcoholic liver disease. *Alcohol Alcohol, 39*, 297–302.

Finn, P., Sharkansky, E., Brandt, K., & Turcotte, N. (2000). The effects of familial risk, personality, and expectancies on alcohol use and abuse. *J Abnorm Psychol, 109*, 122–133.

Folkman, S., & Lazarus, R. (1980). An analysis of coping in middle aged community sample. *J Health Soc Behav, 21*, 219–239.

Golden, C. J. (1981). A standardized version of Luria's neuropsychological tests. In S. Filskov & T. J. Boll (Eds.), *Handbook of clinical neuropsychology*. New York: Wiley-Interscience.

Goldstein, G., Tarter, R., Shelly, C., & Hegedus, A. (1983). The Pittsburgh Initial Neuropsychological Testing System (PINTS): A neuropsychological screening battery for psychiatric patients. *J Behav Assess, 5*, 227–238.

Grant, I., Adams, K., & Reed, R. (1979). Normal neuropsychological abilities of alcoholic men in their late thirties. *Am J Psychiatry, 136*, 1263–1269.

Haertzen, C. A. (1974). *An overview of Addiction Research Center Inventory scales (ARCI): An appendix and manual of scales* (DHEW Publication No. ADM 74-92). Rockville, MD: National Institute on Drug Abuse.

Handelsman, L., Cochran, K. J., Aronson, M. J., Ness, R., Rubinstein, K. J., & Kanof, P. D. (1987). Two new rating scales for opiate withdrawal. *Am J Drug Alcohol Abuse, 13*, 293–308.

Hathaway, S. R., & McKinley, J. C. (1951). *The Minnesota Multiphasic Personality Inventory manual* (rev.). New York: Psychological Corporation.

Helzer, J. E., & Pryzbeck, T. R. (1988). The co-occurrence of alcoholism with other psychiatric disorders in the general population and its impact on treatment. *J Stud Alcohol, 49*, 219–224.

Henly, G., & Winters, K. (1988). Development of problem severity scales for the assessment of adolescent alcohol and drug abuse. *Int J Addict, 23*, 65–85.

Hunt, S. M., McEwen, J., & McKenna, S. P. (1985). Measuring health status: A tool for clinicians and epidemiologists. *J R Coll Gen Pract, 35*, 185.

Jacobson, G., Pisani, V., & Berenbaum, H. (1970). Temporal stability of field dependence among hospitalized alcoholics. *J Abnorm Psychol, 76*, 10–12.

Kaminer, Y., Bukstein, O. G., & Tarter, R. E. (1991). The Teen Addiction Severity Index: Rationale and reliability. *Int J Addict, 26*, 219–226.

Kandel, D. (1975). Stages in adolescent involvement in drug use. *Science, 190*, 912–914.

Karp, S., Kissin, B., & Hustmeyer, F. (1970). Field-dependence as a predictor of alcoholic therapy dropouts. *J Nerv Ment Dis, 15*, 77–83.

Khantzian, E. J. (1985). The self-medication hypothesis of addictive disorders: Focus on heroin and cocaine dependence. *Am J Psychiatry, 142*, 1259–1264.

Kirisci, L., Hsu, T., & Tarter, R. (1994). Fitting a two-parameter logistic item response model to clarify the psychometric properties of the Drug Use Screening Inventory for adolescent alcohol and drug abusers. *Alcohol Clin Exp Res, 18*, 1335–1341.

Kissin, B., Platz, A., & Su, W. (1970). Social and psychological factors in the treatment of chronic alcoholism. *J Psychiatr Res, 8*, 13–27.

Lezak, M., Howieson, D., & Loring, D. (2004). *Neuropsychological assessment* (4th ed.). New York: Oxford University Press.

Loney, J., & Milich, R. (1982). Hyperactivity, inattention, and aggression in clinical practice. In M. Wolraich & D. Routh (Eds.), *Advances in developmental and behavioral pediatrics*. Greenwich, CT: JAI Press.

Mann, R. E., Sobell, L. C., Sobell, M. B., & Pavan, D. (1985). Reliability of family tree questionnaire for assessing family history of alcohol problems. *Drug Alcohol Depend, 15*, 61–67.

Manuzza, S., Fryer, A. J., Endicott, J., & Klein, D. F. (1985). *Family Informant Schedule and Criteria (FISC)*. New York: New York State Psychiatric Institute.

McClain, C., Potter, T., Krombout, J., & Zieve, L. (1984). The effect of lactulose on psychomotor performance tests in alcoholic cirrhotics without evert encephalopathy. *Clin Gastroenterol, 6*, 325–329.

McFarlane, A. H., Neale, K. A., Norman, G. R., Roy, R. G., & Steiner, D. L. (1981). Methodological issues in developing a scale to measure social support. *Schizophrenia Bull, 7*, 90–100.

McLellan, A. (1986). "Psychiatric severity" as a predictor of outcome from substance abuse treatments. In R. E. Meyer (Ed.), *Psychopathology and addictive disorders* (pp. 97–139). New York: Guilford Press.

McLellan, A., Luborsky, L., Woody, G., & O'Brien, C. (1980). An improved diagnostic evaluation instrument for substance abuse patients: The Addiction Severity Scale Index. *J Nerv Ment Dis, 168*, 26–33.

Moos, R. (1974). *Combined preliminary manual for the family, work, and group environment Scales*. Palo Alto, CA: Consulting Psychologists Press.

Moos, R., & Moos, B. (1981). *Family Environment Scale manual*. Palo Alto, CA: Consulting Psychologists Press.

Morral, A., McCaffrey, D., & Paddock, S. (2002). Reassessing the marijuana gateway effect. *Addiction, 97*, 1493–1504.

Nixon, S. J. (1999). Neuropsychological assessment. In P. Ott, R. Tarter, & R. Ammerman (Eds.), *Sourcebook on assessment and treatment* (pp. 227–235). Boston: Allyn & Bacon.

Oetting, E., Beauvais, F., Edwards, R., & Waters, M. (1984). *The drug and alcohol assessment system*. Fort Collins, CO: Rocky Mountain Behavioral Sciences Institute.

Olson, D. H., McCubbin, H. I., Barnes, H. L., Larsen, A. S., Muxen, M. J., & Wilson, M. A. (1989). *Families: What makes them work* (updated ed.). Newbury Park, CA: Sage.

Olson, D. H., Russell, C. S., & Sprenkle, D. H. (1980). Circumplex model of marital and family systems: II. Empirical studies and clinical intervention. In J. Vincent (Ed.), *Advances in family intervention, assessment and theory* (Vol. I, pp. 129–179). Greenwich, CT: JAI Press.

Olson, D. H., Russell, C. S., & Sprenkle, D. H. (1983). Circumplex model of marital and family systems: VI. Theoretical update. *Fam Process, 22*, 69–83.

Orvaschel, H., Puig-Antich, J., Chambers, W., Tabrizi, M. A., & Johnson, R. (1982). Retrospective assessment of prepubertal major depression with the Kiddie-SADS-E. *J Am Acad Child Adolesc Psychiatry, 21*, 392–397.

Parkerson, G. R., Gehlbach, S. H., Wagner, E. H., James, S. A., Clapp, N. E., &

Muhlbaier, L. H. (1981). The Duke–UNC Health Profile: An adult health status instrument for primary care. *Med Care, 19,* 806–809.

Parsons, A., & Farr, S. (1981). The neuropsychology of alcohol and drug abuse. In S. Filskov & T. Boll (Eds.), *Handbook of clinical neuropsychology* (pp. 320–365). New York: Wiley.

Peace, K., & Mellsop, G. (1987). Alcoholism and psychiatric disorder. *Aust NZ J Psychiatry, 21,* 94–101.

Pelham, W. E., & Murphy, D. A. (1987). *The DBD rating scale: A parent and teacher rating scale for the disruptive behavior disorders of childhood in DSM-III-R.* Unpublished manuscript, University of Pittsburgh.

Reitan, R. (1955). An investigation of the validity of Halstead's measures of biological intelligence. *AMA Arch Neurol Psychiatry, 73,* 28–35.

Robins, L., Helzer, J., Croughan, J., & Ratcliff, K. (1981). National Institute of Mental Health Diagnostic Schedule: Its history, characteristics and validity. *Arch Gen Psychiatry, 38,* 381–389.

Rounsaville, B. J. (1993). Overview: Rationale and guidelines for using comparable measures to evaluate substance abusers. In B. J. Rounsaville, F. M. Tims, A. M. Horton, & B. J. Sowder (Eds.), *Diagnostic source book on drug abuse research and treatment* (pp. 1–10). Rockville, MD: National Institute on Drug Abuse.

Schooler, C., Zahn, T., Murphy, D., & Buchsbaum, M. (1978). Psychological correlates of monoamine oxidase activity in normals. *J Nerv Ment Dis, 166,* 177–186.

Selzer, M. (1971). The Michigan Alcoholism Screening Test: The quest for a new diagnostic instrument. *Am J Psychiatry, 127,* 1653–1658.

Shaffer, H. J. (1992). The psychology of stage change: The transition from addiction to recovery. In J. H. Lowinson, P. Ruiz, & R. B. Millman (Eds.), *Substance abuse: A comprehensive textbook* (pp. 1019–1033). Baltimore: Williams & Wilkins.

Skinner, H. A. (1982). The Drug Abuse Screening Test. *Addict Behav, 7,* 363–371.

Skinner, H. A., Steinhauer, P. D., & Santa Barbara, J. (1983). The Family Assessment Measure. *Can J Commun Ment Health, 2,* 91–105.

Spear, L. (2000). The adolescent brain and age-related behavioral manifestations. *Neurosci Biobehav Rev, 24,* 417–463.

Spitzer, R. L., Endicott, J., & Robins, E. (1975). Clinical criteria for psychiatric diagnosis and DSM-III. *Am J Psychiatry, 132,* 1187–1192.

Spitzer, R. L., Williams, J. B. W., & Gibbon, M. (1987, April 1). *Instruction manual for the Structured Clinical Interview for DSM-III-R* (rev.). New York: New York State Psychiatric Institute.

Steinglass, P., Bennett, L., Wolin, S., & Reiss, D. (1987). *The alcoholic family.* New York: Basic Books.

Steinhauer, P. D., Santa-Barbara, J., & Skinner, H. A. (1984). The process model of family functioning. *Can J Psychiatry, 29,* 77–88.

Stewart, A. L., Hays, R. D., & Ware, J. E. (1988). The MOS short form general health survey: Reliability and validity in a patient population. *Med Care, 27,* S12–S26.

Sugerman, A., & Schneider, D. (1976). Cognitive styles in alcoholism. In R. Tarter & A. Sugerman (Eds.), *Alcoholism: Interdisciplinary approaches to an enduring problem* (pp. 395–433). Reading, MA: Addison-Wesley.

Tarter, R. (1990). Evaluation and treatment of adolescent substance abuse: A decision tree method. *Am J Drug Alcohol Abuse, 16,* 1–46.

Tarter, R., Alterman, A., & Edwards, K. (1985). Vulnerability to alcoholism in men: A behavior genetic perspective. *J Stud Alcohol, 46*, 329–356.

Tarter, R., & Edwards, K. (1985). Neuropsychology of alcoholism. In R. Tarter & D. Van Thiel (Eds.), *Alcohol and brain: Chronic effects.* New York: Plenum Press.

Tarter, R., & Edwards, K. (1987). Brief and comprehensive neuropsychological assessment of alcoholism and drug abuse. In L. Hartlage, M. Ashen, & L. Hornsby (Eds.), *Essentials of neuropsychological assessment* (pp. 138–162). New York: Springer.

Tarter, R., Edwards, K., & Van Thiel, D. (1986). Hepatic encephalopathy. In G. Goldstein & R. Tarter (Eds.), *Advances in clinical neuropsychology* (Vol. 3, pp. 243–263). New York: Plenum Press.

Tarter, R., & Kirisci, L. (1997). The Drug Use Screening Inventory for adults: Psychometric structure and discriminative sensitivity. *Am J Drug Alcohol Abuse, 23*, 207–219.

Tarter, R., & Kirisci, L. (2001). Validity of the Drug Use Screening Inventory for predicting DSM-III-R substance use disorder. *J Child Adolesc Subst Abuse, 10*, 45–53.

Tarter, R., Kirisci, L., Habeych, M., Reynolds, M., & Vanyukov, M. (2004). Neurobehavior disinhibition predisposes to early age onset substance use disorder: Direct and mediated etiologic pathways. *Drug Alcohol Depend, 73*, 121–132.

Tarter, R., Kirisci, L., Mezzich, A., Cornelius, J., Pajer, K., Vanyukov, M., Gardner, W., & Clark, D. (2003). Neurobehavior disinhibition in childhood predicts early age onset substance use disorder. *Am J Psychiatry, 160*, 1078–1085.

Tarter, R., & Ryan, C. (1983). Neuropsychology of alcoholism: Etiology, phenomenology, process and outcome. In M. Galanter (Ed.), *Recent developments in alcoholism* (pp. 449–469). New York: Plenum Press.

Tarter, R., Van Thiel, D., & Moss, H. (1988). Impact of cirrhosis on the neuropsychological test performance of alcoholics. *Alcohol Clin Exp Res, 12*, 619–621.

Tarter, R., Vanyukov, M., Giancola, P., Dawes, M., Blackson, T., Mezzich, A., & Clark, D. (1999). Etiology of early age onset substance abuse: A maturational prospective. *Dev Psychopathology, 11*, 657–683.

Tellegen, A. (1982). *A manual for the Differential Personality Questionnaire.* Unpublished manuscript.

Tellegen, A. (1985). Structures of mood and personality and their relevance to assessing anxiety with an emphasis on self-report. In A. H. Tuma & J. D. Maser (Eds.), *Anxiety and the anxiety disorders.* Hillsdale, NJ: Erlbaum.

Tellegen, A., Lykken, D., Bourchard, T., Wilcox, K., Segal, N., & Rich, S. (1988). Personality similarity in twins reared apart and together. *J Pers Soc Psychol, 54*, 1031–1039.

Van Hasselt, V. B., Hersen, M., & Milliones, J. (1978). Social skills for alcoholics and drug addicts: A review. *Addict Behav, 3*, 221–233.

Vanuyukov, M., Tarter, R., Kirisci, L., Kirillova, G., Maher, B., & Clark, D. (2003). Liability to substance use disorders: 1. Common mechanisms and manifestations. *Neurosci Biobehav Rev, 27*, 507–515.

Vernon, P., Lee, D., Harris, J., Jang, K. (1996). Genetic and environmental contributions to individual differences in alcohol expectancies. *Pers Individ Dif, 21*, 183–187.

Von Knorring, A., Bohman, M., Von Knorring, L., & Oreland, L. (1985). Platelet

MAO activity as a biological marker in subgroups of alcoholism. *Acta Psychiatr Scand, 72,* 51–58.

Wanberg, K., & Horn, J. (1985). *The Alcohol Use Inventory: A guide to the use of the paper and pencil version.* Fort Logan, CO: Multivariate Measurement Consultants.

Weissman, M. (1988). Anxiety and alcoholism. *J Clin Psychiatry, 49,* 17–19.

Wellner, Z., Reich, W., Herjanic, B., Jung, D., & Amado, K. (1987). Reliability, validity and parent–child agreement studies of the Diagnostic Interview for Children and Adolescents (DICA). *J Am Acad Child Adolesc Psychiatry, 26,* 649–653.

Wilkinson, D., & Carlen, P. (1980). Relationship of neuropsychological test performance to brain morphology in amnesic and non-amnesic chronic alcoholics. *Acta Psychiatr Scand, 62,* 89–102.

Woody, G. E., Luborsky, L., McLellan, A. T., O'Brien, C. P., Beck, A. T., Blaine, J., et al. (1983). Psychotherapy for opiate addicts: Does it help? *Arch Gen Psychiatry, 40,* 639–645.

Zuckerman, M., Bone, R., Neary, R., Mangelsdorff, D., & Brastman, B. (1972). What is the sensation seeker?: Personality and trait experience correlates of the Sensation Seeking Scales. *J Consult Clin Psychol, 39,* 308–321.

CHAPTER 4

Laboratory Testing
for Substances of Abuse

DAVID A. BARON
D. ANDREW BARON
STEVEN H. BARON

For the professional working in clinical settings and in consultative roles (including sports, criminal/forensic, and occupational settings), there will always be a need for corroborative sources of information. Testing of human tissues usually provides invaluable, albeit not definitive, information in working with substance-using individuals. This information may assist in diagnostic or in therapeutic decisions, which are especially important in this population, because drugs are illegal and drug-abusing individuals often present in denial of their problem. Furthermore, this is particularly relevant when comorbid psychiatric symptoms are present. Drug testing can also aid in determining whether presenting symptoms are primarily psychiatric or substance-induced. Drug testing may be utilized as part of an initial treatment contract between the patient and treating clinician. Coercion often helps to improve treatment outcomes. This is especially so in methadone maintenance programs, where testing is typically mandatory. There is evidence to suggest that testing deters use. For example, prior to testing in 1981, 48% of military personnel used drugs, but this rate declined to 5% after 3 years of testing, and this appears to have occurred among athletes as well.

A number of questions must be contemplated before settling on a final decision:

1. For what drugs ought we to test?
2. What biological sample should be tested: urine, blood, sweat, saliva, hair, and so forth?
3. How fast do we want to see the results?
4. How much of our resources should be spent on testing?

This chapter reviews testing methodologies and the fundamental aspects of planning effective testing procedures in both clinical and consultative settings.

TESTING METHODOLOGIES

A multitude of methods are available to aid in the detection of drug use in humans. The most common drug testing technologies are listed in Table 4.1. The most popular initial test screen is an enzyme immunoassay (EIA) analysis of a urine sample. If this is positive, a confirmatory gas chromatography–mass spectroscopy (GC-MS) test is performed on the split sample. Given the greater sensitivity of GC-MS over EIA, the cutoff levels are reduced. The most commonly used analytic technique for a "comprehensive drug screen," thin-layer chromatography (TLC), is the least expensive test available. TLC utilizes the differences in polarity and chemical interaction with developing solvents to produce different visualizations on a thin-layer coating. The visualizations are highlighted using ultraviolet (UV) or fluorescent lighting, or by color reactions created after being sprayed with chemical dyes. Identical molecules cluster in the same area, yielding specific color reactions. Unfortunately, TLC is somewhat insensitive to detection of controlled substances.

Of all the available tests, how does a clinician decide on which test to administer? If there is no clinical indication to test for a specific compound, a "comprehensive drug screen" may be performed. There are settings and instances when it is important to contact the laboratory to ensure that there is a means to test for the substance, or to prompt the laboratory to test for the sub-

---

TABLE 4.1. Most Common Drug Testing Technologies

- Thin-layer chromatography
- Radio immunoassay, enzyme immunoassay, fluorescent polarization immunoassay, enzyme-linked immunosorbent assay
- Gas chromatography
- Gas chromatography–mass spetroscopy
- Liquid chromatography

---

stance. It is common for general hospital laboratories to screen only for a limited number of substances. For example, many do not screen for gamma-hydroxybutyric acid (GHB) (although methods for testing for GHB continue to undergo refinement; Chappell, Meyn, & Ngim, 2004). A drug screen done using TLC will only detect high levels of the following compounds: amphetamine, barbiturates, cocaine, codeine, dextromethorphan, diphenylhydantoin, morphine, phenylpropanolamine, methadone, propoxyphene, or quinine (a heroin diluent). TLC does not detect the following compounds: 3, 4-methlyenedioxyamphetamine (MDA), 3, 4-methylenedioxymethamphetamine (MDMA), fentanyl, D-lysergic acid diethylamide (LSD), marijuana, mescaline, and phencyclidine (PCP).

Although urine analysis is the most widely used and best overall body fluid to screen for drug use, other body fluids can be measured as well. Hair testing is growing in popularity but is not as sensitive to marijuana use as urine. Despite commercial success, the scientific foundation for using hair analysis is limited. Its primary utility might be as a tool in the diagnosis and treatment of drug abuse disorders, particularly cocaine dependence. Salivary measurements offer the advantage of ease of collection but only detect recent drug use, limiting their utility. A number of drugs, including cocaine, morphine, amphetamine, and ethanol, have been detected in sweat. Unfortunately, there is a wide intersubject variability of drug concentration in sweat. This results in a significant disadvantage when sweat is compared with other body fluids. To add to the problem, sweat collection takes several days to several weeks and requires the use of a sweat patch (Cone, 1996).

For some substances, other tests can be helpful in determining qualitative or quantitative aspects of use. For example, likely alcohol use may be detected by liver enzymes or by the new test for carbohydrate-deficient transferrin (CDT), and some investigators are studying whether certain combinations of these tests have varying specificities or sensitivities (see Chapter 5 on alcohol, this volume). And, certain blood or urine tests are vital in determining the presence of dangerous effects of substances, such as muscle breakdown leading to rhabdomyolysis and a high creatine kinase among users of cocaine and PCP.

For the consultant who works in the "field," requiring on-the-spot testing, a number of kits can be used. Most of these are the "on-site" screening immunoassays. "On-site" testing has a variety of features that make it better suited for companies than its counterpart, TLC. "On-site" testing can produce results in as little as 10 minutes, with significant accuracy. Thus, "on-site" screening is the preferred method outside of the hospital. Despite the popularity of "on-site" kits and the fact that these kits have demonstrated a greater than 97% agreement with GC/MS tests, it must be stressed that these kits provide only *preliminary* results. For best results, it is recommended that a more thorough analysis on the sample be performed.

INTERPRETATION

In an ideal world, testing biological samples should lead to definitive answers. However, test results sometimes lead to more questions than answers. Adept interpretation of results will lead to improved clinical care or to more surety in consultative cases. Interpretation depends on awareness of which test was used and its meaning to the situation.

In most settings, the primary purpose of drug testing is to identify individuals who are using illegal or illicit drugs. Falsely accusing someone of using drugs is highly problematic and undermines the testing program. Similarly, not being able to identify active drug users because of false-negative results renders a program of limited value. It does not deter use or identify users. This is so both for the emergency room physician wondering if the agitated patient used PCP, and for the consultant to the local college track team. For these situations, highly sensitive qualitative screening tests should be employed, even if this leads to some false-positive results. On the other hand, definitive tests should have the highest level of specificity: They should exclude as many true negatives as possible. For nonusers who are subjected to drug testing, issues related to false-positive results are of great concern. Questions addressing which foods, prescribed medications, dietary supplements, or potentially secondhand marijuana smoke could result in a positive test are common, and some laboratories have responded by raising the level required in order to render a positive test result.

With the proliferation of private laboratories and commercially manufactured kits, there has grown to be some interlaboratory variation in standards and thresholds for results. The industry even has its own trade organization, the Drug and Alcohol Testing Industry Association (DATIA). The major concern in drug testing occurs with the reporting of laboratory results. Unlike National Institute on Drug Abuse (NIDA)–certified testing of the Standard Drug Panel (see Table 4.2), clinical drug testing for drugs of abuse currently has no standard technical criteria, no standard screening cutoffs for positive tests, no confirmation cutoffs, no chain-of-custody requirements, no blind proficiency submission requirements, and no certification programs. As a result, a sample testing posi-

TABLE 4.2. "NIDA 5" or the DOT Standard Drug Panel 1990

Drug	Cutoffs (ng/ml)
Cocaine	300/150
Cannabinoids	50/15
PCP	25/25
Opiates	2,000/2,000
Amphetamines	1,000/500

tive in laboratory A may be reported as negative by laboratory B, based on different cutoff levels. This is not a new development (Hansen, Caudill, & Boone, 1985). Unfortunately, little progress has been made in correcting it over the past 17 years. The issue is not the type of test administered, or poor-quality laboratories, but rather the nonstandardized threshold for reporting a test as positive.

Evasion of True Positive Results

For obvious reasons, drug users are highly motivated to "produce" a clean sample. In response to this need, a black market has emerged to provide products with the sole purpose of creating a false-negative test result. These products include pretested and certified drug-free urine substitution kits, and a variety of adulterants. These include the "Whizzinator" (an artificial penis used to deliver a known drug-free urine under direct observation conditions) and *passingpisstest.com*, which provides a nontechnical description of how blood and urine drug tests work.

Those who interpret test results should be aware that addicts can be highly creative in their efforts to thwart detection and monitoring. As an example, adulterants are substances placed in a sample to alter the results of a drug test. They accomplish this by physically altering the characteristics of the sample, such as temperature, pH, and specific gravity, which disrupts the mechanisms of the assay. Adulterants range from inexpensive household products, such as soap, salt, bleach, lemon juice, or vinegar, to expensive additives specifically marketed to produce a negative test. One Internet product selling for over $100 comes with a 300% money-back guarantee. As a result of adulterant use, drug testers must now employ techniques to screen for these additives. If the sample does not fall within established physiological parameters at the time of collection, it is voided on the spot, and another sample must be produced, which is then sent to the laboratory for analysis. One "do-it-yourself" kit, available on the Internet, includes a concealed IV bag with tubing (to be strapped to the lower abdomen or upper thigh) and two heating elements with temperature strips, all in an attempt to mask the use of adulterants. One study demonstrated the ability of one adulterant to create false negative tests (Cody & Valtier, 2001).

MECHANICS OF DRUG TESTING PROGRAMS

Chain of Custody and the Medical Review Officer

A critical component of all drug testing protocols (sports and workplace) is chain of custody, which refers to the policy whereby the collected sample (usually urine) never leaves the direct observation of a member of the drug testing team until it arrives at the laboratory. Once collected, the processed sample remains under the direct observation of the testing team until it is hand-delivered to the shipping company, which also maintains direct observation until the sample is hand-delivered to the certified laboratory. The goal is to eliminate any potential tampering with the specimen. The MRO (medical review officer) is responsible for reviewing the chain of custody form to ensure no potential tampering. If chain of custody cannot be verified, the test result is considered invalid. The overarching goal and philosophy of the Drug-Free Workplace (DFW) program is to *deter*, not merely detect, drug use in the workplace. The role of the MRO physician is to advocate for the employee–athlete donor and ensure the ongoing integrity of the testing program.

Testing Programs for Athletes

Unlike drug use in the general workplace, drugs have been used for thousands of years to enhance athletic performance, increase work endurance, recreate, and to self-medicate pain and psychopathology. *Doping*, the term used to describe the use of drugs to increase athletic performance, has been documented back to the ancient Greeks. Throughout history, the use of drugs to gain an advantage over one's competitors has been considered morally wrong and worthy of severe sanctions. Fair competition was, in theory, the keystone of competitive sports. In fact, the Creed of the Olympics states that the most important factors are taking part and giving one's best effort, not winning. Fighting well and honorably took precedence over conquering the opponent, thus separating sport from war (where all was fair). Cheaters disgraced not only themselves and their families but also the sport itself. Dopers in ancient times were stripped of their winnings and often ended up as slaves, attempting to pay back their debt to the sporting world. These drastic measures, including using victory awards from cheaters to build statues to honor the gods ringing the Olympic Stadium, were intended to deter drug use and other forms of cheating (e.g., casting spells on competitors) by producing a constant reminder to every athlete who entered the arena of the potential perils of attempting to gain an unfair advantage. Unfortunately, the spoils of victory and the cost of defeat, combined with an overwhelming drive to win at any cost, have kept doping a major issue in sports at every age and level of competition.

Despite the long history of drug abuse in sports and in the workplace, laboratory testing to detect drug use is a modern phenomenon. Only since 1967 has the International Olympic Committee Medical Commission banned certain drugs and tested for their use. Full-scale drug testing for doping by athletes began in the 1972 Munich Games. Since 1967, the number of banned substances has grown every year, and the sophistication of laboratory analysis and testing protocols has advanced.

Sports doping control is not federally regulated in the United States, as it is in Australia, but typically is closely monitored by the specific sports governing bodies. For example, the National Collegiate Athletic Association (NCAA) closely monitors the testing of collegiate athletes while the U.S. Anti-Doping

Agency (USADA) monitors and conducts all Olympic-related events in the United States. In sports testing, as in DFW programs, there are two types of testing: in-competition and out-of-competition programs. No advanced notice (NAN) out-of-competition testing is the preferred method of USADA and is reported by athletes themselves to be the best deterrent of drug use. As its name implies, this form of testing consists of approaching an athlete at any time, without prior notice, and obtaining a urine sample. Olympic caliber athletes must consent to participate in the program, which includes providing a personal log of their whereabouts at all times. Failure to comply leads to sanctions by the individual sport governing body (track and field, swimming, etc.).

Testing Programs in Occupational Settings

There are two types of workplace testing: regulated and nonregulated. Regulated testing refers to programs conducted under the Federal Testing Guidelines and includes industries working with the Department of Transportation (DOT), Federal employees, and companies with Federal contracts over $25,000 per year. Nonregulated programs are typically private sector employers who are not federally required to have a DFW program but voluntarily choose to drug-test employees. These programs are not required to have an MRO and are not federally regulated.

Drug testing in the workplace has seen dramatic growth since 1988. Former President Ronald Reagan proclaimed the need for a drug-free workplace in America during his years in office. This initiative resulted in the Drug-Free Workplace (DFW) Act signed into law in November 1988. This legislation (HR-5210-124 Section 5152) laid the groundwork for the existing regulations (49-CFR-40) for virtually all of the drug-testing policies and protocols currently enforced in the workplace today. Interestingly, the DFW legislation was a significant extension of the preexisting "catastrophe-driven" testing, in which testing was only done after a catastrophic event, such as a serious work-related accident. This new policy offered a proactive deterrent philosophy.

Each DFW program is mandated to include five elements: (1) a formal written policy, (2) an Employee Assistance Program, (3) formal training for supervisors, (4) formal employee education, and (5) a drug-testing protocol. Five participants are involved with every DFW drug test: (1) the employer, (2) the donor/employee, (3) the specimen collection site, (4) the laboratory analyzing the sample, and (5) the MRO. The employer is responsible for informing the employee in writing of the Drug-Testing Policy, including all policies and procedures of the test, circumstances warranting testing in addition to preemployment testing, and consequences of a positive test. Employees must sign a form acknowledging that they are aware of the program and the existence of an Employee Assistance Program, and participate in a DFW educational presentation. They must also sign an informed consent document, agreeing to be tested under the circumstances described in the policy handbook. The collection site must also conform to specifications described in the policy handbook. The laboratory used must be certified by the Department of Health and Human Services (DHHS). There are over 80 certified laboratories throughout the United States. An up-to-date list is published regularly in the Federal Register. The laboratory is responsible for verifying appropriate chain of custody of the sample (Universal Chain of Custody forms became effective in January, 1995) and conducting a valid and reliable analysis of the specimen. The laboratory must report any breach in protocol it discovers, including any suspicion of tampering with the sample.

The MRO plays a unique and important role in the drug-testing process. Positive tests are reported to the MRO, who then evaluates the facts in the test. For example, if a worker was taking a prescribed stimulant for a medical condition with appropriate preauthorized permission, the MRO can reverse a positive test. The MRO is an "independent agent" in the testing process and is responsible for investigating all positive tests before reporting to the employer.

The five substances routinely tested for include marijuana, cocaine, amphetamines, opiates, and PCP. Other drugs, such as alcohol, may be added to the panel if suspected by the employer from objective evidence (i.e., slurred speech, alcohol on the breath). Keeping with the "Rule of Fives," there are five situations in which drug testing is conducted: (1) preemployment, (2) random, (3) postaccident, (4) probable cause, and (5) return to work/follow-up. The employer may request testing for additional substances in the case of postaccident, reasonable suspicion, and return-to-work situations. In order to undergo this additional testing, the employee must be notified via an official Employee Drug Policy document. Recognizing the high prevalence of alcohol abuse, ethanol testing was mandated in a 1994 amendment. There are separate regulations for alcohol testing, including not requiring MRO participation.

The program is designed always to give the employee the benefit of the doubt, and the benefit of the MRO's advocacy. In workplace testing, the safety of the public, as well as the individual, is at stake. Impaired judgment and hand–eye coordination resulting from intoxication have potentially devastating consequences for professional drivers, pilots, and operators of heavy equipment. Virtually every job performance, with the *possible exception* of rock stars, will be adversely affected by drug use at the workplace. The highest rates of current and past-year drug use were reported in construction workers, food preparation workers, waiters, and waitresses. Excessive alcohol consumption was observed in these groups, as well as auto mechanics, vehicle repairmen, light truck drivers, and laborers (Hoffman, Brittingham, & Larison, 1996). NIDA (1989) has estimated that if every employee/worker between the ages of 18 and 40 years old were drug tested randomly on any given day, between 14 and 25% would test positive. The cost to society is staggering, not to mention the impact on the user's life. Schwab and Syne (1997) estimates workplace drug use costs between $60 and 100 billion a year in lost and diminished productivity.

CONCLUSION

Despite the legitimate concern with false-positive and false-negative test results, the weakest link in the "chain" of drug testing is chain-of-custody violations. Regardless of the sophistication of laboratory technology, human error in completing the requisite paperwork at the drug-testing site remains the single most important inconsistent aspect of the testing process. Given the variety of available methods to cheat, it is likely that drug testing will not catch all drug users.

As is the case in all aspects of clinical medicine, an accurate diagnosis of substance abuse is based on a comprehensive clinical workup; drug testing is only one, albeit important, component of the process. Workplace drug testing hopefully will not only deter drug use by employees while on the job (eliminating costly accidents and errors) but may also assist in initially identifying individuals with drug use disorders. In the world of sports, drug testing is intended to create a level playing field for all competitors and promote the health of athletes by deterring the use of potentially harmful agents. The role of educating the public, particularly those at highest risk for drug use, cannot be overstated and needs to be the keystone of any drug-free program.

REFERENCES

Chappell, J. S., Meyn, A. W., & Ngim, K. K. (2004). The extraction and infrared indentification of gamma-hydroxybutyric acid (GHB) from aqueous solutions. *J Forensic Sci, 49*(1), 52–59.

Cody, J., & Valtier, S. (2001). Effects of stealth adulterant on immunoassay testing for drugs of abuse. *J Anal Toxicol, 25,* 466–470.

Cone, E. J. (1996). Mechanisms of drug incorporation into hair. *Ther Drug Monit, 18,* 438–443.

Hansen, H. J., Caudill, S. P., & Boone, D. J. (1985). Crisis in drug testing: Results of CDC blind study. *JAMA, 253,* 2382–2387.

Hoffman, J. P., Brittingham, A., & Larison, C. (1996). *Drug use among U.S. workers: Prevalence and trends by occupation and industry categories* (DHHS Publication No. [SMA] 96–3089). Rockville, MD: SAMHSA Office of Applied Studies.

National Institute on Drug Abuse. (1989). *Drug abuse curriculum for employee assistance program professionals* (DHHS Publication No. ADM 89-1587, pp. i–vi, 98). Washington, DC: U.S. Government Printing Office.

Schwab, M., & Syne, S. L. (1997). On paradigms, community participation, and the future of public health. *Am J Public Health, 87,* 2049–2052.

PART III

SUBSTANCES OF ABUSE

CHAPTER 5

Alcohol

EDGAR P. NACE

Alcohol dependence continues to be one of the most costly health care problems in American society. The estimated social cost of alcoholism includes treatment costs, productivity costs associated with alcohol-related morbidity and mortality, and costs associated with alcohol-related crime and traffic crashes. The yearly dollar costs for alcoholism is projected to be more than $185 billion (Harwood, 2000). Violence is commonly associated with alcohol use, with an estimated 26% of offenders using alcohol at the time of their crime (Greenfield & Henneberg, 2001).

Epidemiology helps us understand the percentage of United States adults who experience either alcohol abuse or alcohol dependence. The National Comorbidity Study (Kessler et al., 1997) found that 2.5% of those interviewed could be classified as having abused alcohol during the past 12 months (see section on diagnosis for definitions of abuse and dependence). The same study determined that 7.2% could be diagnosed as alcohol-dependent during the previous 12 months. The Epidemiologic Catchment Area study (Regier et al., 1990) determined that 3.5% of Americans met criteria for alcohol abuse at some point in their lives, and an additional 7.9% met criteria for alcohol dependence at some point in their lifetime.

The age at which drinking is initiated has become earlier over the past decades. The earlier the age of onset, the greater the risk for dependence, as well as antisocial behavior.

Current dietary guidelines for Americans recommend that men consume no more than two drinks per day and women, no more than one drink per day

(Dufour, 2001). Consumption of more than five drinks per day is consistently associated with acute and chronic adverse consequences (Midanik, Tam, Greenfield, & Caetano, 1996) Cross-sectional surveys of drinking behavior in the United States have determined that at least 65% of Americans are current drinkers and average 88 drinking days per year. The average number of heavy drinking days per year is 13 (Greenfield, 2000).

DIAGNOSIS

Alcohol use may lead to two alcohol-use disorders (abuse or dependence) and 11 alcohol-induced disorders (see section on clinical features). The fourth text revised edition of the *Diagnostic and Statistical Manual of Mental Disorders* (DSM-IV-TR; American Psychiatric Association, 2000) requires that three or more criteria for dependence occur at any time within a 12-month period. The necessity for occurrence of three or more criteria within a 12-month time frame is more diagnostically rigorous than the criteria of the DSM-III-R. In contrast to DSM-III-R, DSM-IV-TR lists only seven criteria under dependence; a former criterion—"substance often taken to relieve or avoid withdrawal symptoms"—has been subsumed under the withdrawal criteria; and the criteria on failure to fulfill major role obligations at work, school, or home have been shifted to the abuse criteria.

Alcohol abuse criteria have been expanded from two criteria in DSM-III-R to four criteria in DSM-IV-TR. Alcohol abuse requires at least one of the criteria to have occurred within a 12-month period.

Proper diagnosis requires adherence to these criteria. The distinctions between alcohol abuse and alcohol dependence (alcoholism) are clinically useful. For example, if only criteria for abuse are met, it can be assumed that the patient is not alcohol-dependent (and is, therefore, not an "alcoholic"). Such an individual is more likely to benefit from controlled drinking strategies and to be able to return to nonpathological use of alcohol than is the person who reaches criteria for dependence, where abstinence would be the preferred treatment goal. Higher rates of remission can be expected for clients with alcohol abuse compared to clients with alcohol dependence, even in the presence of a severe mental disorder.

The symptoms associated with alcohol abuse and alcohol dependence are far-ranging and involve biological, psychological, and social domains. The presenting symptoms vary from patient to patient, and such heterogeneity should be appreciated by the clinician making a diagnosis.

In assessing a patient for alcoholism, the clinician should consider problems related to the drinker, the family, and the community. Problems for the drinker may include declining job performance, joblessness, divorce, arrests (especially for driving while intoxicated and public intoxication), accidents, withdrawal symptoms, broken relationships, and associated medical and psychiatric illnesses. Assessment of family functioning may reveal marital discord, spousal abuse, child abuse, financial problems, depression or anxiety syndromes, child neglect, child developmental problems, school dropout, and delinquency. At the community level, manifestations may include violence, accidents, property damage, economic costs of welfare or health services, and decreased work productivity.

A diagnosis does not have to be rushed. Interviews with collateral sources are often necessary. Some patients will fall into a "gray zone," which means that it is unclear whether an alcohol use disorder is present. In such circumstances, obtaining further information and following the patient over time should clarify the diagnosis.

Screening

Several instruments and interviewing techniques enable the clinician to screen for an alcohol use disorder. Interview techniques include the CAGE (Ewing, 1984) and the TWEAK (Russell et al., 1991). CAGE is a mnemonic device: (Cut down: "Has anyone ever recommended that you cut back or stop drinking?" Annoyed: "Have you ever felt annoyed or angry if someone comments on your drinking?" Guilt: "Have there been times when you've felt guilty about or regretted things that occurred because of drinking?" Eye-Opener: "Have you ever used alcohol to help you get started in the morning, to steady your nerves?"). Positive answers to three of these four questions strongly suggest alcoholism. "TWEAK," a similar mnemonic device is more useful than the CAGE in interviews with women. T assesses tolerance: "How many drinks can you hold or how many drinks does it take to get high? (If it takes more than two drinks to get "high" or six drinks to feel drunk, tolerance can be assumed to be present). W: "Have close friends or relatives worried about your drinking?" Eye-Opener: "Do you sometimes take a drink in the morning to wake up?" Amnesia: "Has a friend or family member ever told you things you said or did while you were drinking that you could not remember?" K (cut): "Do you sometimes feel the need to cut down on your drinking?" Positive answers to three or more points suggest alcoholism.

Laboratory tests are useful for detecting heavy drinking. Serum gamma-glutamyltransferase (GGT) has been established as a sensitive test of early liver dysfunction. GGT has a sensitivity of 50% and a specificity of 80% (Bean & Daniel, 1996), meaning that 50% of patients with drinking problems will be missed by the GGT. However, 80% of people with an elevated GGT do have an alcohol problem (therefore, 20% of people with elevated GGTs are normal drinkers).

Another useful screening test is increased erythrocyte mean corpuscular volume (MCV), which was elevated in 26% of the patients in a Mayo Clinic study. In both male and female alcoholics, the combinations of elevated GGT and MCV identified 90% of alcoholic patients (Skinner, 1981). Other tests that may be elevated are triglycerides, serum alkaline phosphates, serum bilirubin, and uric acid.

A relatively new test with clinical utility is carbohydrate-deficient transferrin (CDT). Consuming more than 60 grams (5 drinks) of alcohol per day will increase CDT. Normal CDT levels can be expected to return after 2–4 weeks of abstinence (Allen & Anthnelli, 2003).

COMORBIDITY

The Epidemiologic Catchment Area (ECA) study that involved 20,000 adults in the general public determined that 7.3% had an alcohol use disorder within the 12 months prior to the interview (Regier et al., 1993). The National Comorbidity Survey (NCS) involved a sample of over 8,000 individuals, ages 15–54 years, in the noninstitutionalized civilian population of the United States. The 1-year prevalence rates for any alcohol use disorder (i.e., either abuse or dependence) was 9.9%. Alcohol abuse was found in 2.5% of the population within the previous 12 months, and alcohol dependence in 7.2% of the sample within the past 12 months (Kessler et al., 1994). More recently, these statistics have been revised to address the issue of clinical significance (Narrow, Rae, Robins, & Regier, 2002). Clinical significance was assessed by determining whether a physician or other professional was told about the symptoms, whether medicine was taken more than once for the symptoms, or whether the symptoms interfered a lot with one's life or activities. When these aspects of clinical significance were factored in, the prevalence rates for any alcohol use disorder went from 9.9% of the sample to 6.5% in the sample in the NCS and from 7.3% of the sample to 7.2% of the sample in the ECA study.

For each psychiatric disorder assessed in these epidemiological studies, the prevalence rates of psychiatric disorders were higher among people diagnosed with alcohol dependence or alcohol abuse. Furthermore, those with alcohol dependence were more likely to have a psychiatric disorder than those diagnosed with alcohol abuse.

In the NCS study, the median age for onset of a comorbid psychiatric disorder preceded the median age of onset for all addictive disorders by about 10 years. The majority of individuals who had both a psychiatric disorder and an addictive disorder reported that they had experienced the symptoms of the psychiatric disorder before the addictive disorder started. One exception to this order of onset was that nearly 72% of alcohol-abusing males reported that their alcohol abuse preceded the onset of a mood disorder (Petrakis, Gonzales, Rosenheck, & Krystal, 2002).

Drug Abuse–Dependence

A common comorbidity associated with alcohol use disorders is co-occurring drug use disorders. In 2001, the National Household Survey on Drug Abuse found that among teenagers who binge drink, two-thirds were also abusing drugs. In contrast, one in 20 teenagers who did not drink abused drugs. Drawing upon the ECA and NCS data, it has been determined that one in five individuals with an alcohol use disorder will also have a drug use disorder. A breakdown of the NCS data indicates that those with either alcohol abuse or alcohol dependence in 40% of cases have either drug abuse or drug dependence.

The more serious the drug use disorder, the more likely it is that alcohol abuse–dependence will be found. For example, the ECA data indicate that if no drug problem exists, the rate of alcohol abuse–dependence is 11% (compared to 13% for the total population). When tetrahydrocannabinol abuse–dependence is present, the prevalence of alcohol abuse–dependence rises to 36%. The rates of alcohol abuse–dependence rise even further with amphetamines (62%), opioids (67%), barbiturates (71%), and cocaine (84%) (Helzer & Pryzbeck, 1988).

An additional drug use comorbidity associated with drinking is that of tobacco dependence. Smoking rates among alcoholics are estimated to be as high as 90%, with approximately 70% of alcoholics smoking heavily, that is, at least one pack of cigarettes per day. Smokers who are dependent on nicotine have an approximately three times greater risk of becoming alcohol-dependent than nonsmokers (National Institute on Alcohol Abuse and Alcoholism, 1998). It is well known that the smoking rate in the general population has gradually declined over past decades, but the smoking rates among those with alcohol dependence have remained persistently high (Hays et al., 1999).

Mood Disorders

When corrected for clinical significance (Narrow et al., 2002) 1-year major depression prevalence rates are approximately 5%. Women are twice as likely as men to experience major depression. Major depression will be found nearly four times more commonly in individuals with alcohol dependence compared to the non-alcohol-dependent population. Those with a diagnosis of alcohol abuse (rather than alcohol dependence) have only a slight increased risk of major depression compared to the general population. There is a strong sex difference in order of onset. For example, in males, alcoholism precedes depression in 78% of cases, whereas for women, the reverse is true (i.e., depression precedes alcohol dependence in about 66% of cases) (Helzer & Pryzbeck, 1988).

Bipolar disorder and alcohol use disorders have a strong association. Bipolar I patients have alcohol dependence in approximately 31% of cases, and another 15% meet criteria for alcohol abuse. Patients with bipolar II illness have a rate of alcohol dependence at approximately 21% and an alcohol abuse pattern of 18%. Non-substance-abusing patients with bipolar illness have a more favorable course of treatment than do those who are using alcohol or other drugs. For example, the patients with comorbid substance use and bipolar disorders have more frequent hospitalizations for mood symptoms, earlier onset of bipolar disorder, more rapid cycling, and a greater prevalence of mixed mania. It is more common for bipolar disorder to precede alcoholism, although the reverse situation is certainly found. In either case, it is critical that the alcohol use disorder and the mood disorder be treated in a synchronous fashion, because failure to address one is likely to aggravate the occurrence of the other.

Anxiety Disorders

Compared to depressive disorder, it is usually easier to determine whether or not an anxiety disorder is independent of alcohol use. For example, posttraumatic stress disorder (PTSD) does require a specific traumatic event. Panic attacks are typically clearly recalled by individuals and are therefore easier to separate from possible anxiety symptoms that have resulted from alcohol use, intoxication, or withdrawal. There is a strong comorbidity between alcohol use disorders and anxiety disorders; nearly 37% of individuals with alcohol dependence have met criteria for an anxiety disorder during the previous year. Generalized anxiety disorder accounts for 11.6%, panic disorder for 3.9%, and PTSD for 7.7%. Another way to appreciate these comorbidities is that the alcohol-dependent person is 4.6 times more likely to have generalized anxiety disorder, 2.2 times more likely to have PTSD, and 1.7 times more likely to have panic disorder than the non-alcoholic-dependent individual. The prevalence of social anxiety disorder has been found to range from 2 to 13%, with the latter figure determined through the NCS. Typically, social anxiety disorder (social phobia) is present before the development of an alcohol use disorder, because individuals with social phobia are typically shy or behaviorally inhibited as small children. Conservative estimates of co-occurring social anxiety disorder and alcohol use disorders indicate that 15% of people receiving alcoholism treatment have both disorders, and 20% of patients seeking treatment for social anxiety disorder also have a comorbid alcohol use disorder (Randall, Thomas, & Thevos, 2001). Generally, anxiety disorders develop prior to an alcohol use disorder, and alcohol is typically seen to achieve, at least briefly, tension reduction.

Schizophrenia

Other than nicotine, alcohol is the most commonly abused drug in patients with schizophrenia. Schizophrenia occurs in about 1% of the population, but ECA data revealed that 33.7% of people with schizophreniform disorder (same symptoms as schizophrenia but lasting less than 6 months) or schizophrenia have a diagnosis of alcohol abuse or alcohol dependence at some time in their lives. The high rate of alcohol use disorders in patients with schizophrenia may be related to biological factors, such as self-medication to alleviate symptoms of schizophrenia, or side effects of antipsychotic medications; underlying abnormalities of dopamine regulation may provide a common basis for the high rate of co-occurrence; or patients with schizophrenia may be particularly vulnerable to the negative effects of substance use due to the impaired thinking and impaired social judgment that are part of the schizophrenic syndrome, thus increasing their vulnerability for a substance use disorder. It is critical that the treatment for schizophrenia and alcohol use disorders be integrated. This involves multidisciplinary treatment teams that provide outreach and comprehensive services. Osher and Kofoed (1989) describe four stages that are effective with patients with comorbid schizophrenia and alcohol use disorders: (1) developing a trusting relationship; (2) motivating the patient to manage both illnesses and pursue recovery goals; (3) providing active treatment that includes development of skills and supports needed for illness management and recovery; and (4) developing relapse prevention strategies to avoid and minimize the effects of relapse.

Eating Disorders

Over the past decades, numerous studies among patients in treatment have indicated the co-occurrence of eating disorders and substance use disorders. However, these studies are often methodologically limited, and have provided a wide range of estimates of eating disorders in patients with substance use disorders, from 2 to 41%. More recently, improved methodological approaches have determined that (1) substance use disorders do not have a significantly greater co-occurrence with eating disorders compared to other psychiatric controls, and (2) although eating disorders are frequently diagnosed among inpatients with substance use disorders, they are also frequently diagnosed in other psychiatric inpatients. At this time, there is no strong relationship between eating disorders and substance use disorders, and studies that report strong associations typically involve patients who have additional psychiatric disorders that frequently co-occur with eating disorders and substance use disorders (Dansky, Brewerton, & Kilpatrick, 2000).

Personality Disorders

The assumption that alcoholism and personality traits are linked in some fashion has a long history. Earlier editions of the DSM (DSM-I and DSM-II) classified alcoholism along with personality disorders. By 1980, with publication of DSM-III, substance use disorders (including alcoholism) were understood as entities independent of the personality disorders.

Generally, antisocial personality disorder (APD) is the most prevalent personality disorder associated with alcoholism when samples from public treatment centers are studied, and borderline personality disorder (BPD) is the most common disorder in studies from private treatment facilities. In a private psychiatric hospital sample, 57% of substance-abusing patients met DSM-III-R criteria for a personality disorder; with BPD being the most commonly occurring personality disorder (Nace, Davis, & Gaspari, 1991).

Personality disorder occurs more commonly in alcoholics than in the general population. A prospective long-term study of a nonclinical sample (Drake & Vaillant, 1985) determined that by age 47, 23% of males met criteria for a personality disorder. However, the alcoholic males in the sample met criteria for a personality disorder in 37% of cases. In a review of over 2,400 psychiatric patients (Koenigsberg, Kaplan, Gilmore, & Cooper, 1985), 36% were found to have a personality disorder. The alcoholics in this clinical sample, however, had a personality disorder in 48% of cases. ECA study data document APD in 15% of alcoholic men and 4% of alcoholic women. These prevalences exceed the rate of APD in the total population four times for men and 12 times for women (Helzer & Pryzbeck, 1988).

Cloninger (1987) has empirically determined type I, or milieu-limited alcoholism, that affects both men and women typically after age 25. Type II, or male-limited alcoholism, occurs predominately in males, develops before age 25, and is associated with severe medical and social consequences. In an extensive review, Howard, Kivlahan, and Walker (1997) determined that novelty-seeking traits predict early-onset criminality, alcoholism, and other forms of substance abuse. Furthermore, children of alcoholic parents tend to be higher in novelty seeking and lower in reward dependence than children of non-alcoholic parents. The traits of reward dependence and harm avoidance are more typical of the type I milieu-limited alcoholic and high novelty seeking, with low scores on reward dependence and harm avoidance being found more commonly in the aggressive early-onset type II male form of alcoholism.

ETHNICITY AND ALCOHOLISM

Ethnic minorities made up 29% of the U.S. population in 2000. Cultural attitudes exert a powerful influence on drinking behaviors and response to treatment. It has been shown that although cultural approval may increase the accessibility of alcohol, ritualistic use of the drug by the culture may help to inhibit abuse or dependence (Westermeyer, 1986). The lower rates of drinking problems among Italian Americans, Italians, and Jews have been explained by the traditional use of wine in these groups; integration of drinking into family life; and, in the Jewish drinkers, the religious significance attached to alcohol. However, even ethnic groups with ritualistic use patterns do not consistently show low incidences of alcoholism or alcoholic complications. For example, the French have relatively high rates of alcoholism and cirrhosis.

Native Americans

Many Native American tribal groups have high rates of alcohol-related problems (Westermeyer, 1986). However, attitudes toward drinking vary considerably from tribe to tribe. Westermeyer noted increasing rates of alcoholism and medical complications secondary to alcohol as Native American tribes have moved from their rural tribal areas to cities. Those living on reservations drink less frequently but are more likely to binge drink and to consume more alcohol per drinking occasion (May & Gossage, 2001). A recent study that contradicted the "firewater myth" theory that Native Americans are more sensitive to the effects of alcohol (Garcia-Andrade, Wall, & Ehlers, 1997) found that the Mission Indian men were generally less sensitive to alcohol effects, a physiological characteristic shown to be associated with a greater risk for alcoholism in white populations.

Alcohol-related motor vehicle fatalities are highest in the Native American population, with a 68.1% rate compared to 44.2% for whites (National Highway Traffic Safety Administration, 1999). Cirrhosis is the sixth leading cause of death in Native Americans (Stinson, Grant, & Dufour, 2001).

African Americans

A 1996 report by the Group for the Advancement of Psychiatry (GAP) on alcohol abuse among African Americans found little difference in the lifetime prevalence of alcoholism between African Americans and whites. The alcoholism prevalence for African Americans is low in the young adult group and then increases, in contrast to the alcoholism prevalence for whites, which starts at moderately high levels in the young group and then decreases. Deaths from alcohol-induced causes are about 2.5 times higher in the black population than in the white population. Cirrhosis death rates for African American males are 45.3% compared to 34.7% for whites (Caeteno & Clark, 1998b). Motor vehicle fatalities are essentially equal between blacks (45.2) and whites (44.2%) (National Highway Traffic Safety Administration, 1999).

Asian Americans

Asians have the lowest rates of cirrhosis (11.5 per 100,000 males) and the lowest percentage of motor vehicle fatalities (28.2%). A variant of aldehyde dehydrogenase-2 is found in Asians (e.g., in 48% of college students of Chinese ancestry and 35% of those of Korean background) (Luczak et al., 2001). This genetic variant changes the way alcohol is metabolized and leads to the aversive symptoms of headache, nausea, dizziness, and facial flushing.

Hispanic Americans

Hispanic American men drink more than Hispanic American women regardless of age. Mexican American men drink more and abstain less than either Puerto Rican or Cuban American men. Hispanic American men and women drink more as their income increases (Group for Advancement of Psychiatry, 1996). Surveys in 1984 and 1995 revealed that alcohol-related problems increased in Hispanic males but remained stable in women of all ethnicities, and stable in black males and white males (Caetano & Clark, 1998b). Mexican Americans have a motor vehicle alcohol-related mortality rate of 54.6%, while that of Cuban Americans is 36.6% (National Highway Traffic Safety Administration, 1999). Cirrhosis rates for Hispanic males are 61.8 per 100,000, which is higher than that found in black or white males. The notion that *machismo* is related to drinking in Mexican American males is dispelled by statistics showing equal *machismo* influences in white and non-Hispanic minorities (Caetano & Clark, 1998a).

PHARMACOLOGY OF ALCOHOL

Alcohol refers to compounds with a hydroxyl group, that is, an oxygen and hydrogen (-OH) bonded to a carbon atom. Beverage alcohol consists of ethanol, which occurs naturally as a fermentation product of sugars and grains. The ethyl alcohol molecule is hydrophilic and affects all cells of the body.

Alcohol is absorbed from the stomach and the proximal part of the small bowel. Ninety-five percent of alcohol is metabolized in the liver by alcohol dehydrogenase (ADH), which converts alcohol to the toxic substance acetaldehyde. The stomach contains at least three isoenzymes of alcohol dehydrogenase. Women have less gastric ADH and may therefore metabolize alcohol less efficiently. If gastric emptying is slowed, as with ingestion of food or with drugs having anticholinergic properties, more metabolism of alcohol by gastric ADH occurs, resulting in a lower blood alcohol concentration (Wedel, Pieters, Pikaar, & Ockhuizen, 1991). Alternatively, aspirin and cimetidine inhibit gastric ADH and may lead to an increased blood alcohol concentration.

The principal route of metabolism of alcohol is through the ADH pathway, which eliminates approximately one drink (13 g of alcohol) per hour. The major product is the toxic substance acetaldehyde. Acetaldehyde is further broken down to acetic acid via the enzyme aldehyde dehydrogenase (ALDH), and subsequently goes through the citric acid cycle to become carbon dioxide and water. Both ADH and ALDH possess several distinct isoenzymes that may reflect a genetic predisposition to alcoholism. Another pathway for oxidation, the microsomal ethanol-oxidizing system (MEOS), is induced by chronic ingestion of alcohol. An increase in the activity of the MEOS pathway can increase the rate of elimination by 50–70%. The MEOS may be responsible for the increased metabolic tolerance seen in chronic alcoholics for other hypnotic/sedative drugs, as well as for alcohol.

One action of ethanol is the disruption of the phospholipid molecular chain in the nerve cell membrane. The result is an increased "fluidity" of the membrane. This disturbance in the structure of the membrane affects the functional protein system (enzymes, receptors, and ionophores), which is attached to the membrane. For example, adenylate cyclase and monoamine oxidase activity are lower in alcoholics than in controls. Adenylate cyclase is important in the formation of cyclic adenosine monophosphate (cAMP), which in turn influences metabolism within the cytoplasm. Of particular interest is the finding that adenylate cyclase remains inhibited in alcoholics 12–48 months following abstinence (Tabakoff et al., 1988).

More important than the disruption of the cell membrane is the effect of alcohol on the gamma-aminobutyric acid (GABA) system and glutamate system of the brain. The brain has three types of GABA receptors: A, B, and C. GABA A receptors are the targets for alcohol, benzodiazepines, barbituates, and neurosteroids. Stimulation of the GABA receptor by the binding of these compounds causes an ion channel to open temporarily and emit chloride ions into the cell. Alcohol enhances the influx of chloride ion, and the result is sedative and anxiolytic effects. Chronic use of alcohol down-regulates the GABA system, and the neuron eventually becomes dependent on alcohol to enable GABA to function. If alcohol is withdrawn, the opening of the chloride ion channel fails, because GABA is no longer capable of performing the task secondary to the cell, having adapted to the role of alcohol. Thus, the cell becomes hyperexcitable, leading to irritability, insomnia, hypertension, tachycardia, and possibly hallucinations and seizures.

The second major neurotransmitter system involving alcohol is the glutamate system, and in particular the glutamate receptor N-methyl-D aspartate (NMDA). Ethanol is a potent inhibitor of the NMDA receptor and most likely blocks NMDA-stimulated calcium uptake. The NMDA receptor is involved in memory formation, neuronal excitability, and seizures. Alcohol's acute actions on this receptor leads to sedative, amnestic, and anxiolytic effects. However, when alcohol is withdrawn, the NMDA receptor becomes abnormally excited, and seizure activity and hypoxic damage may result.

Low doses of alcohol activate the norepinephrine system via the reticular activating system in the brainstem. This action stimulates behavior and arousal, and as the concentration of alcohol in the brain increases, the dopamine pathways in the mesolimbic system assume importance as a reward center. This system, which involves the ventral tegmental area and projections to the nucleus accumbens, is the same system activated by opiates and stimulants.

It has also been demonstrated that individuals with family histories that are positive for alcoholism show increased beta-endorphin release and increased euphoria after drinking alcohol. Similarly, serotonin function might predispose to alcoholism, as evidenced by the fact that some alcoholics have been found to have reduced serotonergic function and, although inconsistent, some serotonin medications have attenuated drinking behavior (Dackis & O'Brien, 2002; Pettinati, 2001)

CLINICAL FEATURES

DSM-IV (American Psychiatric Association, 1994) lists, in addition to the syndromes of alcohol abuse and alcohol dependence, 11 alcohol-induced disorders. Alcohol idiosyncratic intoxication ("pathological intoxication") was deleted in DSM-IV.

Alcohol Intoxication

Alcohol intoxication is the most common alcohol-induced disorder. It is a reversible syndrome characterized by slurred speech, impaired judgment, disinhibition, mood lability, motor incoordination, cognitive impairment, and impaired social or occupational functioning. These effects vary according to setting, mental set, dose, and tolerance of the individual, and are a result of a direct stimulant effect of alcohol on norepinephrine and dopamine systems, combined with inhibition of the stimulating effect of the glutamate-mediated NMDA receptor and facilitation of the inhibiting function of the GABA system.

A blood alcohol level of 30 mg% will produce a euphoric effect in most individuals who are not tolerant. At 50 mg%, the central nervous system (CNS) depressant effects of alcohol become prominent, with associated motor coordination problems and some cognitive deficits. In most states, the legal level of intoxication is 80 mg%. At levels greater than 250 mg%, significant confusion and a decreased state of consciousness may occur. Alcoholic coma may occur at this level, and at greater than 400 mg%, death may result. Because of tolerance, some heavy drinkers may not show these effects even at high blood levels.

Alcohol Withdrawal

With prolonged exposure to ethanol, the brain adapts by down-regulating (i.e., reducing) the inhibitory GABA A receptors—especially the alpha 1 subunit of GABA A. Ethanol also inhibits the excitatory NMDA glutamate receptors, and the brain adapts by increasing or up-regulating NMDA receptors. Therefore, when alcohol use is discontinued there is a relative decrease in inhibiting (GABA) mechanisms and a relative increase in excitatory (NMDA) mechanisms. The symptoms of alcohol withdrawal then emerge and commonly include tremor, sweating, anxiety or agitation, elevated blood pressure, increased pulse, increased respiration, headaches, nausea, vomiting, and light and sound sensitivity. If the withdrawal is more severe, grand mal seizures (usually only one) may occur 24–48 hours after the last drink.

Alcohol withdrawal may be accompanied by perceptual disturbances and is coded accordingly if the perceptual disturbance occurs with intact reality testing (i.e., the person knows that the perceptions are caused by alcohol). The perceptual disturbances may be auditory, visual, or tactile hallucinations or illusions. They are transitory and usually develop within 48 hours of cessation of drinking. "Alcohol hallucinosis" is a clinical term commonly applied to these perceptual disturbances.

Delirium

An alcohol-induced delirium may occur during intoxication (alcohol intoxication delirium) or during withdrawal (delirium tremens, or DTs).

Alcohol intoxication delirium (unlike delirium from stimulants or hallucinogens, which may emerge in hours) requires days of heavy use of alcohol to occur. Evidence for a delirium would include a disturbance in consciousness manifested by inability to shift, sustain, or focus one's attention; reduced awareness of the environment; and cognitive impairment, such as disorientation, memory deficits, and language disturbance (e.g., mumbling). The symptoms would fluctuate during the course of a day and would be linked by history and physical or laboratory data to the use of alcohol (American Psychiatric Association, 1994).

DTs are most likely to develop if the patient has had an alcohol withdrawal seizure or a concomitant medical disorder, such as an infection, hepatic insufficiency, pancreatitis, subdural hematoma, or a bone fracture. Onset is usually 2–3 days after cessation of alcohol use and usually lasts 3–7 days, but can be prolonged. DTs must be considered a medical emergency (Goforth, Primeau, & Fernandez, 2003) and are characterized by visual, auditory, and/or tactile hallucinations, gross tremor, tachycardia, sweating, and, possibly, fever, as well as the disturbances of consciousness described earlier.

Alcohol-Induced Persisting Amnestic Disorder

Alcohol-induced persisting amnestic disorder constitutes a continuum involving Wernicke's acute encephalopathy, the amnestic disorder per se (commonly known as Korsakoff's psychosis), and cerebellar degeneration. Alcohol-induced persisting amnestic disorder typically follows an acute episode of Wernicke's encephalopathy. The latter consists of ataxia, sixth cranial nerve (abducens) paralysis, nystagmus, and confusion. Wernicke's often clears with vigorous thiamine treatment, but 50–65% of patients show persistent signs of amnesia. If untreated, the mortality rate is about 15%.

The amnesia is characterized by anterograde amnesia (inability to form new memories due to failure of information acquisition), retrograde amnesia (loss of previously formed memories), and cognitive deficits, such as loss of concentration and distractibility.

The etiology is based on nutritional factors, specifically, the thiamin deficiency present with chronic alcohol use, either through intestinal malabsorption or poor dietary intake associated with alcohol. Other factors, such as familial transketolase deficiency may be important in the pathogenesis of this syndrome in a subgroup of individuals.

The disorder in memory that persists is correlated with microhemorrhages in the dorsomedial nucleus of the thalamus, in the mammillary bodies, and in the periventricular gray matter.

In contrast to other dementias, intellectual function is typically preserved. In a review of Wernicke–Korsakoff syndrome, McEvoy (1982) points out that 20% of patients show complete recovery over a period of months to years, 60% show some improvement, and 20% show minimal improvement. Previously believed to be a distinct clinical entity, alcoholic cerebellar degeneration may be indistinguishable clinically and pathophysiologically from the cerebellar dysfunction seen with Wernicke–Korsakoff syndrome.

Alcoholic amnestic disorder should not be confused with "blackouts," which are periods of retrograde amnesia during periods of intoxication. Blackouts, caused by high blood alcohol levels, may occur in nonalcoholics, as well as at any time in the course of alcoholism.

Alcohol-Induced Persisting Dementia

This disorder develops in approximately 9% of alcoholics (Evert & Oscar-Berman, 1995) and consists of memory impairment combined with aphasia, apraxia, agnosia, and impairment in executive functions, such as planning, organizing, sequencing, and abstracting. These deficits are not part of a delirium and persist beyond intoxication and withdrawal. The dementia is caused by the direct effects of alcohol, as well as by vitamin deficiencies.

Models of cognitive impairment in alcoholics include "premature aging," which means that alcohol accelerates the aging process, and/or that vulnerability to alcohol-induced brain damage is magnified in people over the age of 50; the "right-hemisphere model," which is derived from the evidence that nonverbal skills (reading maps, block design tests, etc.) are more profoundly impaired in alcoholics than left-hemisphere tasks (language functions); and the "diffuse brain dysfunction" model, which proposes that chronic alcoholism leads to widespread brain damage (Ellis & Oscar-Berman, 1989).

Personality changes, irritability, and mild memory deficits in an abstinent individual with a history of alcoholism are early clues suggestive of alcohol-induced persisting dementia.

Alcohol-Induced Anxiety, Affective, or Psychotic Disorder

If symptoms of an anxiety disorder, affective disorder (depressive, manic, or mixed), or psychotic disorder (hallucinations or delusions) develop during or within 1 month of intoxication or withdrawal, an alcohol-induced anxiety, affective, or psychotic disorder may be diagnosed. If the patient has insight that hallucinations are alcohol-induced, an alcohol-induced psychotic disorder is not diagnosed. The anxiety and affective symptoms must exceed the usual presentation of such symptoms as they commonly occur during intoxication or withdrawal (DSM-IV).

These disorders must be distinguished from comorbid psychiatric disorders (see section on comorbidity). A careful history eliciting the onset and the course of symptoms during abstinence or reexposure to alcohol will help distinguish alcohol-induced syndromes from psychiatric comorbidity.

Alcohol-Induced Sleep Disorder

Alcohol consumed at bedtime may decrease the time required to fall asleep but typically disrupts the second half of the sleep cycle, resulting in subsequent daytime fatigue and sleepiness. Even a moderate dose of alcohol consumed within 6 hours prior to bedtime can increase wakefulness during the second half of sleep (Vitiello, 1997). Alcohol use prior to bedtime will also aggravate obstructive sleep apnea, and heavy drinkers or those with alcoholism are at increased risk for sleep apnea. Patients with severe obstructive sleep apnea are at a five-fold increased risk for fatigue-related traffic crashes if they consume two or more drinks per day compared to obstructive sleep apnea patients who consume little or no alcohol (Bassetti & Aldrich, 1996).

In alcoholics, heavy drinking eventually leads to increased time required to fall asleep, frequent awakenings, and a decrease in subjective quality of sleep. Slow-wave sleep is interrupted, and during periods of withdrawal there is pronounced insomnia and increased rapid eye movement (REM) sleep. Following withdrawal from alcohol, sleep patterns may be abnormal, even following years of abstinence.

Alcohol-Induced Sexual Dysfunction

Sexual dysfunction refers to impairment in sexual desire, arousal, or orgasm, or presence of pain associated with intercourse as a result of alcohol use. Alcohol-induced sexual dysfunction differs from a primary sexual disorder in that improvement would be expected with abstinence from alcohol.

Alcohol consumption has been found to have a negative relationship to physiological arousal in women. Although women state that they felt more aroused, the physical responses tend to be depressed when alcohol is consumed. Inhibition of ovulation, decrease in gonadal mass, and infertility may follow chronic heavy alcohol use.

In males, erectile dysfunction may occur transiently with alcohol use, especially at blood alcohol levels above 50 mg/100 ml. Decreased libido, erectile dysfunction, and gonadal atrophy are reported in chronic alcoholics (Adler, 1992).

Chronic male alcoholics, even without liver dysfunction, commonly demonstrate primary hypogonadism, as evidenced by decreased sperm count and motility, and altered sperm morphology. Increases in luteinizing hormone and a decrease in the free androgen index were reported in noncirrhotic males and related to lifetime quantity of ethanol intake (Villalta et al., 1977).

However, a controlled study of abstinent alcohol males selected for absence of physical illness and use of medications found that sexual dysfunction, level of lutenizing hormone, and level of bioavailable testosterone did not differ between the controls and the alcoholics (Schiave, Stimmel, Mandeli, & White, 1995).

Normal sexual functioning in abstinent alcoholic men can be expected in the absence of sexually impairing medications (e.g., disulfiram), liver disease, or gonadal failure.

MEDICAL COMPLICATIONS OF ALCOHOLISM

Gastrointestinal Tract and Pancreas

Secondary to vitamin deficiencies, alcoholics suffer from inflammation of the tongue (glossitis), inflammation of the mouth (stomatitis), caries, and periodontitis. A low-protein diet, associated with alcoholism, can lead to a zinc deficiency, which impairs the sense of taste and further curbs the appetite of the alcoholic. Parotid gland enlargement may be noted.

Alcohol causes decreased peristalsis and decreased esophageal sphincter tone, which leads to reflux esophagitis with pain and stricture formation (Bor et al., 1998). The Mallory–Weiss syndrome refers to a tear at the esophageal–gastric junction caused by intense vomiting. Another source of bleeding from the esophagus is esophageal varices secondary to the portal hypertension of cirrhosis.

Alcohol decreases gastric emptying and increases gastric secretion. As a result, the mucosal barrier of the gastrium is disrupted, allowing hydrogen ions to seep into the mucosa, which release histamine and may cause bleeding. Acute gastritis is characterized by vomiting (with or without hematemesis), anorexia, and epigastric pain. It remains unclear whether chronic alcohol abuse increases the risk of ulcer disease.

The small intestine shows histological changes and contractual pattern changes even with adequate nutrition. Acute alcohol consumption impairs absorption of folate, vitamin B_{12}, thiamine, and vitamin A, as well as some amino acids and lipids. Intestinal enzyme activity is altered as well (Hauge, Nilsson, Persson, & Hultberg, 1998).

Alcohol consumption and gallstones are the two most common causes of acute pancreatitis. Alcohol in moderate amounts does not increase the risk for acute pancreatitis, but consumption of 35 or more drinks per week increases the odds ratio to 4.1 (Blomgren et al., 2002). Acute pancreatitis presents as a dull, steady epigastric pain that may radiate to the back. Bending or sitting may partially relieve the pain, confirming its retroperitoneal origin. Pain may be precipitated or aggravated by meals and relieved by vomiting. A serum amylase of 1.5 to 2.0 times the upper limit of normal has a sensitivity of 95% and a specificity of 98% for acute pancreatitis. Ethanol-induced acute pancreatitis is the result of the toxic effect of ethanol on pancreatic acinar cells, leading to inflammation and release of proteolytic enzymes. Chronic pancreatitis is caused most commonly by alcoholism. The common presenting symptoms are abdominal pain, weight loss, nausea, vomiting, jaundice, and diarrhea. Surgical procedures are available for treatment of chronic pancreatitis, with favorable long-term results (Sohn et al., 2000).

Liver

Three histological distinct lesions occur in the evaluation of alcohol-induced liver disease. The most common, occurring in 90% of heavy drinkers, is fatty liver (hepatic steatosis); 10–35% of heavy drinkers acquire alcoholic hepatitis, and 10–20% acquire alcohol cirrhosis (fibrosis, nodules, loss of normal structure).

Alcohol leads to liver damage by several mechanisms: the production of acetaldehyde, free radicals, and cytokines as alcohol is metabolized; the passage of bacterial endotoxins through the intestinal wall is enhanced by the presence of alcohol; and alcohol-induced cell death and inflammation, which lead to scarring (Lieber, 1998).

Hepatic steatosis is a common, reversible condition that may progress to cirrhosis in about 7% of cases (Gish, 1996). Signs and symptoms of alcoholic steatosis include nausea, vomiting, hepatomegaly, right-upper-quadrant pain, and tenderness. Ascites and jaundice are uncommon. Laboratory data may reveal mild elevation of transaminases, alkaline phosphatase, or bilirubin. Clinically, fatty liver may mimic or coexist with alcoholic hepatitis. Symptoms of alcoholic fatty liver, as well as alcoholic hepatitis, should resolve with abstinence.

Alcoholic hepatitis frequently coexists with fatty liver and cirrhosis. Symptoms include anorexia, nausea, vomiting, fever, chills, and abdominal pain. Hepatomegaly and right-upper-quadrant tenderness are common.

Transaminase levels rarely exceed 500 international units (IU), with a typical ratio of aspartate aminotransferase to alanine aminotransferase of 2:1 to 5:1. Liver biopsy can be helpful in distinguishing fatty liver from hepatitis and from cirrhosis. Ascites, encephalopathy, high bilirubin levels, and prolongation of the prothrombin time are poor prognostic indicators that portend an increased mortality. Treatment consists of abstinence and nutritional support. Treatment with steroids, propylthiouracil, and colchicines has yielded mixed results. There is a relative-risk increase of 14–20 for individuals who drink more than five drinks per day, although wine drinkers are at a lower risk than beer or liquor drinkers (Becker, Gronbaek, Johansen, & Sorensen, 2002). Women have a higher incidence of alcoholic hepatitis and cirrhosis than men, although the mechanisms underlying these gender differences is not known. Alcoholic cirrhosis develops as a result of prolonged hepatocyte damage, leading to centrilobular inflammation and fibrosis. The latter pathology causes portal hypertension and the development of varices. Esophageal varices may bleed spontaneously, or bleeding may be precipitated by respiratory tract infections, nonsteroidal anti-inflammatory drugs, and alcohol. Cirrhosis also leads to ascites, clotting deficiencies, secondary malnutrition, and hepatic encephalopathy (Sutton & Shields, 1995).

Nutrition

Alcoholics are especially susceptible to deficiencies of thiamine, folate, B vitamins, and ascorbic acid. Alcohol intake leads to negative nitrogen balance, increased protein turnover, and inhibition of lipolysis (Bunout, 1999). Deficiencies in folate, vitamin B_6, and vitamin B_{12} play a role in elevated levels of homocysteine, which in turn promotes atherosclerosis and thrombosis formation (Cravo & Camilo, 2000). Ethanol can suppress appetite through its effect on the CNS. Gastric, hepatic, and pancreatic disease my further decrease enteral intake and contribute to maldigestion or malabsorption. Signs of malnutrition include thinning of the hair, ecchymosis, glossitis, abdominal distention, peripheral edema, hypocalcemic tetany, and neuropathy. Nutritional management consists of abstinence and institution of a well-balanced diet and multivitamins, plus thiamine and vitamin B supplements when indicated.

Cardiovascular System

It is well established that alcoholic heart muscle disease is a complication of long-term alcoholism and not malnutrition or other possible causes of dilated cardiomyopathy. In a dose-dependent fashion, left ventricular systolic function declines, implicating alcohol in at least 30% of all dilated cardiomyopathies (Lee & Regan, 2002). The contractility of heart muscle is decreased through alcohol's effect of increased calcium flow into muscle cells, decreased protein synthesis (possibly secondary to increased acetaldehyde), and mitochondrial disruption (e.g., depressed adenosine triphosphate (ATP) level, leakage of enzymes, and accumulation of glycogen) (Davidson, 1989).

Alcoholic cardiomyopathy should not be confused with heart disease occasionally resulting from congeners, as occurred in the 1960s when cobalt was added to beer to stabilize the foam. The symptoms are similar to other forms of congestive heart failure, and begin with shortness of breath and fatigue. Abstinence is necessary for recovery: A 54% morality rate from this disease is reported in those who continue to drink compared to 9% who abstain (Regan, 1990).

Transient hypertension is noted in nearly 50% of alcoholics undergoing detoxification and is related to quantity of drinking and severity of other withdrawal symptoms. Epidemiological studies have demonstrated that alcohol elevates blood pressure independently of age, body weight, or cigarette smoking (Klatsky, Friedman, & Armstrong, 1986). A 10-year follow-up study found even moderate intake of alcohol (<23 grams/day) significantly increased the risk for hypertension in men, independent of age and body mass index. The risk of hypertension was increased for women, but not significantly, when age and body mass index were controlled (Ohmori et al., 2002).

Heavy alcohol intake (>60 grams/day) is associated with increased risk of ischemic and hemorrhagic stroke. Mechanisms involved include alcohol-induced hypertension, coagulation disorders, atrial fibrillation, and reduction in cerebral blood flow (Reynolds, Lewis, Nolen, Kinney, & Sathya, 2003). Alcohol has been shown directly to cause vasoconstriction of cerebral blood vessels, and this effect can be reversed or prevented by calcium-channel blocking drugs and by magnesium (Altura & Altura, 1989).

Thus far, the effects of alcohol on the cardiovascular system are distinctly negative—cardiomyopathy, hypertension, and strokes. Yet beneficial effect has been observed, in that people who drink low to moderate amounts of alcohol are at lower risk for coronary artery disease. Light drinkers (two drinks per day) have a 20% reduction in risk for coronary artery disease (Klatsky, Friedman, & Armstrong, 1986). The protective effect of alcohol seems to follow a U-shaped curve, with nondrinkers and heavy drinkers showing greater risk for coronary artery disease (Criqui, 1990).

The mechanism by which alcohol provides some protective effect against coronary artery disease is in the elevation of high-density lipoproteins, decreased platelet aggregation, and fibrinolytic activity (Zakari, 1997).

Nervous System

Ethanol damages the CNS and peripheral nervous system by altering both neurotransmitter levels and cell membrane fluidity and function. Among the neurological effects, alcoholic dementia and Wernicke–Korsakoff syndrome were discussed earlier. Hepatic encephalopathy occurs in the setting of severe liver failure as a result of either severe alcoholic hepatitis or cirrhosis. Early manifestations of encephalopathy include inappropriate behavior, agitation, depression, apathy, and sleep disturbance. Confusion, disorientation, and depressed mental status develop in the advanced stages of encephalopathy. Physical examination may demonstrate asterixis, tremor, rigidity, hyperreflexia, and fetor hepaticus. Treatment requires the elimination of the offending condition, dietary protein restriction, and removal of nitrogenous waste from the gut with osmotic laxatives and antibiotics (lactulose and neomycin, respectively) (Adams & Victor, 1989).

The most frequent neurological consequence of chronic alcohol intake is a toxic polyneuropathy, which results from inadequate nutrition, mainly deficiency of thiamine and other B vitamins. Additionally, there is a relationship to total lifetime dose of ethanol. Signs and symptoms are (1) distal sensory disturbances, with pain, paresthesia, and numbness in a glove-and-stockings pattern; (2) weakness and atrophy of distal muscles, pronounced in the lower limbs; (3) loss of tendon jerks; and (4) dysfunction of autonomic fibers. As a result, therapy consists of alcohol abstinence, high-calorie nutrition, parenteral thiamine, and other vitamins. For paresthesia and pain, carbamazepine, salicylates, and amitrytiline are effective. The prognosis of alcoholic polyneuropathy is favorable with alcohol abstinence. In chronic alcoholic patients, peripheral nerves frequently are injured by compression during alcohol intoxication. Peroneal nerve lesions result from compression in the region of the neck of the fibula during a prolonged lying position, and the radial nerve is injured during sitting with the upper arm placed on the backrest of a bench. Usually, pressure palsies resolve spontaneously (Schuchardt, 2000).

Hematology

Anemia can result from hemorrhage, hemolysis, or bone marrow hypoplasia. Megaloblastic anemia, usually a result of folate deficiency, has been observed in 20–40% of seriously ill, hospitalized alcoholic patients and in up to 4% of ambulatory alcoholics. Alcohol inhibits absorption of folate. There is not a strong correlation between megaloblastic anemia and the presence of liver disease. Alcohol also has a direct toxic effect on the bone marrow, which results in a transient sideroblastic anemia. Reticulocytosis commonly occurs as part of recovery from alcohol toxicity (Lee, 1999). Transient thrombocytopenia is found after consumption of large quantities of alcohol, especially in binge drinkers (Hardin, 2001).

Leukopenia is less common, resulting from the same mechanisms of toxic and nutritional factors already mentioned. Hypersplenism, an irreversible complication, may also contribute to leukopenia, thrombocytopenia, and anemia.

Bone marrow recovery with resolution of leukopenia usually occurs after 1–2 weeks of abstinence.

Alcohol also affects both thrombotic and coagulation functions. In particular, the cascade of clotting proteins is impeded as a result of diminished production of the vitamin K–dependent clotting factors (prothrombin, VII, IX, and X). Fibrinolysis, and occasionally disseminated intravascular coagulation may also occur. Transient thrombocytopenia is found after consumption of large quantities of alcohol, especially in binge drinkers (Hardin, 2001).

Endocrine System

Alcohol interferes with gonadal function even in the absence of cirrhosis by inhibiting normal testicular, pituitary, and hypothalamic function. Testicular atrophy, low testosterone levels, decreased beard growth, diminished sperm count, and a loss of libido result. However, testicular atrophy does not occur in all male alcoholics but is associated with alcohol dehydrogenase polymorphism in the testes, as reflected by the genetic variant of an increased frequency of the ADH21 allele (Yanauchi et al., 2001).

Thyroid dysfunction is common in alcoholics. Consistent findings indicate reduced thyroxine, and total and free triodothyronine concentrations in early abstinence. A blunted thyroid stimulation test is found in one-third of alcoholics during detoxification and into the early weeks of abstinence. A direct toxic effect of alcohol on the thyroid is likely, which in turn induces a compensatory activation of the hypothalamic–pituitary (HP) axis (Hermann, Heinz, & Mann, 2002).

Alcohol intoxication activates the HP axis and results in elevated glucocorticoid levels. Elevated levels of these stress hormones may contribute to alcohol's pleasurable effects. With chronic alcohol consumption, however, tolerance may develop to alcohol's HP axis–activating effects. Chronic alcohol consumption, as well as chronic glucocorticoid exposure, can result in premature aging (Spencer & Hutchison, 1999).

Musculoskeletal System

Acute alcoholic myopathy (rhabdomyolysis) may cause painful, tender swelling of one or more large muscle groups. Diagnosis depends on a high index of clinical suspicion, elevation of serum creatine phosphokinase, and myoglobinuria. Chronic alcoholic myopathy may accompany alcoholic polyneuropathy, presenting as painless, progressive muscle weakness and wasting.

The development of osteoporosis in middle-age men is uncommon except in male alcoholics, where decreased bone mass has been documented (Turner, 2000). In women, improvement in bone mass has been shown with moderate alcohol use, especially in postmenopausal women (Laitinen et al., 1993).

Immune System

Alcoholics often have impaired immune response, placing them at risk for frequent and severe infections. Alcohol increases hepatitis C virus (HCV) replication and inhibits the anti-HCV effect of interferon-alpha therapy. Alcohol's effect is most pronounced during the early phase of the immune response and interferes with the antigen-presenting cells (not directly on T-cells). The result is a decreased response from immunoglobulins (Latif, Peterson, & Waltenbaugh, 2002). People who abuse alcohol are more likely to participate in behaviors that put them at risk to develop human immunodeficiency virus (HIV), and alcohol use disorders are associated with an increased incidence of HIV, as well as opportunistic infections.

Skin

Skin disorders can serve as early markers of alcohol misuse. Florid facies and flushing are common. Psoriasis in men has been associated with alcohol abuse, and the treatment responsiveness of psoriasis is significantly reduced when daily alcohol use exceeds 80 g per day (Gupta, Schork, Gupta, & Ellis, 1993). Other early skin markers of excessive alcohol use include discoid eczema (coin-shaped, scaly lesions, usually on the lower legs), rosacea, and skin infections such as tinea pedis, pityriasis, and onychomycosis (Higgins & du Vivier, 1992).

Immunosuppression secondary to alcohol intake is the likely mechanism for the increased incidence of skin infections. Squamous cell carcinoma of the oral cavity is increased with heavy alcohol consumption (Smith & Fenske, 2000). Late stages of alcoholism may reveal cigarette burns, bruises, acne, and cutaneous stigmata of liver disease, such as spider nevi and palmer erythema.

Cancer

Alcohol increases the risk for developing some types of cancer in a dose-dependent fashion. Alcohol is most strongly associated with increased risk for cancer of the oral cavity and pharynx (relative risk [RR] = 5.7), esophagus (RR = 4.2), and larynx (RR = 3.2). Statistically significant increases in risk also are found for cancers of the stomach, colon, rectum, liver, female breast, and ovaries (Bagnardi, Blangiardo, La Vecchia, & Corras, 2001).

Alcohol has not been demonstrated to be a carcinogen per se, but is likely to act as a co-carcinogen, or cancer-promoting effect, when known cancer-inducing agents are present. For example, smoking heavily and drinking heavily synergistically increase the risk factors for some cancers, as does the combination of high alcohol consumption and low consumption of fruits and vegetables. The synergism between tobacco use and alcohol is highest for cancers of the oral cavity, pharynx, larynx, and esophagus.

Female breast cancer shows a dose-dependent increased risk with alcohol consumption (e.g., RR = 1.3 with use of two drinks per day) but an increased RR of 2.7 if alcohol consumption averages over eight drinks per day (Bagnardi et al., 2001). The mechanism of alcohol's interaction with breast cancer is most likely related to increased estrogen levels associated with drinking. The increased risk of breast cancer with alcohol use may be limited to women with a family history of breast cancer (Vachon, Cerhan, Vierkant, & Sellers, 2001).

Fetal Effects

Fetal alcohol syndrome (FAS) is the leading known preventable cause of mental retardation. FAS is defined by maternal drinking during pregnancy, growth retardation, a pattern of facial abnormalities, and brain damage characterized by intellectual difficulties or behavioral problems (Stratton, Howe, & Battaglia, 1996). The fetus is most vulnerable to alcohol during the first trimester. Facial abnormalities are characterized by a thin upper lip, absence of a philtrum, midfacial hypoplasia, and short palpetral fissures. Behavioral and intellectual problems include difficulty in shifting attention, slower reaction time, poorer memory, language problems, and deficits in executive functions such as planning and organization (Olson, Feldman, Streissguth, Sampson, & Bookstein, 1998).

No safe limit of alcohol use has been determined, but infants born to women who drink more than 150 grams of alcohol per day during pregnancy have a 33% chance of having FAS (Greenfield, Weiss, & Mirin, 1997). About 3.1 per 1,000 first-grade students may show evidence of FAS in the United States (Clarren, Randels, Sanderson, & Fineman, 2001).

TREATMENT PRIORITIES

Establishing a trusting *therapeutic relationship* is integral to treating the alcoholic patient. A psychiatrist is in a strong position to develop a nonjudgmental, empathic relationship with alcoholic patients but, in addition, must be prepared to challenge denial and confront pathological behavior or regression. The physician's awareness of the continuing incentive to drink, mediated by chronic stimulation of dopamine-rich pathways in the mesocortical system, will assist him or her in tolerating relapses and encouraging the patient to learn from relapses rather than either the patient or the clinician succumbing to a sense of defeat. Alcoholism leads to impaired impulse control and an impaired priority system; that is, the salience or importance of alcohol has become dominant for the alcoholic patient, and the reversal of this priority is a slow, steady, day-by-day process.

Demoralization is always a potential factor, but it can be effectively countered by the doctor–patient relationship, combined with utilization of a support system such as Alcoholics Anonymous. The development of negative countertransference on the part of the physician needs to be guarded against to the extent possible. Work with a sufficient number of alcoholic patients will demonstrate the heterogeniety of those who develop alcoholism and lead to the physician's ability to assist in recovery and witness the restoration of health, the reestablishment of effective work patterns, and the gratification of renewed relationships.

Detecting relapse is a treatment priority. The patient may report relapse, but often this is not the case. Family members, employers, or other collateral sources may provide information that suggests relapse. Observations made by the physician may indicate relapse. Biomarkers may be very useful in detecting relapse—for example, an increase of 30% or more in GGT above a previously obtained value is likely to reflect relapse (Anton, Lieber, & CDTect Study Group, 2002). CDT may rise before other signs of relapse are apparent. There are few sources of false-positive results. An elevation can be expected if alcohol is consumed for 2 weeks at a level of five drinks (60 grams) per day (Schmidt et al., 1997). Early detection of relapse offers the potential to prevent a return to harmful or dependent drinking, as well as an opportunity to identify "triggers" that render an individual susceptible to relapse.

Comorbidity with other psychiatric disorders is common in alcoholic patients. This potential multiplicity of clinical problems raises questions about what condition is treated first, which setting, and what modalities. Several guidelines can be offered.

1. The issues of acuity and safety must receive priority (Nace, 1995). A patient who presents as acutely suicidal would necessarily be placed in an inpatient setting capable of offering close or constant observation. An acutely delusional patient would require the intensity of an inpatient psychiatric unit as well. Addressing recovery issues would await psychotic stabilization.

2. Alcohol-related and co-occurring disorders should be treated in parallel or synchronously. For example, a suicidal patient requiring the protection of a locked psychiatric unit may also require detoxification, simultaneous with efforts to protect him or her from self-harm.

3. Sufficient time free of alcohol may clarify the issue of comorbidity. Alcohol-related anxiety and affective or psychotic disorders are expected to resolve in about 4 weeks, although clinical judgment is more appropriate than fixed time intervals in determining whether symptoms are alcohol-related or part of a comorbid condition. If symptoms abate as alcohol is withdrawn, the likelihood of a co-occurring disorder diminishes. If symptoms persist, or if new symptoms emerge in the absence of alcohol, a co-occurring disorder is likely.

tion and management. Panic attacks occurring in association with alcohol may require relief with alprazolam or other suitable drugs. Addressing acute symptoms pharmacologically does not imply that an additional dependence will be established, or that alcohol dependence will be prolonged.

5. Each disorder requires treatment. Severely depressed patients cannot be expected to respond to 12-step programs or rehabilitation efforts if they are not simultaneously receiving appropriate pharmacology and psychotherapy. Nor will a bipolar patient be likely to achieve stabilization if his or her alcoholism or alcohol abuse is not arrested. See Chapter 26, "Psychopharmacological Treatments," for the mechanism and utility of the agents used in alcohol use disorders, including disulfiram, naltrexone, and acamprosate, all recently approved for use in the United States.

CONCLUSION

Alcoholism is a disease that manifests itself through social, medical, legal, and family consequences. Alcohol dependence and alcohol abuse are amenable to reliable diagnostic criteria. Subjectively, the alcoholic struggles with prolonged cravings for the substance, fear of functioning without alcohol, and doubts about his or her ability to abstain, and hence to recover. Concomitant with the ambivalent struggle to change, the alcoholic endures remorse, regret, guilt, and shame.

The physician, if not cognizant of the protean manifestations of this disease, or if blinded to the suffering of the patient by the alcoholic's often outrageous behavior, may miss or decline to take the opportunity for a life-changing clinical encounter. On the other hand, the physician prepared for the diagnosis and treatment of addictive disorders will find clinical experiences that contradict the pessimism often instilled during training years.

The psychiatrist's role in the treatment of alcoholism is especially pertinent given the significant issue of comorbidity and the biopsychosocial orientation of modern psychiatry. With an understanding of the overlapping relationships between substance use disorders and other psychiatric disorders, and an ability to establish treatment priorities, the psychiatrist is in a unique position to provide medical leadership to treat effectively this complex biopsychosocial disorder.

REFERENCES

Adler, R. A. (1992). Clinically important effect of alcohol on endocrine function. *J Clin Endocrinol Metab, 74,* 957–960.

Allen, J. O., & Anthenelli, R. M. (2003). Problem drinking: The case for routine screening. *Curr Psychiatry, 2*(6), 27–44.

Altura, B. A., & Altura B. T. (1989). Cardiovascular functions in alcoholism and after acute administration of alcohol: Heart and blood vessels. In H. W. Goedde & D. P. Agarwal (Eds.), *Alcoholism: Biochemical and genetic aspects* (pp. 167–215). New York: Pergamon Press.

American Psychiatric Association. (1994). *Diagnostic and statistical manual of mental disorders* (4th ed.). Washington, DC: Author.

American Psychiatric Association. (2000). *Diagnostic and statistical manual of mental disorders* (4th ed., text rev.). Washington, DC: Author.

Anton, R. F., Lieber, C., Tabakoff, B., and CDTect Study Group. (2002). Carbohydrate-deficient transferrin and gamma-glutamyltransferase for the detection and monitoring of alcohol use: Results from a multi-site study. *Alcohol Clin Exp Res, 26*(8), 1215–1222.

Bagnardi, V., Blangiardo, M., La Vecchia, C., & Corras, G. (2001). Alcohol consumption and the risks of cancer: A meta-analysis. *Alcohol Res Health, 25*, 263–270.

Bassetti, C., & Aldrich, M. S. (1996). Alcohol consumption and sleep apnea in patients with transient ischemic attack and ischemic stroke: A prospective study of 59 patients. *Neurology, 47*, 1167–1173.

Bean, P., & Daniel, P. (1996). CDT current facts and future projections for the insurance industry. *On the Risk, 12*, 43–48.

Becker, U., Gronbaek, M., Johansen, D., & Sorensen, T. I. (2002). Lower risk for alcohol-induced cirrhosis in wine drinkers. *Hepatology, 35*, 868–875.

Blomgren, K. B., Sundstrom, A., Steineck, G., Genell, S., Sjostedt, S., & Wikohm, B. E. (2002). A Swedish case–control network for studies of drug-induced morbidity–acute pancreatitis. *Eur J Clin Pharmacol, 58*, 275–283.

Bor, S., Caymaz-Bor, C., Tobey, N. A., Abdulmour-Nakhoul, S., Marten, E., & Orlando, R. C. (1998). The effect of ethanol on the structure and function of rabbit esophageal epithelium. *Am J Physiol, 274*, G819–G826.

Bunout, D. (1999). Nutritional and metabolic effects of alcoholism: Their relationship with alcoholic liver disease. *Nutrition, 15*, 583–589.

Caetano, R., & Clark, C. L. (1998a). Trends in alcohol consumption patterns among Whites, Blacks and Hispanics: 1984–1995. *J Stud Alcohol, 59*, 659–668

Caetano, R., & Clark, C. L. (1998b). Trends in alcohol-related problems among Whites, Blacks, and Hispanics: 1984–1995. *Alcohol Clin Exp Res, 22*, 534–538.

Clarren, S. K., Randels, S. P., Sanderson, M., & Fineman, R. M. (2001). Screening for fetal alcohol syndrome in primary schools: A feasibility study. *Teratology, 63*, 3–10.

Cloninger, C. R. (1987). Neurogenetic adaptive mechanisms in alcoholism. *Science, 236*, 410–416.

Cravo, M. L., & Camilo, M. E. (2000). Hyperhomocysteinemia in chronic alcoholism: Relations to folic acid and vitamin B (6) and B (12) status. *Nutrition, 16*, 296–302.

Criqui, M. H. (1990). The reduction of coronary heart disease with light to moderate alcohol consumption: Effect or artifact. *Br J Addict, 85*, 854–857.

Dackis, C. A., & O'Brien, C. P. (2002). The neurobiology of alcoholism. In S. Gershon & R. Soires (Eds.), *Handbook of psychiatric disorders* (pp. 563–580). New York: Marcel Dekker.

Dansky, D. S., Brewerton, T. D., & Kilpatrick, D. G. (2000). Comorbidity of bulimia nervosa and alcohol use disorders: Results from the National Women's Study. *Int J Eat Disord, 27,* 180–190.

Davidson, D. M. (1989). Cardiovascular effects of alcohol. *West J Med, 151*(4), 430–439.

Drake, R. E., & Vaillant, G. E. (1985). A validity study of Axis II of DSM-III. *Am J Psychiatry, 142,* 553–558.

Dufour, M. C. (2001). If you drink alcoholic beverages do so in moderation: What does this mean? *J Nutr, 131,* 552–561.

Ellis, R. J., & Oscar-Berman, M. (1989). Alcoholism, aging, and functional cerebral asymmetries. *Psychol Bull, 106*(1), 128–147.

Evert, D. L., & Oscar-Berman, M. (1995). Alcohol-related cognitive impairments: An overview of how alcohol may effect the workings of the brain. *Alcohol Health Res World, 19*(2), 189–196.

Ewing, J. A. (1984). Detecting alcoholism: The CAGE questionnaire. *JAMA, 252*(14), 1905–1907.

Garcia-Andrade, C., Wall, T. L., & Ehlers, C. L. (1997). The firewater myth and response to alcohol in Mission Indians. *Am J Psychiatry, 154,* 983–988.

Gish, R. (1996, November 30). *Rational evaluation of liver dysfunction of the chemically dependent patient and diagnosis and treatment of hepatitis C.* Audiotape presentation at the 7th annual meeting and symposium of the American Academy of Addiction Psychiatry, San Francisco.

Goforth, H. W., Primeau, M., & Fernandez, F. (2003). Alcohol and HIV/AIDS. In B. Johnson, P. Ruiz, & M. Galanter (Eds.), *Handbook of clinical alcoholism treatment* (pp. 249–257). Baltimore: Lippincott/Williams & Wilkins.

Greenfield, L. A., & Henneberg, M. A. (2001). Victim and offender self-reports of alcohol involvement in crime. *Alcohol Res Health, 25,* 20–31.

Greenfield, S. F., Weiss, R. D., & Mirin, S. M. (1997). Psychiatric substance use disorder. In A. J. Gelenberg & E. L. Bassuk (Eds.), *The practitioner's guide to psychoactive substances* (pp. 243–316). New York: Plenum Press.

Greenfield, T. K. (2000). Ways of measuring drinking patterns and the difference they make: Experience with graduated frequencies. *J Subst Abuse, 12,* 33–49.

Group for the Advancement of Psychiatry. (1996). *Alcoholism in the United States: Racial and ethnic considerations* (Report No. 141, VII–X). Washington DC: American Psychiatric Press.

Gupta, M. A., Schork, N. J., Gupta, A. K., & Ellis, C. N. (1993). Alcohol intake and treatment responsiveness of psoriasis: A prospective study. *J Am Acad Dermatol, 5*(1), 730–732.

Hardin, R. I. (2001). Disorders of the platelet and vessel wall. In E. Braunwald, A. Fuuci, D. Kasper, S. Hauser, D. Longo, & J. Jameson (Eds.), *Harrison's principles of internal medicine* (15th ed., pp. 745–750). New York: McGraw-Hill.

Harwood, H. (2000). *Updating estimates of the economic costs of alcohol abuse in the United States: Estimates, update methods, and data* [Report prepared by the Lewin Group for the National Institute on Alcohol Abuse and Alcoholism]. Washington, DC: U.S. Department of Health & Human Services.

Hauge, T., Nilsson, A., Persson, J., & Hultberg, B. (1998). Gamma-glutamyl transferase, intestinal alkaline phosphatase and beta-hexoaminidase activity in duodenal biopsies of chronic alcoholics. *Hepatogastroenterology, 45,* 985–989.

Hays, J. T., Schroeder, D. R., Offord, K. P., Croghan, T. T., Patten, C. A., Hurt, R. D., et al. (1999). Response to nicotine dependence treatment in smokers with current and past alcohol problems. *Ann Behav Med, 21,* 244–250.

Helzer, J. E., & Pryzbeck, T. R. (1988). The co-occurrence of alcoholism with other psychiatric disorders in the general population and its impact on treatment. *J Stud Alcohol, 49*(3), 219–224.

Hermann, D., Heinz, A., & Mann, K. (2002). Dysregulation of the hypothalamice–pituitary–thyroid axis in alcoholism. *Addiction, 97*(11), 1369–1381.

Higgins, E. M., & du Vivier, A. W. P. (1992). Alcohol and the skin. *Alcohol, 27,* 595–602.

Howard, M. O., Kivlahan, D., & Walker, R. D. (1997). Cloninger's tri-dimensional theory of personality and psychopathology: Applications to substance use disorders. *J Stud Alcohol, 58,* 48–66.

Kessler, R. C., Crum, R. M., Warner, L. A., Nelson, C. B., Schulenberg J., & Anthony J. C. (1997). Lifetime co occurrence of DSM-III-R alcohol abuse and dependence with other psychiatric disorders in the National Comorbidity Survey. *Arch Gen Psychiatry, 54,* 313–321.

Kessler, R. C., McGonagle, K. A., Zhao, S., Nelson, C. B., Hughes, M., Eshleman, S., et al. (1994). Lifetime and 12 month prevalence of DSM-III-R psychiatric disorders in the United States. *Arch Gen Psychiatry, 51,* 8–19.

Klatsky, A. L., Friedman, G. D., & Armstrong, M. A. (1986). Relationships between alcoholic beverage use and other traits to blood pressure: A new Kaiser Permanente study. *Circulation, 73*(4),628–636.

Koenigsberg, H. W., Kaplan, R. D., Gilmore, M. M., & Cooper, A. M. (1985). The relationship between syndrome and personality disorder in DSM-III: Experience with 2,462 patients. *Am J Psychiatry, 142*(2), 207–212.

Laitinen, K., Karkkainen, M., Lalla, M., Lamberg-Allardt, C., Tunninen, R., Tahtela, R., & Volamaki, M. (1993). Is alcohol an osteoporosis-inducing agent for young and middle-aged women? *Metabolism, 42,* 875–881.

Latif, O., Peterson, J. D., & Waltenbaugh, C. (2002). Alcohol-mediated polarization of type I and type II immune responses. *Front Biosci, 7,* 135–147.

Lee, G. R. (1999). Folate deficiency: Causes and management. In G. R. Lee, J. Foerster, J. Lukens, F. Paraskeras, J. Greer, & G. Rodgers (Eds.), *Wintrole's clinical hematology* (10th ed., pp. 965–972). Baltimore: Williams & Wilkins.

Lee, W. K., & Regan, T. J. (2002). Alcoholic cardiomyopathy: Is it dose dependent? *Congest Heart Fail, 8*(6), 303–306, 312.

Lieber, C. S. (1998). Hepatic and other medical disorders of alcoholism: From pathogenesis to treatment. *J Stud Alcohol, 59*(1), 9–25.

Luczak, S. E., Wall, T. L., Shea, S. H., Byun, S. M., & Carr, L. G. (2001). Binge drinking in Chinese, Korea, and White college students: Genetic and ethnic group differences. *Psychol Addict Behav, 15,* 306–309.

May, P., & Gossage, J. (2001). The epidemiology of alcohol consumption among American Indians living on four reservations and in nearby border towns. *Drug Alcohol Depend, 63*(Suppl 1), S100.

McEvoy, J. P. (1982). The chronic neuropsychiatric disorders associated with alcohol. In E. M. Pattison & E. Kauknan (Eds.), *Encyclopedic handbook of alcoholism* (pp.167–179). New York: Gardner Press.

Midanik, L. T., Tam, T. W., Greenfield, T. K., & Caetano, R. (1996). Risk functions for alcohol-related problems in a 1988 US national sample. *Addiction, 91,* 1427–1437.

Nace, E. P. (1995). *Achievement and addiction: A guide to the treatment of professionals.* New York: Brunner/Mazel.

Nace, E. P., Davis, C., & Gaspari, J. D. (1991). Personality disorders in substance abusers. *Am J Psychiatry, 148,* 118–120.

Narrow, W. E., Rae, D. S., Robins, L. N., & Regier, D. A. (2002). Revised prevalence estimates of mental disorders in the United States: Using a clinical significance criteria to reconcile two surveys estimates. *Arch Gen Psychiatry, 59,* 115–123.

National Highway Traffic Safety Administration. (1999). An analysis of alcohol-related motor vehicle fatalities by ethnicity. *Annals Emerg Med, 34,* 550–553.

National Institute on Alcohol Abuse and Alcoholism. (1998). *Alcohol and tobacco* (Alcohol Alert No. 39). Rockville, MD: Author.

Ohmoris, S., Kiyohara, Y., Kato, I., Kubo, M., Tanzaki, Y., Iwamoto, H., et al. (2002). Alcohol intake and future incidents of hypertension in a general Japanese population: The Hisayoma study. *Alcohol Clin Exp Res, 26,* 1010–1016.

Olson, H. C., Feldman, J. J., Streissguth, A. P., Sampson, P. D., & Bookstein, F. L. (1998). Neuropsychological deficits in adolescents with fetal alcohol syndrome: Clinical findings. *Alcohol Clin Exp Res, 22,* 1998–2012.

Osher, F. C., & Kofoed, L. L. (1989). Treatment of patients with psychiatric and psychoactive substance abuse disorders. *Hosp Community Psychiatry, 40,* 1025–1030.

Petrakis, I. L., Gonzales, G., Rosenheck, R., & Krystal, J. H. (2002). Comorbidity of alcoholism and psychiatric disorders: An overview. *Alcohol Res Health, 26,* 81–89.

Pettinati, H. N. (2001). The use of selective serotonin reuptake inhibitors in treating alcoholic subtypes. *J Clin Psychiatry, 62*(Suppl 20), 26–31.

Randall, C. L., Thomas, S., & Thevos, A. K. (2001). Concurrent alcoholism and social anxiety disorder: A first step towards developing effective treatments. *Alcohol Clin Exp Res, 25,* 210–220.

Regan, R. J. (1990). Alcohol and the cardiovascular system. *JAMA, 264,* 377–381.

Regier, D. A., Farmer, M. E., Rae, D. S., Locke, B. Z., Keith, S. J., Judd, L. L., & Goodwin, K. K. (1990). Comorbidity of mental disorders with alcohol and other drug abuse. *JAMA, 264,* 2511–2518.

Regier, D. A., Narrow, W. E., Rae, D. S., Manderscheid, R. W., Lock, B. Z., & Goodwin, F. K. (1993). The defacto US mental and addictive disorder service system: Epidemiologic Catchment Area perspective one-year prevalence rates of disorders and services. *Arch Gen Psychiatry, 50,* 85–94.

Reynolds, K., Lewis, L. B., Nolen, J. D. L., Kinney, G. L., Sathya, B., & He, J. (2003). Alcohol consumption and risk of stroke: A meta-analysis. *JAMA, 289,* 579–588.

Russell, M., Martier, S. S., Sokol, R. J., Jacobson, S., Jacobson, J., & Bottoms, S. (1994). Screening for pregnancy risk-drinking: TWEAKING the tests. *Alcohol Clin Exp Res, 18*(5), 1156–1161.

Schiave, R. C., Stimmel, B. B., Mandeli, J., & White, D. (1995). Chronic alcoholism and male sexual function. *Am J Psychiatry, 152,* 1045–1051.

Schmidt, L. G., Schmidt, K., Dufeu, P., Ohse, A., Rommelspacher, H., & Muller, C. (2000). Superiority of carbohydrate-deficient transferrin to gamma-glutamyltransferase in detecting relapse in alcoholism. *Am J Psychiatry, 154*(1), 75–80.

Schuchardt, V. (2000). Alcohol and the peripheral nervous system. *Ther Umsch, 57*(4), 196–199.

Skinner, H. (1981). Early identification of alcohol abuse. *Can Med Assoc J, 124,* 1279–1295.

Smith, K. E., & Fenske, N. A. (2000). Cutaneous manifestations of alcohol abuse. *J Am Acad Dermatol, 43*(1), 1–25.

Sohn, T. A., Campbell, K. A., Pitt, H. A., Sauter, P. K., Coleman, J. A., Lillemo, K. D., Yeo, C. J., & Cameron, J. L. (2000). Quality of life and long-term survival after surgery for chronic pancreatitis. *J Gastrointest Surg, 4*(4), 355–364.

Spencer, R. L., & Hutchinson, K. E. (1999). Alcohol, aging and the stress response. *Alcohol Res Health, 23,* 272–283.

Stinson, F. S., Grant, B. F., & Dufour, M. C. (2001). The critical dimension of ethnicity in liver cirrhosis mortality statistics. *Alcohol Clin Exp Res, 25,* 1181–1187.

Stratton, K., Howe, C., & Battaglia, F. (Eds.). (1996). *Fetal alcohol syndrome: Diagnosis, epidemiology, prevention and treatment.* Washington, DC: National Academy Press.

Sutton, R., & Shields, R. (1995). Alcohol and esophageal varices. *Alcohol, 30*(5), 581–589.

Tabakoff, B., Hoffman, P. L., Lee, J. M., Saio, T., Willard, B., & Deleon-Jones, R. (1988). Differences in platelet enzyme activity. *N Engl J Med, 313,* 134–139.

Turner, R. T. (2000). Skeletal response to alcohol. *Alcohol Clin Exp Res, 24,* 1693–1701.

Vachon, C. M., Cerhan, J. R., Vierkant, R. A., & Sellers, T. A. (2001). Investigation of an interaction of alcohol intake and family history on breast cancer risk in the Minnesota Cancer Family Study. *Cancer, 92,* 240–248.

Victor, M. (1989). Alcohol and alcoholism. In R. D. Adams (Ed.), *Principles of neurology* (pp. 870–888). New York: McGraw-Hill.

Villalta, F., Ballesca, J. L., Nicholas, J. M., Martinez di Osaba, M. J., Antunez, E., & Pimentel, C. J. (1977). Testicles function in asymptomatic chronic alcoholics: Relation to ethanol intake. *Alcohol Clin Exp Res, 21*(1), 128–133.

Vitiello, M. V. (1997). Sleep, alcohol and alcohol abuse. *Addict Biol, 2,* 151–158.

Wedel, M., Pieters, J. E., Pikaar, N. A., & Ockhuizen, T. (1991). The application of a three-compartment model to a study of the effects of sex, alcohol dose and concentration, exercise, and food consumption on the pharmacokinetics of ethanol in healthy volunteers. *Alcohol, 26*(3), 329–336.

Westermeyer, J. (1986). *A clinical guide to alcohol and drug problems.* New York: Praeger.

Yanauchi, M., Takeda, K., Sakamoto, K., Searaski, Y., Vetake, S., Kenichi, H., & Toda, G. (2001). Association of polymorphism in the alcohol dehydrogenase 2 gene with alcohol-induced testicular atrophy. *Alcohol Clin Exp Res, 25*(Suppl 6), 165–185.

Zakari, S. (1997). Alcohol and the cardiovascular system: Molecular mechanisms for beneficial and harmful actions. *Alcohol Health Res World, 21,* 21–29.

CHAPTER 6

Tobacco

NORMAN HYMOWITZ

HISTORY AND OVERVIEW OF THE PROBLEM

Early Beginnings

The use of tobacco (*Nicotine tobaccum*) has been traced to early American civilizations, where it played a prominent role in religious rites and ceremonies. Among the ancient Maya, tobacco smoke was used as "solar incense" to bring rain during the dry season. Shooting stars were believed to be burning butts cast off by the rain god. The Aztecs employed tobacco (*Nicotine rustica*) as a power that was used in ceremonial rites as well as chewed as a euphoric agent with lime (Schultes, 1978).

In 1492, Columbus and his crew observed natives lighting rolls of dried leaves, which they called *tobacos* (cigars), and "swallowing" the smoke (Schultes, 1978). Twenty years later, Juan Ponce de Leon brought tobacco back to Portugal, where it soon was grown on Portuguese soil. Sir Walter Raleigh introduced smoking to England in 1565, and the English, too, successfully grew tobacco (Vogt, 1982). The growth of world trade led to the spread of tobacco to every corner of the globe.

The popular "weed" was not without its detractors. James I of England published a *counterblaste to tobacco* in 1604, and he arranged a public debate on the effects of tobacco in 1605. Pope Urban III condemned tobacco use in 1642, threatening excommunication of offenders. In Russia, a decree in 1634 punished tobacco users by nose slitting, castration, flogging, and banishment. These harsh measures were abolished by Peter the Great, who took to smoking a pipe in an effort to open a window to the West. It is believed that the smok-

105

ing of cigarettes first occurred in Mexico, where chopped tobacco was wrapped in corn husks (Van Lancker, 1977).

The 19th Century

The most popular forms of tobacco used in the United States in the past were chewing tobacco and dipping snuff, as evidenced by spittoons in homes and public places. In the late 1800s, cigarette smoking grew in popularity. James Buchanan Duke brought Polish and Russian Jews to the United States to manufacture cigarettes in 1867, and he used advertising to enlighten Americans about the pleasures of smoking. Cigarettes were first mass-produced in Durham, North Carolina, in 1884. Washington Duke used a newly invented cigarette machine to produce some 120,000 cigarettes per day, thus ushering in the era of cheap, abundant tobacco products for smoking, and setting the stage for 20th-century epidemics of lung cancer, emphysema, and coronary heart disease (Vogt, 1982).

The "Cigarette Century"

In 1900, the total consumption of cigarettes in the United States was 2.5 billion (U.S. Department of Health and Human Services, 1989b). Major advances in agriculture, manufacturing, and marketing, the Great Depression, two world wars, and changing cultural norms led to a marked increase in consumption. Total consumption increased from 2.5 billion in 1900 to 631.5 billion in 1980 (U.S. Department of Health and Human Services, 1989b). Cigarette consumption peaked in 1981 (640 billion) but declined in 1987 to an estimated 574 billion, the equivalent of more than 6 trillion doses of nicotine (Jones, 1987). An estimated 430 billion cigarettes were consumed in 2000 (U.S. Department of Agriculture, 2001).

Early Warning Signs

The decline in per capita cigarette consumption during the latter part of the 20th century was due in large part to growing concerns about the adverse health consequences of cigarette smoking and the growth of the anti-smoking movement. Early case reports and case studies called attention to the likely role of smoking and chewing tobacco as a cause of cancer (Samet, 2001). Key initial observations were made in epidemiological studies carried out to examine changing patterns of disease in the 20th century, particularly the dramatic rise in lung cancer, coronary heart disease, and chronic obstructive lung disease (Samet, 2001). Dr. Luther Terry, who served as Surgeon General of the U.S. Public Health Service from 1961 to 1965, noted that the landmark 1964 Surgeon General's Advisory Committee Report, *Smoking and Health*, was the culmination of growing scientific concern over a period of more than 25 years (Terry, 1983). The report also recognized the "habitual" nature of tobacco use but stopped short of recognizing tobacco use as an addiction.

The Leading Preventable Cause of Death

According to the Centers for Disease Control and Prevention (2002), tobacco causes approximately 440,000 deaths in the United States each year, making it the leading preventable cause of death. Cigarette smoking accounts for about 30% of all cancer deaths (87% of lung cancers) and is a major cause of heart disease, cerebrovascular disease, chronic bronchitis, and emphysema (American Cancer Society [ACS], 2003). Tobacco use costs the U.S. economy nearly $150 billion in health costs and lost productivity each year (American Lung Association [ALA], 2003). Smoking-related diseases cost the Medicare system $20.5 billion and Medicaid, the federal insurance program for the poor, $17 billion in 1997 (American Lung Association, 2003).

Nicotine Addiction

It was not until 1988 that the addictive nature of cigarette smoking was formally recognized. Major conclusions from the 1988 Surgeon General's report (U.S. Department of Health and Human Services, 1988) were as follows: (1) Cigarettes and other forms of tobacco are addicting; (2) nicotine is the drug in tobacco that causes addiction; and (3) the pharmacological and behavioral processes that determine tobacco addiction are similar to those that determine addiction to drugs such as heroin and cocaine.

The Anti-Smoking Movement

Key events that contributed to the decline in the per capita consumption of cigarettes in the United States were the banning of cigarette advertisements on the air waves, increases in the excise tax on cigarettes, and evidence that secondhand smoke harms nonsmokers. Mounting evidence of the dangers of environmental tobacco smoke (ETS; Environmental Protection Agency [EPA], 1992) served as a stimulus to advocate for smoke-free environments, and to support policies and legislation to protect young people and adults from secondhand smoke.

The EPA report officially categorized ETS as a known human carcinogen, placing ETS in the Class A (most dangerous) category reserved for only a few toxic substances, including radon, benzene, and asbestos (Carlson, 1997). The report also identified ETS as a cause of serious respiratory illness in children, including bronchitis, asthmatic episodes, new cases of asthma, and sudden infant death syndrome (SIDS). Nonsmokers exposed to ETS at work were 39% more likely to get lung cancer than nonexposed, nonsmoking workers (Carlson, 1997).

A Worldwide Problem

While tobacco consumption declined in the United States, global tobacco consumption increased, particularly in developing countries. According to the World Health Organization (WHO; 1999), cigarette smoking in developing countries increased at a rate of about 3.4% per year. Worldwide tobacco-related deaths are expected to increase from about 4 million per year in 1999 to about 10 million per year by the 2030s, with 70% of those deaths occurring in developing nations. This is a higher death toll than is expected from malaria, maternal and major childhood conditions, and tuberculosis combined (American Cancer Society, 2003).

Big Tobacco

In response to mounting health concerns and declining demand, Big Tobacco spared little expense to fend off criticism and to assuage public concern. Cigarette advertising expenditures in the United States were estimated at more than $2 billion for 1985—twice the annual expenditures of the National Cancer Institute (American Cancer Society, 1986). In 1999, the five largest cigarette manufacturers in the United States spent $8.24 billion on advertising and promotional expenditures (Federal Trade Commission, 2001), with additional expenditures for promoting and marketing cigarettes abroad.

Safe Cigarettes

Big Tobacco used its vast resources to keep alive debates about whether cigarette smoking is harmful or addictive, and whether secondhand smoke poses a danger to nonsmokers. Tobacco companies also responded to mounting health concerns by designing and marketing safer cigarettes. They introduced cigarette filters, menthol flavoring, light and ultralight brands, and, most recently, high technology cigarettes, such as Omni, Advance, Eclipse, Accord, Quest, and, soon to be released, the Phillip Morris product, SCOR. Innovations in manufacturing and design were heralded by expensive marketing campaigns, fostering the impression that new and improved cigarettes offered satisfaction, flavor, and peace of mind (Burns & Benowitz, 2001). Today, more than 80% of the cigarettes sold in the United States are of the low-tar and low-nicotine variety (Myers, 2002), and most smokers believe light and ultralight cigarettes are less harmful than regular cigarettes (Giovino et al., 1996).

Smokers are wrong about the safety of low-tar and low-nicotine cigarettes (Burns & Benowitz, 2001), and the new high-technology cigarettes similarly are likely to fall far short of the mark (Slade, Connolly, & Lymperis, 2002). A 20-year study by the American Cancer Society showed that smokers who smoked *light* and *ultralight* cigarettes experienced the same rates of lung cancer and heart disease as smokers who smoked regular cigarettes (Burns & Benowitz, 2001). This was due in part to compensatory smoking patterns by smokers seeking to regulate nicotine intake, the *elastic* nature of newly designed cigarettes that facilitate compensation, differences in machine-measured and biologically measured yields of tar and nicotine, and deceptive marketing and labeling practices (Kozlowski, O'Connor, & Sweeney, 2001).

The tactic of heralding new cigarette designs by sophisticated marketing campaigns proved equally effective with youthful smokers. R. J. Reynolds carried out a highly successful campaign in the 1980s and 1990s to promote the Camel brand among young people. The combination of a less harsh cigarette, *sweetened* to appeal to youthful tastes, and the *Smooth Moves* Joe Camel advertising campaign led to demonstrated share growth, moving progressively from 2.5% of the market in 1987, to 4.0% in 1988, to 4.4% in 1989, and to 6.1% in 1990 (Wayne & Connolly, 2002). Ultimately, Camel became one of the three leading brands, along with Marlboro and Newport, which today account for more than 80% of adolescent smoking.

The Challenge Ahead

By the end of the 20th century, the stage was set for a *life or death* struggle between *Big Tobacco* and the public health community over the fate of the next generation of smokers. Both parties are aware that most adults begin smoking as youth, and if people do not start smoking by their late teens, they are unlikely to smoke as adults (Lynch & Bonnie, 1994). *Big Tobacco* must recruit another generation of young people to stay in business, and the public health community must thwart its efforts.

While smoking rates in the United States have declined since the mid-1960s, much work remains. The United States failed to meet the *Healthy People 2000* goals for tobacco prevention and control, and smoking initiation rates among middle and high school students increased dramatically in the 1990s (Bonnie, 2001). In 1996, more than 1.8 million people became daily smokers in the United States, two-thirds of them (1.2 million) under age 18 (Bonnie, 2001). Rates of cigarette smoking and use of other forms of tobacco also increased among college students (18–21 years old), the youngest legal target for tobacco advertising dollars (Rigotti, Lee, & Wechsler, 2000). According to a recent survey, 46% of college students reported using tobacco products in the past year, and more than 25% of them started smoking for the first time while in college (Wechsler, Kelley, Seibring, Kuo, & Rigotti, 2001).

DEFINITIONS

Henningfield (1986) compared tobacco dependence to other forms of drug dependence and concluded that there are more similarities than differences. He noted that (1) tobacco dependence, like other forms of drug dependence, is a complex process, involving interactions between drug and nondrug factors; (2) tobacco dependence is an orderly and lawful process governed by the same factors that control other forms of drug self-administration; (3) tobacco use, like other forms of drug use, is sensitive to dose manipulation; (4) development of tolerance (diminished response to repeated doses of a drug or the requirement for increasing the dose to have the same effect) and physiological dependence (termination of nicotine followed by a syndrome of withdrawal phenomena) when nicotine is repeatedly administered is similar to the development of tolerance and dependence of other drugs of abuse; and (5) tobacco, like many other substances of abuse, produces effects often considered a utility or benefit to the user (e.g., relief of anxiety or stress, avoidance of weight gain, alteration in mood).

Although the similarities between tobacco or nicotine dependence and other forms of drug dependence are noteworthy, there are features of tobacco use that make it unique. In contrast to many other drugs of abuse, tobacco products are legal and readily available. When used as intended, tobacco products lead to disease and death. Unlike alcohol, a legal drug that can be consumed socially and in moderation without ill effects, all levels of tobacco use are harmful (U.S. Department of Health and Human Services, 1988).

Large sums of money are spent each year to advertise and market tobacco products, particularly cigarettes. This adds an important dimension to tobacco dependence not present to the same degree with other substances, with the possible exception of alcohol. Few children in our society grow up free of *Big Tobacco's* reach, which provides unique opportunities for the tobacco companies to teach them about the virtues of tobacco, the manner in which it should be used, and the role it should play in their daily lives. So pervasive is the positive imagery associated with cigarette smoking that it is almost impossible to distinguish between the reinforcing qualities of cigarettes that derive from past conditioning and learning and those that derive solely from nicotine.

DIAGNOSIS

According to the fourth edition of the *Diagnostic and Statistical Manual of Mental Disorders* (DSM-IV; American Psychiatric Association, 1994), nicotine dependence is considered to be a substance-related disorder. The key features of substance dependence are a cluster of cognitive, behavioral, and physiological symptoms indicating that the individual continues use of the substance despite significant substance-related problems. There is a pattern of repeated self-administration that usually results in tolerance, withdrawal, and compulsive drug-taking behavior (American Psychiatric Association, 2000).

The diagnosis of nicotine dependence in DSM-IV is fairly straightforward. Information needed to make the diagnosis can be obtained through interview and questionnaire, and can readily be collected along with other medical history data. Two National Institutes of Health publications (U.S. Department of Health and Human Services, 1986, 1989a), a report prepared by the American Psychiatric Association (1996), and a recently published clinical practice guideline (Fiore et al., 2000) are available to help physicians inquire about smoking, assess their patients' needs, and encourage patients to quit smoking.

Most of the criteria for psychoactive substance dependence are characteristic of cigarette smoking and other forms of tobacco use. Cigarette smokers often smoke more than they intend to, have difficulty quitting or simply cutting down, spend a great deal of time procuring cigarettes and smoking them, persist in smoking despite known risk and/or current illness, and readily develop tolerance, enabling them to smoke a larger number of cigarettes per day than they did when they first started smoking. The fact that most smokers who quit smoking in the past did so on their own, without formal treatment, seems to be somewhat at odds with the popular notion of addiction. However, it is important to note that most former heroin users also gave up heroin without formal treatment (Johnson, 1977).

When smokers, adolescents as well as adults, stop smoking, they may experience nicotine withdrawal as defined by DSM-IV-TR (American Psychiatric Association, 2000). About 50% of adults who attempt to stop smoking will meet DSM-IV criteria for nicotine dependence (American Psychiatric Association, 1996), and young smokers show signs of addiction within several months of taking up the habit (DiFranza et al., 2002). Diagnostic criteria for nicotine withdrawal are presented in DSM-IV-TR. Associated features include craving, a desire for sweets, and impaired performance on tasks requiring vigilance (American Psychiatric Association, 2000). Depression and difficulty sleeping are not uncommon. Associated laboratory findings include a slowing on electroencephalograph, decreases in catecholamine and cortisol levels, rapid eye movement (REM) changes, impairment on neuropsychological testing, and decreased metabolic rate (American Psychiatric Association, 2000). Nicotine withdrawal also may be associated with a dry or productive cough, decreased heart rate, increased appetite or weight gain, and a dampened orthostatic response (American Psychiatric Association, 2000).

When smokers quit smoking, there is a fairly high probability that they will return to smoking (relapse). Smokers often quit many times before they succeed in remaining abstinent. Relapse is most likely to occur soon after quitting. Studies of quit-smoking programs show that most smokers relapse within about 3 months (Hunt & Bespalec, 1974). Although ex-smokers are less likely to relapse after they have been abstinent for 3 months, the potential for relapse remains present for many years (Ockene, Hymowitz, Lagus, & Shaten, 1991).

CLINICAL FEATURES

Under normal circumstances, cigarette smoking and other forms of tobacco use do not cause obvious states of intoxication, nor does their chronic use lead to organic brain damage, although acute effects of nicotine may affect vigilance and memory (U.S. Department of Health and Human Services, 1988). Overdose typically is not a problem, and acute effects of nicotine on health have received less attention than chronic effects in the medical literature.

A number of poisonings and deaths from ingestion of nicotine, primarily involving nicotine-containing pesticides, have been reported, and acute intoxication has been observed in children after swallowing tobacco materials (U.S. Department of Health and Human Services, 1988). The lethal oral dose of nicotine in adults has been estimated at 40–60 mg (U.S. Department of Health and Human Services, 1988). Nicotine intoxication produces nausea, vomiting, abdominal pain, diarrhea, headaches, sweating, and pallor. More severe intoxication results in dizziness, weakness, and confusion, progressing to convulsions, hypotension, and coma. Death is usually due to paralysis of respiratory muscles and/or central respiratory control (U.S. Department of Health and Human Services, 1988).

As noted previously, the chronic effects of cigarette smoking take a massive toll. The role of cigarette smoking in the pathogenesis of coronary heart disease, lung and other cancers, and chronic obstructive lung disease, as well as many other forms of illness, has been dramatically documented in a series of reports by U.S. surgeons general dating back to 1964 (U.S. Public Health Service, 1964). Cigarette smoking has been cited as the chief avoidable cause of death and morbidity in our society, and the number one public health problem of our time (U.S. Department of Health and Human Services, 1989b).

The problems of cigarette smoking and tobacco-related diseases are not limited to the United States. Worldwide, approximately 1.1 billion people ages 15 and older smoke; 300 million live in developed countries, and 800 million in developing countries. About one-third of the world's adults smoke. Four million people die yearly from tobacco-related disease, one death every 8 seconds. If current trends continue, the toll will rise to 10 million by 2030, one death every 3 seconds (World Health Organization, 1999).

The acute effects of nicotine also are important, having been implicated in sudden heart attack death and stroke (Black, 1990). Cigarette smoking and other forms of tobacco use are contraindicated in patients with heart disease, hypertension, diabetes, chronic obstructive lung disease, and diseases of the gastrointestinal tract, for fear that nicotine and other components of tobacco will exacerbate existing illness as well as contribute to progressive pathogenesis, according to the U.S. Department of Health, Education, and Welfare (DHEW; 1979). Direct effects of nicotine on heart rate, cerebral blood flow, blood pressure, platelet aggregation, and fibrinogen are just a few of the mechanisms by which nicotine and cigarette smoking exert acute influences on health and well-being (Black, 1990).

Evidence of the harmful effects of cigarette smoking also may be observed in smokers in whom frank disease has not yet developed. Shortness of breath, cough, excessive phlegm, and nasal catarrh are common symptoms that readily subside when smokers stop smoking (U.S. Department of Health, Education, and Welfare, 1979). Smokers often report a dulling of the senses of taste and smell, and smokers, as well as their family members, generally experience more colds and illness than nonsmokers (U.S. Department of Health, Education, and Welfare, 1979). Tobacco smoke and products may interact with other drugs that patients are taking (Pharmacists' "Helping Smokers Quit" Program, 1986). Drugs that show the most significant interactions with tobacco smoke include oral contraceptives, theophylline, propranolol, and other antianginal drugs. Drugs with moderately significant clinical interactions with smoking include propoxyphene, pentazocine, phenylbutazone, phenothiazine, tricyclic antidepressants, benzodiazepines, amobarbital, heparin, furosemide, and vitamins (Pharmacists' "Helping Smokers Quit" Program, 1986).

Bansil, Hymowitz, and Keller (1989) showed that outpatients with schizophrenia who smoked cigarettes required significantly more neuroleptic medication to control psychiatric symptoms than comparable nonsmokers, despite the fact that the patients were identical with respect to initial severity of illness. Multivariate analyses showed that the difference between the groups was not due to age, weight, sex, alcohol consumption, or tea–coffee intake. In view of the side-effects profile of many drugs used in psychiatry, and the fact that the prevalence of tardive dyskinesia may be higher in mentally ill patients who smoke than in patients who do not smoke (Yassa, Lal, Korpassy, & Ally, 1987), it is important to achieve clinical effectiveness with as low a dose as possible. Cigarette smoking compromises this important goal.

Cigarette smoking, other forms of tobacco use, and ETS adversely affect the health and vitality of the young (American Academy of Pediatrics, 2001). Smoking by pregnant women may lead to low birthweight, preterm delivery, birth defects, and death of the fetus, and exposure to ETS following birth increases the risk of SIDS, respiratory distress, ear infections, and asthma (American Academy of Pediatrics, 2001). The initiation of cigarette smoking predisposes youth to a lifetime of addiction and tobacco-related disease (Samet, 2001).

The evidence clearly indicates that smokers benefit in many ways when they stop smoking (U.S. Department of Health and Human Services, 1990). Carbon monoxide is eliminated from their systems within 24 hours, and within a few months, ex-smokers report a lessening of pulmonary symptoms, such as shortness of breath, cough, phlegm, and nasal catarrh. Their senses of taste and smell return, peripheral vascular circulation improves, and ex-smokers may experience an improvement in small-airway disease and a slowing in the rate of decline of pulmonary function. Most important, risk of serious disease and premature death declines markedly over the course of several years following smoking cessation, and in people already disabled by frank disease, prospects for recovery improve greatly (U.S. Department of Health, Education, and Welfare, 1979).

COURSE

Cigarette smoking starts at an early age, usually in response to peer pressure and/or curiosity (Lynch & Bonnie, 1994). The younger the age of initiation, the greater the risk of habitual smoking (Burt, Dinh, Peterson, & Sarason, 2000). Social and environmental factors, personal characteristics, expectations of personal effects of smoking, and biological factors influence the initiation of smoking (U.S. Department of Health and Human Services, 2001). A sizable proportion (one-third or more) of children as young as 9 years old have engaged in experimental "puffing," and there is a steady rise with age in the proportion of children who report smoking (Oei & Fea, 1987). Among American children age 13 years and older, only about one-third of those surveyed had not at least puffed a cigarette (Chassin et al., 1981).

The rate of progression from experimentation to established smoking is about 32% (Choi, Ahluwalia, Harris, & Okuyemi, 2002). Receptivity to tobacco advertisements and promotions (Sargent et al., 2000), the belief that "I can quit smoking whenever I want" (Choi et al., 2002), and a propensity to risk taking and rebelliousness (Burt et al., 2000) are among a host of variables that distinguish between youth who progress to established smoking and those who do not. Other risk factors for youth progressing to regular smoking include relatively low grades in school, low behavioral self-control, high susceptibility to peer influence, and the belief that they would not be in trouble if their parents knew they were smoking (Jackson, Henricksen, Dickinson, Messer, & Robertson, 1998).

By age 14 or 15, cigarette smoking is an established pattern, and little experimentation takes place thereafter (Aitken, 1980). Approximately 60% of high school smokers report that they tried to stop smoking in the past year (Centers for Disease Control and Prevention, 2001). Unfortunately, they suffer failure and relapse rates that exceed those of adults (Ershler, Leventhal, Fleming, & Glynn, 1989). Most adolescent smokers will smoke well into adulthood before they are able to quit (Pierce & Gilpin, 1996).

Substance use, in general, increases between adolescence and young adulthood, then declines in the mid-20s. Individuals may discontinue substance use in adulthood, because the responsibilities and demands of marital, occupational, and parental roles are incompatible with substance use (Yamaguchi & Kandel, 1985). Chassin, Presson, Rose, and Sherman (1996) reported that age-related trends for cigarette smoking paralleled those for other drugs in showing a significant increase between adolescence and young adulthood. However, unlike other forms of drug use, there was no significant decline in cigarette smoking in the late 20s. The persistence of cigarette smoking into the late 20s (and beyond) may be due to three factors: (1) Nicotine dependence may contribute to low cessation rates; (2) the negative health impact of cigarette smoking may not be encountered until later ages; and (3) because smoking is a legal behavior whose pharmacological effects are not incompatible with the day-to-day demands of adult roles, role socialization pressure for cessation may be less intense (Chassin et al., 1996).

Although psychosocial factors play a major role in smoking onset and progression to established smoking in adolescence, addiction to nicotine also is of paramount importance. Recent studies (DiFranza et al., 2002) suggest that children show signs of nicotine dependence within a matter of months of exposure, far quicker than heretofore imagined. Like adults, young people have difficulty stopping smoking (Burt & Peterson, 1998; Green, 1980). The reasons for this difficulty—social pressure, urges, and withdrawal symptoms—implicate behavioral factors and dependence on tobacco (Biglan & Lichtenstein, 1984). Hansen (1983) studied abstinence and relapse in high-school-age smokers (16–18 years old) who smoked an average of 15–20 cigarettes per day. Most students who quit smoking relapsed within 3 months. Variables that predicted relapse were the number of cigarettes smoked per day and the regularity of a teenager's smoking pattern—findings indicative of tobacco dependence.

The early initiation of smoking is of considerable concern to the public health community. The pathogenesis of diseases such as chronic obstructive lung disease and atherosclerotic heart disease begins early in life, and duration of exposure to tobacco contributes to the likelihood of suffering adverse consequences as an adult (U.S. Department of Health, Education, and Welfare, 1979). However, it is not necessary to wait until adulthood to see signs of impaired health. Seely, Zuskin, and Bouhuys (1971) reported that cough, phlegm, and shortness of breath were more common among high school students who smoked than among nonsmokers, with no significant differences between sexes. Pulmonary function testing showed that maximum ventilation (V_{max}) at both 50% and 25% vital capacity (midmaximal flow rates, respectively) were significantly below expected levels in boys who smoked more than 15 cigarettes per day and in girls who smoked more than 10 cigarettes per day (Seely et al., 1971). The authors concluded that regular smoking for 1–5 years is sufficient to cause demonstrable decreases in lung function (see also U.S. Department of Health and Human Services, 1994a).

After high school, there is a gradual transition to regular adult smoking levels, and the relative influence of dependence on nicotine increases (Sachs, 1986). For most, smoking rates will hover around one pack per day and remain quite stable for most of their adult lives. Others will progress to higher smoking rates, again revealing marked day-to-day stability in nicotine ingestion.

Tobacco dependence shows many features of a chronic disease (Fiore et al., 2000). Although a minority of tobacco users achieves permanent abstinence in an initial quit attempt, the majority persists in tobacco use for many years and typically cycle through multiple periods of relapse and remission. More than 70% of the 50 million smokers in the United States in 2000 had made at least one prior quit attempt, and approximately 46% try to quit each year (Fiore et al., 2000). About 2% per year succeed (U.S. Department of Health and Human Services, 1989b), with most making a number of attempts before succeeding. Nearly half of all living adults who ever smoked have quit (U.S. Department of Health and Human Services, 1989b), and most did so "on their own" (Schachter, 1982).

DIFFERENTIAL DIAGNOSIS

The diagnosis of nicotine dependence is relatively straightforward, particularly in adults. Most adults admit that they smoke cigarettes, and they typically smoke on a daily basis. For adolescents and teens, smoking may not occur on a daily basis. The physician should ask them if they ever smoked and how frequently they smoke. If they do not smoke, or smoke only on occasion, the physician should inquire about expectations for smoking in the future. Older teens, of course, are more likely to report that they smoke on a daily basis, although the number of cigarettes smoked per day may be fewer than those smoked by adults.

The clinician often wishes to determine the severity of tobacco dependence, because such information provides insight into how difficult it will be for the smoker to quit and what kind of quitting strategy will be most effective. Fagerstrom (1978) developed a brief nicotine dependence questionnaire. Among the most discriminating questions are the following: "How soon after you wake up do you smoke your first cigarette?", "How many cigarettes a day do you smoke?", and "Have you stopped smoking or tried to stop smoking in the past?" (Kozlowski et al., 1989).

Heavy smokers, those who smoke soon after waking, and those who have never quit smoking in the past are least likely to quit smoking on their own or with assistance (cf. Hymowitz et al., 1997). They are the smokers who are most likely to benefit from nicotine replacement therapy (NRT) and other pharmacological aids (Fagerstrom, 1988). Smokers with psychiatric illness such as schizophrenia, alcoholism, and depression also have an extremely difficult time quitting smoking (Glassman, 1993; American Psychiatric Association, 1996), and for smokers who succeed in quitting, negative affect and stress play a major role in smoking relapse (Shiffman, 1986).

ETHNICITY

Youth Smoking Rates

Findings from the Year 2000 National Youth Tobacco Survey indicate that current tobacco use ranges from 15.1% among middle school students (17.6%, male; 12.7%, female) to 34.5% among high school students (39.1% male; 29.8%, female; Centers for Disease Control and Prevention, 2001). Cigarette smoking is the most prevalent form of tobacco use, followed by cigar smoking and smokeless tobacco use.

Approximately one-half of current cigarette smokers in middle school and high school reported that they smoked Marlboro cigarettes. Black students were most likely to smoke Newport (Centers for Disease Control and Prevention, 2001). White (14.3%), black (17.5%), and Hispanic (16.0%) middle school students were significantly more likely than Asian (7.5%) middle school students to use any tobacco products. Among current users, cigarettes were the most prevalent form of tobacco used (11.0% of students). White (10.8%), black (11.2%), and Hispanic (11.4%) middle school students were significantly more likely than Asian (5.3%) middle school students to smoke cigarettes. There was little difference in rates of cigarette smoking for male (11.7%) and female (10.2%) students (Centers for Disease Control and Prevention, 2001).

Nationally, 34.5% of high school students were current users of any tobacco product. White students (38.0%) were significantly more likely than black (26.5%), Hispanic (28.4%), or Asian (22.9%) students to use tobacco products (Centers for Disease Control and Prevention, 2001). Cigarettes were the most prevalent form of tobacco (28.0%), with white students (31.8%) significantly more likely than blacks (16.8%), Hispanics (22.6%), or Asians (20.6%) to smoke cigarettes. Male (28.8%) and female (27.3%) high school students smoked about the same number of cigarettes per day (Centers for Disease Control and Prevention, 2001).

Adult Smoking Rates

In 2000, an estimated 46.5 million adults (23.3%) were current smokers (Centers for Disease Control and Prevention, 2002). The prevalence of smoking was higher among men (25.7%) than among women (21.0%). Among racial/ethnic groups, Asians (14.4%) and Hispanics (18.6%) had the lowest prevalence of adult cigarette use. Native Americans/Alaska Natives had the highest prevalence (36.0%). The smoking rates for whites and blacks were 24.1% and 23.2%, respectively, and the rates of smoking among adult men and women were similar (white: 25.9% and 22.4%, respectively; black: 26.1% and 20.9%, respectively). For Hispanics and Asians, adult men smoked at considerably higher rates than adult women (24.0%, Hispanic men; 13.3%, Hispanic women; 21.0%, Asian men; 7.6%, Asian women). For Native Americans/Alaska Natives, the opposite relationship held (29.1%, men; 42.5%, women; Centers for Disease Control and Prevention, 2002).

Adults who had earned a General Educational Development (GED) diploma had the highest prevalence of smoking (47.2%). Persons with master's, professional, and doctoral degrees had the lowest prevalence (8.4%). The prevalence of current smoking was higher among adults living below the poverty level (31.7%) than those at or above the poverty level (22.9%) (CDC, 2002).

In 2000, an estimated 44.3 million adults (22.2%) were former smokers, representing 24 million men and 19.7 million women (Centers for Disease Control and Prevention, 2002). Among smokers, 70.0% reported that they wanted to quit smoking completely; an estimated 15.7 million (41.0%) had stopped smoking for one or more days during the preceding months because they were trying to quit; and 4.7% of smokers who had smoked every day or some days during the preceding year quit and maintained abstinence for 3–12 months in 2000. The percentage of ever smokers who had quit varied sharply by demographic group. By race/ethnicity, the percentage of persons who had ever smoked and had quit was highest for whites (51.0%) and lowest for non-Hispanic blacks (37.3%; Centers for Disease Control and Prevention, 2002).

Although blacks have not quit smoking at the same rate as the general population (cf. Fiore, Novotny, Pierce, et al., 1990), data from large smoking intervention studies (e.g., Multiple Risk Factor Intervention Trial [MRFIT]; Hymowitz, Sexton, Ockene, & Grandits, 1991; Community Intervention Trial for Smoking Cessation [COMMIT]; Hymowitz et al., 1995) revealed comparable quit rates for blacks and whites. Variables that emerged as significant predictors of smoking cessation in these studies were older age, higher income, less frequent alcohol intake, lower levels of daily cigarette consumption, longer time to first cigarette in the morning, initiation of smoking after age 20, more than one previous quit attempt, a strong desire to stop smoking, absence of other smokers in the household, and male gender.

PHARMACOLOGY

Nicotine is a tertiary amine composed of a pyridine and a pyrolidine ring (DHHS, 1988). Absorption of nicotine across biological membranes depends on pH. Modern cigarettes produce smoke that is suitably flavored and sufficiently nonirritating to be inhaled deeply into lung alveoli (Jones, 1987). When tobacco smoke reaches the small airways and alveoli of the lung, the nicotine is readily absorbed. The rapid absorption of nicotine from cigarette smoke in the lung occurs because of the huge surface area of the alveoli and small airways, and because of the dissolution of nicotine at physiological pH, which facilitates transfer across cell membranes. Concentrations of nicotine in blood rise quickly during cigarette smoking and peak at its completion (U.S. Department of Health and Human Services, 1988).

Chewing tobacco, snuff, and nicotine polacrilex gum have an alkaline pH as a result of tobacco selection and/or buffering with additives by the manufacturer. The alkaline pH facilitates absorption of nicotine through mucous membranes. The rate of nicotine absorption from smokeless tobacco depends on the product and the route of administration. With fine-ground nasal snuff, blood levels of nicotine rise almost as fast as after cigarette smoking. The rate of nicotine absorption with the use of oral snuff, chewing tobacco, and nicotine polacrilex gum is more gradual (U.S. Department of Health and Human Services, 1988). Transdermal nicotine provides a stable source of nicotine, while new products, such as the nicotine nasal spray and inhaler, deliver a quicker bolus of nicotine to the brain that more closely matches what happens when a cigarette is inhaled. Swallowed nicotine is poorly absorbed because of the high acidity of the gut.

Nicotine inhaled in tobacco smoke enters the blood very rapidly, with uptake into the brain occurring within 1–2 minutes. After smoking, the action of nicotine on the brain occurs very quickly. The rapid onset of effects after a puff is believed to provide optimal reinforcement for the development of drug dependence (U.S. Department of Health and Human Services, 1988). The effects of nicotine decline after it is distributed to other tissues. The distribution half-life, which describes the movement of nicotine from the blood and rapidly perfused tissues to other body tissues, is approximately 9 minutes (U.S. Department of Health and Human Services, 1988).

After absorption into the blood, which is at pH 7.4, about 69% of the nicotine is ionized and 31% is nonionized. Binding to plasma protein is less than 5%. The drug is distributed to body tissues with a steady-state volume of distribution averaging 180 liters. Spleen, liver, lungs, and brain have a high affinity for nicotine, whereas the affinity of adipose tissue is very low (U.S. Department of Health and Human Services, 1988). Nicotine-binding sites or receptors in the brain have been identified and differentiated as very-high-affinity, high-affinity, and low-affinity types (U.S. Department of Health and Human Services, 1988). The most intense localization of labeled nicotine has been found in the interpeduncular nucleus and medial habenula.

Nicotine is extensively metabolized, primarily in the liver, but also to a small extent in the lung. Renal excretion of unchanged nicotine depends on urinary pH and urine flow, and may range from 2 to 35% but typically accounts for 5–10% of elimination (U.S. Department of Health and Human Services, 1988).

The relationship between the dose of nicotine and the resulting response (dose–response relationship) is complex and varies with the specific response that is measured. Nicotine is commonly thought of as an example of a drug that in low doses causes ganglionic stimulation and in high doses causes ganglionic blockade (U.S. Department of Health and Human Services, 1988). At very low doses, similar to those seen during cigarette smoking, cardiovascular effects appear to be mediated by the central nervous system, either through activation of chemoreceptor afferent pathways or by direct effects on the brainstem. The net result is sympathetic neural discharge, with an increase in blood pressure and heart rate. At higher doses, nicotine may act directly on the peripheral nervous system, producing ganglionic stimulation and the release of adrenal catecholamine. With high doses or rapid administration, nicotine produces hypotension and slowing of heart rate, mediated by either peripheral vagal activation or direct central depressor effects (U.S. Department of Health and Human Services, 1988).

Humans and other species readily develop tolerance of the effects of nicotine. Studies of tolerance to nicotine on *in vitro* tissue preparations may be summarized as follows: (1) With repeated dosing, responses diminish to nearly negligible levels; (2) after tolerance occurs, responsiveness can be restored by increasing the size of the dose; and (3) after a few hours without nicotine, responsiveness is partially or fully restored (U.S. Department of Health and Human Services, 1988). It is apparent that cigarette smokers reveal evidence for both acute tolerance (tachyphylaxis) and chronic tolerance to nicotine. This is consistent with the fact that smokers increase their tobacco consumption and intake of nicotine with experience (chronic tolerance). When smokers abstain for a while, the first few cigarettes they smoke produce a variety of bodily symptoms. Thereafter, they quickly become less sensitive (acute tolerance). Tolerance may be related to an increase in central nicotine-binding sites or to a decrease in the sensitivity of the sites (U.S. Department of Health and Human Services, 1988).

ACTIONS OF NICOTINE ON THE BRAIN

The nicotine molecule is shaped like acetycholine (Benowitz, 2001). Nicotine activates certain cholinergic receptors in the brain that would ordinarily be activated by acetylcholine. By activating cholinergic receptors, nicotine enhances the release of neurotransmitters and hormones, including acetylcholine, norepinephrine, dopamine, vasopressin, serotonin, and beta-endorphin. The cholinergic activation leads to behavioral arousal and sympathetic neural activation. The release of specific neurotransmitters has been specifically linked to particular reinforcing effects of nicotine. Enhanced release of dopamine, norepinephrine, and serotonin may be associated with pleasure, mood elavation, and appetite suppression. Release of acetycholine may be associated with improved performance on behavioral tasks and improvement of memory, and the release of beta-endorphin may be associated with the reduction of anxiety and tension (Benowitz, 2001).

CLINICAL PRACTICE GUIDELINES

Physicians have a unique role to play in the anti-smoking arena (Sullivan, 1991). Past reviews (Orleans, 1993), monographs (U.S. Department of Health and Human Services, 1994b), and guidelines (American Psychiatric Association, 1996) underscore the importance of physician intervention on smoking in a variety of medical settings. The Public Health Service–sponsored Clinical Practice Guideline, *Treating Tobacco Use and Dependence* (Fiore et al., 2000), provides clinical and systems interventions that are intended to increase the likelihood of successful quitting. The major findings and recommendations may be summarized as follows:

1. Tobacco dependence is a chronic condition that often requires repeated intervention. However, existent effective treatments can produce long-term or even permanent abstinence.

2. Because effective tobacco dependence treatments are available, every patient who uses tobacco should be offered at least one of these treatments:

- Patients *willing* to try to quit tobacco should be provided treatments identified as effective.
- Patients *unwilling* to try to quit tobacco use should be provided a brief intervention designed to increase their motivation to quit.

3. It is essential that clinicians and health care delivery systems institutionalize the consistent identification, documentation, and treatment of every tobacco user seen in a health care setting.

4. Brief tobacco treatment is effective, and every patient who uses tobacco should be offered at least brief treatment.

5. There is a strong dose–response relation between the intensity of tobacco counseling and its effectiveness. Treatments involving person-to-person contact (via individual, group, or proactive telephone counseling) are consistently effective, and their effectiveness increases with treatment intensity (e.g., minutes of contact).

6. Three types of counseling and behavioral therapies were found to be especially effective and should be used with all patients attempting tobacco cessation:

- Provision of practical counseling (problem-solving/skills training).
- Provision of social support as part of treatment (intratreatment social support).
- Help in securing social support outside of treatment (extratreatment social support).

7. Numerous effective pharmacotherapies for smoking cessation now exist. Except in the presence of contraindications, these should be used with all patients attempting to quit smoking.

Five *first-line* pharmacotherapies were identified that reliably increase long-term smoking abstinence rates: bupropion SR (slow release), nicotine gum, nicotine inhaler, nicotine nasal spray, and nicotine patch. The guidelines also concluded that combining the nicotine patch (a passive form of dosing that produces relatively stable levels of drug in the body) with a self-administered form of nicotine replacement (nicotine gum or nasal spray) is more efficacious than a single form of NRT.

Two *second-line* pharmacotherapies were identified as efficacious and may be considered by clinicians if first-line pharmacotherpies are not effective: clonidine and nortriptyline.

PREVENTION OF SMOKING

The prevention of tobacco use in children and adolescents requires a multi-pronged approach that targets the social environment, as well as individual behaviors (Bonnie, 2001; Lantz et al., 2000; Lynch & Bonnie, 1994; U.S. Department of Health and Human Services, 1994a). Individual behavior change strategies include school-based prevention programs, computer-based systems, and peer-based interventions (Lantz et al., 2000). Pediatricians and other health professionals also have an important role to play in preventing smoking initiation (Hymowitz, Schwab, & Eckholdt, 2001). Sussman, Lichtman, Ritt, and Pallonen (1999) reported that average reductions in smoking onset among youth generated by school-based prevention programs was about 6%, with a range of 0 to 11%. Programs that focused on teaching young people *resistance* skills to deal with social and other influences to smoke were most successful and had a longer lasting impact (Lantz et al., 2000). At the environmental level, mass media campaigns and policies aimed at restricting access to cigarettes, increasing the price of cigarettes, restricting cigarette advertising, and creating smoke-free facilities decrease smoking initiation in young people (Lantz et al., 2000).

Community interventions target multiple systems, institutions, or channels simultaneously to influence individual behaviors and community norms.

The results of a small number of controlled trials of community intervention attest to their ability to have a positive effect on youth smoking behavior. The effectiveness of school-based interventions is enhanced when they are included in a broad-based community effort, and the impact of community interventions may be enhanced if they are combined with strong advocacy, taxation, media, and policy interventions (Lantz et al., 2000).

PSYCHOPHARMACOTHERAPY

General Considerations

There are numerous approaches to smoking cessation and many comprehensive reviews of the literature (e.g., Hymowitz, 1999; Lando, 1993; Leventhal & Cleary, 1980; Schwartz, 1987). Although many approaches to smoking cessation have been successful in the short run, few, if any, have proved satisfactory in the long term. This is true for traditional group and individual counseling programs, hypnosis and acupuncture, self-help stop-smoking strategies, multi-component behavioral interventions, and pharmacological therapies (Hunt & Bespalec, 1974; Hymowitz, 1999; Yudkin et al., 2003). The tendency of smokers to quit, relapse, and quit highlights the cyclic nature of the quitting process and serves as a reminder that as much care and effort must go into helping smokers remain cigarette-free as into helping them stop smoking in the first place.

Youth Smoking Cessation

Efforts to help adolescents quit smoking have received relatively little attention. Studies suggest that teenagers who smoke on a daily basis; who were unable to quit in the past for an extended period of time; who have parents who smoke, particularly mothers, and a number of friends who smoke; who do poorly in school and score high on a depression scale are least likely to quit smoking (Burt & Peterson, 1998; Zhu, Sun, Billings, Choi, & Malarcher, 1999). The more risk factors, the less likely adolescents are to quit (Zhu et al., 1999).

Reviews of quit-smoking programs for adolescents painted a bleak picture (Burton, 1994; Digiusto, 1994; Sussman, et al., 1999). Retention and recruitment of students were problematic, and end-of-group quit rates were modest. Many studies failed to use appropriate control groups, objective measures of smoking status, and long-term follow-up of graduates (Sussman et al., 1999). Teenage focus groups have provided insight into the nature of smoking cessation programs that appeal to youth (Balch, 1998). Some suggestions were to (1) highlight the seriousness of quitting smoking before becoming an adult; (2) include mood control and stress management; (3) help teen smokers deal with smoking peers; (4) avoid lecturing, preaching, or nagging; and (5) ensure confidentiality from parents.

Sussman, Dent, and Lichtman (2000) designed an innovative school quit-smoking program that featured interactive activities, such as "games" and "talk shows," alternative medicine techniques (i.e., yoga, relaxation, and meditation), and behavioral strategies for smoking cessation. Two hundred and fifty-nine students enrolled in the program at 12 schools and another 76 students served as "standard care" controls (smoking status surveyed at baseline and at 3 months). Objective measures of cigarette smoking were used. Elective class credit and class release time were offered for participation in the program.

Only 54% of the students (n = 141) completed the program, and only 14% of them were abstinent for 30 days at the end of group. Comparable outcome data for controls were not obtained, nor was the end-of-group quit rate based on an *intent-to-treat* analysis (students who did not complete the group were not included in the immediate outcome data).

A total of 128 (49%) of the clinic enrollees were contacted at 3 months, including 40 (42%) of the clinic dropouts (those who did not complete four sessions). Forty-four (58%) standard care controls were successfully contacted. The 30-day quit rate (no smoking in the past 30 days) for students who completed the program was 30%, compared to 16% for students assigned to the standard care condition. This difference was statistically significant. An *intent-to-treat* analysis, which assumed that students who were not contacted at follow-up still were smoking, yielded more modest, although still significantly different, quit rates of 17% and 8% for the program and control conditions, respectively.

Hurt and colleagues (2000) studied the effects of nicotine replacement patch therapy plus minimal behavioral intervention on smoking cessation in adolescents who expressed a desire to stop smoking. Out of 101 adolescents, 71 completed the entire 6 weeks of patch therapy. Biochemical tests confirmed that 7-day point-prevalence smoking abstinence rates were 10.9% at 6 weeks (end of patch therapy), 5% at 12-week follow-up, and 5% at 6-month follow-up. These outcomes are much poorer than those obtained for adults in similar studies.

Adult Smoking Cessation

Nonpharmacological Approaches

Of the many nonpharmacological approaches to smoking cessation, here, behavioral approaches are the most germane. They have undergone the most extensive experimental study, are suitable for office and clinic-based physician interventions, and often are used in combination with pharmacological approaches to smoking cessation (Fagerstrom, 1988; Hymowitz, 1999). Multi-component behavioral programs, whether in group, individual, or "self-help" formats, typically include a number of strategies (self-monitoring, stimulus–control procedures, behavioral contracting, alternative behaviors, aversive conditioning, relaxation training, diet and exercise, self-management skill training for relapse prevention, etc.) to motivate smokers, to help them gain control over smoking, and to eliminate smoking systematically from their behavioral repertoire. Once smokers stop smoking, many of the very same behavioral skills that helped them quit smoking are used to help them prevent relapse. Schwartz (1987) reported that 1-year quit rates for multicomponent behavioral group quit-smoking programs average 40%. Initial end-of-treatment quit rates may be considerably higher.

The MRFIT employed diversified behavioral strategies for initial smoking cessation and long-term smoking abstinence (Hughes, Hymowitz, Ockene, Simon, & Vogt, 1981). The reported quit rates for special intervention (SI) men were 43.1% at year 1 and 50% at year 6. These quit rates were significantly superior to those for usual care (UC) participants (13% and 29% at years 1 and 6, respectively). When serum thiocyanate, a breakdown product of hydrogen cyanide, was used as an objective measure of smoking, the quit rate at year 6 for SI participants was reduced to 46% (Hymowitz, 1987).

The Lung Health Study, like the MRFIT, was a large-scale, multicenter, multiyear study in which smokers were exposed to comprehensive behavioral interventions for initial cessation and long-term follow-up (Anthonisen et al., 1994). In addition, SI participants in the Lung Health Study received NRT (nicotine gum, 2 mg). Five-year cross-sectional quit rates, confirmed by expired air carbon monoxide and cotinine, were close to 40% for SI and 20% for UC participants, a highly significant difference.

The MRFIT and the Lung Health Study generated excellent long-term smoking cessation results. Each study featured a multicomponent treatment *package* for initial smoking cessation, behavioral strategies for active relapse prevention, and comprehensive and sustained approaches to long-term abstinence. While few programs have the resources necessary to provide comparable sustained intervention and follow-up, it is important to incorporate strategies to help successful quitters remain abstinent. Booster sessions, reunions, telephone contact, hot lines, mailings, and the Internet have been tried with varying degrees of success (Hymowitz, 1999).

Nicotine Replacement Therapy

Pharmacotherapies include several forms of NRT and several antidepressants, among which only bupropion SR has been sponsored and approved by the U.S. Food and Drug Administration (FDA; Sweeney, Fant, Fagerstrom, McGovern,

& Henningfield, 2001). Four NRT medications have been approved by the FDA (gum, transdermal patch, nasal spray, and oral inhaler), and a lozenge has recently entered the U.S. market (Shiffman et al., 2002).

Nicotine replacement medications enable the tobacco-dependent person to abstain from tobacco by replacing, at least partially, the nicotine obtained from tobacco. As noted by Sweeney and colleagues (2001), there appear to be at least three major mechanisms by which NRT medications enhance smoking cessation. They (1) reduce either general withdrawal symptoms, or at least prominent ones, enabling people to function normally while they learn to live without a cigarette; (2) reduce the reinforcing effects of tobacco-delivered nicotine; and (3) provide some effects for which the patient previously relied on cigarettes, such as sustaining desirable mood and attention states, and making it easier to handle stressful or boring situations.

The efficacy of NRT products for smoking cessation has been demonstrated in a number of placebo-controlled studies. The gum, transdermal patch, nasal spray, and oral inhaler yield initial and long-term quit rates that more than double those generated by placebo products, and, when combined with behavioral counseling and follow-up, quit rates as high as 40–50 after 1 year have been reported (Fiore et al., 2000). Physicians in a busy office setting, with minimal time available for counseling and follow-up, may generate 1-year quit rates as high as 10% (Hughes, Gust, Keenan, Fenwick, & Healey, 1989), and over-the-counter (OTC) sales of the gum, patch, and lozenge have markedly increased the number of quit-smoking attempts and the number of people using NRT (Shiffman et al., 1997). Although a recent meta-analysis suggests that OTC NRT products yield initial quit rates of the same magnitude as NRT products prescribed by a physician, and twice the quit rate obtained by use of placebo products (Hughes, Shiffman, Callas, & Zhang, 2003), other analyses have questioned the long-term efficacy of OTC NRT products (Pierce & Gilpin, 2002). A survey in California showed that smokers who reported using NRT products to quit smoking were just as likely to relapse after 1 year as those who did not use NRT products (Pierce & Gilpin, 2002; Walsh & Penman, 2000).

In 20 cities that participated in COMMIT, 12.8% of smokers (1 out of 8) used the transdermal nicotine patch, making it the most popular method for stopping smoking (Cummings, Hyland, Ockene, Hymowitz, & Manley, 1997). By comparison, 1 out of 10 smokers used nicotine gum, 1 out of 13 attended a stop-smoking program, 1 out of 16 went to a hypnotist or acupuncturist, and 1 out of 20 used some other commercially available stop-smoking device. Among smokers who made an attempt to quit smoking, the likelihood of successful quitting was more than twice as high among patch users than among nonusers. Among patch users, the highest quit rates were observed among those who used the patch between 1 and 3 months (Cummings et al., 1997).

Compared to nonusers, patch users in COMMIT were more likely to be female and white, to have higher annual incomes, to be more motivated to stop smoking, and to smoke more heavily. Among low-income smokers, nicotine patch use was significantly higher among those who lived in a state where the public insurance program (i.e., Medicaid or MediCal) included the patch as a benefit (Cummings et al., 1997).

Hall, Tunstall, Rugg, Jones, and Benowitz (1985) studied the effects nicotine gum and intensive behavioral treatment. They assigned 122 subjects to (1) intensive behavioral treatment, (2) nicotine gum (2 mg) in a low-contact treatment, or (3) intensive behavioral treatment plus nicotine gum. Gum was available for 6 months from the start of treatment. Subjects met in groups of five to six with experienced psychologists serving as group leaders. The behavioral treatment consisted of aversive smoking, relapse prevention skills training, relaxation training, and written exercises to increase commitment to stopping smoking. Group sessions were held 14 times in an 8-week period. The low-contact treatment had fewer sessions (four times over a 3-week period), paper-and-pencil exercises on reasons for smoking, educational material, and group discussions.

Assessments were held at 0, 2, 12, 26, and 52 weeks. Reports of abstinence were verified by measurement of expired air carbon monoxide and serum thiocyanate, as well as reports from significant others (Hall et al., 1985). Differences between the combined condition and the other two conditions were significant at weeks 3, 12, and 26, but not at week 52. For the combined condition, abstinence rates were 95, 73, 59, and 44% at weeks 3, 12, 26, and 52. Corresponding abstinence rates for the low-contact condition were 81, 58, 47, and 37%. For the behavioral condition, the quit rates were 78, 47, 31, and 28% for weeks 3, 12, 26, and 52, respectively. Smokers with high blood cotinine levels (i.e., highly dependent smokers) were more likely to be helped by nicotine gum than were less dependent smokers (Hall et al., 1985).

With NRT strongly endorsed as an effective therapy for smoking cessation, attention has shifted toward ways of enhancing its effectiveness, particularly for the heavily addicted smokers. Options include increasing the dose of NRT product, extending the duration of use, and combination therapy (e.g., two or more forms of NRT or NRT plus bupropion SR). For heavily addicted smokers, higher doses of nicotine gum (4 mg) led to higher quit rates than 2 mg gum (Herrara et al., 1995). In another study, the 21-mg nicotine patch yielded superior quit rates than 14-mg and placebo patches (Transdermal Nicotine Study Group, 1991). However, no advantage was gained by using a 44-mg patch over a 21-mg patch (Jorenby et al., 1995).

Sims and Fiore (2002) noted that extending the use of pharmacotherapy beyond the recommended time frame may be an effective strategy for helping tobacco users achieve abstinence and for preventing relapse to tobacco use, especially for those who are highly nicotine dependent or concerned about weight gain. Their review suggests that long-term use is not harmful and is an acceptable alternative to continued smoking.

Another approach to enhancing efficacy entails combining an NRT medication that allows for passive nicotine delivery (e.g., transdermal patch) with a form of NRT that permits *ad libitum* nicotine delivery (e.g., gum, nasal spray, inhaler; Sweeney et al., 2001). The rationale for combining NRT medications is that smokers may need both a slow delivery system to achieve a constant concentration of nicotine to relieve cravings and tobacco withdrawal symptoms, and a faster acting preparation that can be administered on demand for immediate relief of *breakthrough* cravings and symptoms.

Sweeney and colleagues (2001) identified five published studies that tested the combined use of different nicotine delivery systems. All of the studies used a nicotine patch as one of the study medications, with four of the five studies supplementing nicotine patch treatment with nicotine gum, and the fifth study supplementing patch treatment with nicotine nasal spray. For two of the five studies, the suppression of nicotine withdrawal symptoms was the primary outcome of interest, while the remaining three studies tested the impact of combination therapy on smoking abstinence rates. On the basis of their review, Sweeney and colleagues concluded that there are conditions under which combinations of NRT products provide greater efficacy in relieving withdrawal and fostering cessation than monotherapy. However, the findings are not robust (mean odds ratio = 1.9; Fiore et al., 2000), and additional research is warranted to understand better the magnitude and generality of the benefits of combination therapy.

Bupropion SR

Bupropion SR is the first non-nicotine medication shown to be effective for smoking cessation and approved by the FDA for that use (Fiore et al., 2000). Its mechanism of action may be mediated by its capacity to block neural reuptake of dopamine and/or norepinephrine. Bupropion SR is available exclusively as a prescription medication, with an indication for smoking cessation (Zyban) and an indication for depression (Wellbutrin) (Fiore et al., 2000).

Hurt and colleagues (1997) conducted a double-blind, placebo-controlled trial of bupropion SR for smoking cessation. Six hundred and fifteen subjects were assigned randomly to receive placebo or 100, 150, or 300 mg of bupropion SR per day for 7 weeks. The target quit date was 1 week after the beginning of treatment. Brief counseling was provided at baseline, weekly during treatment, and at 8, 12, 26, and 52 weeks. Self-reported abstinence was confirmed by expired air carbon monoxide (≤ 10 ppm).

At the end of 7 weeks of treatment, the rates of confirmed smoking cessation were 19% for the placebo group and 28.8, 38.6, and 44.2% for the 100-, 150-, and 300-mg bupropion SR groups, respectively. At 1 year, the respective rates were 12.4, 19.6, 22.9, and 23.1% for the placebo, 100-, 150-, and 300-mg bupropion SR groups, respectively. The quit rates for the 150-mg group (p =

.02) and the 300-mg group (p = .01)—but not the 100-mg group (p = .09)—were significantly higher than those for the placebo group (Hurt et al., 1997).

Bupropion SR is effective for women and men (Gonzalez et al., 2002) and for both blacks and whites (Ahluwalia, Harris, Catley, & Okuyemi, 2002). Bupropion SR minimizes weight gain associated with stopping smoking and reduces withdrawal symptoms (Hurt et al., 1997). Multivariate predictors of successful end-of-treatment outcomes include fewer cigarettes per day, longest duration quit in the past, and male gender (Dale et al., 2001).

While bupropion SR may lower seizure thresholds and cause hypersensitivity reaction (Ferry & Johnston, 2003), clinical studies and 32 million patient exposures (9 million for smoking) show that it is generally well tolerated. The most common adverse event in clinical trials or clinical practice is insomnia, which can also be a symptom of nicotine withdrawal. Tonstad and colleagues (2003) showed that bupropion SR was efficacious and safe for use with patients with cardiovascular disease. One-year continuous abstinence rates for bupropion SR were more than double the rates obtained with placebo (22 vs. 9%).

Bupropion SR may be safely combined with NRT to enhance 12-month quit rates (Gold, Rubey, & Harvey, 2002; Jorenby et al., 1999), although support for this strategy is weak. In one study, weight gain following the combination treatment was significantly less than with bupropion SR alone, although the difference in 12-month quit rates (30.3 vs. 35.5%) did not achieve statistical significance (Jorenby et al., 1999). In a study involving primary care smoking cessation clinics (Gold et al., 2002), the 6-month self-reported abstinence rate for nicotine patch alone was 14.8%, for bupropion SR alone, 27.7%, and for patch plus bupropion SR, 34.4%. Quit rates for both forms of bupropion SR treatments were significantly superior to patch treatment, although they were not significantly different from one another.

Hays and colleagues (2001) studied the efficacy of bupropion SR for prevention of smoking relapse. Participants (n = 784 healthy community volunteers) received open-label bupropion SR, 300 mg, for 7 weeks. Participants who were abstinent throughout week 7 of open-label treatment were randomly assigned to placebo or bupropion SR, 300 mg, for 45 weeks, and were subsequently followed for an additional year after the conclusion of the medication phase.

At the end of initial treatment, 58.8% of the participants were abstinent. The point prevalence smoking abstinence rates were significantly higher in the bupropion SR group than in the placebo group at weeks 52 (55.1 vs. 42.3%) and 78 (47.7 vs. 37.7%). The two groups did not differ at the final week of follow-up (week 104) (41.4 vs. 40.0%). The continuous abstinence rate was higher in the bupropion SR group than in the placebo group at study week 24 (17 weeks after randomization) (52.3 vs. 42.3%), but did not differ between groups after week 24. The median time to relapse was significantly greater for bupropion SR recipients than for placebo recipients (156 vs. 65 days), and weight gain was significantly less in the bupropion SR group at study weeks 52 (3.8 vs. 5.6 kg) and 104 (4.1 vs. 5.4 kg). Predictors of successful relapse prevention (in addition to assignment to bupropion SR treatment) were lower baseline smoking rates, a Fagerstrom Tolerance Questionnaire score < 6, and initiation of smoking at an older age (Hurt et al., 2002).

Hurt and colleagues (2003) studied the efficacy of bupropion SR (1) for preventing relapse in adult smokers who quit smoking with transdermal nicotine patch therapy and (2) for quitting smoking in smokers who failed to quit on the patch. At completion of nicotine patch therapy, nonsmoking participants were assigned to bupropion SR or placebo for 6 months (relapse prevention), and smoking participants were assigned to bupropion SR or placebo for 8 weeks of treatment. Of 578 subjects, 31% were abstinent at the end of nicotine patch therapy. Of those not smoking at the end of initial patch treatment, 28 and 25% were not smoking at 6 months (end of medication phase) for bupropion SR and placebo, respectively. For those still smoking at the end of nicotine patch therapy, 3.1 and 0.0% stopped smoking with bupropion SR and placebo, respectively. Hurt and colleagues concluded that bupropion SR neither reduced relapse to smoking in smokers who stopped smoking with the nicotine patch nor initiated abstinence among smokers who failed to stop smoking on the patch.

REFERENCES

Ahluwalia, J. S., Harris, K. J., Catley, D., Okuyemi, K. S., & Mayo, M. S. (2002). Sustained release bupropion for smoking cessation in African-Americans: A randomized controlled trial. JAMA, 228, 468–474.

Aitken, P. (1980). Peer group pressures, parental controls and cigarette smoking among ten- to- fourteen year olds. Br J Soc Clin Psychol, 19, 141–146.

American Academy of Pediatrics Committee on Substance Abuse. (2001). Tobacco's toll: implications for the pediatrician. Pediatrics, 107, 794–798.

American Cancer Society. (1986). Facts and figures on smoking, 1976–1986 (Publication No. 5650-LE). New York: Author.

American Cancer Society. (2003). Cancer facts and figures 2003. Atlanta: Author.

American Lung Association. (2003). Key facts about tobacco use. Retrieved on April 15, 2003, from www.lungusa.org

American Psychiatric Association. (1994). Diagnostic and statistical manual of mental disorders (4th ed.). Washington, DC: Author.

American Psychiatric Association. (1996). Practice guidelines for the treatment of patients with nicotine dependence. Am J Psychiatry, 153(Suppl), 1–31.

American Psychiatric Association. (2000). Diagnostic and statistical manual of mental disorders (4th ed., text rev.). Washington, DC: Author.

Anthonisen, N. R., Connett, J. E., Kiley, J. P., Altose, M. D., Bailey, W. C., Buist, A. S., et al. (1994). Effects of smoking intervention and use of an inhaled anticholinergic bronchodilator on the rate of decline of FEV: The Lung Health Study. *JAMA, 272,* 1497–1505.

Balch, G. I. (1998). Exploring perceptions of smoking cessation among high school smokers: Input and feedback from focus groups. *Prev Med, 27,* A55–A63.

Bansil, R. K., Hymowitz, N., & Keller, S. (1989, May). *Cigarette smoking and neuroleptics.* Paper presented at the annual meeting of the American Psychiatric Association, San Francisco.

Benowitz, N. L. (2001). The nature of nicotine addiction. In P. Slovic (Ed.), *Smoking risk, perception, and policy* (pp. 159–187). Thousand Oaks, CA: Sage.

Biglan, O., & Lichtenstein, E. (1984). A behavior–analytic approach to smoking acquisition: Some recent findings. *J Appl Soc Psychol, 14,* 207–223.

Black, H. R. (1990). Smoking and cardiovascular disease. In J. H. Laragh & B. M. Brenner (Eds.), *Hypertension: Pathophysiology, diagnosis, and management* (pp. 1917–1936). New York: Raven Press.

Bonnie, R. J. (2001). Tobacco and public health policy. In P. Slovic (Ed.), *Smoking risk, perception, and policy* (pp. 277–300). Thousand Oaks, CA: Sage.

Burns, D. M., & Benowitz, N. L. (2001). Public health implications of changes in cigarette design and marketing. In National Cancer Institute (Ed.), *Risks associated with smoking cigarettes with low machine yields of tar and nicotine* (Smoking and Tobacco Control Monograph No. 13, NIH Publication No. 02-5074, pp. 1–12). Bethesda, MD: U.S. Department of Health and Human Services, National Institutes of Health, National Cancer Institute.

Burt, R., Dinh, K., Peterson, A. V., Jr., & Sarason, I. G. (2000). Predicting adolescent smoking: A prospective study of personality variables. *Prev Med, 30,* 115–125.

Burt, R., & Peterson, A. V., Jr. (1998). Smoking cessation among high school seniors. *Prev Med, 27,* 319–327.

Burton, D. (1994). Tobacco cessation programs for adolescents. In R. Richmond (Ed.), *Interventions for smokers: An international perspective* (pp. 95–105). Baltimore: Williams & Wilkins.

Carlson, R. (1997). *Smoke free air everywhere.* Summit: New Jersey Group Against Smoking Pollution.

Centers for Disease Control and Prevention. (2001). Youth tobacco surveillance—United States, 2000. *Morb Mortal Wkly Rep, 50*(SS04), 1–84.

Centers for Disease Control and Prevention. (2002). Annual smoking-attributable mortality, years of potential life lost, and economic costs—United States, 1995–1999. *Morb Mortal Wkly Rep, 51,* 300–303.

Chassin, L., Presson, C. C., Bensenberg, M., Corty, E., Olshavsky, R., & Sherman, S. J. (1981). Predicting adolescents' intentions to smoke cigarettes. *J Health Soc Behav, 22,* 445–455.

Chassin, L., Presson, C. C., Rose, J. S., & Sherman, S. J. (1996). The natural history of cigarette smoking from adolescence to adulthood: Demographic predictors of continuity and change. *Health Psychol, 15,* 478–484.

Choi, W., Ahluwalia, J., Harris, K., & Okuyemi, K. (2002). Progression to established smoking—the influence of tobacco marketing. *Am J Prev Med, 22,* 228–233.

Cummings, K.M., Hyland, A., Ockene, J. K., Hymowitz, N., & Manley, M. (1997). Use of the nicotine skin patch by smokers in 20 United States communities, 1992–1993. *Tob Control, 6*(Suppl 2), S63–S70.

Dale, L. C., Glover, E. D., Sachs, D. P., Schroeder, D. R., Offord, K. P., Croghan, I. T., & Hurt, R. D. (2001). Bupropion for smoking cessation: Predictors of successful outcome. *Chest, 119,* 1357–1364.

DiFranza, J. R., Savageau, J. A., Rigotti, N. A., Fletcher, K., Ockene, J. K., McNeill, A. D., et al. (2002). Development of symptoms of tobacco dependence in youths: 30 month follow up data from the DANDY study. *Tob Control, 11,* 228–235.

Digiusto, E. (1994). Pros and cons of cessation interventions for adolescent smokers at school. In R. Richmond (Ed.), *Interventions for smokers: An international perspective* (pp. 107–136). Baltimore: Williams & Wilkins.

Environmental Protection Agency. (1992). *Respiratory health effects of passive smoking: Lung cancer and other disorders.* Washington, DC: Office of Health and Environmental Assessment. Office of Research and Development.

Ershler, J., Leventhal, H., Fleming, R., & Glynn, K. (1989). The quitting experience for smokers in sixth through twelfth grades. *Addict Behav, 14,* 365–378.

Fagerstrom, K. O. (1978). Measuring degree of physical dependence to tobacco smoking with reference to individualization of treatment. *Addict Behav, 3,* 235–241.

Fagerstrom, K. O. (1988). Efficacy of nicotine chewing gum: A review. In O. F. Pomerleau & C. S. Pomerleau (Eds.), *Nicotine replacement* (pp. 109–128). New York: Alan R. Liss.

Federal Trade Commission. (2001). *Federal Trade Commission Cigarette Report for 1999.* Retrieved on April 13, 2003, from *http://www.ftc.gov/opa/2001/03/cigarette.htm*

Ferry, L., & Johnston, J. (2003). Efficacy and safety of bupropion SR for smoking cessation: Data from clinical trials and five years of post marketing experience. *Int J Clin Pract, 57,* 224–230.

Fiore, M. C., Bailey, W. C., Cohen, S. J., Dorfman, S. F., Goldstein, M. G., Gritz, E. R., et al. (2000). *Treating tobacco use and dependence: Clinical practice guideline.* Rockville, MD: U.S. Department of Health and Human Services, Public Health Service.

Fiore, M. C., Novotny, T. E., Pierce, J. P., Giovino, G. A., Hatziandreu, E. J., Newcomb, P. A., et al. (1990). Methods used to quit smoking in the United States: Do cessation programs help? *JAMA, 263,* 2760–2765.

Giovino, G. A., Tomar, S., Reddy, M., Peddicord, J. P., Zhu, B. P., Escobedo, L. G., & Eriksen, M. P. (1996). Attitudes, knowledge, and beliefs about low-yield cigarettes among adolescents and adults. In *The FTC Cigarette Test Method for determining tar, nicotine, and carbon monoxide yields of U.S. cigarettes* (Smoking and Tob Control Monograph No. 7, NIH Publication No. 96-4028, pp. 39–57). Bethesda, MD: U.S. Department of Health and Human Services, National Institutes of Health, National Cancer Institute.

Glassman, A. H. (1993). Cigarette smoking: Implications for psychiatric illness. *Am J Psychiatry, 150,* 546–553.

Gold, P., Rubey, R., & Harvey, R. (2002). Naturalistic, self-assignment comparative trial of bupropion SR, a nicotine patch, or both, for smoking cessation treatment in primary care. *Am J Addict, 11,* 315–331.

Gonzales, D., Bjornson, W., Durcan, M., White, J. D., Johnston, J. A., Buist, A. S., et al. (2002). Effects of gender on relapse prevention in smokers treated with bupropion SR. *Am J Prev Med, 22,* 234–239.

Green, D.E. (1980). Beliefs of teenagers about smoking and health. In R. M. Leauer & R. B. Shekelle (Eds.), *Childhood prevention of atherosclerosis and hypertension* (pp. 223–228). New York: Raven Press.

Hall, S. M., Tunstall, C., Rugg, D., Jones, R. T., & Benowitz, N. (1985). Nicotine gum and behavioral treatment in smoking cessation. *J Consult Clin Psychol, 53,* 256–258.

Hansen, W. B. (1983). Behavioral predictors of abstinence: Early indicators of a dependence on tobacco among adolescents. *Int J Addict, 18,* 913–920.

Hays, J. T., Hurt, R. D., Rigotti, N. A., Niaura, R., Gonzalez, D., Durcan, M. J., et al. (2001). Sustained-release bupropion for pharmacologic relapse prevention after smoking cessation: A randomized controlled trial. *Ann Intern Med, 135,* 423–433.

Henningfield, J. E. (1986). How tobacco produces drug dependence. In J. K. Ockene (Ed.), *The pharmacologic treatment of tobacco dependence: Proceedings of the World Congress* (pp. 19–31). Cambridge, MA: Institute for the Study of Smoking Behavior and Policy.

Herrara, N., Franco, R., Herrara, L., Partidas, A., Rolando, R., & Fagerström, K. O. (1995). Nicotine gum, 2 and 4 mg, for nicotine dependence. *Chest, 108,* 447–451.

Hughes, G.H., Hymowitz, N., Ockene, J. K., Simon, N., & Vogt, T. M. (1981). The Multiple Risk Factor Intervention Trial (MRFIT): V. Intervention on smoking. *Prev Med, 10,* 476–500.

Hughes, J. R., Gust, S. W., Keenan, R. M., Fenwick, J. W., & Healey, M. L. (1989). Nicotine vs placebo gum in general medical practice. *JAMA, 261,* 1300–1306.

Hughes, J. R., Shiffman, S., Callas, P., & Zhang, J. (2003). A meta-analysis of the efficacy of over-the-counter nicotine replacement. *Tob Control, 12,* 21–27.

Hunt, W. A., & Bespalec, D. A. (1974). An evaluation of current methods of modifying smoking behavior. *J Clin Psychol, 30,* 431–438.

Hurt, R. D., Croghan, G., Beede, S., Wolter, T. D., Croghan, I. T., & Patten, C. A. (2000). Nicotine patch therapy in 101 adolescent smokers. *Arch Pediatr Adolesc Med, 154,* 31–37.

Hurt, R. D., Krook, J., Croghan, I., Loprinzi, C. L., Sloan, J. A., Novotny, P. J., et al. (2003). Nicotine patch therapy based on smoking rate followed by bupropion for prevention of relapse to smoking. *J Clin Oncol, 21,* 914–920.

Hurt, R. D., Sachs, D. P., Glover, E. D., Offord, K. P., Johnston, J. A., Dale, L. C., et al. (1997). A comparison of sustained-release bupropion and placebo for smoking cessation. *N Engl J Med, 337,* 1195–1202.

Hurt, R. D., Wolter, T. D., Rigotti, N., Hays, J. T., Niaura, R., Durcan, M. J., et al. (2002). Bupropion for pharmacologic relapse prevention to smoking, predictors of outcome. *Addict Behav, 27,* 493–507.

Hymowitz, N. (1987). Community and clinical trials of disease prevention: Effects on cigarette smoking. *Public Health Rev, 15,* 45–81.

Hymowitz, N. (1999). Smoking cessation. In N. S. Cherniack, M. D. Altose, & I. Homma (Eds.), *Rehabilitation of the patient with respiratory disease* (pp. 319–353). New York: McGraw-Hill.

Hymowitz, N., Corle, D., Royce, J., Hartwell, T., Corbett, K., Orlandi, M., & Piland, N. (1995). Smokers' baseline characteristics in the COMMIT Trial. *Prev Med, 24,* 503–508.

Hymowitz, N., Cummings, K. M., Hyland, A., Lynn, W. R., Pechacek, T. F., & Hartwell, T. D. (1997). Predictors of smoking cessation in a cohort of adult smokers followed for five years. *Tob Control*, 6(Suppl 2), S57–S62.

Hymowitz, N., Schwab, J., & Eckholdt, H. (2001). Pediatric residency training on tobacco: Training Director Tobacco Survey. *Prev Med*, 33, 688–698.

Hymowitz, N., Sexton, M., Ockene, J., & Grandits, G. (1991). Baseline factors associated with smoking cessation and relapse. *Prev Med*, 20, 590–601.

Jackson, C., Henriksen, L., Dickinson, D., Messer, L., & Robertson, S. B. (1998). A longitudinal study predicting patterns of cigarette smoking in late childhood. *Health Educ Behav*, 25, 436–447.

Johnson, B. D. (1977). The race, class, and irreversibility hypotheses: Myths and research about heroin. In J. D. Rittenhouse (Ed.), *The epidemiology of heroin and other addictions* (NIDA Research Monograph No. 16, pp. 51–60). Washington, DC: U.S. Government Printing Office.

Jones, R. T. (1987). Tobacco dependence. In H. Y. Meltzer (Ed.), *Psychopharmacology: The third generation of progress* (pp. 1589–1595). New York: Raven Press.

Jorenby, D. E., Leischow, S. J., Nides, M. A., Rennard, S. I., Johnston, J. A., Hughes, A. R., et al. (1999). A controlled trial of sustained-release bupropion, a nicotine patch, or both for smoking cessation. *The N Engl J Med*, 340, 685–691.

Jorenby, D. E., Smith, S. S., Fiore, M. C., Hurt, R. D., Offord, K. P., Croghan, I. T., et al. (1995). Varying nicotine patch dose and type of smoking cessation counseling. *JAMA*, 274, 1347–1352.

Kozlowski, L., O'Connor, R. J., & Sweeney, C. T. (2001). Cigarette design. In National Cancer Institute (Ed.), *Risks associated with smoking cigarettes with low machine yields of tar and nicotine* (Smoking and Tobacco Control Monograph No. 13, NIH Publication No. 02-5074, pp. 13–37). Bethesda, MD: U.S. Department of Health and Human Services, National Institutes of Health, National Cancer Institute.

Kozlowski, L. T., Wilkinson, P. A., Skinner, W., Kent, C., Franklin, T., & Pope, M. (1989). Comparing tobacco cigarette dependence with other drug dependencies. *JAMA*, 261, 898–901.

Lando, H. A. (1993). Formal quit smoking treatments. In C. T. Orleans & J. Slade (Eds.), *Nicotine addiction: Principles and management* (pp. 221–244). New York: Oxford University Press.

Lantz, P., Jacobson, P., Warner, K., Wasserman, J., Pollack, H. A., Berson, J., & Ahlstrom, A. (1999). Investing in youth tobacco control: A review of smoking prevention and control strategies. *Tob Control*, 9, 47–63.

Leventhal, H., & Cleary, P. P. (1980). The smoking problem: A review of the research and theory in behavioral risk modification. *Psychol Bull*, 88, 370–405.

Lynch, B. S., & Bonnie, R. J. (1994). *Growing up tobacco free*. Washington, DC: National Academy Press.

Myers, M. L. (2002). Star Scientific's phase out of "light" and similar terms is significant step if extended to all its cigarette brands. Retrieved April 20, 2003, from *www.tobaccofreekids.org/script/displaypressrelease.php3?display+479*

Ockene, J. K., Hymowitz, N., Lagus, J., & Shaten, B. J. (1991). Comparison of smoking behavior change for special intervention and usual care groups. *Prev Med*, 20, 564–573.

Oei, T. S., & Fea, A. (1987). Smoking prevention program for children: A review. *J Drug Educ*, 17, 11–42.

Orleans, C. T. (1993). Treating nicotine dependence in medical settings: A stepped care model. In C. T. Orleans & J. Slade (Eds.), *Nicotine addiction: Principles and management* (pp. 145–161). New York: Oxford University Press.

Pharmacists' "Helping Smokers Quit" Program. (1986). *Am Pharm, NS26,* 25–33.

Pierce, J. P., & Gilpin, E. A. (1996). How long will today's new adolescent smoker be addicted to cigarettes? *Am J Public Health, 86,* 253–256.

Pierce, J. P., & Gilpin, E. A. (2002). Impact of over-the-counter sales on effectiveness of pharmaceutical aids for smoking cessation. *JAMA, 288,* 1260–1264.

Rigotti, N. A., Lee, J. E., & Wechsler, H. (2000). U.S. college students use of cigarettes, cigars, pipes, and smokeless tobacco. *JAMA, 284,* 699–705.

Sachs, D. P. L. (1986). Nicotine polacrilex: Clinical promises delivered and yet to come. In J. K. Ockene (Ed.), *The pharmacologic treatment of tobacco dependence: Proceedings of the World Congress* (pp. 120–140). Cambridge, MA: Institute for the Study of Smoking Behavior and Policy.

Samet, J. M. (2001). The risks of active and passive smoking. In P. Slovic (Ed.), *Smoking, risk, perception, and policy* (pp. 3–28). Thousand Oaks, CA: Sage.

Sargent, J. D., Dalton, M., Beach, M., Bernhardt, A., Heatherton, T., & Stevens, M. (2000). Effect of cigarette promotions on smoking uptake among adolescents. *Prev Med, 30,* 320–327.

Schachter, S. (1982). Recidivism and self-cure of smoking and obesity. *Am Psychol, 37,* 436–444.

Schultes, R. E. (1978). Ethnopharmacological significance of psychotropic drugs of vegetal origin. In W. G. Clark & J. del Giudice (Eds.), *Principles of psychopharmacology* (pp. 41–70). New York: Academic Press.

Schwartz, J. L. (1987). *Smoking cessation methods: The United States and Canada, 1978–1985* (DHHS Publication No. NIH 87-2940). Washington, DC: U.S. Government Printing Office.

Seely, J. E., Zuskin, E., & Bouhuys, A. (1971). Cigarette smoking: Objective evidence for lung damage in teen-agers. *Science, 172,* 741–743.

Shiffman, S. (1986). A cluster-analytic typology of smoking relapse episodes. *Addict Behav, 11,* 295–307.

Shiffman, S., Dresler, C. M., Hajek, P., Gilburt, S. J., Targett, D. A., & Strahs, K. R. (2002). Efficacy of a nicotine lozenge for smoking cessation. *Arch Intern Med, 162,* 1267–1276.

Shiffman, S., Gitchell, J., Pinney, J. M., Burton, S. L., Kemper, K. E., & Lara, E. A. (1997). Public health benefit of over-the-counter nicotine medications. *Tob Control, 6,* 306–310.

Sims, T. H. & Fiore, M. C. (2002). Pharmacotherapy for treating tobacco dependence: What is the ideal duration of therapy? *CNS Drugs, 16,* 653–662.

Slade, J., Connolly, G. N., & Lymperis, D. (2002). Eclipse: Does it live up to its health claims? *Tob Control, 11,* 64–70.

Sullivan, L. W. (1991). To thwart the tobacco companies. *JAMA, 266,* 2131.

Sussman, S., Dent, C. W., & Lichtman, K. (2000). Project EX outcomes of a teen smoking cessation program. *Addict Behav, 25,* 1–14.

Sussman, S., Lichtman, K., Ritt, A., & Pallonen, U. E. (1999). Effects of thirty-four adolescent tobacco use cessation and prevention trials on regular users of tobacco products. *Subst Use Misuse, 34,* 1469–1503.

Sweeney, C. T., Fant, R. V., Fagerstrom, K. O., McGovern, J. F., & Henningfield, J. E. (2001). Combination nicotine replacement therapy for smoking cessation. *CNS Drugs, 15,* 453–467.

Terry, L. L. (1983). The Surgeon General's first report on smoking and health. *NY State J Med, 83,* 1254–1255.

Tonstad, S., Farsang, C., Klaene, G., Lewis, K., Manolis, A., Perruchoud, A. P., et al. (2003). Bupropion SR for smoking cessation in smokers with cardiovascular disease: A multicentre randomised study. *Eur Heart J, 24,* 946–955.

Transdermal Nicotine Study Group. (1991). Transdermal nicotine for smoking cessation. *JAMA, 266,* 3133–3138.

U.S. Department of Agriculture. (2001). *Tobacco situation and outlook.* Retrieved on April 13, 2003, from *www.ers.usda.gov/briefing/tobacco*

U.S. Department of Health, Education, and Welfare. (1979). *Smoking and health: A report of the Surgeon General.* (DHEW Publication No. PHS 79-500066). Washington, DC: U.S. Government Printing Office.

U.S. Department of Health and Human Services. (1986). *Clinical opportunities for smoking intervention: A guide for the busy physician* (NIH Publication No. 86-2178). Washington, DC: U.S. Government Printing Office.

U.S. Department of Health and Human Services. (1988). *The health consequences of smoking: Nicotine addiction: A report of the Surgeon General* (DHHS Publication No. CDC 88-8406). Washington, DC: U.S. Government Printing Office.

U.S. Department of Health and Human Services. (1989a). *How to help your patients stop smoking: A National Cancer Institute manual for physicians* (NIH Publication No. 89-3064). Washington, DC: U.S. Government Printing Office.

U.S. Department of Health and Human Services. (1989b). *Reducing the health consequences of smoking: 25 years of progress* (DHHS Publication No. CDC 89-8411). Washington, DC: U.S. Government Printing Office.

U.S. Department of Health and Human Services. (1990). *The health benefits of smoking cessation. A report of the Surgeon General* (DHHS Publication No. CDC 90-8416). Washington, DC: U.S. Government Printing Office.

U.S. Department of Health and Human Services. (1994a). *Preventing tobacco use among young people: A report of the Surgeon General.* Atlanta: U.S. Department of Health and Human Services, Public Health Service, Centers for Disease Control and Prevention, National Center for Chronic Disease Prevention and Health Promotion, Office on Smoking and Health, U.S. Government Printing Office.

U.S. Department of Health and Human Services. (1994b). *Tobacco and the clinician* (NIH Publication No. 94-3693). Bethesda, MD: National Institutes of Health.

U.S. Department of Health and Human Services. (2001). *Women and smoking: A report of the Surgeon General.* Washington, DC: Public Health Service, Office of the Surgeon General, U.S. Government Printing Office.

U.S. Public Health Service. (1964). *Smoking and health* (Report of the Advisory Committee to the Surgeon General of the Public Health Service, U.S. Department of Health, Education, and Welfare, Public Health Service, Centers for Disease Control, PHS Publication No. 1103). Washington, DC: U.S. Government Printing Office.

Van Lancker, J. (1977). Smoking and disease. In M. E. Jarvik, J. W. Cullen, E. R. Gritz, T. M. Vogt, & L. J. West (Eds.), *Research on smoking behavior* (NIDA Research

Monograph No. 17, DHEW Publication No. ADM 78-581, pp. 230–283). Washington, DC: U.S. Government Printing Office.

Vogt, T. M. (1982). Cigarette smoking: History, risks, and behavior change. *International Journal of Mental Health, 11*, 6–43.

Walsh, R. A., & Penman, A. G. (2000). The effectiveness of nicotine replacement therapy over-the-counter. *Drug Alcohol Rev, 19*, 243–247.

Wayne, G. F., & Connolly, G. N. (2002). How cigarette design can affect youth initiation into smoking: Camel cigarettes 1983–93. *Tob Control, 11*, i32–i39.

Wechsler, H., Kelley, K., Seibring, M., Kuo, M., & Rigotti, N. A. (2001). College smoking policies and smoking cessation programs: Results of a survey of college health directors. *J Am Coll Health, 49*, 205–212.

World Health Organization. (1999). Worldwide trends in tobacco consumption and mortality. Retrieved on April 13, 2003, from *www.druglibrary.org/schaffer/tobacco/who-tobacco.htm*

Yamaguchi, K., & Kandel, D. B. (1985). On the resolution of role incompatibility: A life event history analysis of family roles and marijuana use. *Am J Sociol, 90*, 1284–1325.

Yassa, R., Lal, S., Korpassy, A., & Ally, J. (1987). Nicotine exposure and tardive dyskinesia. *Biol Psychiatry, 22*, 67–72.

Yudkin, P., Hey, K., Roberts, S., Welch, S., Murphy, M., & Walton, R. (2003). Abstinence from smoking eight years after participation in randomized controlled trial of nicotine patch. *Br Med J, 327*, 28–29.

Zhu, S., Sun, J., Billings, S. C., Choi, W. S., & Malarcher, A. (1999). Predictors of smoking cessation in U.S. adolescents. *Am J Prev Med, 16*, 202–207.

CHAPTER 7

Opioids

STEPHEN L. DILTS, JR.
STEPHEN L. DILTS

Opioids constitute the group of compounds whose pharmacological effects duplicate those of morphine. They are commonly used medically as an adjunct to anesthesia, for the relief of pain, for the prevention of an abstinence syndrome, and for cough suppression. Opioids also are abused for their intoxicating effects.

The history of opioid use goes back thousands of years in human history. The Ebers Papyri from approximately 7000 B.C. refer to the use of opium in children suffering from colic (Deneau & Mule, 1981). In the Victorian era, the use of laudanum was socially acceptable. In the present day, opioids use is stringently regulated, especially in the United States; however, demand by addicts results in the existence of a "black market" characterized by crime, disease, poverty, and loss of personal and social productivity. The sexually promiscuous intravenous heroin user is at high risk to contract and effectively spread the deadly acquired immune deficiency syndrome (AIDS) virus, as well as venereal and other infectious diseases, such as hepatitis C. High overall death rates are associated with opioid abuse, approximately 10–15 per 1,000 in the United States (Jaffe, 1989). The Drug Abuse Warning Network (Substance Abuse and Mental Health Services Administration, 1995) indicates an alarming increase in the use of opioids, especially prescription drugs such as oxycodone.

DEFINITIONS

The opioids are addicting; that is, they produce a well-defined syndrome of repeated self-administration over time, tolerance to the effects of the drug, and an abstinence syndrome when the drug is no longer available. "Cross-tolerance" refers to the ability of any drug in the opioid class to produce similar effects and to block the abstinence syndrome associated with opioids in general. The primary effects of opiates are mediated through their action at the opioid mu, kappa, and delta receptors. Morphine, codeine, and thebaine are naturally occurring phenanthrene alkaloids in opium, the milky exudate from the unripe capsule of the poppy plant, *Papaver somniferum*. Raw opium contains 4–21% morphine and 0.7–2.5% codeine, and is refined to produce these medically useful products. In practice, most codeine is actually converted directly from morphine, which also can be used to produce hydromorphone (Dilaudid). Thebaine, found in very small concentrations in raw opium, is similar to morphine. It is converted into medically useful compounds such as codeine, hydrocodone (Vicodin), oxycodone (Percodan, Percocet, Tylox), oxymorphone (Numorphan), nalbuphine (Nubain), and diacetylmorphine (heroin). Naloxone (Narcan) is also produced from morphine but lacks euphoric and analgesic properties; its use in humans is discussed later in this chapter. Etorphine (M99), which is produced from thebaine, is a potent opioid useful mainly in the immobilization of large animals. Raw opium, morphine, codeine, and thebaine are referred to as naturally occurring opioids or opiates, whereas those compounds mentioned previously, which are produced directly from these naturally occurring compounds, are called semisynthetic opioids or opiates.

Attempts to synthesize opioid-like compounds have produced a variety of agents that are chemically distinct from morphine yet seem to act via similar mechanisms and also exhibit cross-tolerance. These include meperidine (Demerol), propoxyphene (Darvon), methadone (Dolophine), and levo-alpha-acetyl methadol (LAAM). Fentanyl (Sublimaze) and sufentanil (Sufenta) are very potent short-acting opioids used mainly in anesthesia. Buprenorphine, a partial mu agonist, is useful in the treatment of heroin addiction. These compounds are collectively referred to as the synthetic opioids.

With the exception of methadone and LAAM, most opiates have short half-lives. Extended release preparations of oxycodone (Oxycontin) and morphine (MSContin) have become increasingly popular in pain management, because they offer fewer peaks and troughs over 24 hours. Most opioids are legitimately used medically for pain relief; however, the addicting properties of opiates have prompted the search for a nonaddicting analgesic with the same potent pain-relieving properties as the opioids; unfortunately, this has not come to pass, and the following examples are known to produce dependence along with analgesia. Pentazocine (Talwin) and butorphanol (Stadol) produce analgesia in the opioid-free individual but are addicting, and when given to someone who is opioid dependent produce an abstinence syndrome. The semisynthetic compound nalbuphine, mentioned earlier, has similar properties. Tramadol (Ultram), a synthetic aminocyclohexanol, binds to mu opioid receptors and also inhibits reuptake of norepinephrine and serotonin; there have been increasing reports of tramadol abuse.

Despite their similarities, opioids may have varying effects on opioid receptors. For example, the mu receptor is occupied preferentially by the classic morphine-like opioids, but butorphanol (Stadol) and nalbuphaine (Nubain) prefer the kappa receptor. Both receptors are highly specific, and an abstinence syndrome mediated by the kappa receptor will not be relieved if a mu receptor compound is administered. Like pentazocine, butorphanol, and tramadol, buprenorphine (Subutex) is a mixed opiate agonist–antagonist, with partial mu receptor agonism and full kappa agonism. Partial agonists show a "ceiling effect"; unlike full agonists, dose escalation does not produce ever-increasing pharmacological effects. There are also compounds that bind selectively to the receptor site, yet produce no agonistic action. These compounds are antagonistic in nature, because they occupy the receptor site and exclude agonist opioids; examples include naloxone (Narcan) and naltrexone (ReVia). These opioid antagonists, useful for the treatment of opioid intoxication and addiction, are discussed later. Relative to full agonists, partial agonists may act as antagonists. Also of interest is the discovery and description of endogenous opioid substances in humans, operating at the kappa receptor site along the spectrum from agonistic to antagonistic function. To date, no endogenous mu receptor opioid has been discovered (Jaffe, 1989).

DIAGNOSIS

In the framework provided by the fourth edition of the *Diagnostic and Statistical Manual of Mental Disorders* (DSM-IV-TR; American Psychiatric Association, 2000), the problem of opioid misuse is divided into four categories, among which there may be some overlap. Opioid intoxication and opioid withdrawal are specifically defined in DSM-IV-TR. Facility in making these diagnoses requires a clear understanding of the clinical features associated with opioids, as discussed later in this chapter. In addition to intoxication or withdrawal, it is important to characterize the individual's relationship to the use of opioids over time.

Initial assessment always includes a thorough history of the individual's substance use over time, with corroboration from outside sources if possible. This corroboration of the individual's history is essential because of the nearly universal presence of denial in the nonrecovered substance abuser. Minimization of the frequency and amounts of opioid use is common, as is the illusion of control characterized by the often-heard phrase, "I can stop anytime I want to." Progression in the pattern of usage is the rule, as the reinforcing qualities of the opioid and tolerance exert their powerful influence. Critical to the initial assessment is an accurate answer to this question: "When did you last use and how much did you use?" With this information, the clinician can begin to assess the impact of intoxication or withdrawal upon the immediate clinical presentation. It is also necessary to understand the crises or events precipitating contact with the health care system to assess whether the patient has truly "hit bottom" or merely experienced a temporary loss of ability to obtain opioids. This information may be useful in predicting readiness to accept treatment interventions.

A family history of substance abuse provides data reflective of the genetic influences in opioid dependence, as well as the contribution of learned behavior and sanction of substance abuse within the family structure. This information is particularly useful in planning a strategy for recovery and relapse prevention. Returning an individual to contact with family members and/or friends who are still using opioids and other drugs will virtually guarantee a quick relapse.

Also important are inquiries into the individual's functioning in the workplace, at home, and in the social arena. Trouble may occur in each area because of the competition between dependence-driven, drug-seeking behavior and the demands of everyday living. It is important to ask specifically about legal difficulties, arrests, convictions, or restrictions of freedom (e.g., loss of professional licensure).

A medical review of systems in tandem with a thorough physical examination, including a neurological examination and a mental status examination, may reveal signs of intoxication or withdrawal, as outlined later. Stigmata of opioid use, such as fresh or old needle marks (tracks) around superficial veins in the extremities and neck, are readily observed. These often appear as increased lines of pigmentation. There may be evidence of old and new skin abscesses, clotted or thrombosed veins, an enlarged and tender liver, swollen lymph nodes, a heart murmur caused by endocarditis, hypo- or hyperactive bowel sounds, and pupillary abnormalities, which depend on the stage of intoxication or withdrawal. Significant weight loss is common, though weight gain is occasionally reported.

Useful laboratory studies include serum liver function studies, which may show inflammation in the form of elevated serum aspartate aminotransferase (AST), serum alanine aminotransferase (ALT), bilirubin, alkaline phosphatase, and reduction in total protein, clotting factors, and immunoglobulins. Blood urea nitrogen may also be elevated, though the meaning of this finding is unclear. Further testing may include hepatitis A, B, and C screening; human immunodeficiency virus (HIV) testing; complete blood count; and urine and/or serum analyses for the presence of opioids, cocaine metabolites, marijuana, alcohol, benzodiazepines, barbiturates, other stimulants, and hallucinogens. If possible, the collection of urine samples should be actively observed to ensure that the samples are not falsified in some manner by the individual. "Scams" for avoiding detection of illicit drugs in urine are diverse and imaginative: Some men have provided "clean" urine from a small tube alongside the penis, and some women have concealed a balloon of "clean" urine in the vagina to be lacerated with a fingernail, while apparently positioning the specimen cup near the urethral meatus as the sample is collected.

As evidence of opioid abuse or dependence grows, the clinician can mount a firm but respectful confrontation of the individual, who will frequently admit the problem because he or she now recognizes that there may exist an opportunity for treatment. The "addiction as an illness" concept can be useful at this critical juncture in the physician's interactions with an opioid-dependent person. If the patient's denial prevents engagement in treatment, leverage on his or her behavior may be gained by involving significant others, employers, or the legal system.

CLINICAL FEATURES AND PHARMACOLOGY

Clinical features of opioid use are logically divided into three categories: intoxication, withdrawal, and overdose. These features are outlined in Tables 7.1, 7.2, and 7.3, respectively. The features listed in these tables are directly related to the pharmacological actions of the opiates and are uniform in humans, with the occasional exception of the individual who experiences an idiosyncratic reaction.

TABLE 7.1. Signs of Opioid Intoxiciation

1. Euphoria immediately following ingestion; profound relief from anxiety and tension.
2. Apathy following euphoria.
3. An initial mild-to-moderate burst of energy in the minutes following ingestion, ultimately replaced with psychomotor retardation.
4. "Nodding," a "twilight state" in between alertness and sleep, during which the individual is quiescent but arousable.
5. Pupillary constriction (miosis).
6. Hypoactive bowel sounds.
7. Slow regular respiration.
8. Slurred speech.
9. Impaired judgment, attention, concentration, and memory.
10. Physical evidence of recent use, including needle marks, hyperemic nasal mucosa, if insufflation was the route of administration, and positive opioid blood or urine screen.

TABLE 7.2. Opioid Withdrawal

Stage I—begins within hours of last dose and peaks at 36–72 hours:

1. Craving for the drug.
2. Tearing (lacrimation).
3. "Runny nose" (rhinorrhea).
4. Yawning.
5. Sweating (diaphoresis).

Stage II—begins at 12 hours and peaks at 72 hours:

1. Mild-to-moderate sleep disturbance.
2. Dilated pupils (mydriasis).
3. Loss of appetite (anorexia).
4. "Goose flesh" or "cold turkey" (piloerection).
5. Irritability.
6. Tremor.

Stage III—begins at 24–36 hours and peaks at 72 hours:

1. Severe insomnia.
2. Violent yawning.
3. Weakness.
4. Nausea, vomiting, and diarrhea.
5. Chills and fever.
6. Muscle spasms or "kicking the habit" (especially in the lower extremities).
7. Flushing.
8. Spontaneous ejaculation.
9. Abdominal pain.

TABLE 7.3. Opioid Overdose

1. Signs of recent ingestion.
2. Profoundly decreased respirations or apnea.
3. Pale skin and blue mucous membranes.
4. Pinpoint pupils, unless prolonged cerebral apnea has caused some brain damage, in which case pupillary dilatation may occur.
5. Pulmonary edema resulting in characteristic gasping and audible rhonchi; occasional froth in the upper airway.
6. Cardiovascular collapse.
7. Cardiac dysrhythmias.
8. Convulsions, especially with meperidine, propoxyphene, or codeine.
9. Semicoma or coma.

Analgesia is the principal useful effect of the opioids. It seems not to matter whether the pain is physical or emotional: Relief is significant. The addiction potential of a given opioid appears to be at least partly related to the analgesic affect. Analgesia from full opioid agonists increases in a dose-related manner, to a point beyond which larger doses cause greater side effects but no greater analgesia (Deneau & Mule, 1981). Contravening side effects include respiratory depression, sedation, seizures, and loss of motor control. Heroin, morphine, and hydromorphone are among the best analgesics because of rapid absorption into the central nervous system and a relatively higher threshold for side effects. Meperidine and codeine are less effective in this regard. Route of administration significantly affects analgesia. Parenteral use is the most efficient, because oral administration subjects the opioid to erratic absorption in the gastrointestinal tract, as well as passage through the portal system before reaching the central nervous system. Codeine and methadone are reliably absorbed orally; morphine and meperidine are not.

Opioids are potent suppressors of the cough reflex, and this antitussive action is most often accomplished with codeine or hydrocodone. A related phenomenon is that of respiratory depression. Opioids cause the central respiratory center to become less sensitive to carbon dioxide, which in rising concentrations ordinarily stimulates breathing. The mechanism of death in acute opioid overdose usually is respiratory arrest.

Opioids have pronounced gastrointestinal effects. Initially the user may experience nausea and emesis due to central stimulation; however, this is followed by depression of the central structures controlling emesis, and even emetic agents frequently fail to produce vomiting. The intestinal smooth muscle is stimulated to contract by opioids, thus reducing peristalsis. Although this action may be desirable in preventing loss of water through diarrhea, the related undesirable effect of constipation routinely appears with repeated administration.

Smooth muscle contraction in the urinary bladder is also stimulated by opioids, sometimes resulting in an unpleasant sensation of nearly constant urinary urgency. Although uterine muscle is not significantly affected by opioids, labor is frequently prolonged. Because opioids do cross the placental barrier, newborn infants can show all the adult signs of intoxication, withdrawal, and overdose.

Blood vessels in the periphery are generally dilated as a result of opioid-induced histamine release; this sometimes causes a blush of the skin, with itching, especially in the face. By a separate mechanism, reflex vasoconstriction is inhibited, resulting in significant orthostasis. Some endocrine effects have also been noted. Thyroid activity, output of gonadotropins, and adrenal steroid output are all reduced. These effects are caused by opioid actions on the pituitary gland.

The concept of tolerance has been previously mentioned. Repeated administration of opioids results in decreasing levels of euphoria and analgesia over time. The user also becomes less affected by respiratory depression, nausea and emesis, and impairment of consciousness. Less tolerance develops to orthostasis and very little to miosis, constipation, and urinary urgency; however, these side effects may be counteracted by the euphoric and analgesic properties of opioids, in which individuals remain aware of unpleasant physical sensations but insist that they are no longer bothered by these. Tolerance is reversed during periods of abstinence.

Tolerance is the direct result of neuroadaptive change at the opioid receptor site during a period of continuous occupation by an exogenous opioid. A state of physical dependence is reached when removal of the opioid from its receptor site produces an abstinence syndrome. A more sudden removal of the opioid from its receptor site produces a more intense abstinence syndrome. The most rapid removal of opioid from its receptor site is accomplished by the opioid antagonists, which selectively compete for the site but have no agonist properties. Shorter acting opioids exit the receptor site more quickly than do opioids with longer half-lives. Thus, heroin and morphine produce intense abstinence syndromes with relatively rapid onset and progression, whereas methadone produces an abstinence syndrome of less overall intensity, but with slower progression through the stages of acute abstinence to resolution, which, for a short-acting drug such as heroin, arrives at 5–10 days. Abrupt methadone withdrawal produces an abstinence syndrome that may not resolve for 14–21 days. Following resolution of the acute abstinence syndrome, a more subtle abstinence syndrome may occur and last for many months. Symptoms include hyposensitivity to the respiratory stimulant effect of carbon dioxide, disturbed sleep, preoccupation with physical discomfort, poor self-esteem, and diminished ability to tolerate stress. Risk of relapse is higher during this period (Martin & Jasinski, 1969).

COURSE

Many complex factors influence the natural history of opioid addiction. Overall, the course is one of relapse and remission. Attempts to define opioid abusers as a group have been limited, because long-term contact with these frequently itinerant persons is difficult, and only a minority of opioid abusers can be studied effectively (i.e., those who elect to enter treatment). Given these obstacles to accurate understanding, some generalizations can still be made. The vast majority of active opioid abusers are between the ages of 20 and 50 years. Age at first use is usually in the teens or 20s. Race, ethnicity, and socioeconomic status variables are important. Though opioid addiction affects persons from all groups in the United States, black or Hispanic poor persons are overrepresented. True iatrogenic opioid dependence rarely persists to become chronic, although the risk exists for those with chronic, painful medical or surgical problems. Although men and women seek treatment in roughly equal numbers, women who are mothers of dependent children may benefit from a more favorable prognosis.

Opioid addiction follows a relapsing and remitting course until middle age, when its relentless grip on the individual seems to abate slowly and spontaneously. Some experts have estimated 9 years as the average duration of active opioid addiction (Jaffe, 1989). Criminal activity, usually in support of addiction, is very common during periods of active use. In periods of remission, criminal activity drops off significantly. The overall death rate in opioid abusers is estimated to be as much as 20 times that of the general population. The proximate cause of death is usually overdose, use-related infections, suicide, homicide, or accidental death.

Significant psychiatric comorbidity has been observed; depression and personality disorder are the most frequent diagnoses. Polysubstance abuse is common in opioid addicts. Many are nicotine addicted, and many have serious alcohol-related problems as well. Benzodiazepine use is common and probably underestimated, because it may not be specifically assayed in urine specimens. Sporadic use of cocaine and other stimulants is common, as is the use of marijuana. A few opioid addicts also use hallucinogens or inhalants.

The medical complications of opioid abuse are many and diverse. They stem most commonly from (1) the failure to use aseptic techniques during injection, (2) the presence of particulate contaminants in the injected solution, and (3) the direct pharmacological actions of the drug. The consequences of infection are the most frequently encountered medical complications of opioid abuse. Skin abscesses, lymphadenopathy, osteomyelitis, septic emboli in the lungs, endocarditis, septicemia, glomerulonephritis, meningitis, and brain abscesses are encountered with regularity when "dirty needles" are used. A low-level immunodeficiency may exist in chronic opioid addicts, causing them to be more susceptible to infectious processes such as tuberculosis, syphilis, malaria, tetanus, and hepatitis (Senay, 1983). HIV infection may result from sharing needles with an infected individual. Risk of this complication is highest in the northeastern United States, where a survey of opioid addicts in methadone treatment programs showed seropositivity in 60% of those who reported sharing needles (Jaffe, 1989). Fortunately, the percentage drops dramatically in most other parts of the country, and aggressive efforts at education of both addicts and those who treat them in clinics and elsewhere have helped slow the spread of this deadly virus.

Addicts frequently inject opioid solutions contaminated with adulterants such as talc and starch; these substances are used to increase the bulk of the illicit powder, thus increasing profits for the drug dealer. Addicts mix the powder with water, heat it, and use cotton or a cigarette filter to block the entry of undissolved particles as the solution is drawn into the syringe. As a result, fibers enter the venous bloodstream and lodge in the lungs, where conditions become favorable for the development over time of pulmonary thrombosis (emboli arise at distant sites), pulmonary hypertension, and right-side heart failure. Opioid abusers are at further risk of compromised pulmonary function if they use cigarettes and marijuana, as they often do. The antitussive effect of opioids also compromises pulmonary function, contributing to frequent pneumonia and other respiratory tract infections.

A number of lesions may occur in the central nervous system of those persons who have survived overdoses that featured anoxia and coma. The residual effects of such trauma include partial paralysis, parkinsonism, intellectual impairment, personality changes, peripheral neuropathy, acute transverse myelitis, and blindness.

Psychiatric comorbidity caused by opioid dependence occurs most frequently in the form of depression. When depression is observed during the recovery period, treatment with antidepressants and psychotherapy is indicated and frequently helpful if the individual is abstinent from illicit drug use. Dysphoria is common during with withdrawal interval, and is not helped by antidepressants, but rather by appropriate treatment of withdrawal symptoms.

The following disorders also are seen in association with opioid dependence:

1. Bipolar disorder.
2. Antisocial personality disorder.
3. Anxiety disorders.
4. Other personality disorders, including paranoid, schizoid, schizotypal, histrionic, narcissistic, borderline, dependent, obsessive–compulsive, and mixed.
5. Delirium and dementia (rare).
6. Schizophrenia (very rare).

Mood disorders may be diagnosable in many opioid addicts (Mirin, Weiss, Michael, & Griffin, 1989). Major depression is the most common mood disorder, diagnosed at almost 16% (Brooner, King, Kidorf, Schmidt, & Bigelow, 1997); it may have preceded the onset of drug abuse as chronic, episodic low-grade depression or dysthymia, and a full-blown major depressive episode may develop in the stressful and traumatic context of opioid addiction. Depression occurs more frequently in women than in men. Depression coexisting with opioid dependence is more strongly associated with a history of concomitant polydrug abuse. More attention is being paid to the complicating presence of attention-deficit/hyperactivity disorder (ADHD; King, Brooner, Kidorf, Stoller, & Mirsky, 1999).

Of the personality disorders, antisocial personality disorder is the most commonly diagnosed and can be seen in as many as 25% of opioid abusers seeking treatment; this is noted in men the vast majority of the time (Brooner et al., 1997). It is inaccurate to assume that drug-seeking behavior learned during years of addiction is responsible for the high percentage of antisocial personalities among opioid addicts. Antisocial personality disorder can be reliably diagnosed historically in most individuals at a young age, prior to the onset of opioid dependence. The relationship between opioid abuse and antisocial personality is complicated and appears to be influenced by a non-sex-linked genetic factor. When antisocial personality and opioid dependence are found together, the treatment course is frequently challenging, and the overall outcome is poor with regard to adequate length of time in treatment, relapse, criminal behavior during treatment, and ability to establish rapport with a therapist or counselor. The one exception appears to be the antisocial addict who also has a diagnosable depression. This group responds much better to treatment, on a par with the average opioid addict without significant psychiatric comorbidity (Woody, McLellan, Luborsky, & O'Brien, 1985).

Anxiety disorders, such as panic disorder, obsessive–compulsive disorder, generalized anxiety disorder, and phobia, are seen in approximately 10% of opioid addicts. Members of this group are typically somewhat younger in age and higher in socioeconomic status, and their drug use histories are not as extensive.

Delirium, dementia, and psychotic disorders such as schizophrenia, mania, and psychotic depression are not usually seen in opioid clinic populations. The presence of both a DSM-IV Axis I diagnosis (depression or an anxiety disorder) and an Axis II diagnosis (a personality disorder) in the same opioid-dependent individual is frequently observed; the proportion of such patients may approach 50% in clinic populations (Khantzian & Treece, 1985).

TREATMENT

The various nonpharmacological treatment modalities used to treat other types of substance abusers are also useful in treating opioid addicts, and are discussed in Chapter 19. The focus of this chapter is on pharmacotherapy of situations commonly found in the context of opioid use, including overdose, withdrawal, detoxification, and maintenance.

Intoxication

The management of opioid overdose is best accomplished in a medical facility with the availability of sophisticated expertise and technology. These can be brought to bear on the potential "worst-case scenario," for example, opioid overdose in a pregnant female with septicemia, pulmonary edema, and coma. In addition to intensive physiological support needed in opioid overdose, the use of an opioid antagonist can be life saving. Naloxone is the drug of choice, because it does not further depress respiratory drive (Berger & Dunn, 1986). A regimen of 0.4–0.8 mg, administered intravenously several times over the course of 20–30 minutes, is usually effective. If after 10 mg of naloxone there is no improvement in the patient's condition, one must question the diagnosis of opioid overdose. Other drugs may be involved, or other central nervous system processes may exist. One also must remember that the action of naloxone almost always will be shorter than the action of the opioid, necessitating close attention to the reemergence of the opioid's physiological effects (Wilford, 1981). The use of opiate antagonists in tolerant individuals will precipitate opiate withdrawal.

Withdrawal

The opioid withdrawal syndrome can easily be suppressed by administering any opioid with significant same-receptor agonism as the drug that originally produced the addiction. However, it is more useful to prevent opioid withdrawal symptoms pharmacologically with a nonaddicting drug. This approach furthers the goals of detoxification and abstinence. When circumstances force addicts to treat their withdrawal symptoms without opioids, they most commonly use alcohol and/or benzodiazepines. The main disadvantage to this approach is that because of the lack of cross-tolerance between opioids and alcohol/benzodiazepines, blockade of withdrawal symptoms requires the ingestion of large amounts of these sedatives to achieve suppression. Clonidine, a presynaptic alpha$_2$ agonist originally marketed as an antihypertensive, represents an effective and safer alternative for the treatment of opiate withdrawal symptoms (Koob & Bloom, 1988; O'Connor et al., 1995). It can partially suppress many (but not all) elements of opioid withdrawal, so that the risk of immediate relapse is reduced (Jasinski, Johnson, & Kocher, 1985). Clonidine is most effective for those motivated persons who are involved in their overall treatment program and are using small amounts of opioid (Kleber et al., 1985). Outpatients who are on less than 20 mg of methadone per day and detoxifying at rates approaching 1 mg per day make ideal candidates for the adjunctive use of clonidine. These individuals can be given 0.1 to 0.3 mg up to three or four times a day throughout the withdrawal period, with good effect. Sometimes only small amounts of clonidine (on the order of 0.1 mg per day) may be useful, to be administered at the time of day that is most difficult for the patient. Clonidine is not generally useful beyond 2 weeks after the last dose of methadone (Gold, Pottash, Sweeney, & Kleber, 1980). A transdermal delivery system (Catapres-TTS), which is active over a 7-day period, is useful in the outpatient setting, because the indiscriminate use of large amounts of clonidine by the individual can be avoided, thus limiting the risk of adverse reactions (Spencer & Gregory, 1989). Hypotension and bradycardia are major side effects of clonidine, and can be profound. Lethargy is also common, but this effect can be useful at night.

In a hospital setting, clonidine has been used in concert with abstinence and an opioid antagonist to produce tolerable withdrawal and detoxification in a short period (5–6 days) for persons on methadone doses of 50 mg or less; various protocols exist (Charney, Heninger, & Kleber, 1986). This treatment can be complicated by delirium and/or psychosis (Brewer, Rezae, & Bailey, 1988). The treatment involves sudden cessation of opioid ingestion, precipitation of an acute abstinence syndrome with an opioid antagonist, and aggressive treatment of the withdrawal symptoms with large doses of clonidine throughout the day and benzodiazepines at night. Over the 5- to 6-day course, the clonidine and opioid blocker are tapered. Naltrexone with buprenorphine has been used successfully (Cheskin, Fudala, & Johnson, 1994; Gerra et al., 1995), and this combination produces the shortest and least severe withdrawal interval. Benzodiazepines are not routinely used after the second or third night, and there is a risk of synergistic respiratory suppression in the coadministration of benzodiazepines and full or partial opiate agonists. A more time-consuming approach would involve abstinence not precipitated suddenly by an opioid blocker and more aggressive use of clonidine than would be practical in an outpatient setting. These approaches are appropriate for those individuals who are highly motivated to become drug-free quickly in a controlled manner, for reasons related to employment or to impending incarceration.

It is generally recognized that abrupt withdrawal from opioids is almost always followed by relapse. The risk of relapse is less with a rational plan for detoxification, using decreasing amounts of an opioid over time. In this way, the withdrawal syndrome is minimized, rendering the individual more responsive to other, nonpharmacological therapies during this high-risk phase of treatment. In the United States, the usual first step toward detoxification is to switch the addicted individual to a longer acting opioid. Methadone is the obvious choice, with a half-life of 15–25 hours in comparison to 2–3 hours for morphine, heroin, and many other commonly available opioids. In addition to methadone, LAAM was approved in 1993 as a maintenance treatment agent for opioid dependence; however, because of growing awareness of life-threatening arrhythmias, it is no longer used. Generally speaking, for every 2 mg of heroin, 1 mg of methadone may be substituted. The same is true for 4 mg of morphine, 20 mg of meperidine, 50 mg of codeine, and 12 mg of oxycodone. Other equivalencies are available in standard pharmacology texts.

Usually, it is not possible to know how much heroin a user is actually administering in a 24-hour period because of the impure nature of the product available on the street. Experience shows that an initial dose of 20–30 mg of methadone will block most withdrawal symptoms in moderate to heavy users who may inject from four to 12 or more times in 24 hours. For those who inject two to three times per day, a starting dose of 10–20 mg of methadone is usually sufficient. Methadone may be given every 24 hours, and the dose may be adjusted daily up or down by 5- to 10-mg increments, based on observable symptoms of withdrawal or intoxication. The peak plasma levels from methadone occur between 2 and 6 hours after ingestion. Over time, methadone becomes tissue-bound throughout the body, creating a buffer against significant withdrawal in those persons who occasionally miss a daily dose. This phenomenon also facilitates a smooth detoxification over time as daily dosage is reduced. Stabilization on methadone can usually be accomplished with 20–50 mg daily. Detoxification may then begin. Federal law allows the use of opiates for detoxification only when doses are dispensed directly by the provider. Of course, methadone may only be dispensed for the treatment of opiate addiction by a licensed clinic.

For the hospitalized patient, federal law allows the administration of opiates for a maximum of 3 days, or longer as required, if the patient is primarily admitted for a general medical condition. Any opiate may be selected, but common choices are methadone, buprenorphine, or propoxyphene.

Regulations at the various levels of government historically mandated that outpatient detoxification be accomplished within 21 days. Unfortunately, this period was too short for all but the most minimally addicted individuals and frequently resulted in relapse. Fortunately, the regulations have been liberalized, largely because of recognition that HIV/AIDS is spread very rapidly among intravenous drug abusers who share needles. Changes in the regulations are intended to allow more addicts to enter and stay in treatment. As a practical matter, 30 days is the minimum amount of time required for successful detoxification, and often 45 days or more may be needed; relapse still is a definite risk. For those individuals with long abuse histories and high doses of opioids, 6 months or more may be required. Veteran opioid users are extremely sensitive to even small reductions in their daily dose of methadone. The critical stage of detoxification occurs below 20 mg of methadone daily, and the use of clonidine is helpful in blocking withdrawal symptoms. In some individuals, detoxification is successful, but symptoms of insomnia, malaise, irritability, fatigue, gastrointestinal hypermotility, and even premature ejaculation may persist for months. Clonidine is less effective in this situation.

Ultrarapid detoxification (URD) under anesthesia, which has received a great deal of recent attention and controversy, is not generally accepted as cost-effective in the long term but may be useful in special cases (Hensel & Kox, 2000). Naltrexone maintenance, which probably is underutilized as a general treatment technique, has been utilized in follow-up after URD (Rabinowitz, Cohen, & Atias, 2002).

Acupuncture may be helpful in detoxification, as well as maintenance, although scientific studies are limited (Otto, 2003).

Maintenance

After detoxification, relapse prevention must be actively addressed with whatever treatment interventions are available.

Unfortunately, a large percentage of addicts seem unable to tolerate acute withdrawal, to succeed at controlled detoxification, or to remain drug free. Methadone maintenance may then become the treatment of choice. Administered on a once-a-day schedule, methadone in appropriate doses blocks opioid withdrawal, thus reducing compulsive drug-seeking behavior and use. The individual may then focus energy and attention on more productive behaviors. Indications for the use of methadone maintenance include (1) a history of chronic, high-dose opioid abuse; (2) repeated failures at abstinence; (3) history of prior successful methadone maintenance; (4) history of drug-related criminal convictions or incarcerations; (5) pregnancy, especially first and third trimesters; and (6) HIV seropositivity.

Relative contraindications to methadone maintenance include (1) age less than 16 years, (2) the expectation of incarceration within 30–45 days, and (3) history of abuse of methadone maintenance, including diversion of methadone to "the street" and failure to cease illicit use despite adequate doses.

The administration of methadone, as noted earlier, is heavily regulated by Federal and state governments. Specific requirements must be met by individuals and clinics offering this service. Generally, after the individual's history and physical condition are assessed, methadone dosing begins according to the protocol previously described. A period of 4–10 days may be required to stabilize the patient at an appropriate dose. When stabilization has occurred, the individual's illicit drug use should cease, as evidenced by regular, monitored urinalysis showing only methadone. Methadone maintenance programs that maintain an overall average dose of 60–100 mg a day yield consistently better results in decreasing illicit opioid use. Doses in excess of 120 mg a day are seldom needed (Gerstein, 1990). A pitfall here is that individuals may supplement their maintenance dose with "black market" methadone. Urinalyses will not be helpful in detecting this behavior, since quantification techniques are not generally employed. Dosage requirements should not change after stabilization, unless something has occurred to change the body's absorption, metabolism, distribution, or excretion of methadone. Emesis within 20–30 minutes after the oral ingestion of methadone is an obvious example of disruption to absorption. Metabolism of methadone may be increased by the use of phenytoin, rifampin, barbiturates, carbamazepine, and some tricyclic antidepressants, all of which can precipitate withdrawal symptoms by reducing methadone plasma levels. Concealed regular use of other opiates in addition to methadone will result in the user's asking for more methadone, because the development of tolerance has outpaced current stable dosing. Abusive use of alcohol and/or benzodiazepines with methadone maintenance will also cause individuals to request more methadone, possibly because of enhanced hepatic metabolism and/or significant withdrawal symptoms from these agents that do not share cross-tolerance with methadone. Administering disulfiram with methadone is a common and highly useful therapeutic approach.

Some individuals report that heavy labor with much perspiration reduces the effectiveness of methadone in a 24-hour period. This phenomenon is usually easily addressed with a small increase in dose, unless the individual is not being truthful. After months or years of methadone maintenance, most individuals are able to tolerate a slow taper of a few milligrams per week or month. For those persons who become suspicious or psychologically unstable as their dose is lowered, a "blind" detoxification schedule may be used, in which the individual never knows the exact amount of methadone he or she is receiving.

Pregnancy is a special situation for which continued methadone maintenance is recommended, because any withdrawal symptoms place the fetus at risk for spontaneous abortion (Finnegan, 1979). In addition, relapse to street drugs after detoxification also places the fetus at risk. Therefore, maintenance at a level of 20 mg is the safest plan. Slow detoxification down to this level can be achieved safely during the second trimester.

Other agents may be useful in maintenance of opioid users. Safety, regulatory, and political concerns unfortunately have limited the availability of methadone maintenance, so that a significant number of opiate dependent individuals who might benefit from this therapy fail to receive it. Because of these problems, the federal government in 2003 approved buprenorphine for use in the treatment of opiate withdrawal and maintenance. As previously discussed, buprenorphine is a long half-life (24 hours), mixed opiate agonist–antagonist. A dose of 8–16 mg of sublingual buprenorphine (Subutex) administered daily for 2–4 days can be extremely effective in ameliorating withdrawal symptoms (Bickel et al., 1988). For maintenance treatment, this same dose of sublingual buprenorphine (in combination with naltrexone to prevent street value, marketed as Suboxone) has been shown to be equivalently effective to methadone and LAAM in preventing relapse (Johnson et al., 2000; Mattick et al., 2003; Petitjean et al., 2001). Unlike methadone and LAAM, buprenorphine may be prescribed in the general office setting by practitioners specially qualified through the Drug Enforcement Agency. Currently, candidates for qualification are those practitioners who are either subspecialty boarded in addiction psychiatry, or who have received 8 hours of training through the American Academy of Addiction Psychiatry or the American Society of Addiction Medicine.

A pharmacological agent in the form of an opioid antagonist can be a useful adjunct in relapse prevention. A long-acting antagonist such as naltrexone (ReVia) is effective in blocking the euphoric effects of opioids and ultimately leads to the extinction of operantly conditioned drug-seeking behaviors. Naltrexone is given orally in the opioid-free individual three times a week in doses of 50–150 mg, and it blocks the effects of relatively large doses of opioids (Johnson & Strain, 1999). This adjunctive therapy works best in the context of ongoing treatment and support. Its administration should be monitored over time, because compliance with voluntary, unsupervised self-administration of naltrexone is notoriously poor. Length of treatment with this agent is a therapeutic issue having mainly to do with the individual's ability to embrace a drug-free lifestyle consistently over time. Because of the significant risk of developing hepatitis during naltrexone treatment, monitoring of liver function tests is important.

Psychosocial Treatments

Although this chapter has presented only pharmacotherapies for opioid addiction, it is crucial that psychosocial interventions be used to help these patients change their lifestyles. It is generally accepted that escape from drug seeking and the accompanying antisocial impulses requires a change in deeply rooted behavioral patterns. Individual and group psychotherapy may be useful in approaching this goal. Contingency management may be very helpful (Robles, Stitzer, Strain, Bigelow, & Silverman, 2002). The various 12-step programs such as Narcotics Anonymous are also useful adjuncts to treatment and facilitate significant degrees of change. For those persons who continue to relapse in less restrictive treatment settings, a "therapeutic community" may be the appropriate next step (O'Brien & Biase, 1981); these nonhospital, community-based, 24-hour, live-in programs are geared to subject the addict to continuous treatment pressure for as long as 1 or 2 years. Personal freedom is severely curtailed, and community rules are rigorously enforced. The goal is to use nonviolent but highly confrontational tactics, in the context of peer pressure, for the purpose of breaking down denial and exposing destructive attitudes and behaviors that formerly led to drug use (Rosenthal, 1989). A growth process may then occur, allowing the individual to achieve a degree of personal integrity that is unrelated to the former identity of drug abuser. When successful, this type of personal transformation can lead to permanent recovery. However, this form of treatment requires total commitment, which many opioid addicts are unable to make; thus, the dropout rate is high. As with any treatment modality, selection of appropriate candidates leads to greater success.

REFERENCES

American Psychiatric Association. (2000). *Diagnostic and statistical manual of mental disorders* (4th ed., text rev.). Washington, DC: Author.

Berger, P. A., & Dunn, M. J. (1986). The biology and treatment of drug abuse. In S. Arieti (Ed.), *American handbook of psychiatry* (Vol. 8, pp. 811–822). New York: Basic Books.

Bickel, W. K., Stitzer, M. L., Bigelow, G. E., Liebson, I. A., Jasinski, D. R., & Johnson, R. E. (1988). A clinical trial of buprenorphine: Comparison with methadone in the detoxification of heroin addicts. *Clin Pharmacol Ther, 43,* 72–78.

Brewer, C., Rezae, H., & Bailey, C. (1988). Opioid withdrawal and naltrexone induction in 48–72 hours with minimal drop-out, using a modification of the naltrexone–clonidine technique. *Br J Psychiatry, 153,* 340–343.

Brooner, R. K., King, V. L., Kidorf, M., Schmidt, C. W. Jr., & Bigelow, G. E. (1997). Psychiatric and substance use comorbidity among treatment-seeking opioid abusers. *Arch Gen Psychiatry, 54,* 71–80.

Charney, D. S., Heninger, G. R., & Kleber, H. D. (1986). The combined use of clonidine and naltrexone as a rapid, safe, and effective treatment of abrupt withdrawal from methadone. *Am J Psychiatry, 143,* 831–837.

Cheskin, L. J., Fudala, P. J., & Johnson, R. E. (1994). A controlled comparison of buprenorphine and clonidine for acute detoxification from opioids. *Drug Alcohol Depend, 36,* 115–121.

Deneau, G. A., & Mule, S. J. (1981). Pharmacology of the opiates. In J. H. Lowinson & P. Ruiz (Eds.), *Substance abuse: Clinical problems and perspectives* (pp. 129–139). Baltimore: Williams & Wilkins.

Finnegan, L. P. (Ed.). (1979). *Drug dependency in pregnancy: Clinical management of mother and child.* Rockville, MD: National Institute on Drug Abuse.

Gerra, G., Marcato, A., Caccavari, R., Fontanesi, B., Deisignore, R., Fertonani, G., et al. (1995). Clonidine and opiate receptor antagonists in the treatment of heroin addiction. *J Subst Abuse Treat, 12,* 35–41.

Gerstein, D. R. (1990). The effectiveness of treatment. In D. R. Gerstein & H. J. Harwood (Eds.), *Treating drug problems* (Vol. 1, pp. 132–199). Washington, DC: National Academy Press.

Gold, M. S., Pottash, A. C., Sweeney, D. R., & Kleber, H. D. (1980). Opiate withdrawal using clonidine. *JAMA, 243*(4), 343–346.

Hensel, M., & Kox, W. J. (2000). Safety, efficacy, and long-term results of a modified version of rapid opiate detoxification under general anesthesia: A prospective study in methadone, heroin, codeine, and morphine addicts. *Acta Anaesthsiol Scand, 44*(3), 326–333.

Jaffe, J. H. (1989). Psychoactive substance use disorders. In H. I. Kaplan & B. J. Sadock (Eds.), *Comprehensive textbook of psychiatry* (5th ed., pp. 642–698). Baltimore: Williams & Wilkins.

Jasinski, D. R., Johnson, R. E., & Kocher, T. R. (1985). Clonidine in morphine withdrawal: Differential effects on signs and symptoms. *Arch Gen Psychiatry, 42,* 1063–1066.

Johnson, R. E., Chutuape, M. A., Strain, E. C., Walsh, S. L., Stitzer, M. L., & Bigelow, G. E. (2000). A comparison of levomethadyl acetate, buprenorphine, and methadone for opioid dependence. *N Engl J Med, 343,* 1290–1297.

Johnson, R. E., & Strain, E. C. (1999). Other medications for opioid dependence. In E. C. Strain & M. L. Stitzer (Eds.), *Methadone treatment for opioid dependence* (pp. 281–321). Baltimore: Johns Hopkins University Press.

Khantzian, E. J., & Treece, C. (1985). DSM-III psychiatric diagnosis of narcotic addicts: Recent findings. *Arch Gen Psychiatry, 42,* 1067–1071.

King, V. L., Brooner, R. K., Kidorf, M. S., Stoller, K. B., & Mirsky, A. F. (1999). Attention deficit hyperactivity disorder and treatment outcome in opioid abusers entering treatment. J Nerv Ment Dis, 187(8), 487–495.

Kleber, H. D., Riordan, C. E., Rounsaville, B., Kosten, T., Charney, D., Gaspari, J., et al. (1985). Clonidine in outpatient detoxification from methadone maintenance. Arch Gen Psychiatry, 42, 391–394.

Koob, G. F., & Bloom, F. E. (1988). Cellular and molecular mechanisms of drug dependence. Science, 242, 715–723.

Martin, W. R., & Jasinski, D. R. (1969). Physiological parameters of morphine dependence in men: Tolerance, early abstinence, protracted abstinence. J Psychiatr Res, 7, 9–17.

Mattick, R. P., Ali, R., White, J. M., O'Brien, S., Wolk, S., & Danz, C. (2003). Buprenorphine versus methadone maintenance therapy: A randomized double blind trial with 405 opioid-dependent patients. Addiction, 98, 441–452.

Mirin, S. M., Weiss, R. D., Michael, J., & Griffin, M. L. (1989). Psychopathology in substance abusers: Diagnosis and treatment. Am J Drug Alcohol Abuse, 14, 139–157.

O'Brein, W. B., & Biase, D. V. (1981). The therapeutic community: The family-milieu approach to recovery. In J. H. Lowinson & P. Ruiz (Eds.), Substance abuse: Clinical problems and perspectives (pp. 303–316). Baltimore: Williams & Wilkins.

O'Connor, P. G., Waugh, M. E., Carroll, K. M., Rounsaville, B. J., Diagkogiannis, I. A., & Schottenfeld, R. S. (1995). Primary care-based ambulatory opioid detoxification: The results of a clinical trial. J Gen Intern Med, 10, 255–260.

Otto, K. C. (2003). Acupuncture and substance abuse: A synopsis, with indications for further research. Am J Addict, 12(1), 43–51.

Petitjean, S., Stohler, R., Deglon, J. J., Livoti, S., Waldvogel, D., Uehlinger, C., & Ladenwig, D. (2001). Double-blind randomized trial of buprenorphine and methadone in opiate dependence. Drug Alcohol Depend, 62, 97–104.

Rabinowitz, J., Cohen, H., & Atias, S. (2002). Outcome of naltrexone maintenance following ultra rapid opiate detoxification versus intensive inpatient detoxification. Am J Addict, 11(1), 52–56.

Robles, E., Stitzer, M. I., Strain, E. C., Bigelow, G. E., & Silverman, K. (2002). Voucher-based reinforcement of opiate abstinence during methadone detoxification. Drug Alcohol Depend, 65(2), 179–189.

Rosenthal, M. S. (1989). The therapeutic community: Exploring the boundaries. Br J Addict, 84, 141–150.

Senay, E. C. (1983). Substance abuse disorders in clinical practice. Littleton, MA: John Wright/PSG.

Spencer, L., & Gregory, M. (1989). Clonidine transdermal patches for use in outpatient opiate withdrawal. J Subst Abuse, 6, 113–117.

Substance Abuse and Mental Health Services Administration. (1995, November). Preliminary estimates from the Drug Abuse Warning Network (Advance Report No. 11). Washington, DC: Author.

Wilford, B. B. (1981). Drug abuse for the primary care physician. Chicago: American Medical Association.

Woody, G. E., McLellan, A. T., Luborsky, L., & O'Brien, C. P. (1985). Sociopathy and psychotherapy outcome. Arch Gen Psychiatry, 42, 1081–1086.

CHAPTER 8

Marijuana, Hallucinogens, and Club Drugs

DAVID McDOWELL

Hallucinogens consist of a disparate group of psychoactive substances, and include 3,4-methylenedioxyamphetamine (MDMA), hallucinogens, ketamine, and marijuana. They differ in terms of administration, mechanism of action, and effect. In many cases, they are used by groups of younger people and are taken in various combinations with each other and other classes of substances, usually in social settings (often at "raves" [see Bellis, Hale, Bennett, Chaudry, & Kilfoyle, 2000] or other parties). At some of these events, a substantial majority of rave participants are using MDMA, ketamine, gamma-hydroxy-butyric acid (GHB), or other drugs, such as marijuana and D-lysergic acid diethylamide (LSD). In addition, at times inhalants are used at these events (Lee & McDowell, 2003; McDowell & Kleber, 1994; Winstock, Griffiths, & Stewart, 2001). Polysubstance might be considered the norm at such events, with over 80% of participants using more than one substance (Boys, Lenton, & Norcross, 1997; Winstock et al., 2001). Although the demographics and settings of use have changed, these substances remain significant clinical problems.

MARIJUANA

Marijuana refers to the dried-out leaves, flowers, stems, and seeds of the hemp plant, *Cannabis sativa*. The plant is a common weed that grows freely in most areas of the world. Marijuana, also known as cannabis, is also probably the most commonly used, abusable substance in the world, with the U.N. World Drug Report (1997) estimating 140 million daily users. It is most frequently smoked in small, hand-rolled cigarettes called "joints" (Schwartz, 2002). Alternatively, users employ regular pipes or water pipes called "bongs." The resin from the flowering tips, hashish, is more potent and may also be smoked (Abel, 1980). Marijuana can also be ingested; usually this occurs when it's baked into lipid-rich foods, such as brownies.

Peak popularity occurred in the late 1970s, then steadily declined until 1992. Since that time, marijuana's use has been on the rise, and whether its current level of use has reached a plateau phase is still a subject of debate. Marijuana has many purported uses; in recent years, the debate over its controversial role as a medicine has been revived.

History

Marijuana has been used since antiquity, and it can be found in numerous ancient texts. The oldest known reference to marijuana is in a 15th-century B.C. Chinese text on herbal remedy (Walton, 1938). Also, Assyrian cuneiform tablets from 650 B.C. that contain references to people smoking marijuana "are generally regarded as obvious copies of much older texts," according to Walton. Although archeological findings in Berlin, Germany, suggest that marijuana was in Western Europe by 500 B.C., an exact date or extent of use is unknown. However, hemp-based clothing was widespread in central and southern Italy, and the intoxicating effects of marijuana were also recorded in Renaissance texts. In Europe, it was quite popular in 19th-century high society. In the United States, in the beginning of this century, it was popular principally in the West and was mostly associated with ethnic groups and jazz musicians. Marijuana's social stigma, epitomized in the now-popular classic cult film *Reefer Madness*, led Congress to enact the Marijuana Tax Act of 1937 (Bonnie & Whitebread, 1974). This legislation calls for the requirement of a federally approved stamp for commerce with marijuana. No such stamps were ever issued, however.

Marijuana, considered benign by many, became more popular as a mainstream drug in late the1960s, coinciding with the growing drug subculture. Its peak use was in 1979, when approximately 51% of high school seniors admitted to having tried it (Johnson, O'Malley, & Bachman, 2002). Perhaps due to the public's exposure to individuals who used the drug frequently and suffered lethargy and impairment from it, as well as pressure from the newly emerging law in drugs, marijuana use declined substantially through the 1980s, bottoming out at 22% in 1992 (Johnson et al., 2002). The mid-1990s, however, saw substantial increase in the popularity of the drug, with 1996 being the peak year for 8th graders, and 1997 for 10th and 12th graders. Coinciding with this resurgence of drug use, mainstream iconographic representations of the marijuana plant also began appearing on numerous articles of clothing (from such companies as *www.happyhippie.com* or *www.hempstyle.com*), worn by both adolescents and adults, thereby attesting to widespread renewed interest among marijuana users.

Mechanism of Action

Marijuana smokers usually inhale deeply, with the user keeping the smoke in his or her lungs for as long as possible. This allows for 25–50% of the delta-9-tetrahydrocannabinol (THC) in the marijuana cigarette to be absorbed. THC is the most potent, but by no means the only, active ingredient in marijuana. THC is the psychoactive substance of most studies, and the one that most literature agrees is responsible for its psychoactive property. THC is to marijuana as nicotine is to tobacco. The THC level in the blood is quickly distributed throughout the body, especially in areas with high fat content, such as the brain and testes for men. THC then leaches out, and small levels of the drug can be detected in the bloodsteam. This effect lasts for 2–4 days in a naive user and as long as 2 months in a heavy daily user. It should be noted that though the urine test would be positive in such a person, the marijuana would not be intoxicating, unless the person had used additional doses. As with other drugs of abuse, it is the rise in concentration of THC that is intoxicating, and this residual amount that leaches out into the bloodsteam probably does not have much effect on the user.

While the effects of the drug can be felt almost immediately, usually heralded by the giggles of the new initiator, the peak effect occurs after about 20 minutes. The user feels a mild euphoria, an alternation of sensory acuity, and a distortion of time perception. These effects gradually diminish over the next 3–4 hours. For persons who ingest marijuana, the effects also begin in 20–30 minutes but peak at about 2 hours. The effects of the orally ingested drug usually last for up to 8 hours. Most users of the oral form cite it as reinforcing, but describe the subjective effect as "heavy." The molecular bases of THC's actions are only now being understood. It has a number of physiological properties that act like a barbiturate, and it has anticonvulsant activity, as well as opioid properties, causing weak analgesia and antidiarrheal action. In addition, it suppresses rapid eye movement (REM) nondream sleep. Smokers of marijuana usually report an increase in nonrestorative sleep. It increases brain limbic stimulation and is thought to activate the pleasure/reward system in the brain. It is for this reason that it is an addictive agent.

In recent years, a specific receptor in the mammalian and hence the human brain has been discovered and, in fact, cloned (Sugiura & Waku, 2002). There are at least two subtypes of this receptor. Along with it, a natural ligand in marijuana, anandamide, has been identified. Substances of abuse mimic molecules that naturally occur in the brain. Such compounds (the naturally occurring ones), called ligands, have an effect on the receptors to which they have an affinity. This effect may be to stimulate, to inhibit, or a variety of in-between effects. The natural ligand for marijuana is called anandamide, and its receptor is the anandamide receptor. Interestingly, the term "anandamide" is derived from the Hindi word for bless. At present, pharmaceutical companies have synthesized both agonists and antagonists to the receptor. Much research has been conducted to identify the properties of these compounds, but it is still unclear what function they serve in mammalian and human brains. Cannabinoid receptors have been described in various regions of the brain, with the greatest abundance in the basal ganglia and hippocampus, areas involved with memory function.

The hemp plant synthesizes at least 400 chemicals, of which more than 60 are cannabinoid. Pyrolyzing the plant can create even more molecules. Very little is known about the vast majorities of these molecules or their effects on human. The most psychologically and physiologically active compound is THC. In the pyrolyzed form, it actually becomes delta-11-tetrahydrocanbonol. This molecule is believed to account for most of marijuana's effects. There are, however, numerous compounds whose effects remain completely unknown. For instance, it is known that marijuana use raises the seizure threshold overall and makes it more difficult to have a seizure (Zagnoni & Albano, 2002). THC alone decreases the seizure threshold. This property of marijuana, therefore, is not the result of THC, but rather some other cannabinoid. The two most abundant cannabinoids are cannabinol and cannabidiol. Much research is currently underway regarding the possible use of marijuana in clinical or other settings.

Physiological Effects

Cannabis intoxication commonly heightens the user's sensitivity to external stimuli, thus making colors seem brighter and smells more pungent. It also distorts, sometimes severely, the user's sense of time. The term "temporal disintegration" (Mathew, Wilson, Humphreys, Lowe, & Weithe, 1993) has been coined to describe this slowing of subjective time after use of marijuana. In addition, at least in low doses, marijuana causes mild euphoria and feelings of relaxation. It is also know to increase appetite. There is some controversy over whether individuals intoxicated with cannabis pose a hazard, as they seem to be attracted to thrill-seeking behavior and are usually subdued. Some people have argued that individuals who smoke marijuana are less likely to drive fast; however, reaction time to complex and unforeseen situations is slowed, and muscle strength and hand–eye coordination is decreased. Because it delays reaction time, alters time perception, and for many other reasons, marijuana must be considered a danger to those who would operate a motor vehicle or use complex machinery or equipment, thus putting themselves and others in danger.

At higher dose levels and with chronic patterns of use, cannabis can induce panic attacks (Deas, Gerding, & Hazy, 2000). This is especially common in first-time users or in older experimenters who have not used marijuana for a long time. Hypervigilance, sometimes resembling frank paranoia, is seen with higher doses. Cannabis-induced psychosis is rare but does occur, especially in countries where heavy smoking is more common and the THC concentration of the plant is higher (Chopra & Smith, 1974). The term "hemp insanity" refers to this type of psychosis. The question of whether the drug causes long-term psychotic disorders is more difficult to answer. Clearly, first-break psychotic episodes are commonly associated with marijuana ingestion, but again, whether they are causal is a matter of debate. More probably, individuals who are prone to psychosis are attracted to the drug. In a population that is prone to psychosis, such as individuals with schizophrenia, marijuana is a risk factor for relapse and psychosis (Arseneault, Cannon, Witton, & Murray, 2004; Verdoux, Gindre, Sorbara, Tournier, & Swendsen, 2003).

Much has been written about the amotivational syndrome, and it has remained a controversial entity (Lynskey & Hall, 2000). It is marked by apathy, poor concentration, social withdrawal, and loss of interest in achievements (Solowij, 1998). Because research in the topic is contradictory, it is unclear at this time whether marijuana induces amotivational attitudes and behavior or causes permanent, irreversible impairment in cerebral function. However, the general consensus is that it likely does not cause permanent cognitive damage. Still, individuals who are chronic users tend to smoke marijuana often and in high doses; cannabis has a long half-life, and users can be thought to be chronically under the influence of marijuana or "stoned." So marijuana clearly causes impairment in the acquisition of short-term memory, at least for the time an individual is intoxicated, although there is evidence of specific residual effects (Block, 1996; Pope & Yurgelun-Todd, 1996; Schwartz, 1991). If an individual, especially a young person, is "stoned" nearly all the time, his or her accumulation of knowledge will be seriously impaired (Lynskey & Hall, 2000; Solowij, Michie, & Fox, 1995). If the intoxication continues long enough during critical growing time, it may have permanent consequences. This is the most dangerous and insidious aspect of marijuana use. A high school student who is constantly "stoned" will not learn to the degree to which he or she is capable of functioning. For many people, this will lead to a lifetime deficit that can never be completely repaired.

Treatment

Marijuana withdrawal has been demonstrated in laboratory animals, as well as in humans, and is now well documented. Chronic heavy users of cannabis may experience some withdrawal in the form of irritability, general discomfort, disrupted sleep, and decreased appetite (Budney, Moore, Vandrey, & Hughes, 2003). This syndrome is not as painful as that with heroin, as dangerous as that with alcohol, or as long-lasting as that with cocaine. It may contribute to relapse in some individuals.

The clinician is confronted with a wider range of marijuana users. At one end is the individual who uses the drug only rarely, but whose use is detected on a routine drug screen and brought to the clinician's attention, perhaps for an evaluation. Brief assessment, to make sure the problem is not more serious than it appears, is always necessary in this case. Subsequent follow-up, to ensure that the initial impression was correct, is part of a thorough assessment. In this instance, the user is usually embarrassed and repentant, and has no objection to future monitoring. Users who do not have a problem with marijuana do not have a problem giving it up. They may be able to use it in the future, once they have demonstrated the capacity for voluntary nonuse.

On the other end of spectrum is the person, most predictably the adolescent, who uses the drug both daily and heavily. In this case, the individual may need much more intensive rehabilitation and may need to be admitted to a residential drug treatment facility. In any case, the clinician must be alert to any underlying comorbid condition and treat it appropriately. Many researchers believe that marijuana is administered as a form of self-medication (Marmor, 1998).

The comorbid conditions that have been suggested to be associated with marijuana use range from the personality disorders to psychotic spectrum illness. In certain personality disorders, the drug's sedating and anxiolytic properties may be used to reduce painful affects. In some mode disorders, marijuana may be a form of self-medication for agitation, even manic or hypomanic states. This hypothesis is still quite intriguing and controversial; at the present time, there is only anecdotal and circumstantial evidence for its existence.

In recent years, there has been increased interest in "medicinal marijuana" (Iversen & Snyder, 1999) as an advocacy issue for such conditions as glaucoma (American Academy of Opthalmology, 1992; Hepler & Petrus, 1976; National Eye Institute, 1997), epilepsy (Feeney, 1976), nausea and other symptoms associated with cancer and chemotherapy (Kris et al., 1996; Maurer, Henn, Dittrich, & Hofmann, 1990; Nelson et al., 1994; Sallan, Zinberg, & Frei, 1975; Tramer et al., 2001; Vinciguerra, Moore, & Brennan, 1988). In general, there are better and safer agents for such medical conditions. Marijuana may, however, have some use, and the issue has been subject to much debate within the public arena, such as California voters' passing of the Compassionate Use Act (Proposition 215) (Marmor, 1998). Although the possible medicinal benefits of marijuana have been a matter of perennial debate within the medical community as well (Grinspoon & Bakalar, 1995; Kassirer, 1999), with articles and commentary frequently appearing in the *Journal of the American Medical Association* and the *New England Journal of Medicine*, the issue has yet to have been satisfactorily resolved through sound, scientifically methodical research (National Institutes of Health, 1997).

MDMA

MDMA has many names, but is perhaps best known as Ecstasy. It is sometimes classified as a stimulant and does have similar properties to the amphetamines, although it also has some unique effects that distinguish it (Hermle et al., 1993; Shulgin, 1986). MDMA was legal in this country until 1985, when it was made a Schedule I drug. Prior to that, its use was unregulated and therefore legal.

The primary appeal of MDMA is its psychological effect, a dramatic and consistent ability to induce a profound feeling of attachment and connection in the user. The compound's street name is perhaps a misnomer; the Los Angeles drug dealer who coined the term "Ecstasy" originally wanted to call the drug "Empathy," but asked, "Who would know what that means?" (Eisner, 1968).

MDMA has long been known to damage brain serotonin (5-HT) neurons in laboratory animals (McCann & Ricaurte, 1993; Montoya, Sorrentino, Lucas, & Price, 2002). Although a minority of researchers disagree with the conclusion, it has become increasingly apparent over the past decade that MDMA is neurotoxic to humans. Furthermore, the neurotoxicity has real and functional implications (McCann, Eligulashvili, & Ricaurte, 2000; Montoya et al., 2002; Morgan, 2000; Sprague, Everman, & Nichols, 1998). Ecstasy use is associated with sleep, mood, and anxiety disturbances, elevated impulsiveness, memory deficits, and attention problems. Many of these disturbances appear to be permanent and seem likely to depend on the overall amount of MDMA consumed over time, but may be caused by as little as a single dose (Rodgers, 2000; Turner & Parrott, 2000).

History

A synthetic process for the creation of MDMA was patented in 1914 by Merck in Darmstadt, Germany (Shulgin, 1990). MDMA was not, as is sometimes thought, intended as an appetite suppressant. It was most likely developed as an experimental compound. Except for a minor chemical modification mentioned in a patent in 1919, there is no other known historical record of MDMA until the 1950s. At that time, the United States Army experimented with MDMA. The resulting information was declassified and became available to the general public in the early 1970s. These findings consisted primarily of a number of LD_{50} (median lethal dose) determinations for a variety of laboratory animals.

Humans probably first used MDMA in the late 1960s. It was discovered as a recreational drug by free-thinking individualists (New Age seekers), people who liked its properties of inducing feelings of well-being and connection (Watson & Beck, 1986). MDMA does induce feelings of warmth and connectedness, and using this rationale, its use was promulgated by therapists in the 1970s (Shulgin, 1990). Before the compound became illegal in 1985, it was used extensively for this purpose (Beck, 1990).

Although for an organic chemist, the synthesis of MDMA is reasonably simple, most supplies in the United States are imported and then distributed by organized crime networks. Its price, usually $25–40 for a 125-mg tablet, the amount producing the sought-after effect in most intermittent users (Green, Cross, & Goodwin, 1995), has remained remarkably stable over the past two decades. This high price makes adulteration attractive to the criminal element. Such adulteration can be dangerous when the substance used is something that is physiologically dangerous. Paramethoxymethamphetamine (PMA) has been sold as MDMA, and in those unfortunate enough to consume both substances, appears to be highly dangerous.

Physiological Effects

MDMA is almost exclusively available in pill form. Often the pills are stamped with clever images. The usual single dose is 100–150 mg. The onset of effect begins about 20–40 minutes after ingestion and is experienced with immediacy. Often this "rush" is accompanied by nausea and an urgent need to defecate (*disco dump*).

The plateau stage of drug effects lasts 3–4 hours. The principal desired effect, according to most users, is a profound feeling of relatedness to the rest of the world. Most users experience this feeling as a powerful connection to those around them, as well as to the universe (Leister, Grob, Bravo, & Walsh, 1992). Although the desire for sex can increase, the ability to achieve arousal and orgasm is greatly diminished in both men and women (Buffum & Moser, 1986). MDMA has thus been termed a sensual, not a sexual, drug. The prescription drug sildenafil (Viagra) may be taken in order to counteract this effect, and may be sold along with MDMA (Weir, 2000); the successor medications involving sexual enhancement can be expected to be used in this manner. The array of physical effects and behaviors produced by MDMA is remarkably similar across mammalian species (Green et al., 1995) and includes mild psychomotor restlessness, bruxism, trismus, anorexia, diaphoresis, hot flashes, tremor, and piloerection (Peroutka, Newman, & Harris, 1998).

Aftereffects associated with MDMA are common and can be pronounced. People using MDMA once, or on multiple occasions, may experience any number of symptoms, including lethargy, anorexia, decreased motivation, sleepiness, depression, and fatigue. Combining MDMA with PMA has been associated with a number of serious adverse events and deaths (Ling, Marchant, Buckley, Prior, & Irvine, 2001). Another acute adverse event, hyponatremia, followed by seizure and coma, appears be a result of the law of unintended consequences. The "harm reduction" admonition of advising MDMA users to adopt the strategy of ingesting copious amounts of water prior to and while taking MDMA appears, in some instances, to have backfired and has caused these severe physiological adverse events (Ajaelo, Koenig, & Snoey, 1998; Holmes, Banerjee, & Alexander, 1999).

Severe, immediate effects appear to be rare, but they do occur: altered mental status, convulsions, hypo- or hyperthermia, severe changes in blood pressure, tachycardia, coagulopathy, acute renal failure, hepatotoxicity, rhabdomyolysis, and death have all occurred (Demirkiran, Jankovic, & Dean, 1996; Khalant, 2001). There are numerous case reports of a single dose of MDMA precipitating severe psychiatric illness. MDMA probably induces a range of depressive symptoms and anxiety in some individuals; for that reason, people with affective illness should be specifically cautioned about the dangers of using MDMA (Cohen, 1998; McCann, Ridenour, Shaham, & Ricaurte, 1994; McDowell, 1998).

Mechanism of Action

MDMA is a "dirty drug," affecting many neurotransmitter systems. It is primarily serotonergic, and its principal mechanism of action is as an indirect serotonergic agonist (Ames & Wirshing, 1993; Rattray, 1991; Sprague et al., 1998). The drug's effects, and side effects (an arbitrary distinction), including anorexia, psychomotor agitation, difficulty in achieving orgasm, and profound feelings of empathy, can be explained as a result of the flooding of the serotonin system (Beck & Rosenbaum, 1994). After ingestion, MDMA is taken up by the serotonin cells through active channels, effecting the release of serotonin stores. MDMA also blocks reuptake of serotonin, and this contributes to its length of action. Although it inhibits the synthesis of new serotonin, this does not contribute to the intoxication phase, but it may contribute to sustained feelings of depression reported by some users and to a diminished magnitude of subjective effects when the next dose is taken within a few days of the first dose.

Most people who use MDMA on a regular basis tend not to increase their use as time goes on (Cohen, 1998; Peroutka, 1990). Because of its mechanism of action (the drug depletes serotonin stores and inhibits synthesis of new serotonin), subsequent doses produce a diminished high and a worsening of the drug's undesirable effects, such as psychomotor restlessness and teeth gnashing. MDMA users most typically become aware of the benefits of periodic, even rare use. First-time users are often instant advocates of MDMA, only to have their enthusiasm dampen with time. An adage about Ecstasy captures this succinctly: "Freshmen love it, sophomores like it, juniors are ambivalent, and seniors are afraid of it" (Eisner, 1993).

MDMA's effects may be arbitrarily divided into short- and long-term categories (McKenna & Peroutka, 1990). The short-term effects presumably result from the acute release of serotonin and are associated with decreases in serotonin and 5-hydroxyindoleacetic acid (5-HIAA), and in tryptamine hydroxylase (TPH) activity. The long-term effects are manifested by a steady, slow decrease in serotonin and 5-HIAA after initial recovery, persistently depressed TPH activity, and a decrease in serotonin terminal density (Demirkiran et al., 1996; Ricaurte, McCann, Szabo, & Scheffel, 2000). 5-HIAA levels most typically recover to baseline levels within 24 hours.

Neurotoxicity

The most important individual and public health danger posed by the widespread use of MDMA is the likelihood that it causes the permanent destruction of serotonin axons in humans who use it. The ingestion of MDMA in laboratory animals causes a decrease in the serum and spinal fluid levels of 5-HIAA in a dose-dependent fashion (McCann et al., 2000; Shulgin, 1990) and damages brain serotonin neurons (Burgess, McDonoghoe, & Gill, 2000; McCann & Ricaurte, 1993; Montoya, Sorrentino, Lucas, & Price, 2002). The dosage necessary to cause permanent damage to most rodent species is many times greater than that normally ingested by humans (Shulgin, 1990). In nonhuman primates, the neurotoxic dosage approximates the recreational dosage taken by humans (McCann & Ricaurte, 1993). A recent study by Ricaurte and McCann (2001), which reported an alarmingly small dose necessary for the neurotoxicity to occur, has subsequently been retracted due to a human error in the laboratory (Walgate, 2003). Nevertheless, like its close structural relative methylenedioxyamphetamine (MDA, or "Eve"), MDMA has been found to damage serotonin neurons in all animal species tested to date (McCann, Slate, & Ricaurte, 1996), and the same is likely to occur in humans.

MDMA produces a 30–35% drop in serotonin metabolism in humans (McCann et al., 1994). Even one dose of MDMA may cause lasting damage to the serotonin system. There are many reports of individuals with lasting neuropsychiatric disturbances after MDMA use (Cohen, 1998; Creighton, Black, & Hyde, 1991; McCann & Ricaurte, 1991; Schifano, 1991). Such damage might become apparent only with time or under conditions of stress. Users with no initial complications may manifest problems over time (McCann et al., 1996).

For obvious reasons of safety and ethics, human studies are more difficult to execute, and those that are done offer legitimate and ample room for criticism. The bulk of evidence that MDMA is neurotoxic in humans is indirect but convincing (Burgess et al., 2000; Green et al., 1995). This evidence includes metabolite studies, which quantify the levels of serotonin and metabolites in populations of Ecstasy users. An increasing number of investigations demonstrate that metabolite levels of serotonin are much lower in chronic users, even when abstinent for long periods of time. The difficulties of the studies notwithstanding, the available clinical evidence suggests that repeated ingestion of high doses of MDMA produces long-term reductions in serotonergic activity and degeneration of serotonergic terminals in humans (Montoya et al., 2002).

Extensive cognitive studies in individuals using MDMA, though rife with methodological problems, show a consistent pattern of cognitive dysfunction seen in the frontal cortex and the hippocampus. This phenomenon is consistent with that found in animals exposed to MDMA (Fox, Parrott, & Turner, 2001; Montoya et al., 2002). Psychiatric problems, such as depression, anxiety, panic, increased impulsiveness, and sleep disturbances, are significantly higher in MDMA users, even when users are abstinent and the last use is remote. In a symposium ("Is MDMA a Human Neurotoxin?"), Turner and Parrott (2000) concluded: "Novel studies . . . confirmed and extended the range of cognitive, behavioral, EEG, and neurological deficits, displayed by drug-free Ecstasy users. Moreover, these deficits often remained when other illicit drug use was statistically controlled. In conclusion: If MDMA neurotoxicity in humans is a myth, then it is a myth with a heavy serotonergic component." A recent study by Ricaurte, Yuan, Hatzidiitrious, Cord, and McCann (2002) implicated MDMA as causal of dopaminergic neurotoxicity as well. The involvement of the dopamine system has important implications in terms of increased vulnerability to a variety of motor and cognitive functions. Some of the more dramatic results of the work of Ricaurte have recently been thrown into doubt and are controversial, but the basic results of his and others' work are still considered consistent. This is a general chapter dealing with all aspects of club drugs and MDMA. The reader is directed to several excellent and extensive reviews of the particular subject of MDMA and neurotoxicity (McCann et al., 2000; Montoya et al., 2002; Verkes et al., 2001).

Treatment

The treatment of MDMA abuse may be divided into the treatment of acute reactions to the drug and the treatment of those who abuse the drug chronically.

Urgent Treatments

Fatalities from Ecstasy use and overdose, although rare, do occur. Because polydrug use is the norm in many of the venues where Ecstasy is popular (Lee & McDowell, 2003), it is sometimes difficult to ascertain the contribution of MDMA versus those other substances. Fatalities can be caused by hyperpyrexia, rhabdomyolysis, intravascular coagulopathy, hepatic necrosis, cardiac arrhythmias, cerebrovascular accidents, as well as by a variety of behaviors associated with confusion and impaired judgment (Khalant, 2001).

Ecstasy has many chemical similarities to amphetamine, and drug detection products may indicate a positive presence of amphetamine after use. MDMA intoxication or overdose may be suspected in any individual with alterations of sensorium, hyperthermia, muscle rigidity, and/or fever. Because the drug is used in specific settings and by specific subgroups, the level of suspicion should take into account the user and the circumstance involved. If an individual patient has been to a rave, or to some club event, this should raise the clinician's suspicion that MDMA was ingested. In addition, the clinician should have a high degree of suspicion that the patient may have taken multiple drugs. Drugs that may have been substituted for Ecstasy tablets, such as ephedrine, Ma-Huang (herbal ecstasy), and caffeine, should be considered.

Tachycardia, agitation, tremor, mydriasis, and diaphoresis may occur with MDMA intoxication. Ecstasy ingestion may mimic LSD or other classic hallucinogen ingestion. In addition, MDMA overdose may mimic the ingestion of an anticholinergic agent (Shannon, 2000). Anticholinergic agents induce dry, hot skin, however; this result is in contrast to MDMA, which, except in the case of dehydration, causes diaphoretic skin.

Ecstasy overdose would most likely involve the ingestion of multiple doses and also occur in an environment that induced dehydration. MDMA overdose or toxic reaction is a diagnosis by exclusion. Supportive measures, such as effective hydration using intravenous fluids and lowering the temperature of the patient with cooling blankets or an ice bath, are often necessary. Standard gastric lavage should be employed (Schwartz & Miller, 1997). Physical restraint may be necessary for agitated patients but should be used sparingly. Benzodiazepines are the preferred choice as sedating agent (Shannon, 2000). Hypertension often resolves with sedation. If it persists, nitroprusside, or a calcium-channel blocker, is preferred over a beta-blocker, which may worsen vasospasm and hypertension (Holland, 2001).

Nonurgent Treatment

MDMA ingestion may be associated with a number of adverse psychiatric symptoms, notably, anxiety, panic, and depression. These symptoms usually subside in a matter of hours or days. Support and reassurance are often all that is needed. If the symptoms are severe, brief pharmacotherapy to alleviate symptoms is recommended.

Although classical physiological dependence on MDMA does not occur, some individuals use the drug compulsively. For these people, the standard array of treatments, based on a thorough assessment of internal and external resources, should be employed.

Adolescents are frequent users of MDMA and the population most likely to present with this as the drug causing the most problems for them (McDowell & Spitz, 1999). Furthermore, they are more likely to be involved with the subculture that is enmeshed with MDMA, and that views the drug as harmless at worst, and life-transforming at best (Beck & Rosenbaum, 1994; Winstock et al., 2001). Clinicians are cautioned against adopting a knee-jerk, negative attitude that may inadvertently preclude the initiation of a therapeutic alliance.

KETAMINE

Special K, Super K, Vitamin K, or just plain *K,* are all names for the nonanalgesic anesthetic ketamine. Ketamine was first manufactured in 1965. Veterinarians and pediatric surgeons still legally manufacture it, primarily for therapeutic use; recent crackdowns on the illegal distribution of ketamine from these sources have led to the increased smuggling of it from foreign sources. The recreational use of ketamine probably began in the 1960s and was first described in detail by Lilly (1978). Since that time, its popularity has continued to rise (Cooper, 1996; Dotson, Ackerman, & West, 1995; Graeme, 2000).

Ketamine is classified as a dissociative anesthetic. As this classification implies, the drug causes a dose-dependent dissociative episode, with feelings of fragmentation, detachment, and what one user has described as "psychic/physical/spiritual scatter." Use of ketamine imparts a disconnection from awareness of stimuli from the general environment. This includes but is not limited to pain.

History

Ketamine was first manufactured in 1965 at the University of Michigan and marketed under the name of Ketalar. It is most commonly available in 10-ml (100 mg/ml) liquid-containing vials (Fort Dodge Laboratories, 1997). It is a close chemical cousin of phencyclidine, also known as PCP or angel dust. PCP has physiological properties that made it advantageous as an anesthetic. PCP does not cause the kind of cardiac arrhythmias and respiratory depression inherent in classical anesthetics. PCP also had a number of severe limitations as an anesthetic, most significantly, that it causes a high degree of psychotic and violent reactions (National Institute on Drug Abuse, 1979). These effects occur at an alarmingly high rate (50%) and may persist for as long as 10 days (Crider, 1986; Meyer, Greifenstein, & DeVault, 1959). Ketamine produces minimal cardiac and respiratory effects, and its anesthetic and behavioral effects remit soon after administration (Moretti, Hassan, Goodman, & Meltzer, 1984; Pandit, Kothary, & Kumar, 1980). The medication continues to have therapeutic usefulness, principally with children and animals.

Since the 1970s, ketamine has been a drug used for "recreational" purposes. Although the distinction is by no means complete, ketamine users cluster into two distinct subtypes. The first type uses ketamine in a solitary fashion; the second type uses the drug in a social setting, although the effects of the drug do not promote sociability. These are the young clubgoers and "ravers" (Weir, 2000). Ketamine is especially popular at circuit parties and thus a favorite of gay urbanites (Lee & McDowell, 2003).

Ketamine is commercially available as a liquid. About 90% of ketamine comes from diverted veterinary sources (National Institute on Drug Abuse,

2002). The liquid form is easily evaporated into a powder, the form in which it is most often sold. Ketamine can be administered in a variety of ways. At clubs, most people snort lines of the powder. Ketamine may also be dabbed on the tongue or mixed with a liquid and imbibed.

Physiological Effects

Ketamine has been studied extensively in humans. It is a noncompetitive N-methyl-D-aspartate (NMDA) antagonist (Curran & Monaghan, 2001). Recreational users of ketamine report feeling anesthetized and sedated in a dose-dependent manner (Krystal et al., 1994). Ketamine can influence all modes of sensory function (Garfield et al., 1994; Óye, Paulsen, & Maurset, 1992). At typical dosages, ketamine distorts sensory stimuli, producing illusions (Garfield et al., 1994). In higher than typical dosages, hallucinations and paranoid delusions can occur (Malhotra et al., 1996).

Ketamine substantially disrupts both attention and learning. In human research subjects, ketamine affects the ability to modify behavior, to learn new tasks, and to remember (Curran & Monaghan, 2001; Krystal et al., 1994). The recreational dosage of ketamine is approximately 0.4 mg/kg, and the anesthetic dosage is almost double that. The median lethal dose (LD_{50}) is nearly 30 times the anesthetic dosage, which makes overdose from ketamine very rare.

One dose of ketamine creates a "trip" that lasts about 1 hour (Delgarno & Shewan, 1996). Larger doses last longer and have a more intense effect (Malhotra et al., 1996). The user feels physical tingling, followed by a feeling of removal from the outside sensory world. Tolerance develops rapidly to ketamine, and dependence, though rare, is well known. Flashbacks have been reported, and their incidence may be higher than with many other hallucinogens (Siegel, 1984). Ketamine works in a dose-dependent fashion. Mild doses involve an autistic stare and a paucity of thinking. Higher doses result in the K-hole phenomenon, which is characterized by social withdrawal, autistic behavior, and an inability to maintain a cognitive set. Such individuals may be described as zombie-like (Gay Men's Health Crisis, 1997).

Mechanism of Action

Ketamine is chemically similar to PCP but has important differences (Jansen, 1990). Ketamine binds to the NMDA receptor complex on the same site as PCP, located inside the calcium channel. It works by inhibiting several of the excitatory amino acid neurotransmitters (Cotman & Monaghan, 1987; Hampton et al., 1982). Ketamine works globally, affecting numerous neurotransmitter systems, but its action, as an NMDA antagonist, is likely the cause of its schizotypal and dissociative symptoms. NMDA blockade causes an increase in dopamine release in the midbrain and prefrontal cortex as well

(Bubser Keseberg, Notz, & Griffiths, 1992), and this is likely the cause of its ability to reinforce and cause dependence. Furthermore, persisting memory deficits have been demonstrated (Curran & Monaghan, 2001).

Treatment

The most dangerous effects of ketamine are behavioral. Individuals may become withdrawn, paranoid, and physically sloppy. In the event of dealing with an individual who is intoxicated on ketamine, the physician must treat the individual symptomatically. Calm reassurance and a low-stimulation environment are usually most helpful. The patient should be placed in a part of the clinic or emergency room with the least amount of light and stimulation. If necessary, the patient may be given benzodiazepines to control the associated anxiety (Graeme, 2000). Neuroleptics should be avoided, because the side-effect profile may cause discomfort and possibly exacerbate the patient's agitated state.

Ketamine is an addictive drug. There are numerous reports of individuals who have become dependent on the drug and use it daily (Galloway et al., 1997; Jansen, 1990). Such dependence should be treated in the same manner as any other chemical dependence. The clinician should do a careful evaluation in order to discern other psychological conditions. These should be dealt with in the most clinically expeditious manner.

GHB

History

GHB was first synthesized in the mid-1970s by Dr. H. Laborit, a French researcher interested in exploring the effects of gamma-aminobutyric acid (GABA) in the brain. Laborit was attempting to manufacture a GABA-like agent that would cross the blood–brain barrier (Vickers, 1969). During the 1980s, GHB was widely available in health food stores. It came to the attention of authorities in the late 1980s as a drug of abuse, and the Food and Drug Administration (FDA) banned it in 1990, after reports of several poisonings with the drug (Chin, Kreutzer, & Dyer, 1992). In the past decade, it has become more widely known as a drug of abuse associated with nightclubs and raves.

GHB is known as "liquid Ecstasy," and in Great Britain as GBH, or "grievous bodily harm." It can be found, occurring naturally, in many mammalian cells. In the brain, the highest amounts are found in the hypothalamus and basal ganglia (Gallimberti et al., 1989). It is likely that it is itself a neurotransmitter (Galloway et al., 1997). GHB is closely linked to GABA and is both a precursor and a metabolite of GABA (Chin et al., 1992).

In the 1970s, GHB was available commercially as a sleep aid. It has some demonstrated therapeutic efficacy, particularly in the treatment of narcolepsy (Lammers et al., 1993; Mamelak, Scharf, & Woods, 1986; Scrima, Hartman, Johnson, Thomas, & Hiller, 1990). In 1990, after reports indicated that GHB might have contributed to the hospitalization of several California youth, the FDA banned it. GHB has an extremely small therapeutic index, and as little as double the euphorigenic dose may cause serious central nervous system (CNS) depression. In recent years, it has been associated with numerous incidents of respiratory depression and coma. Increasing numbers of deaths have been linked to GHB (Li, Stokes, & Woeckner, 1998).

The legal status of GHB is complicated. Recently, GHB, under the brand name Xyrem, was classified as a Schedule III controlled substance, but with special regulations. The company that makes and markets the medication has developed a rigorous system that makes Xyrem available to patients from a single specialty pharmacy. Both physicians and patients must receive an education program from the manufacturer, Orphan Medical, before obtaining Xyrem. Orphan Medical has worked closely with the FDA, the Drug Enforcement Administration (DEA), and law enforcement agencies to develop strict distribution and risk-management controls designed to restrict access to Xyrem to the intended patient population (Tunnicliff & Raess, 2002). Illicit use of Xyrem is subject to penalties reserved for Schedule I drugs.

Most of the GHB sold in the United States is of the bootleg variety, manufactured by nonprofessionals. In fact, it is relatively easy to manufacture, and Internet sites devoted to explaining the process can be found readily, although they are sometimes cleverly concealed.

Physiological Effects

GHB is ingested orally, absorbed rapidly, and reaches peak plasma concentrations in 20–60 minutes (Vickers, 1969). The typical recreational dosage is 0.75–1.5 g; higher dosages result in increased effects. The high lasts for no more than 3 hours and reportedly has few lasting effects. Repeated use of the drug can prolong its effects.

Users of the drug report that GHB induces a pleasant state of relaxation and tranquility. Frequently reported effects are placidity, mild euphoria, and an enhanced tendency to verbalize. GHB, like MDMA, has also been described as a sensual drug. Its effects have been likened to alcohol, another GABA-like drug (McCabe, Layne, Sayler, Slusher, & Bessman, 1971). Users report a feeling of mild numbing and pleasant disinhibition. This effect may account for the reports that GHB enhances the experience of sex. The dose–response curve for GHB is exceedingly steep. The LD_{50} is estimated at perhaps only five times the intoxicating dosage (Vickers, 1969). Furthermore, the drug has synergistic effects with alcohol and probably other drugs as well. Therefore, small increases in the amount ingested may lead to significant intensification of the effects and to the onset of CNS depression. Overdose is a real danger. Users who drink alcohol, which impairs judgment and with which synergy is likely, are at greater risk.

The most commonly experienced side effects of GHB are drowsiness, dizziness, nausea, and vomiting. Less common side effects include weakness, loss of peripheral vision, confusion, agitation, hallucinations, and bradycardia. The drug is a sedative and can produce ataxia and loss of coordination. As doses increase, patients may experience loss of bladder control, temporary amnesia, and sleepwalking. Clonus, seizures, and cardiopulmonary depression can occur. Coma and persistent vegetative states, and death may result from overdose (Chin et al., 1992; Gallimberti et al., 1989; Takahara et al., 1977; Vickers, 1969).

Mechanism of Action

Several lines of evidence support the hypothesis that GHB is a neurotransmitter. GHB temporarily suppresses the release of dopamine in the mammalian brain. This is followed by a marked increase in dopamine release, accompanied by the increased release of endogenous opioids (Hechler, Goebaille, & Maitre, 1992). GHB also stimulates pituitary growth hormone (GH) release, although the mechanism by which GHB stimulates GH release is not known. Dopamine activity in the hypothalamus stimulates pituitary release of GH, but GHB inhibits dopamine release as it stimulates GH release. While GH is being released, serum prolactin levels also rise in a similar, time-dependent fashion. GHB has several different actions in the CNS, and some reports indicate that it antagonizes the effects of marijuana (Galloway et al., 1997). The consequences of these physiological changes are unclear, as are the overall health consequences for individuals who use GHB.

Treatment

GHB is not detectable by routine drug screening; thus, history is that much more important. Clinicians should remember to ask about GHB use, especially in younger people, for whom it has become a drug of choice. In cases of acute GHB intoxication, physicians should provide physiological support and maintain a high index of suspicion for intoxication with other drugs. A recent review (Li et al., 1998) suggested the following features for the management of GHB ingestion with a spontaneously breathing patient:

1. Maintain oxygen supplementation and intravenous access.
2. Maintain comprehensive physiological and cardiac monitoring.
3. Attempt to keep the patient stimulated.
4. Use atropine for persistent symptomatic bradycardia.

5. Admit the patient to the hospital if he or she is still intoxicated after 6 hours.
6. Discharge the patient if he or she is clinically well in 6 hours (with plans for follow-up, and a suggestion that therapy may be appropriate).

Patients whose breathing is labored should be managed in the intensive care unit. Most patients who overdose on GHB recover completely, if they receive proper medical attention.

Individuals may develop physiological dependence on GHB. The symptoms are similar to those of alcohol withdrawal: anxiety, tremor, insomnia, and "feelings of doom," which may persist for several weeks after cessation of use (Galloway et al., 1997). There is anecdotal evidence, such as the proliferation of support groups and help lines for GHB-dependent individuals, that the numbers of GHB-dependent individuals is rising.

The complex symptoms suggest that benzodiazepines may be useful in treating GHB withdrawal. Because data are lacking, clinicians must exercise their most prudent judgment regarding what will be most helpful in a given situation.

HALLUCINOGENS

Hallucinogens produce a wide range of effects depending on the properties, dosage, and potency of the drug, the personality and mood of the drug taker, and the immediate environment. Visually, perception of light and space is altered, and colors and detail take on increased significance. If the eyes are closed, the drug taker often sees intense visions of different kinds. Nonexistent conversations, music, odors, tastes, and other sensations are also perceived. The sensations may be either very pleasant or very distasteful and disturbing. The nature of this effect is often random and not predictable. The drugs frequently alter the sense of time and cause feelings of emptiness. For many individuals, the separation between self and environment disappears, leading to a sense of oneness or holiness.

The effects, sometimes referred to as a "trip," can last from an hour to a few days. "Bad trips," full of frightening images, monsters, and paranoid thoughts, are known to have resulted in accidents and suicides. Flashbacks (unexpected reappearances of the effects) can occur months later.

Physiologically, the drugs act as mild stimulants of the sympathetic nervous system, causing dilation of the pupils, constriction of some arteries, a rise in blood pressure, and increased excitability of certain spinal reflexes. Many hallucinogenic drugs share a basic chemical structural unit, the indole ring, which is also found in the nervous system substance serotonin. Mescaline has chemical similarities to both the indole ring and the adrenal hormone epinephrine. This suggests that, like most psychoactive substances, hallucinogens mimic the action of naturally occurring biological entities (McDowell & Spitz, 1999).

LSD

Lysergic acid diethylamide is an alkaloid synthesized from lysergic acid, which is found in the fungus ergot (*Claviceps purpurea*). It is perhaps the most famous and well known hallucinogenic drug that intensifies sense perceptions and produces hallucinations, mood changes, and changes in the sense of time. It also can cause restlessness, acute anxiety, and, occasionally, depression. Although lysergic acid itself is without hallucinogenic effects, LSD, one of the most powerful drugs known, is weight for weight 5,000 times as potent as the hallucinogenic drug mescaline and 200 times as potent as psilocybin. LSD is usually taken orally from little squares of blotter paper, gelatin "windowpanes," or tiny tablets called "microdots." The period of its effects, or "trip," is usually 8 to 12 hours. Unexpected reappearances of the hallucinations, called "flashbacks," can occur months after taking the drug. The drug does not appear to cause psychological or physical dependence. It can cause psychological dependence in some individuals (Koesters, Rogers, & Rajasingham, 2002). The danger of LSD is that its effects are unpredictable, even in experienced users. These individuals may act in dangerous ways. This is termed behavioral toxicity.

History

LSD was developed in 1938 by Arthur Stoll and Albert Hofmann, Swiss chemists hoping to create a headache cure. Hofmann accidentally ingested some of the drug and discovered its hallucinogenic effect. On his ride home by bicycle, he began to experience the beginnings of what would be a 2-day-long nightmarish "bad trip."

In the 1960s and 1970s, LSD was used by millions of young people in America; its popularity waned as its reputation for bad trips and resulting accidents and suicides became known. In 1967, the federal government classified it as a Schedule I drug (i.e., having a high abuse potential and no accepted medical use), along with heroin and marijuana. In the early 1990s, it again became popular, presumably because of its low cost. It is produced in clandestine laboratories (Graeme, 2000).

Inhalants

Inhalants are substances whose chemical vapors can be intentionally inhaled to produce psychoactive effects. These are used by a variety of individuals, usually adolescents. According to the 2002 National Survey on Drug Use and Health,

4.4% of youth ages 12–17 used inhalants in the past year, compared to 0.5% of adults. Inhalants are often found in legal and easily obtained products.

Inhalants are generally classified into four different groups:

1. Volatile solvents, which include glue, paint thinner, and gasoline. The street names for these are air blast, discorama, hippie crack, moon gas, oz and poor man's pot.
2. Aerosols, which include hair spray and spray paint.
3. Gases, which include nitrous oxide and ether. Nitrous oxide is known as laughing gas or whippets.
4. Nitrites, which include amyl, butyl, and isobutyl nitrites.

Effects

The instant, short-lived high produced after directly inhaling these substances (called huffing) produce an instant, short-lived euphoria, along with disinhibition, impaired judgment, slurred speech, lethargy, nervous system depression, and, in extreme cases, unconsciousness.

Prolonged use may result in neurological impairment and damage to the heart, lungs, and other vital organs. Death may be the result, usually from heart failure, but can also be the result of asphyxiation, suffocation, choking, or behavioral toxicity (CESAR, 2004).

CONCLUSION

MDMA, ketamine, and GHB are by no means the only drugs found at clubs, raves, or circuit parties. They are, however, the most emblematic. Attendees also use more traditional drugs, such as LSD and other hallucinogens. Marijuana is perennially popular, and alcohol use is also common. Furthermore, each week seems to bring a report of some "new" drug of abuse. Often this is just an older, well-known drug, packaged differently or with a new name, but the effect on a new generation of users will be just as devastating.

Drugs such as these are being increasingly used at clubs, often in combination, and often by very young people. This is cause for concern for several reasons. The younger a person is when he or she begins to use drugs, and the more often he or she uses them, the more likely he or she is to develop serious problems with these or other substances. In the future, we are likely to see more and more use of such drugs and the problems that come with their use.

When the evidence of MDMA's neurotoxicity was lacking, and what research existed on GHB and marijuana was not as compelling, individuals concerned with the public's safety could afford to be less alarmed. The mounting bodies of evidence, however, and the possible public health implications, are a call for effective prevention and education interventions.

REFERENCES

Abel, E. L. (1980). *Marijuana: The first twelve thousand years.* New York: Plenum Press.

Ajaelo, I., Koenig, K., & Snoey, E. (1998). Severe hyponatremia and inappropriate antidiuretic hormone secretion following ecstasy use. *Acad Emerg Med, 5,* 939–840.

American Academy of Ophthalmology. (1992, June). *The use of marijuana in the treatment of glaucoma.* Statement by the Board of Directors of the American Academy of Ophthalmology, San Francisco.

Ames, D., & Wirshing, W. (1993). Ecstasy, the serotonin syndrome, and neuroleptic malignant syndrome—a possible link? *JAMA, 269,* 869–870.

Arseneault, L. Cannon, M., Witton, J., & Murray, R. M. (2004). Causal association between cannabis and psychosis: Examination of the evidence. *Br J Psychiatry, 194,* 110–117.

Beck, J. (1990). The public health implications of MDMA use. In S. J. Peroutka (Ed.), *Ecstasy: The clinical, pharmacological and neurotoxicological effects of the drug MDMA* (pp. 77–103). Boston: Kluwer Academic.

Beck, J., & Rosenbaum, M. (1994). *Pursuit of Ecstasy: The MDMA experience.* Albany: State University of New York Press.

Bellis, M. A., Hale, G., Bennett, A., Chaudry, M., & Kilfoyle, M. (2000). Ibiza uncovered: Changes in substance use and sexual behavior amongst young people visiting an international nightlife resort. *Int J Drug Policy, 11,* 235–244.

Block, R. I. (1996). Does heavy marijuana use impair human cognition and brain function? *JAMA, 275,* 560–561.

Bonnie, R. J., & Whitebread, C. H. (1974). *The marijuana conviction: A history of marijuana prohibition in the United States.* Charlottesville: University of Virginia Press.

Boys, A., Lenton, S., & Norcross, K. (1997). Polydrug use at raves by a Western Australian sample. *Drug Alcohol Rev, 16,* 227–234.

Bubser, M., Keseberg, U., Notz, P. K., & Griffiths, P. (1992). Differential behavioral and neurochemical effects of competitive and noncompetitive NMDA receptor antagonists in rats. *Eur J Pharmacol, 229,* 75–82.

Budney, A. J., Moore, B. A., Vandrey, R. G., & Hughes, J. R. (2003). The time course and significance of cannabis withdrawal. *J Abnorm Psychol, 112,* 393–402.

Buffum, J., & Moser, C. (1986). MDMA and human sexual function. *J Psychoactive Drugs, 18,* 355–359.

Burgess, C., O'Donoghoe, A., & Gill, M. (2000). Agony and ecstasy: A review of MDMA effects and toxicity. *Eur Psychiatry, 15,* 287–294.

CESAR, the Center for Substance Abuse Research. (2004). Inhalant abuse: Nothing to sniff at. *CESAR Fax, 13*(12).

Chin, M. Y., Kreutzer, R. A., & Dyer, J. E. (1992). Acute poisoning from gamma-hydroxybutyrate in California. *West J Med, 156,* 380–384.

Chopra, G. S., & Smith, J. W. (1974). Psychotic reactions following cannabis use in East Indians. *Arch Gen Psychiatry, 30,* 24–27.

Cohen, R. (1998). *The love drug: Marching to the beat of Ecstasy.* Binghamton, NY: Hayworth Press.

Cooper, M. (1996, January 28). "Special K": Rough catnip for clubgoers. *New York Times,* p. A-6.

Cotman, C. W., & Monaghan, D. T. (1987). Chemistry and anatomy of excitatory amino acid systems. In H. Y. Meltzer (Ed.), *Psychopharmacology: The third generation of progress* (pp. 194–210). New York: Raven Press.

Creighton, F., Black, D., & Hyde, C. (1991). Ecstasy psychosis and flashbacks. *Br J Psychiatry, 159,* 713–715.

Crider, R. A. (1986). Phencyclidine: Changing abuse patterns. In D. H. Clouet (Ed.), *Phencyclidine: An update* (pp. 163–173). Rockville, MD: U.S. Department of Health and Human Services.

Curran, H. V., & Monaghan, L. (2001). In and out of the K-hole: A comparison of the acute and residual effects of ketamine in frequent and infrequent ketamine users. *Addiction, 96,* 749–760.

Deas, D., Gerding, L., & Hazy, J. (2000). Marijuana and panic disorder. *J Am Acad Child Adolesc Psychiatry, 39,* 1467.

Delgarno, P. J., & Shewan, D. (1996). Illicit use of ketamine in Scotland. *J Psychoactive Drugs, 28,* 191–199.

Demirkiran, M., Jankovic, J., & Dean, J. (1996). Ecstasy intoxication: An overlap between serotonin syndrome and neuroleptic malignant syndrome. *Clin Neuropharmacol, 19,* 157–164.

Dotson, J., Ackerman, D., & West, L. (1995). Ketamine abuse. *J Drug Issues, 25,* 751–757.

Eisner, B. (1986). *Ecstasy: The MDMA story.* Boston: Little, Brown.

Eisner, B. (1993). *Ecstasy: The MDMA story* (2nd ed.). Berkeley, CA: Ronin.

Feeney D. (1976). Marijuana use among epileptics. *JAMA, 235,* 1105.

Fox, H. C., Parrott, A. C., & Turner, J. J. (2001). Ecstasy use: Cognitive deficits related to dosage rather than self reported problematic use of the drug. *J Psychopharmacol, 15,* 273–281.

Fort Dodge Laboratories. (1997). Ketaset [Package insert]. Fort Dodge, IA: Author.

Gallimberti, L., Canton, G., Gentile, N., Ferri, M., Cibin, M., Ferrara, S. D., et al. (1989). Gamma-hydroxybutyric acid for treatment of alcohol withdrawal syndrome. *Lancet, 30,* 787–789.

Galloway, G. P., Frederick, S. L., Staggers, F. E., Jr., Gonzales, M., Stalcup, S. A., & Smith, D. E. (1997). Gamma-hydroxybutyrate: An emerging drug of abuse that causes physical dependence. *Addiction, 92,* 89–96.

Garfield, J. M., Garfield, F. B., Stone, J. G., Hopkins, D., & Johns, L. A. (1994). A comparison of psychologic responses to ketamine and thiopental-nitrous oxide-halothane anesthesia. *Anesthesiology, 36,* 329–338.

Gay Men's Health Crisis (McDowell, D., Consultant). (1997). *Drugs in partyland* [Brochure]. New York: GMHC Press.

Graeme, K. A. (2000). New drugs of abuse. *Emerg Med Clin North Am, 18*(4), 625–636.

Green, A., Cross, A., & Goodwin, G. (1995). Review of pharmacology and clinical pharmacology of 3,4-methylenedioxymethamphetamine (MDMA or "Ecstasy"). *Psychopharmacology, 119,* 247–260.

Grinspoon L., & Bakalar, J. B. (1995). Marijuana as medicine: A plea for reconsideration. *JAMA, 273*, 1875–1876.

Hampton, R. Y., Medzihradsky, F., Woods, J. H., & Dahlstrom, P. J. (1982). Stereospecific binding of ^3H phencyclidine in brain membranes. *Life Sci, 30*, 2147–2154.

Hechler, V., Goebaille, S., & Maitre, M. (1992). Selective distribution pattern of gamma-hydroxybutyrate receptors in the rat forebrain and mid-brain as revealed by quantitative autoradiograph. *Brain Res, 572*, 345–348.

Hepler, R. S., & Petrus, R. J. (1976). Experiences with administration of marijuana to glaucoma patients. In S. Cohen & R. C. Stillman (Eds.), *The therapeutic potential of marijuana* (pp. 63–75). New York: Plenum Medical Books.

Hermle, L., Spitzer, M., Borchardt, D., Kovar, K. A., & Gouzoulis, E. (1993). Psychological effects of MDE in normal subjects. *Neuropsychopharmacology, 8*, 171—176.

Holland, J. (2001). *Ecstasy: The complete guide.* Rochester, VT: Panic Street Press.

Holmes, S. B., Banerjee, A. K., & Alexander, W. D. (1999). Hyponatremia and seizures after ecstasy use. *Postgrad Med J, 75*, 32–43.

Iversen, L. L., & Snyder, S. H. (1999). *The science of marijuana.* New York: Oxford University Press.

Jansen, K. (1990). A review of the non-medical uses of ketamine: Use, uses, and consequences. *J Psychoactive Drugs, 32*, 419–433.

Johnson, L. D., O'Malley, P. M., & Bachman, J. G. (2002). *Monitoring the future national results on adolescent drug use: Overview of key findings, 2001* (NIH Publication No. 02-5105). Bethesda, MD: National Institute on Drug Abuse.

Kassirer, J. P. (1999). Should medical journals try to influence political debates? *N Engl J Med, 340*, 466–467.

Khalant, H. (2001). The pharmacology and toxicology of "Ecstasy" (MDMA) and related drugs. *Can Med Assoc J, 165*, 917–928.

Koesters, S. C., Rogers, P. D., & Rajasingham, C. R. (2002). MDMA ("Ecstasy") and other "club drugs": The new epidemic. *Pediatr Clin North Am, 49*, 415–433.

Kris, M. G., Cubeddu, L. X., Gralla, R. J., Cupissol, D., Tyson, L. B., Venkatraman, E., & Homesley, H. D. (1996). Are more antiemetic trials with a placebo necessary?: Report of patient data from randomized trials of placebo antiemetics with cisplatin. *Cancer, 78*, 2193–2198.

Krystal, J. H., Karper, L. P., Seibyl, J. P., Freeman, G. K., Delaney, R., Bremner, J. D., et al. (1994). Subanesthetic effects of the noncompetitive NMDA antagonist ketamine in humans. *Arch Gen Psychiatry, 51*, 199–214.

Lammers, G. J., Arends, J., Declerck, A. C., Ferrari, M. D., Schouwink, G., & Troost, J. (1993). Gammahydroxybutyrate and narcolepsy: A double blind placebo controlled study. *Sleep, 16*, 216–220.

Lee, S., & McDowell, D. M. (2003). Polysubstance use (GHB, MDMA, and other club drugs) by circuit party attendees. *Am J Addictions*, 181–186.

Leister, M. P., Grob, C. S., Bravo, G. L., & Walsh, R. N. (1992). Phenomenology and sequelae of 3,4-methylenedioxymethamphetamine use. *J Nerv Ment Dis, 180*, 345–354.

Li, J., Stokes, S., & Woeckener, A. (1998). A tale of novel intoxication: A review of the effects of gamma-hydroxybutyric acid with recommendations for management. *Ann Emerg Med, 31*, 729–736.

Lilly, J. C. (1978). *The scientist: A novel autobiography.* New York: Lippincott.

Ling, L. H., Marchant, C., Buckley, N. A., Prior, M., & Irvine, R. J. (2001). Poisoning with the recreational drug paramethoxyamphetamine ("death"). *Med J Aust, 174,* 453–455.

Lynskey, M., & Hall, W. (2000). The effects of adolescent cannabis use on educational attainment: A review. *Addiction, 95,* 1621–1630.

Malhotra, A. K., Pinals, D. A., Weingartner, H., Sirocco, K., Missar, C. D., Pickar, D., & Breier, A. (1996). NMDA receptor function and human cognition: The effects of ketamine in healthy volunteers. *Neuropsychopharmacology, 14,* 301–307.

Mamelak, M., Scharf, M. B., & Woods, M. (1986). Treatment of narcolepsy with gamma-hydroxybutyrate: A review of clinical and sleep laboratory findings. *Sleep, 9,* 285–259.

Marmor, J. B. (1998). Medical marijuana. *West J Med, 168,* 540–543.

Maurer, M., Henn, V., Dittrich, A., & Hofmann, A. (1990). Delta-9-tetrahydrocannabinol shows antispastic and analgesic effects in a single case double-blind trial. *Eur Arch Psychiatry Clin Neurosci, 240,* 1–4.

McCabe, E. R., Layne, E. C., Sayler, D. F., Slusher, N., & Bessman, S. P. (1971). Synergy of ethanol and a natural soporific: Gamma hydroxybutyrate. *Science, 171,* 404–406.

McCann, U. D., Eligulashvili, W., & Ricaurte, G. A. (2000). (+/–) 3,4-Methylentdioxymethamphetamine ("Ecstasy")-induced serotonin neurotoxicity: Clinical studies. *Neuropsychobiology, 42,* 11–16.

McCann, U. D., & Ricaurte, G. (1991). Lasting neuropsychiatric sequelae of methylenedioxymethamphetamine ("Ecstasy") in recreational users. *J Clin Psychopharmacol, 11,* 302–305.

McCann, U. D., & Ricaurte, G. (1993). Reinforcing subjective effects of 3,4-methylenedioxymethamphetamine ("Ecstasy") may be separable from its neurotoxic actions: Clinical evidence. *J Clin Psychopharmacol, 13,* 214–217.

McCann, U. D., Ridenour, A., Shaham, Y., & Ricaurte, G. A. (1994). Serotonin neurotoxicity after (±)3,4-methylenedioxymethamphetamine (MDMA; "Ecstasy"): A controlled study in humans. *Neuropsychopharmacology, 10,* 129–138.

McCann, U. D., Slate, S., & Ricaurte, G. (1996). Adverse reactions with 3,4-methylenedioxymethamphetamine (MDMA: "Ecstasy"). *Drug Safety, 15,* 107–115.

McDowell, D., & Kleber, H. (1994). MDMA, its history and pharmacology. *Psychiatr Ann, 24,* 127–130.

McDowell, D., & Spitz, H. (1999). *Substance abuse: From principles to practice.* New York: Brunner/Mazel.

McDowell, D. M. (1998). Testimony to House Judiciary Committee. Available at *www.house.gov/judiciary/mcdo0615.htm*

McKenna, D., & Peroutka, S. (1990). The neurochemistry and neurotoxicity of 3,4-methylenedioxymethamphetamine, "Ecstasy." *J Neurochem, 54,* 14–22.

Meyer, J. S., Greifenstein, F., & DeVault, M. (1959). A new drug causing symptoms of sensory depravation. *J Nerv Ment Dis, 129,* 54–61.

Moretti, R. J., Hassan, S. Z., Goodman, L. I., & Meltzer, H. Y. (1984). Comparison of ketamine and thiopental in healthy volunteers: Effects on mental status, mood, and personality. *Anesth Analg, 63,* 1087–1096.

Montoya, A., Sorrentino, R., Lucas, S., & Price, B. (2002). Long-term neuropsychiatric consequences of "Ecstasy" (MDMA): A review. *Harv Rev Psychiatry, 10*(4), 212–220.

Morgan, M. J. (2000). Ecstasy (MDMA): A review of its possible persistent psychological effects. *Psychopharmacology, 152*, 230–248.

National Eye Institute. (1997, February 18). *The use of marijuana for glaucoma.* Retrieved February 1, 2004, from *www.nei.nih.gov/news/statements/marij.htm*

National Institute on Drug Abuse. (1979). *Diagnosis and treatment of phencyclidine (PCP) toxicity* [Brochure]. Rockville, MD: Author.

National Institutes of Health. (1997, February 19–20). *Workshop on the medical utility of marijuana.* Retrieved February 1, 2004, from *www.nih.gov/news/medmarijuana/medicalmarijuana.htm*

Nelson, K., Walsh, D., Deeter, P., & Sheehan, F. (1994). A phase II study of delta-9-tetrahydrocannabinol for appetite stimulation in cancer-associated anorexia. *J Palliat Care, 10*, 14–18.

Óye, N., Paulsen, O., & Maurset, A. (1992). Effects of ketamine on sensory perception: Evidence for a role of N-methyl D-aspartate receptors. *J Pharmacol Exp Ther, 260*, 1209–1213.

Pandit, S. K., Kothary, S. P., & Kumar, S. M. (1980). Low dose intravenous infusion technique with ketamine. *Anesthesia, 35*, 669–675.

Peroutka, S. (1990). *Ecstasy: The clinical, pharmacological and neurotoxicological effects of the drug MDMA.* Boston: Kluwer Academic.

Peroutka, S., Newman, H., & Harris, H. (1998). Subjective effects of 3,4-MDMA in recreational abusers. *Neuropsychopharmacology, 11*, 273–277.

Pope, H. G., & Yurgelun-Todd, D. (1996). The residual cognitive effects of heavy marijuana use in college students. *JAMA, 275*, 521–527.

Rattray, M. (1991). Ecstasy: Towards an understanding of the biochemical basis of the actions of MDMA. *Essays Biochem, 26*, 77–87.

Ricaurte, G. A., & McCann, U. D. (2001). Assessing long-term effects of MDMA (Ecstasy). *Lancet, 358*, 1831–1832.

Ricaurte, G. A., McCann, U. D., Szabo, Z., & Scheffel, U. (2000). Toxicodynamics and long-term toxicity of the recreational drug 3,4-methylenedicoxymethamphetamine (MDMA, "Ecstasy"). *Toxicol Lett, 112–113*, 143–146.

Ricaurte, G. A., Yuan, J., Hatzidiitrious, G., Cord, B. J., & McCann, U. D. (2002). Severe dopaminergic neurotoxicity in primates after a common recreational dose regimen of MDMA ("Ecstasy"). *Science, 297*, 2260–2263.

Rodgers, J. (2000). Cognitive performance amongst recreational users of "Ecstasy." *Psychopharmacology, 151*, 19–24.

Sallan, S. E., Zinberg, N. E., & Frei, E. (1975). Antiemetic effect of delta-9-tetrahydrocannabinol in patients receiving cancer chemotherapy. *N Engl J Med, 293*, 795–797.

Schifano, F. (1991). Chronic atypical psychosis associated with MDMA ("Ecstasy") abuse. *Lancet, 338*, 1335.

Schwartz, R. (1991). Heavy marijuana use and recent memory impairment. *Psychiatr Ann, 21*, 80–83.

Schwartz, R. H. (2002). Marijuana: A decade and a half later, still a crude drug with underappreciated toxicity. *Pediatrics, 109*, 284–289.

Schwartz, R. H., & Miller, N. S. (1997). MDMA (Ecstasy) and the rave: A review. *Pediatrics, 100,* 705–708.

Scrima, L., Hartman, P. G., Johnson, F. H., Jr., Thomas, E. E., & Hiller, F. C. (1990). The effects of gamma-hydroxybutyrate on the sleep of narcolepsy patients: A double-blind study. *Sleep, 13,* 479–490.

Shannon, M. (2000). Methylenediocyamphetimine (MDMA, Ecstasy). *Ped Emer Care, 16,* 377–380.

Shulgin, A. (1986). The background and chemistry of MDMA. *J Psychoactive Drugs, 18,* 291–304.

Shulgin, A. (1990). History of MDMA. In S. J. Peroutka (Ed.), *Ecstasy: The clinical, pharmacological and neurotoxicological effects of the drug MDMA* (pp. 1–20). Boston: Kluwer Academic.

Siegel, R. K. (1984). The natural history of hallucinogens. In B. L. Jacobs (Ed.), *Hallucinogens: Neurochemistry, behavioral, and clinical perspectives* (pp. 1–17). New York: Raven Press.

Solowij, N. (1998). *Cannabis and cognitive functioning.* Cambridge, UK: Cambridge University Press.

Solowij, N., Michie, P. T., & Fox, A. M. (1995). Differential impairments of selective attention due to frequency and duration of cannabis use. *Biol Psychiatry, 37,* 731–739.

Sprague, J. E., Everman, S. L., & Nichols, D. E. (1998). An integrated hypothesis for the serotonergic axonal loss induced by 3,4- methylenedioxymethamphetamine. *Neurotoxicology, 19,* 427–441.

Sugiura, T., & Waku, K. (2002). Cannabinoid receptors and their endogenous ligands. *J Biochem, 132,* 7–12.

Takahara, J., Yunoki, S., Yakushiji, W., Yamauchi, J., Yamane, Y., & Ofuji, T. (1977). Stimulatory effects of gamma-hydroxybutyric acid on growth hormone and prolactin release in humans. *J Clin Endocrinol Metab, 44,* 1014–1018.

Tramer, M. R., Carroll, D., Campbell, F. A., Reynolds, D. J. M., Moore, R. A., & McQuay, H. J. (2001). Cannabinoids for control of chemotherapy induced nausea and vomiting: Quantitative systematic review. *Br Med J, 323,* 16–32.

Tunnicliff, G., & Raess, B. U. (2002). Gamma-hydroxybutyrate (orphan medical). *Curr Opin Investig Drugs, 3,* 278–283.

Turner, J. J., & Parrott, A. C. (2000). "Is MDMA a human neurotoxin?": Diverse views from the discussants. *Neuropsychobiology, 42*(1), 42–48.

United Nations. (1997). World drug report. Retrieved February 2, 2004, from *www.un.org/ga/20special/wdr/e_hilite.htm*

Verkes, R. J., Gijsman, H. J., Pieters, M. S., Schoemaker, R. C., de Visser, S., Kuijpers, M., et al. (2001). Cognitive performance and serotonergic function in users of ecstasy. *Psychopharmacology, 153,* 196–202.

Vickers, M. D. (1969). Gamma-hydroxybutyric acid. *Int Anesth Clin, 71,* 75–89.

Vinciguerra, V., Moore, T., & Brennan, E. (1988). Inhalation marijuana as an antiemetic for cancer chemotherapy. *NY State Med J, 88,* 525–527.

Walgate, R. (2003, September 16). Retracted Ecstasy paper "An outrageous scandal." *The Scientist.* Retrieved February 2, 2004, from *www.biomedcentral.com/news/20030916/04*

Walton, R. (1938). *America's new drug problem.* Philadelphia: Lippincott.

Watson, L., & Beck, J. (1986). New Age seekers: MDMA use as an adjunct to spiritual pursuit. *J Psychoactive Drugs, 23,* 261– 270.

Weir, E. (2000). Raves: A review of the culture, the drugs and the prevention of harm. *Can Med Assoc J, 162,* 1843–1848.

Winstock, A. R., Griffiths, P., & Stewart, D. (2001). Drugs and the dance music scene: A survey of current drug use patterns among a sample of dance music enthusiasts in the UK. *Drug Alcohol Depend, 64,* 9–17.

Zagnoni, P. G., & Albano, C. (2002). Psychostimulants and epilepsy. *Epilepsia, 43,* 28– 31.

CHAPTER 9

Cocaine and Stimulants

MICHELLE C. ACOSTA
DEBORAH L. HALLER
SIDNEY H. SCHNOLL

ETHNOGRAPHY

National-level prevalence studies indicate that after a period of recent decline, cocaine use may be rising again, especially among adults. Importantly, cocaine use has recently begun to increase again, with 0.9 million new users in 2000. Data from the 2001 National Household Survey on Drug Abuse (NHSDA; Substance Abuse and Mental Health Services Administration, 2001b) indicate that 1.7 million Americans, or 0.7% of the population age 12 and older, are current cocaine users, and that past year use increased significantly for both powder cocaine (1.5–1.9%) and crack cocaine (0.3–0.5%). Users were more likely to be young adults ages 18–25 (1.9%) than youth ages 12–17 (0.4%) or adults 26 years and older (0.6%). NHSDA data show that current cocaine use among young adults (ages 18–25) grew significantly, from 1.4% in 2000 to 1.9% in 2001, with significant increases in past year use from 4.4 to 5.7% for powder cocaine and 0.7 to 0.9% for crack. For adults age 26 and older, current use was relatively stable (0.4% in 2000 and 0.6% in 2001). However, past year use for adults ages 26–34 rose slightly for both powder cocaine (2.1–2.7%) and crack (0.4–0.6%). A similar 2000 to 2001 trend was found for current use in adults age 35 and older, with powder cocaine use increasing from 0.7 to 0.9% and crack use increasing from 0.2 to 0.3%. Current cocaine use also increased significantly among men (0.7% in 2000 to 1.0% in 2001), while women's use rates stayed approximately the same (0.4–0.5%). In addition, current cocaine use in 2001 was inversely correlated with educational status and was higher among the unemployed (3.6%) than among the employed (1.8%). Because socioeconomically disadvantaged persons are still a minority population, cocaine users are more often white, employed, and high school graduates (Johanson & Schuster, 1995).

Unlike adult levels of use, national-level prevalence studies indicate that adolescent (ages 12–17) levels of cocaine use appear stable and may be declining. According to NHSDA data, adolescents reported that past year cocaine use dropped from 1.7% in 2000 to 1.5 % in 2001, while past year crack use remained the same (0.4%). In 2001, the past year prevalence of cocaine use among youth ages 12–17 years was higher among Hispanic males (0.9%) and white females (0.6%) and males (0.4%) than among blacks (0.1%) and female Hispanics (.1%). The Monitoring the Future study (MTF; Johnston, O'Malley, & Bachman, 2003) demonstrated that past year rates for powder cocaine appear similar (1.9% in 2001 and 1.8% in 2002) for eighth graders, 10th graders (3.0% in 2001 and 3.4% in 2002), and 12th graders (4.4% in 2001 and 2002). Crack cocaine use appeared stable for eighth (1.7% in 2001 and 1.6% in 2002) and 12th graders (2.1% in 2001 to 2.3% in 2002), but increased significantly for 10th graders (1.8% in 2001 to 2.3% in 2002).

Consistent with overall growth in cocaine use, the Drug Abuse Warning Network (DAWN; Substance Abuse and Mental Health Services Administration, 2001a) reports that cocaine continues to be the most frequently mentioned illicit substance reported by hospital emergency departments (EDs) nationwide. The most recent data available regarding the consequences of cocaine use reveal rising ED mentions and declining treatment admissions. Data from DAWN show that the estimated number of cocaine-related ED mentions increased significantly, from 174,881 in 2000 to 193,034 in 2001. In fact, reports of cocaine were present in 30% of the ED drug episodes during 2001 and part of 2002. ED cocaine mentions in 2001 increased 10% from 2000. In a large study conducted in New York City, the rate of overdose deaths for cocaine increased from 1993 to 1998, with cocaine being involved in 69.5% of fatal overdoses. The majority of overdose death rates were attributed to drug combinations of opiates, cocaine, and alcohol. Accidental overdose deaths varied by racial and ethnic group, with overdose deaths among blacks due primarily to cocaine, and overdose deaths among Latinos and whites due to opiates with cocaine (Coffin et al., 2003).

Treatment Episode Data Set (TEDS; Substance Abuse and Mental Health Services Administration, 2002) data also reveal the use of cocaine in combination with other illegal drugs. Marijuana, methamphetamine, and heroin were the secondary drugs of abuse most often mentioned in 1999 TEDS admissions for which cocaine was identified as the primary substance of abuse. Admissions for cocaine taken by routes other than smoking were more likely to be white males (29%), followed by black males (23%), white females (18%), and black females (12%). Admissions for smoked cocaine were more likely to be black males (34%), followed by black females (25%), white males (18%), and white females (14%).

Consistent with NHSDA data, both DAWN ED and TEDS data indicate that the average age of cocaine users is increasing. DAWN data show significant increases between 2000 and 2001 in ED cocaine mentions for patients age 35 and older and for patients age 55 and older. TEDS data further indicate that in 1999, most cocaine-related treatment admissions were in the 35–39 age category, whereas in 1998, most cocaine-related treatment admissions were in the 30–34 age category.

The number of Drug Enforcement Administration (DEA) arrests involving cocaine dropped from 15,767 in 2000 to 12,847 in 2001, and data from the U.S. Sentencing Commission (USSC) show that the percentages of federal drug sentences involving powder and crack cocaine were nearly unchanged from 2000 to 2001. Data from the Arrestee Drug Abuse Monitoring (ADAM; U.S. Department of Justice, 2001) program demonstrated that a median of 29.1% of adult male arrestees and 30.7% of adult female arrestees tested positive for cocaine at arrest in 2001. A median of 18.9% of adult male arrestees and 28.5% of adult female arrestees reported using crack cocaine at least once in the year before being arrested. ADAM data indicate that powder cocaine in adult male arrestees decreased from 13.4% in 2000 to 12.5% in 2001, while crack cocaine in adult male arrestees increased from 17.5% in 2000 to 18.9% in 2001. However, National Drug Threat Survey (U.S. Department of Justice, 2003) data show that 33.1% of state and local law enforcement agencies nationwide identify cocaine as their greatest drug threat; 8.2% identify powder cocaine as their greatest drug threat, while 24.9% identify crack cocaine as their greatest drug threat. In both major urban areas, including Philadelphia and New York City, and rural areas (i.e., St. John Parish, Louisiana), between 31 and 40% of homicide victims tested positive for antemortem cocaine use (Clark, 1996; McGonigal et al., 1993; Tardiff et al., 1994).

PREPARATION AND ROUTES OF ADMINISTRATION

Cocaine is the most potent stimulant of natural origin. It is a benzoylmethylecgonine, an ester of benzoic acid and a nitrogen-containing base. Cocaine occurs naturally in the leaves of *Erythroxylon coca* and other species of *Erythroxylon* indigenous to Peru, Bolivia, Java, and Columbia. There are several basic routes to cocaine administration: chewing the leaves, cocaine sulfate (paste), cocaine hydrochloride, freebase cocaine, and crack cocaine. South American natives who chew coca leaves experience diminished hunger and fatigue, and an improved sense of well-being without evidence of chronic toxicity and dependence. However, other preparations and routes of administration of cocaine have a more rapid onset of action and are more problematic.

Cocaine sulfate (paste) is the intermediate form between the coca leaf and the finished cocaine hydrochloride crystal. The smoking of coca paste, popularly known as "pasta" or "bazooka," is prevalent in South America and also occurs in some parts of the United States. This results in a gray to white or dull brown powder, with a slightly sweet smell, that is 40–85% cocaine sulfate.

Cocaine hydrochloride is a stable, hydrophilic salt. Thus, it is frequently snorted (insufflation) or "tooted" in "lines" or "rails" about one-half to 2 inches long and one-eighth of an inch thick. Users pour the powdered cocaine onto a hard surface such as a mirror, glass, or slab of marble, and arrange it into lines with a razor blade, knife, or credit card. One line is snorted into each nostril via a rolled bill, straw, miniature coke spoon, or a specially grown fingernail. A single gram of cocaine produces about 30 lines averaging 10–35 mg of powder. The actual amount of cocaine hydrochloride present in each line depends on the purity of the drug. Absorption through the nasal mucosa is relatively modest due to a small surface area and the fact that cocaine is vasoconstrictive.

The bioavailability of intranasal cocaine is about 60%. Peak plasma levels occur over a range of 30–120 minutes (Barnett, Hawks, & Resnick, 1981). Cocaine is a topical anesthetic and causes numbness of the nose during snorting. Nasal congestion, with stuffiness and sneezing, may occur after snorting cocaine due to both vasoconstrictive properties and contaminants in the preparation. Users may flush out the inside of the nose with a saltwater mixture after a round of snorting, and they commonly employ decongestants and antihistamines to relieve symptoms.

Cocaine can also be injected intravenously: "shooting" or "mainlining." The cocaine hydrochloride is mixed with water in a spoon or bottle cap to form a solution. Unlike heroin, cocaine hydrochloride may not need to be heated to enter solution. "Kicking" or "booting" refers to drawing blood from the vein back into the syringe and reinjecting it with each cocaine mixture. Injection drug users feel that this produces a heightened drug sensation or "rush," despite the lack of a pharmokinetic basis. Following intravenous administration, users achieve peak plasma levels almost instantaneously.

Freebase cocaine is obtained by extracting cocaine hydrochloride with an alkali, such as buffered ammonia, then mixing it with a solvent, which is usually ether. The solvent fraction is separated and volatilized, leaving very small amounts of residual freebase material. Cocaine freebase is most often smoked in a special freebase glass pipe with a small bowl, into which the freebase cocaine is placed, or in a water pipe with a fine stainless steel screen on which the cocaine is vaporized. Cigarettes are rarely used, because only a small amount of cigarette smoke actually enters the lungs, wasting valuable cocaine. Cocaine hydrochloride is soluble in water and has a melting point of 195°C. In contrast, cocaine freebase is lipid-soluble and has a vaporizing point of 98°C. Thus, cocaine freebase vapors can be smoked, readily crossing the blood–lung barrier

(DePetrillo, 1985), resulting in nearly immediate peak plasma levels that are achieved at a rate similar to that of injecting cocaine hydrochloride.

"Crack" or "rock" is cocaine that has been processed from cocaine hydrochloride to a freebase for smoking. To prepare crack cocaine for injection, the crack cocaine is dissolved in water or alcohol, either by heating the solution or by acidifying it. The resultant viscous solution, which is too thick for use in standard insulin syringes, requires a larger bore needle. Because these needles are considerably harder to obtain, the incidence of needle sharing, along with the risk of HIV infection, is greater.

In the United States, popular street names for cocaine include toot, snow, blow, flake, white lady, snowbirds, paradise, and white. Adulterants commonly found in illicitly purchased cocaine include inert substances such as talc, flour, cornstarch, and various sugars (lactose, inositol, sucrose, maltose, and mannitol). Local anesthetics such as procaine, lidocaine, tetracaine, and benzocaine may be added to replace or enhance the local anesthetic effect of cocaine. Cheaper stimulants, including amphetamines, caffeine, methylphenidate, ergotamine, aminophylline, and strychnine ("death hit"), may also be added to the preparation. Quinine may be added for taste, and other compounds such as thiamin, tyramine, sodium carbonate, magnesium silicate, magnesium sulfate, salicylamide, and arsenic (Lombard, Levin, & Weiner, 1989) may be found. Crack and cocaine are also used frequently in conjunction with tobacco cigarettes and cigars (bananas, coolies, geek joints), 3,4-methylenedioxymethamphetamine (MDMA; "bumping up"), heroin (snow balls, speed balls, smoking gun, dynamite), marijuana (woolas, lace, Sherman stick, champagne, caviar), and amphetamines (snow seals).

Contaminants may include bacteria, fungi, and viruses. Users frequently take cocaine in combination with other drugs, citing the need to take the edge off the abrupt effects and "crash" from cocaine. Intravenous injection of heroin and cocaine mixed together is called "speedballing," and ingesting alcohol in conjunction with cocaine may be referred to as "liquid lady." Any drug combination is possible, and other opioids and depressants, as well as hallucinogens, phencyclidine (PCP), and marijuana, are all frequently used in conjunction with cocaine.

COCAETHYLENE

Simultaneous cocaine and alcohol use produces enhanced euphoria, compared to either substance alone (Farre et al., 1993). This enhanced effect has been attributed to pharmacokinetic factors, such as more rapid absorption and higher plasma concentrations (up to 30% increase) of cocaine (McCance-Katz et al., 1993). Typically, when cocaine and ethanol use coincide, the normal hydrolysis of cocaine to benzoylecgonine by hepatic carboxyesterase enzymes is inhibited, allowing higher levels of cocaine to remain in the body. A portion of this cocaine undergoes hepatic microsomal transesterification and is converted to cocaethylene (Andrews, 1997; Jatlow et al., 1991). Cocaethylene has very similar behavioral and toxicological effects to cocaine, but these effects last much longer (cocaethylene's plasma half-life is three to five times that of cocaine; Jatlow et al., 1991). Cocaethylene causes significant sustained increases in heart rate and blood pressure, myocardial infarctions, arrhythmias, and decreases in heart functioning, possibly due its inhibitory effects on potassium channels in the heart (O'Leary, 2002). In addition, cocaethylene is associated with seizures, liver damage, and immune compromise in adults (Andrews, 1997). Additional toxicological aspects, such as the effects on the exocrine pancreas, remain unexplored (Jatlow et al., 1991).

NEUROTRANSMITTERS AND BEHAVIORAL PHARMACOLOGY

Cocaine is both a stimulant of the central nervous system (CNS) and a local anesthetic, with large abuse liability due to its reinforcing properties. It is widely believed that the cocaine reward system is the mesocorticolimbic pathway, which originates in the ventral tegmental area (VTA) and projects to numerous areas of the forebrain, including the frontal cortex, hippocampus, amygdala, and the striatum (including the nucleus accumbens and the caudate putamen) (Koob, 1992). Recent work examining neurochemical turnover rates suggests that discrete subpopulations of dopamine, serotonin, glutamate, and gamma-aminobutyric acid (GABA)–releasing neurons are responsible for cocaine reward. Data suggest that dopamine in the nucleus accumbens, VTA, septum, lateral hypothalamus, and brainstem; glutamate in the nucleus accumbens and VTA; and serotonin in the medial hypothalamus are implicated in cocaine reward. In addition, surprising findings in the cerebral cortex have included noradrenergic and GABA activation of the somatosensory and anterior cingulate cortices, and glutamate activation of the posterior cingulate and entorhinal and visual cortices in response to cocaine administration (Smith, Koves, & Co, 2003).
Cocaine acts on these brain pathways by blocking the reuptake of dopamine, serotonin, and norepinephrine by binding to their respective neuronal transporters (DAT, SERT, NET), thereby increasing the synaptic concentration of these neurotransmitters. In addition, cocaine is responsible for indirect effects in the glutamate, GABA, and opioid systems, and for activating the stress response in the hypothalamic–pituitary–adrenal (HPA) axis. Research has just begun to elucidate the complex interplay of these direct and indirect effects on both the rewarding and aversive aspects of cocaine use. However, evidence generally suggests that dopamine plays a key role in cocaine reward,

and the many other neurotransmitter systems impact cocaine reward by acting on dopamine.

Corticotropin-releasing factor (CRF) modulates the HPA axis response to stressors. The HPA axis may be implicated in cocaine self-administration, particularly regarding relapse in cocaine use. Inhibition of circulating corticosterone decreases intravenous cocaine self-administration in rats. In addition, data suggest that corticosterone secretion does not play a major role in cocaine-induced reinstatement. However, a minimal level is necessary to achieve both stress-induced and cue-induced cocaine reinstatement, demonstrating an involvement of the HPA axis in the relapse of cocaine use (Goeders, 2002).

CLINICAL FEATURES

Intoxication/Overdose

With intoxication, cocaine blocks monoamine neuronal reuptake, initially leading to increased dopamine serotonin and norepinephrine availability at receptor sites. This stimulation of the endogenous pleasure center results in euphoria, increased energy and libido, decreased appetite, hyperalertness, and increased self-confidence when small initial doses of cocaine are taken. Exaggerated responses such as grandiosity, impulsivity, hyperawareness of the environment, and hypersexuality may also occur. The acute noradrenergic effects of small doses of cocaine include a mild elevation of pulse and blood pressure. Insomnia results from both increased dopamine and norepinephrine concentrations, and decreased serotonin synthesis and turnover.

Higher doses of cocaine are accompanied by increasing toxicity. Not only is there intensification of the "high," but anxiety, agitation, irritability, confusion, paranoia, and hallucinations may also occur. Sympathomimetic effects include dizziness, tremor, hyperreflexia, hyperpyrexia, mydriasis, diaphoresis, tachypnea, tachycardia, and hypertension. These symptoms can be accompanied by a sense of impending doom and may have important ramifications in overdose situations. Overdose complications may become manifest as muscle twitching, rhabdomyolysis, convulsions, cerebral infarction and hemorrhage, cardiac ischemia and arrhythmias, and respiratory failure.

More than any other stimulant, acute intoxication with cocaine is characterized by convulsions and cardiac arrhythmias. Death may be caused by peripheral autonomic toxicity and/or paralysis of the medullary cardiorespiratory centers (Gay, 1982).

Chronic Use

In contrast to acute intoxication, chronic cocaine administration results in neurotransmitter depletion. This is evidenced by a compensatory increase in postsynaptic receptor sensitivity for dopamine and noradrenaline, increased tyrosine hydroxylase activity (a major enzyme in norepinephrine and dopamine synthesis), and hyperprolactinemia. These are expected results for a negative feedback system. Chronic use is also associated with volume losses in the prefrontal cortex and nucleus accumbens. In addition, striatal dopamine response is significantly lower in cocaine abusers during withdrawal than in cocaine nonabusers. Furthermore, lower levels of dopamine receptors in the striatum are associated with lower metabolism in the orbitofrontal cortex and anterior cingulate gyrus in cocaine-addicted subjects (Goldstein & Volkow, 2002).

Clinical features of chronic cocaine use include depression, fatigue, poor concentration, loss of self-esteem, decreased libido, mild parkinsonian features (myoclonus, tremor, bradykinesis), paranoia, and insomnia. Tolerance to the stimulant effects of cocaine, particularly the anorexic effects, develops rapidly. However, repeated phasic use of low-dose cocaine can lead to enhanced sensitivity and potentiation of motor activity, including exaggerated "startle" reactions, dyskinesias, and postural abnormalities. Increased stereotypical behavior and a toxic psychosis can occur after repeated cocaine use. The elimination half-life of cocaine is under 1 hour by the intravenous route, and just over 1 hour by the intranasal route. The physiological and subjective effects due to cocaine correlate well with plasma levels (Javaid, Fischman, Schuster, Dekirmenjian, & Davis, 1978), although, with repeated use, pharmacodynamic tachyphylaxis does occur. Cocaine euphoria is of short duration, with a 10- to 20-second "rush," followed by 15–20 minutes of a lower level of euphoria and the subsequent onset of irritability and craving. Cocaine users who try to maintain the euphoric state readminister the drug frequently, until their supply disappears. Cocaine binges average 12 hours but can last as long as 7 consecutive days.

Withdrawal

A withdrawal syndrome, often referred to as the "crash," consists of strong craving, electroencephalograph abnormalities, depression, alterations in sleep patterns, hypersomnolence, and hyperphagia (Jones, 1984). However, because abrupt discontinuation of cocaine does not cause any major physiological sequelae, cocaine is stopped and not tapered or substituted by a cross-tolerant drug during medically supervised withdrawal. Following the resolution of intoxication and acute withdrawal symptoms, there is a 1- to 10-week period of chronic dysphoria, anergia, and anhedonia. Relapses frequently occur, because the memory of cocaine euphoria is quite compelling in contrast to a bleak background of intense boredom. If patients can remain abstinent from illicit mood-altering drugs during this period, the dysphoria gradually improves. Thereafter, intense cocaine craving is replaced by episodic craving that is frequently triggered by environmentally conditioned cues during an indefinite extinction phase.

Abuse and Addiction

The National Institute on Drug Abuse (NIDA) estimates that of the 30 million Americans who have tried cocaine intranasally, 20% become regular users and 5% develop compulsive use or addiction (Gawin & Ellinwood, 1988). Whether a given recreational cocaine user will become chemically dependent is difficult to predict. Abusers report that controlled use becomes compulsive either when they attain increased access to cocaine and therefore escalate their dosage, or when they switch to a more rapid route of administration (e.g., from intranasal administration to intravenous injection or smoking freebase or crack).

With recreational use, the cocaine user's initial experience of elation and heightened energy, with increased sexuality and self-esteem, appears to be free of negative consequences. Abusers may experience occasional problems associated with their drug use. Unlike dependence on alcohol or opiates, cocaine dependence is frequently characterized by binge use. With chronic and increased use, there is increased drug toxicity, dysphoria, and depression. The addict has irresistible cravings for cocaine. He or she focuses on pharmacologically based cocaine euphoria despite progressive inability to attain this state and adverse physical, psychological, and social sequelae. Loved ones are neglected, responsibility becomes immaterial, financial hardships occur, and nourishment, sleep, and health care are ignored.

GENETIC FACTORS

Studies in rodents suggest that genetic variation influences several aspects of the response to cocaine, including preference, stimulant effects, and sensitization (Miner & Marley, 1995; Schuster, Yu, & Bates, 1977). Cocaine dependence in probands specifically increased the risk of cocaine dependence in siblings (Bierut et al., 1998).

One large-scale twin study of substance use and abuse in male U.S. veterans found that genetic factors played a substantial etiological role in stimulant abuse (Tsuang et al., 1996). However, the effects were generally nonspecific, indicating that the same characteristics that place an individual at risk for cocaine abuse also put that individual at risk for other substance abuse. A second study focusing specifically on cocaine use, abuse, and dependence was conducted in over 800 pairs of female–female twins ascertained from the population-based Virginia Twin Registry (Karkowski, Prescott, & Kendler, 2000). Cocaine use, abuse, and dependence were all found to be strongly influenced by both shared environmental influences and genetic factors, with heritabilities ranging from 69 to 81%. However, both the environmental and genetic factors appeared nonspecific. A third, large-scale twin study examined lifetime history of use and abuse/dependence of cocaine and other drugs in 1,196 male–male twin pairs ascertained by the Virginia Twin Registry (Kendler, Jacobson, Prescott, & Neale, 2003). Ultimately, one must conclude that while cocaine use, abuse, and dependence seem to be strongly influenced by genetic factors, evidence for a cocaine-specific genetic effect is currently lacking.

PSYCHIATRIC COMORBIDITY AND SEQUELAE

More than one-half of all cocaine abusers meet criteria for a current psychiatric diagnosis and nearly three-fourths for a lifetime psychiatric diagnosis (Ziedonis, Rayford, Bryant, Kendall, & Rounsaville, 1994). The most common comorbid psychiatric diagnoses among cocaine abusers include alcohol dependence, affective disorders, anxiety disorders, and antisocial personality disorder (Kleinman et al., 1990; Marlowe, Husband, Lamb, & Kirby, 1995; Mirin, Weiss, Griffin, & Michael, 1991; Rounsaville et al., 1991; Weiss, Mirin, Griffin, Gunderson, & Hufford, 1993). For most cocaine users, co-occurring psychiatric disorders (including agoraphobia, alcohol abuse, alcohol dependence, depression, posttraumatic stress disorder (PTSD), simple phobia, and social phobia) precede cocaine use (Abraham & Fava, 1999; Shaffer & Eber, 2002).

The most frequent co-occurring substance use disorder is alcoholism; 29% of cocaine abusers have a current alcoholism diagnosis, and 62% a lifetime alcoholism diagnosis (Rounsaville et al., 1991). These findings are alarming considering that individuals with comorbid cocaine and alcohol use disorders manifest a more severe form of cocaine dependence, and comorbid alcohol abuse is associated with poorer retention in treatment and poorer treatment outcomes for both disorders (Brady, Sonne, Randall, Adinoff, & Malcolm, 1995). Cocaine use disorders also are common among opioid abusers. In addition, 66% of methadone-maintained patients abuse cocaine (Kosten, Rounsaville, & Kleber, 1987), and 75% of the heroin addicts admitted to methadone programs identify cocaine as their secondary drug of abuse (New York State Division of Substance Abuse Services, 1990). A national survey of 15 clinics (General Accounting Office, 1990) revealed continued cocaine use in as many as 40% of patients after 6 months of treatment. Marijuana is also commonly misused among cocaine-dependent patients. Studies have found that 25–70% of cocaine-dependent patients also abuse marijuana (Higgins, Budney, Bickel, & Badger, 1994). Similarly, 80.5% of cocaine-dependent patients smoke tobacco cigarettes (Patkar et al., 2002), and the heavier the tobacco smoking, the heavier the use of cocaine (Henningfield, Clayton, & Pollin, 1990). In addition, cocaine-dependent individuals who smoke tobacco report an earlier age of onset and more frequent use of cocaine than cocaine-dependent individuals who do not smoke (Budney, Higgins, Hughes, & Bickel, 1993).

Non-substance-related Axis I disorders are also common among cocaine addicts. The rates for current depressive disorders vary between 11 and 55% (Carroll et al., 1994; Griffin, Weiss, Mirin, & Lange, 1989; Haller, Knisely, Dawson, & Schnoll, 1993), whereas those for lifetime depression range from 40 to 60% (Kleinman et al., 1990). Bipolar depression appears to be over-represented among cocaine users. In a large, community-based sample, 42.1% of cocaine abusers were found to have bipolar disorder (Karam, Yabroudi, & Melhem, 2002). Because of the specific actions and effects of cocaine, it is sometimes difficult to determine whether depression is independent of cocaine use or the result of chronic self-administration. However, depression that pre-dates drug use or persists beyond the 1–2 weeks characteristic of cocaine with-drawal may indicate a coexisting disorder. Also, if a cocaine abuser becomes acutely depressed or suicidal after ingesting only very small amounts of the drug, a primary depressive disorder may be indicated (Kosten et al., 1987). In most cases of comorbid depression and cocaine use, depression precedes cocaine use by an average of 7 years (Abraham & Fava, 1999). Panic disorder is prevalent among cocaine abusers, and the literature contains a number of case reports of individuals who developed panic disorder following cocaine use (Aronson & Craig, 1986; Bystritsky, Ackerman, & Pasnau, 1991). Among 122 cocaine-dependent outpatients, 30.2% of women and 15.2% of men met DSM criteria for PTSD (Najavits et al., 1998). Furthermore, in a large epidemiological study, rates of PTSD among cocaine-dependent individuals were 10 times higher than among non-cocaine-dependent individuals. Findings suggest that cocaine de-pendence is a risk factor for PTSD, because it usually precedes the trauma and places individuals in situations where traumatic events are more likely to occur (Cottler, Compton, Mager, Spitznagel, & Janca, 1992).

Attention-deficit/hyperactivity disorder (ADHD) is an important comor-bid condition. In a large longitudinal study, approximately 21% of adults with ADHD were cocaine dependent, compared to 10% of agemate controls (Lam-bert & Hartsough, 1998). Studies indicate that between 12 and 35% of cocaine addicts meet childhood criteria for ADHD (Carroll & Rounsaville, 1993; Levin, Evans, & Kleber, 1998; Rounsaville et al., 1991). Compared to cocaine abusers without comorbid ADHD, those with ADHD are more likely to be male and to also meet criteria for conduct disorder and antisocial personality disorder. Cocaine abusers with ADHD evidence earlier age of onset of use, more frequent and severe use, more alcoholism, and more prior treatment epi-sodes. Men who score high on an ADHD measure also report more use of cocaine for the purpose of self-medication (Horner, Scheibe, & Stine, 1996). Although somewhat controversial, several case reports suggest that stimulants (e.g., magnesium pemoline, and methylphenidate) can be successfully used to treat patients with comorbid cocaine abuse and ADHD (Khantzian, Gawin,

Kleber, & Riordan, 1984; Weiss, Pope, & Mirin, 1985). This treatment effect appears to be selective, because non-ADHD cocaine abusers derive no apparent benefit from stimulants but do manifest cross-tolerance (Gawin, Riordan, & Kleber, 1985).

Studies conducted with both inpatients and outpatients with schizophrenia show prevalence of cocaine use falling between 20 and 93% (Regier et al., 1990; Rosenthal, Hellerstein, Miner, & Christian, 1994; Schwartz, Swanson, & Hannon 2003; Ziedonis & Fischer, 1996). Cocaine-abusing persons with schizophrenia have fewer negative signs (Lysaker, Bell, Beam-Goulet, & Milstein, 1994), but more depression and anxiety at the time of hospital admission (Serper, Alpert, Richardson, & Dickson, 1995); at posttreatment, no differences in negative signs or mood are observed, suggesting that differences result from the effects of cocaine. Persons with schizophrenia who abuse cocaine have increased morbidity, evidenced by higher rates of hospitalization, greater suicidality, and the need for higher doses of neuroleptics than both users of other drugs and nonusers (Seibyl, Satel, Anthoy, & Southwick, 1993). Cocaine use may itself induce noxious psychiatric effects, some of them psychotic in nature. Bruxism, picking at the face and body, and other stereotypical or repetitious behaviors may occur. Cocaine hallucinosis may include visual, tactile, auditory, and olfactory hallucinations, along with delusions. Cocaine users may also perceive "cocaine bugs" on their skin, as well as visual "snow lights." In less severe cases, the user is aware that the hallucinations and delusions are not real. However, in more severe cases, individuals may show a full-blown toxic psychosis with extreme paranoia, hypervigilance, and ideas of persecution. This toxic psychosis can potentially lead to unusual aggressiveness, damaged property, and homicidal or suicidal behavior. Fortunately, these effects are generally limited to the time of cocaine intoxication.

Comorbid Axis II disorders are even more prevalent than Axis I disorders, with rates of personality disorders in cocaine abusers ranging from 30 to 75% in inpatient samples (Kleinman et al., 1990; Kranzler, Satel, & Apter, 1994; Weiss et al., 1993). Cocaine addicts with personality disorders tend to have greater psychiatric severity than those without personality disorders and are also at greater risk for both anxiety and mood disorders (Bunt, Galanter, Lifshutz, & Castaneda, 1990; Stone, 1992). Among cocaine-abusing outpatients, 48% have at least one personality disorder, whereas 18% have two or more (Barber, Frank, Weiss, & Blane, 1996). Even more compelling, 65% of those with a comorbid Axis II diagnosis have a Cluster B disorder, antisocial and borderline personality disorder (BPD) being the most frequent. Patients with BPD have higher levels of polysubstance and cocaine dependence, and also have more personality disorders such as avoidant, antisocial, and dependent personality disorder (Kranzler et al., 1994; Nurnberg, Rifkin, & Doddi, 1993). For cocaine abusers in intensive outpatient treatment, the rates of co-occurring personality disorders are quite high; three-fourths meet criteria for at least one Axis II diagnosis and more than one-third have two or more (Haller et al., 1993; Marlowe et al., 1995). Males are more likely to have comorbid alcohol dependence, stimulant dependence, antisocial personality disorder, and narcissistic personality disorder, whereas females are more likely to be diagnosed with mood disorders and BPD. It is important to evaluate patients routinely for Axis II disorders at point of treatment entry and to design drug treatment programs that provide adequate attention to these comorbid conditions.

Unfortunately, psychiatric comorbidity has negative implications for symptom expression, prognosis, medical compliance, and services utilization (Bartels et al., 1993; Moos, Mertens, & Brennan, 1994; Moos & Moos, 1995; Pristach & Smith, 1990). It is important for substance abuse and mental health clinicians to become aware of patterns of comorbidity among their patients and to develop treatment plans that address dual disorders simultaneously. Awareness of subtypes of cocaine abusers may help to guide treatment in both pharmacological and psychological intervention.

MEDICAL COMPLICATIONS

Direct Results of Cocaine Use

Medical consequences of acute and chronic cocaine abuse may be categorized as those caused directly by cocaine, those due to adulterants, and those related to route of administration. The most common direct medical consequences of cocaine use include cardiovascular and CNS difficulties.

Cocaine use may account for up to 25% of cases of acute myocardial infarction among patients 18–45 years of age (Weber, Hollander, Murphy, Braunwald, & Gibson, 2003). Upon acute administration, cocaine increases blood pressure and heart rate, primarily through an action on the sympathetic nervous system. Through its pharmacological effect at alpha- and beta-adrenergic receptors, cocaine may increase oxygen demand of the myocardium by increasing blood pressure and heart rate. Cocaine also suppresses the baroreflex response and vagal tone, further contributing to its effects on heart rate. At the same time that cocaine is increasing the workload on the heart, it induces coronary artery vasoconstriction and platelet aggregation, potentially leading to coronary spasm and/or cardiac ischemia (Schrank, 1993). In addition, cocaine use is also associated with significantly decreased coronary blood flow velocity, leading to increased microvascular resistance. Slow coronary filling may also suggest the possibility of cocaine use in patients in whom it was not otherwise suspected (Kelly, Sompalli, Sattar, & Khankari, 2003). At higher doses, cocaine can depress ventricular function and slow electrical conduction in the heart. Both these effects appear to be mediated by cocaine's local anesthetic action. Cocaine may potentiate catecholamine activity, impacting voltage-dependent sodium ion channels related to local anesthetic properties.

When cocaine is administered repeatedly over a short period of time, acute tolerance can develop to the sympathomimetic effects of cocaine. In contrast, the effects of cocaine mediated by its local anesthetic action do not appear blunted by anesthesia or susceptible to acute tolerance. In addition to the effects of cocaine alone, the metabolites of cocaine may also contribute to cocaine's acute and chronic cardiovascular toxicity, and both licit and illicit drugs used in combination with cocaine might potentially alter its cardiovascular effects (Schindler, 1996).

With chronic administration, higher cocaine doses appear to induce tolerance, while lower doses may induce sensitization to cocaine's sympathomimetic effects. Chronic cocaine use is associated with multiple cardiovascular conditions, including myocardial infarction, aortic dissection, left ventricular hypertrophy, arrhythmias, sudden death, and cardiomyopathy (Frishman, Del Vecchio, Sanal, & Ismail, 2003).

CNS manifestations of cocaine exposure include seizures, status epilepticus, cerebral hemorrhage, and transient ischemic attacks. Cocaine may produce hyperpyrexia through direct effects on thermoregulatory centers. Depression of the medullary centers may result in respiratory paralysis, and sudden death may be caused by respiratory arrest, myocardial infarction or arrhythmia, or status epilepticus (Cregler & Mark, 1986). Migraine-like headaches have been associated with cocaine withdrawal and may be linked to serotonin dysregulation (Satel & Gawin, 1989). Rhabdomyolysis is a complication of cocaine use. When it is accompanied by acute renal failure, severe liver dysfunction, and disseminated intravascular coagulation, the fatality rate is high (Roth, Alarcon, Fernandez, Preston, & Bourgoignie, 1988).

Other difficulties associated with chronic cocaine use include weight loss, dehydration, nutritional deficiencies (particularly of vitamins B_6, C, and thiamine), and endocrine abnormalities. Neglect of self-care may be evident, including dental caries and periodontitis exacerbated by bruxism. Addicts may medicate their pain with cocaine or other mood-altering drugs and seek medical attention only after prolonged existence of their problem(s).

Adulterants also play a role in the development of medical complications. Local anesthetics and stimulants may increase cocaine's inherent toxicity by increasing the risk of hypertension and cardiovascular complications. Sugars, though relatively benign, may encourage development of bacteria that becomes problematic when injected intravenously.

Other complications of cocaine may be due to the route of administration. Intestinal ischemia caused by vasoconstriction and reduced blood flow in the mesenteric vasculature from catecholamine stimulation of alpha receptors has been reported after oral cocaine ingestion (Texter, Chou, Merrill, Laureton, & Frohlich, 1964). Emergency room patients have required surgical correction of their intestinal perforations, after smoking crack cocaine. The chronological relationship between crack consumption and gastrointestinal perforation indicates that crack may induce ischemic events, causing intestinal ruptures in some people (Muniz & Evans, 2001).

Gastroenterological exposure to cocaine has been studied among drug smugglers, among whom a 58% mortality rate has occurred when swallowed cocaine packets have ruptured (McCarron & Wood, 1983), or among those who swallow cocaine for other reasons. If a packet ruptures, causing severe cocaine intoxication, immediate laparotomy for removal of the packets is the best treatment option (Schaper, Hofmann, Ebbecke, Desel, & Langer, 2003). The treatment for those who swallow cocaine may be less clear, but each group requires medical attention.

Complications of intranasal administration include loss of sense of smell, atrophy and inflammation, and necrosis and perforation of the nasal septum. Snorting cocaine may anesthetize and paralyze the pharynx and larynx, causing hoarseness and predisposing the person to aspiration pneumonia (Estroff & Gold, 1986). Recurrent snorting of cocaine may result in ischemia, necrosis, and infections of the nasal mucosa, sinuses, and adjacent structures.

In terms of pulmonary effects, pneumomediastinum and cervical emphysema have been reported after smoking cocaine due to alveolar rupture with prolonged deep inspiration and Valsalva's maneuver (Aroesty, Stanley, & Crockett, 1986). Other respiratory complications of inhaling or smoking freebase cocaine include abnormal reductions in carbon monoxide diffusing capacity (Itkonen, Schnoll, & Glassroth, 1984), granulomatous pneumonitis (Cooper, Bai, Heyderman, & Lorrin, 1983), pulmonary edema (Allred & Ewer, 1981), thermal airway injury, pulmonary hemorrhage, hypersensitivity reactions, interstitial lung disease, obliterative bronchiolitis, asthma, and persistent gas-exchange abnormalities (Laposata & Mayo, 1993). Respiratory manifestations include shortness of breath, cough, wheezing, hemoptysis, and chest pains. Severe respiratory difficulties have been reported in neonates of abusing mothers. Inhalation of hot cocaine vapors may also result in bilateral loss of eyebrows and eyelashes (Tames & Goldenring, 1986), and preparation of freebase cocaine with solvents such as ether may result in accidental burns and explosions.

Complications of intravenous cocaine use are multiple and include skin abscesses, phlebitis and cellulitis, and septic emboli resulting in pneumonia, pulmonary abscesses, subacute bacterial endocarditis, ophthalmological infections, and fungal cerebritis (Wetti, Weiss, Cleary, & Gyori, 1984). Injected talc and silicate may cause granulomatous pneumonitis with pulmonary hypertension, as well as granulomata of the liver, brain, or eyes (Estroff & Gold, 1986). Hepatitis B, hepatitis C, and delta agent are all too frequently by-products of intravenous drug abuse. In the past several years, concomitant with the increase in HIV infection, there has been an increase in pneumonia, endocarditis, tuberculosis, and hepatitis delta and other sexually transmitted diseases in drug users (see Chapter 19 on HIV and addictions for more information on cocaine and HIV/AIDS).

OBSTETRIC AND DEVELOPMENTAL EFFECTS

In the United States, more than 100,000 babies are exposed prenatally to cocaine each year (Office of the Inspector General, 1990). Increasing evidence indicates that prenatal cocaine exposure is associated with negative perinatal outcomes, including premature delivery, low birthweight, microcephaly, newborn behavioral abnormalities, and possible long-term cognitive and developmental difficulties (Singer et al., 2002). However, the impact of cocaine on the developing fetus is difficult to ascertain, because no confined, homogeneous, syndromic pattern of malformations has been identified, and because the mechanisms by which cocaine impacts on the unborn child are complex; maternal cocaine use may have both indirect and direct effects on a developing fetus (Vidaeff & Mastrobattista, 2003).

Indirect effects of maternal cocaine use include negative health consequences for mothers, which then impact their pregnancies. Women using cocaine are more likely to suffer arrhythmias, cardiac ischemias, and hemorrhagic strokes. In addition, they may develop pregnancy complications similar to preeclampsia, including hypertension, headaches, blurred vision, and placental abruption, as well as vascular damage and uterine vasoconstriction, leading to problems such as spontaneous abortion and premature delivery (Church & Subramanian, 1997). Poor maternal weight gain and increased energy demands are another common effect of cocaine use in pregnant women, often leading to decreased birthweights and poorer prenatal nutrition (Church et al., 1991).

In addition to indirect effects, cocaine readily crosses the placental barrier and can thereby directly influence the unborn child (Moore, Sorg, Miller, Key, & Resnik, 1986; Volpe, 1992). Due to the fetus's immature metabolic systems, the drug is poorly metabolized, increasing its half-life (Chasnoff & Schnoll, 1987). Research has also shown that maternal intake of cocaine results in increased fetal systolic blood pressure, decreased uterine blood flow, and decreased fetal oxygenation (Moore et al., 1986), which may also negatively impact child outcomes.

Cocaine may directly affect early embryonic development by disrupting energy-producing mechanisms for cell metabolism and impact later fetal development by crossing the placenta, causing vascular disruption and changes in neurochemistry. Vascular disruption during a critical developmental period may be responsible for problems such as limb reduction deformities, intestinal atresia, fetal edema, necrotizing enterocolitis, intracranial hemorrhage, stroke, porencephaly, and other cocaine-related problems (Vidaeff & Mastrobasttista, 2003).

A stable, negative, cocaine-specific effect on language functioning was found through age 7, after controlling for sex, age, prenatal exposure to alcohol, marijuana and tobacco, and over 20 other medical and demographic factors (Bandstra et al., 2002). Similarly, Azuma and Chasnoff (1993) reported lower

IQ scores (though still in the normal range) on the Stanford–Binet for children prenatally exposed to cocaine in combination with other drugs; this study also identified mediating variables such as home environment, head circumference, and child behavior. In addition, a large study found that cocaine-exposed children were twice as likely to be significantly delayed developmentally throughout the first 2 years of life and were twice as likely to require intervention as the noncocaine polydrug-exposed comparison group. These cognitive delays were not due to exposure to other drugs or to covariates. Furthermore, poorer cognitive outcomes were related to higher levels of prenatal cocaine exposure (Singer et al., 2002). In addition to cognitive delays, 2-year-olds who had been prenatally exposed to both PCP and cocaine were found to utilize less mature play strategies and to evidence less sustained attention, more deviant behaviors, and poorer quality interactions with caregivers (Beckwith et al., 1994).

In summary, findings on the consequences of prenatal cocaine exposure relative to child development are inconsistent. Early concerns about severe, permanent neurobehavioral deficits appear to have been exaggerations; however, evidence remains that prenatal exposure to cocaine may contribute to the development of more mild or subtle neurobehavioral difficulties, such as poorer language functioning. In studying this population, it will be essential for researchers to control for confounding factors such as age, race, socioeconomic status, and other drug use; this is especially true, because some studies have found environmental factors to be equal even more important determinants of functioning.

ASSESSMENT

Initial evaluation of the cocaine abuser begins with a medical, psychiatric, and psychosocial history, as well as a physical examination. Confirming and augmenting the patient's history through collateral reports of family members and significant others is often helpful. On an emergency basis, the following laboratory tests need to be considered, based on the patient's clinical presentation: complete blood count, chemical profile (SMA-12), urinalysis, urine and/or blood toxicology, electrocardiogram, and chest X-ray. Indications for acute hospitalization include (1) serious medical or psychiatric problems either caused by the stimulant drugs or independently coexisting, and (2) concurrent dependence on other drugs, such as alcohol or sedative hypnotics, necessitating a more closely supervised withdrawal. A validated, widely accepted tool to assess addiction severity specifically to cocaine has not yet been developed. However, DSM-IV-TR (American Psychiatric Association, 2000) diagnostic criteria for cocaine intoxication, withdrawal, delirium, delusional disorder, dependence, and abuse are based on the symptoms described in this chapter. Evaluation to guide addiction treatment needs to address a variety of issues, including the dosage, patterns, chronicity, and method of cocaine use; other drug use; antedating and drug-related medical, social, and psychological problems; the patient's cognitive ability and social skills; and the patient's knowledge, motivation, attitude, and expectations of treatment (Washton, Stone, & Hendrickson, 1988). Additional factors indicating increased severity of addiction that may necessitate inpatient treatment include chronic smoking of freebase or intravenous cocaine use, the demonstrated inability to abstain from use while in outpatient treatment, and the lack of family and social supports.

Once the patient is stabilized and assigned to an appropriate level of care, a more detailed medical, psychiatric, and psychosocial history and physical examination should be performed. Patient motivation and readiness for change may enhance retention and positive treatment outcomes. The search for evidence of medical, neuropsychological, and psychiatric sequelae should be stressed, as well as consequences of self-neglect. The following laboratory tests should be considered supplements to those obtained previously on an acute care basis: pulmonary function testing with diffusing capacity of carbon monoxide (DLCO, DCO) in smokers of freebase and crack cocaine, and purified protein derivative (PPD) tubercular skin testing with controls; rapid plasma reagin agglutination test (RPR; syphilis serology); hepatitis B surface antigen and hepatitis C antigen; and HIV serology in intravenous users. Because these patients generally have poor follow-up rates, immunizations should be given, and general preventive health maintenance should be performed at this time as well.

TREATMENT

Overdose

In the case of a massive cocaine overdose, patients are likely to present with advanced cardiorespiratory distress and seizures. Treatment is performed in an emergency setting, with attention to cardiac function, and with an eye to the presence of other substances. The principles of resuscitation, along with the administration of thiamine, glucose, and naloxone (Narcan), are necessary (Goldfrank & Hoffman, 1993).

Intoxication

Intoxicated persons who seek assistance with less severe cocaine complications are more likely to present with panic, irritability, hyperreflexia, paranoia, hallucinations, and stereotyped repetitive movements. Assurance in a calm, nonthreatening environment is a prerequisite for successful patient management. Psychosis can be treated with haloperidol, although caution is necessary, because this medication can lower the seizure threshold. Monoamine oxidase inhibitors are contraindicated, because they block cocaine degradation. Infectious diseases and other complications need to be treated appropriately. Sodium nitroprusside, phentolamine, and calcium channel blockers are effective therapies for hypertension. Propranolol is controversial due to resultant unopposed alpha-receptor stimulation.

Withdrawal

Benzodiazepines may ameliorate the "crash" or early phase withdrawal from cocaine. However, the high abuse potential of benzodiazepines limits their therapeutic value (Kosten, 1988). The most serious complication of early withdrawal is depression, with the potential for suicide. Patients must be watched closely when manifesting depression and agitation. If symptoms of depression do not remit within 10 days to 2 weeks, despite relative normalization of sleep patterns, underlying major depression requiring psychiatric intervention is suggested. In addition, repeated exposure to cocaine followed by withdrawal leads to an activation of the neuroendocrine stress response, which may increase susceptibility to infection during the initial stages of withdrawal (Avila, Morgan, & Bayer, 2003).

Pharmacological Treatment of Chronic Cocaine Addiction

Clinical researchers have tried to identify drugs to reduce cocaine craving and prevent relapse. Numerous drugs looked promising in initial open-label trials but did not prove efficacious in subsequent placebo-controlled studies. These pharmacological treatments have included dopaminergic agonists (e.g., monamine oxidase inhibitors, amantadine, mazindol, methylphenidate, pemoline, bromocriptine, L-dopa, and pergolide), neurotransmitter precursors (L-tyrosine, L-tryptophan, and multivitamins with B complex), carbamazepine, and antidepressants, including desipramine and fluoxetine. In a meta-analysis examining 45 clinical trials examining mostly antidepressants, carbamazepine, and dopamine agonists, no significant impact of drug treatment was found, regardless of the type of drug or dose used (Lima, Soares, Reisser, & Farrell, 2002).

Clinical trials with bupropion, olanzapine, naltrexone, buprenorphine, and other drugs are ongoing. As our understanding of the neurobiological basis of cocaine addiction becomes further refined, new pharmacological strategies are emerging. Potential targets include specific dopamine, serotonin, and other receptor subtypes, neuroendocrine peptides (i.e., CRF), and biogenic amine transporters, including the dopamine reuptake transporter. These pharmacotherapies and the potential development of a vaccine to prevent cocaine from reaching its CNS site of action are covered in Chapter 26.

Cognitive, Behavioral, and Nonpharmacological Treatments

Cocaine disorders have proven to be refractory to both psychological and pharmacological treatment. Consequently, considerable energy has been directed toward developing and testing the efficacy of new psychotherapeutic approaches in the treatment of cocaine use disorders. Many of these therapies have been adapted from ones originally developed to treat alcoholism. One approach that has received attention is cognitive-behavioral relapse prevention (Marlatt & Gordon, 1985). Relapse prevention strives to teach the addict how to recognize high-risk situations and deal with these using cognitive strategies that have been well rehearsed. Relapse prevention recognizes that with a chronic disorder such as addiction, relapses and remissions are expected. When a relapse occurs, more intense treatment and cognitive restructuring are necessary to help prevent a "slip" from escalating. Reminding patients of their prior progress, focusing on making the "slip" an isolated event, and maximizing the learning value of this experience are constructive ways of handling the situation. The literature on efficacy of relapse prevention in the treatment of cocaine dependence is mixed. In a review of 24 randomized clinical trials of relapse prevention for drug abuse (including cocaine), Carroll (1996) concluded that relapse prevention is superior to no treatment, although superiority to other active therapies is less evident.

Cognitive behavioral therapy (CBT) is also an effective treatment for cocaine addiction, and improves comorbid psychosocial problems (Carroll, 2000). In addition, CBT has demonstrated higher retention rates and improved compliance compared to other forms of individual and group therapy (Crits-Christoph et al., 1999). However, recent findings indicate that patients with cognitive impairments are more likely to drop out of CBT (Aharonovich, Nunes, & Hasin, 2003).

A somewhat different approach has been taken by researchers studying the role of conditioned cues or "reminders" of cocaine use (O'Brien, Childress, Arndt, & McLellan, 1988); this approach attempts to extinguish conditioned responses to these cocaine cues, thereby reducing the chances for relapse. Desensitization training requires that patients be repeatedly exposed to drug stimuli, then given the opportunity to deal with them in real-life situations. Behavioral rehearsal is key to being prepared to deal with the drug-laden situations that exist outside the protection of the treatment center. In one study (O'Brien, Childress, McLellan, & Ehrman, 1990), 30 drug-free cocaine addicts were repeatedly exposed to cocaine cues within a controlled setting. Subjects reported experiencing strong physiological arousal, including cocaine craving, highs, and withdrawal in response to exposure. However, by the sixth hour of extinction (repeated nonreinforced exposure to cocaine cues), highs and withdrawal were no longer reported and, by the 15th hour, craving was no longer experienced. Despite the strong extinction of arousal, these effects diminished over time, unless they were reinforced with repeated cue exposure sessions.

Voucher-based reinforcement strategies have also shown considerable promise (Higgins, Budney, Bickel, & Foerg, 1994; Higgins et al., 1995, 2000). Higgins and colleagues (1994) demonstrated that voucher incentives (in combination with comprehensive behavioral intervention) enhanced retention in the 24-week-long treatment program both for patients receiving interventions (75%) and those receiving behavioral therapy only (40%). In addition, those in the voucher group had greater continuous abstinence and evidenced greater improvements on the Addiction Severity Index (ASI) Drug and Psychiatric scales than those not receiving vouchers. Subsequent follow-up assessments indicated that these gains were maintained 6 months after treatment (Higgins et al., 1995), and as much as 15 months after treatment (Higgins et al., 2000). Other studies of contingent vouchers have yielded similarly positive outcomes in cocaine-dependent outpatients (Kirby, Marlowe, Festinger, Lamb, & Platt, 1998; Silverman et al., 1996). In addition, a study by Rawson and colleagues (2002) compared contingency management (vouchers), CBT, a combination of the two, and a "no-cocaine-treatment condition," which consisted of methadone maintenance for heroin addiction only in patients with heroin and cocaine dependence. They found that contingency management was associated with significantly higher levels of cocaine abstinence than were the CBT or control interventions. However, the CBT group showed improvement at the 6- and 12-month follow-up points that was congruent with the contingency management group.

Unfortunately, not all substance abusers are motivated to change their drug use behavior; this is particularly true of patients with comorbid psychiatric disorders, who may be overwhelmed by their multiple problems and prior treatment failures (Martino, McCance-Katz, Workman, & Boozang, 1995; Ziedonis & Fischer, 1996). Motivational enhancement therapy (MET), or motivational interviewing (MI), a nonconfrontational approach developed by Miller and Rollnick (1991), was originally designed for working with problem drinkers. In numerous trials, the principles of MI have been shown to be effective, sometimes after only one or two sessions (Bien, Miker, & Tonigan, 1993; Brown & Miller, 1993). Because of promising results with alcoholics, MET/MI is currently being adapted for use with drug abusers, including those with cocaine dependence and psychiatric comorbidity. MET/MI works in tandem with the stages-of-change model of Prochaska, DiClemente, and Norcross (1992). The model postulates five distinct stages: precontemplation, contemplation, action, maintenance, and relapse. These stages can be assessed via paper-and-pencil instruments, such as the University of Rhode Island Change Assessment (URICA). Different therapeutic strategies are employed, based on the patient's designated stage of change. MET/MI represents a clear departure from traditional drug abuse counseling strategies. Because acceptance of the addict identity is considered unimportant, patients are less likely to manifest overt resistance. Rather than emphasize powerlessness, this approach assumes that people have within themselves the capacity to change. Although the efficacy of MET/MI for cocaine abusers has yet to be proven, it would appear that its unique focus on readiness should, at minimum, help patients to engage in other forms of therapy. In addition, a few studies have begun to support the use of MET/MI for treatment of cocaine abuse and dependence. In a small study examining 27 female workers with concurrent cocaine or heroin dependence, MI significantly reduced the women's cocaine use (Yahne, Miller, Irvin-Vitela, & Tonigan, 2002). Similarly, compared to patients who only underwent a detoxification program, patients who also received MI were more likely to be abstinent from cocaine following detoxification and demonstrated higher abstinence rates throughout the following relapse prevention treatment. In addition, MI was more effective for those patients with lower initial motivation (Stotts, Schmitz, Rhoades, & Grabowski, 2001). Finally, Brown and colleagues (1998) showed that, compared to patients who received meditation/relaxation, patients who received MI had better retention in treatment, though no differences were found in overall cocaine use. The researchers also found that MI patients who initially reported less motivation for change had higher rates of abstinence at follow-up than did MI patients reporting more motivation for change at baseline. These findings suggest that MET/MI strategies may be most effective for patients who come into drug treatment with low motivation.

The approaches described (i.e., relapse prevention, cue exposure/desensitization, contingency management, and motivational interviewing) are somewhat technical and require specific training and supervision. Research-based interventions such as these appear to be the wave of the future, and most can be adapted for use in community-based programs. Frequently, treatment of cocaine dependence takes place within the context of a comprehensive drug treatment program. Although therapeutic modalities may be the same as for other drug abusers (e.g., education, and individual and group therapy), the intensity of treatment must be greater. Emphasis must be placed on the acquisition of skills that will enable the cocaine abuser to have more internal control, greater self-efficacy, and reduced likelihood of relapse. This means that treatment must have multiple "practical" components.

The first goal of treatment is to interrupt recurrent binges or daily use of cocaine and overcome drug craving. For patients who do not have serious psychiatric comorbidity, a structured outpatient program can be attempted prior to physically removing the person from the drug-using environment for treatment in a residential setting. While attempting to initiate abstinence, treatment should include daily or multiple weekly contacts and urine monitoring, with as many external controls as possible. Explicit practical measures to limit exposure to stimulants and high-risk situations should be individualized but might include monitoring and support by drug-free "significant others," discarding drug supplies and paraphernalia, breaking off relationships with dealers and drug-using comrades, limiting finances, changing one's telephone number and/ or geographic location, and structuring one's time during all waking hours. Instead of simply replacing cocaine's central role in one's existence, emphasizing lifestyle changes such as stress reduction, wellness, exercise, and leisure activities is important. This may be more difficult for persons of lower socioeconomic groups and/or those with an earlier onset of addiction. These persons lack the knowledge, experience, and resources to make these changes. Such patients may need linkage to other social services and habilitation, in addition to the rehabilitation just discussed. The involvement of significant others in the treatment of cocaine use disorders can have a positive impact. For instance, Higgins, Budney, Bickel, and Badger (1994) recently showed that patients who had family involvement were 20 times more likely to complete treatment. Finally, supportive therapies, including self-help groups, may provide positive role models, group spirituality, and the backing needed to assist in change. Special Cocaine Anonymous (CA) groups may be beneficial in addressing issues pertinent to cocaine's strong reinforcing properties and associated lifestyle. On the other hand, CA meetings may have detrimental effects by continuing to foster a sense of cocaine separatism.

METHAMPHETAMINE

According to the NHSDA (Substance Abuse and Mental Health Services Administration, 2001b), approximately 4% of the population (8.8 million people) have tried methamphetamine in their lifetime. Emergency department (ED) mentions of methamphetamine in 2001 (15,000 mentions) were not significantly different from mentions in 1994, 1999, or 2000. However, there was an increase and subsequent decline of ED mentions in 1997 (Substance Abuse and Mental Health Services Administration, 2001a). The highest rates of use are seen in patients 26–29 years of age, followed by patients ages 18–25; 39% of methamphetamine admissions were patients 20–29 years old. In addition, TEDS data reveal that 80% of ED mentions were white (Substance Abuse and Mental Health Services Administration, 2002). Rates of use are highest in Hawaii, San Francisco, San Diego, Phoenix, Seattle, Denver, Los Angeles, and, Minneapolis (Substance Abuse and Mental Health Services Adimnistration, 2001b).

D-Methamphetamine hydrochloride is a stimulant that produces many subjective effects similar to those of cocaine, although its 10- to 12-hour half-life is 6–30 times as long as the 20- to 120-minute duration of cocaine (Gold, Miller, & Jonas, 1992). Its street names include crank, chalk, go-fast, crystal, and crystal meth. Methamphetamine can be snorted, taken orally, injected intravenously, or inhaled, but it must be purified before it can be smoked. The purified form of the d-isomer, often called "ice" or "glass," is frequently sold as large crystals that are smoked. The freebase form of methamphetamine is a liquid at room temperature. Rocks are made by melting, cooling, and cutting the methamphetamine crystals, which is often done in an aluminum turkey roasting pan. Methamphetamine can be smoked by inhaling it from a straw placed on aluminum foil or inhaling it through a glass pipe. Methamphetamine pipes differ from those for crack cocaine, because the drug vaporizes at a much lower temperature (Cook, 1991). Methamphetamine is heated by holding a lighter under a large glass ball at the end of the pipe. A finger placed over a hole on the top of the pipe regulates airflow.

Methamphetamine elevates blood pressure, speeds heart rate, raises body temperature, dilates pupils, reduces food intake, and diminishes sleep. Low doses initially are associated with increased alertness, energy, and vigilance. Higher doses produce intoxication symptoms, including euphoria, enhanced self-esteem, and increased sexual pleasure. Even higher doses result in anxiety, irritability, tremors, paranoia, and stereotypical behavior. Tolerance (needing more drug to achieve a given effect) or sensitization (needing less drug to achieve a given effect) may occur upon continued methamphetamine exposure. Different drug effects may have varying rates of either tolerance or sensitization (Lukas, 1997). Tolerance to methamphetamine euphoria occurs more quickly than tolerance to its tachycardic or anorexic effects. Being more prone to seizures and psychosis after repeated dosing with methamphetamine is an example of sensitization (Koob, 1997). Methamphetamine toxicity can affect many organ systems. Methamphetamine cardiotoxicity is related to catechol excess, and may result in myocardial infarction and/or arrhythmias. Pulmonary hypertension, rhabdomyolysis, acute renal failure, heightened immunosuppression, and idiosyncratic liver necrosis are a few of the morbidities associated with methamphetamine use. Paranoid delusions occur in more than 80% of the cases of toxic psychosis. Acute lead poisoning is also a risk for methamphetamine users, because lead acetate is often used as a reagent in its production. Prenatal exposure to methamphetamine is associated with pregnancy complications, prematurity, problems with reflexes, irritability, and congenital deformities. Finally, injecting methamphetamine places users (increasingly, gay male populations) at increased risk for HIV and hepatitis B and C.

Methamphetamine enters the nerve terminal via the synaptic or membrane transporter, then enters the storage vesicles through vesicular transporters, forcing out neurotransmitters such as dopamine and norepinephrine. Methamphetamine is basic and disrupts the acidic interior of the synaptic vesicles, inactivating the proton pump necessary to transport dopamine back inside the vesicle. The dopamine in the cytoplasm undergoes autooxidation, which produces toxic peroxides, oxygen radicals, and hydroxylquinones, which can cause damage in such dopamine-rich areas of the brain as the ventral tegmentum and substantia nigra (Seiden, 1991; Seiden & Sabol, 1996). Dopamine and seroto-

nin, and their precursor enzymes tyrosine hydroxylase, and tryptophan hydroxylase, are depleted, which in turn affects levels of the major metabolites of
these transmitters, their receptors, and their reuptake transporters. Methamphetamine also affects serotonergic, noradrenergic, and glutamatergic systems
through interactions with dopamine transporters, monoamine transporters, and
N-methyl-D-aspartate (NMDA) receptors. Nitric oxide may have a role in
methamphetamine-induced behavioral sensitization and neurotoxicity.

Chronic methamphetamine abuse can lead to psychotic behavior (particularly paranoia), visual and auditory hallucinations, and violent behavior.
Chronic methamphetamine users also demonstrate deficits in attention, verbal memory, abstract reasoning, task shifting, and spatial abilities (Simon et
al., 2000). Animal studies have demonstrated that chronic administration of
methamphetamine decreases striatal concentrations of dopamine and dopamine metabolites in several regions of the brain (Nordahl, Salo, & Leamon,
2003).

Other than symptomatic treatment of drug-induced sequelae, there are no
specific pharmacological treatments for methamphetamine addiction (Lukas,
1997). Continued progress in understanding the neurobiological basis for methamphetamine addiction, as well as medication development initiatives aimed at
cocaine and other drugs, may benefit methamphetamine pharmacotherapy in
the future. Nonpharmacological therapies for methamphetamine addiction are
similar to those for other chemical dependencies but need to take into account
methamphetamine's longer duration of action, withdrawal period, and potentially longer recovery phase. In addition, methamphetamine users may experience paranoia, psychotic symptoms, and protracted depression and anhedonia,
making them more difficult to treat than the standard drug treatment population. Regarding nonpharmacological treatment, methamphetamine users
and cocaine users respond similarly to manualized behavioral and cognitive-
behavioral treatment strategies (Shoptaw, Rawson, McCann, & Obert, 1994).
In addition, new behavioral treatments under development show promise. The
Matrix Program, a multisite, Center for Substance Abuse Treatment (CSAT)–
funded drug treatment program, demonstrated significantly reduced methamphetamine use from pretreatment levels in a follow-up sample 2–5 years
posttreatment (Rawson et al., 2002). However, continuing high rates of dropout and relapse in this population indicate a need for further treatment research
for this difficult population.

CONCLUSION

Over the past 15 years, much has changed with regard to the use and our understanding of both amphetamines and cocaine. Most notably, cocaine depend-

ence now appears to be differentially affecting poor, minority individuals who live in the inner city. This same population is overrepresented in the AIDS population. This confluence is not surprising, because both sex risk (including sex workers) and needle risk are associated with chronic use of cocaine. It therefore appears that these two epidemics are interconnected in a way that deserves close attention.

At the same time, there may be reason for cautious optimism with regard to the long-term effects of prenatal exposure to cocaine. Some of the early claims of devastating physical consequences to "crack babies" have proven to be exaggerated; experts in the perinatal addiction field now consider that many factors (e.g., poverty, poor maternal nutrition/health, smoking, and exposure to violence) combine to influence development. Molecular mechanisms of developmental neuroadaptation are at the same time beginning to be studied. In the future, we hope to understand better the physiological basis for the observed clinical events.

In the basic sciences area, we have come to understand more about the interactions of various neurotransmitters, drug reinforcement, and the reward pathway. Receptors are being subtyped and cloned. Signal transduction pathways, with their longer range on protein synthesis and genetic regulation, are being explored. We are beginning to make inroads in our understanding of sensitization and tolerance. Although pharmacological treatments for cocaine addiction have not yet proven successful in clinical trials, there are many exciting new avenues of pursuit. These prospects for pharmacological intervention are based on the remarkable advances in neuroscience being made in this decade.

Researchers also have been hard at work testing psychotherapeutic solutions to this complex problem. Cocaine dependence should not be viewed in isolation from other psychiatric conditions and life problems. Rather, we must consider how best to address the problem in the presence of other psychoactive substance use and non-substance-use Axis I and Axis II disorders. Depending on the larger clinical picture, successful treatment may require multiple or highly select therapies that are matched to the patient's pathology and adaptive strengths and resources. It is clear that a "one size fits all" approach to treatment of cocaine dependence is inappropriate; instead, an array of assessment tools is necessary to determine patient needs, along with a menu of cost-effective and readily available therapeutic strategies. Although American Society of Addiction Medicine (Hoffman, Halikas, Mee-Lee, & Weedman, 1991) criteria facilitate patient placement in an appropriate treatment setting based on addiction severity, they provide little guidance in terms of specific interventions to be delivered within those settings. Clinical research aimed at developing therapies for specific subtypes of cocaine addicts in a variety of settings is the most promising approach we now have.

ACKNOWLEDGMENTS

Special thanks to Kenneth S. Kendler, MD, Rachel Brown Banks Distinguished Professor of Psychiatry and Professor of Human Genetics, Medical College of Virginia, Virginia Commonwealth University, Richmond, Virginia, for contributing to the genetic factors section of this chapter on genetic factors.

REFERENCES

Abraham, H. D., & Fava, M. (1999). Order of onset of substance abuse and depression in a sample of depressed outpatients. *Compr Psychiatry, 40,* 44–50.

Allred, R. J., & Ewer, S. (1981). Fatal pulmonary edema following intravenous "free base" cocaine use. *Ann Emerg Med, 10,* 441–442.

American Psychiatric Association. (2000). *Diagnostic and statistical manual of mental disorders* (4th ed., text rev.). Washington, DC: Author.

Andrews, P. (1997). Cocaethylene toxicity. *J Addict Dis, 16*(3), 75–84.

Aroesty, D. J., Stanley, R. B., Jr., & Crockett, D. M. (1986). Pneumomediastinum and cervical emphysema from inhalation of "free based" cocaine: Report of three cases. *Otolaryngol Head Neck Surg, 94,* 372–374.

Aronson, T., & Craig, T. (1986). Cocaine precipitation of panic disorder. *Am J Psychiatry, 143,* 643–645.

Avila, A. H., Morgan, C. A., & Bayer, B. M. (2003). Stress-induced suppression of the immune system after withdrawal from chronic cocaine. *J Pharmacol Exp Ther, 305,* 290–297.

Azuma, S. D., & Chasnoff, I. J. (1993). Outcome of children prenatally exposed to cocaine and other drugs: A path analysis of three-year data. *Pediatrics, 92,* 396–402.

Bandstra, E. S., Morrow, C. E., Vogel, A. L., Fifer, R. C., Ofir, A. Y., Dausa, A. T., et al. (2002). Longitudinal influence of prenatal cocaine exposure on child language functioning. *Neurotoxicol Teratol, 24,* 297–308.

Barber, J., Frank, A., Weiss, R., & Blane, J. (1996). Prevalence and correlates of personality disorder diagnoses among cocaine dependent outpatients. *J Pers Disord, 10,* 297–311.

Barnett, G., Hawks, R., & Resnick, R. (1981). Cocaine pharmacokinetics in humans. *J Ethnopharmacol, 3,* 353–366.

Bartels, S., Teague, G., Drake, R., Clark R., Bush, P., & Noordsy, D. (1993). Service utilization and costs associated with substance abuse among rural schizophrenic patients. *J Nerv Ment Dis, 181,* 227–276.

Beckwith, L., Rodning, C., Norris, D., Phillipsen, L., Khandabi, P., & Howard, J. (1994). Spontaneous play in two-year-olds born to substance-abusing mothers. *Infant Ment Health J, 15,* 189–201.

Bien, T., Miker, W., & Tonigan, S. (1993). Brief interventions for alcohol problems: A review. *Addiction, 8,* 305–325.

Bierut, L. J., Dinwiddie, S. H., Begleiter, H., Crowe, R. R., Hesselbrock, V., Nurnberger, J. I., Jr., et al. (1998). Familial transmission of substance dependence: Alcohol, marijuana, cocaine, and habitual smoking: A report from the Collaborative Study on the Genetics of Alcoholism. *Arch Gen Psychiatry, 55,* 982–988.

Brady, K. T., Sonne, S., Randall, C. L., Adinoff, B., & Malcolm, R. (1995). Features of cocaine dependence with concurrent alcohol abuse. *Drug Alcohol Depend, 39*(1), 69–71.

Brown, J., & Miller, W. (1993). Impact of motivational interviewing on participation and outcome in residential alcoholism treatment. *Psychol Addict Behav, 7,* 211–218.

Brown, R. A., Monti, P. M., Myers, M. G., Martin, R. A., Rivinus, T., Dubreuil, M. E., & Rohsenow, D. J. (1998). Depression among cocaine abusers in treatment: Relation to cocaine and alcohol use and treatment outcome. *Am J Psychiatry, 155,* 220–225.

Budney, A. J., Higgins, S. T., Hughes, J. R., & Bickel, W. K. (1993). Nicotine and caffeine use in cocaine-dependent individuals. *J Subst Abuse, 5,* 117–130.

Bunt, G., Galanter, M., Lifshutz, H., & Castaneda, R. (1990). Cocaine/"crack" dependence among psychiatric inpatients. *Am J Psychiatry, 147,* 1542–1546.

Bystritsky, A., Ackerman, D., & Pasnau, R. (1991). Low dose desipramine treatment of cocaine-related panic attacks. *J Nerv Ment Dis, 179,* 755–758.

Carroll, K. (1996). Relapse prevention as a psychosocial treatment: A review of controlled clinical trials. *Exp Clin Psychopharmacol, 4,* 46–54.

Carroll, K., & Rounsaville, B. (1993). History and significance of childhood attention deficit disorder in treatment-seeking cocaine abusers. *Compr Psychiatry, 34,* 75–82.

Carroll, K., Rounsaville, B., Gordon, L., Nich, C., Jatlow, P., Bisighini, R., & Gawin, F. (1994). Psychotherapy and pharmacotherapy for ambulatory cocaine abusers. *Arch Gen Psychiatry, 51,* 177–187.

Carroll, K. M. (2000). Implications of recent research for program quality in cocaine dependence treatment. *Subst Use Misuse, 35,* 2011–2030.

Chasnoff, I. J., & Schnoll, S. H. (1987). Consequences of cocaine and other drug use in pregnancy. In A. Washton & M. S. Gold (Eds.), *Cocaine: A clinician's handbook* (pp. 241–251). New York: Guilford Press.

Church, M. W., & Subramanian, M. G. (1997). Cocaine's lethality increases during late gestation in the rat: A study of "critical periods" of exposure. *Am J Obstet Gynecol, 176*(4), 901–906.

Church, M. W., Kaufman, R. A., Keenan, J. A., Martier, S. S., Savoy-Moore, R. T., Ostrea, E. M., et al. (1991). Effects of prenatal cocaine exposure. In R. R. Watson (Ed.), *Biochemistry and physiology of substance abuse* (Vol. III, pp. 179–204). Boca Raton, FL: CRC Press.

Clark, T. A. (1996). Prevalence of drugs and alcohol in autopsied homicide cases in St. John Parish, Louisiana. *J La State Med Soc, 148,* 257–259.

Coffin, P. O., Galea, S., Ahern, J., Leon, A. C., Vlahov, D., & Tardiff, K. (2003). Opiates, cocaine and alcohol combinations in accidental drug overdose deaths in New York City, 1990–98. *Addiction, 98,* 739–747.

Cook, C. E. (1991). Pyrolytic characteristics, pharmacokinetics, and bioavailability of smoked heroin, cocaine, phencyclidine, and methamphetyamine. In M. A. Miller & N. J. Kozel (Eds.), *Methamphetamine abuse: Epidemiologic issues and implications* (NIDA Research Monograph No. 115, DHHS Publication No. ADM 91-1836, pp. 6–23). Washington, DC: U.S. Government Printing Office.

Cooper, C. B., Bai, T. R., Heyderman, C., & Lorrin, B. (1983). Cellulose granulomas in the lungs of a cocaine sniffer. *Br Med J, 286,* 2121–2022.

Cottler, L. B., Compton, W. M., III, Mager, D., Spitznagel, E. L., & Janca, A. (1992). Posttraumatic stress disorder among substance users from the general population. *Am J Psychiatry, 149,* 664–670.

Cregler, L. L., & Mark, H. (1986). Special report: Medical complications of cocaine abuse. *N Engl J Med, 315,* 1495–1500.

Crits-Christoph, P., Siqueland, L., Blaine, J., Frank, A., Luborsky, L., Onken, L. S., et al. (1999). Psychosocial treatments for cocaine dependence: National Institute on Drug Abuse Collaborative Cocaine Treatment Study. *Arch Gen Psychiatry, 56,* 493–502.

DePetrillo, P. (1985). Getting to the base of cocaine. *Emerg Med, 8,* 8.

Estroff, T. W., Gold, M. S. (1986). Medical and psychiatric complications of cocaine abuse with possible points of pharmacological treatment. In B. Stimmel (Ed.), *Controversies in alcoholism and substance abuse* (pp. 61–75). New York: Haworth Press.

Farre, M., de la Torre, R., Llorente, M., Lamas, X., Ugena, B., Segura, J., et al. (1993). Alcohol and cocaine interactions in humans. *J Pharmacol Exp Ther, 266,* 1364–1373.

Frishman, W. H., Del Vecchio, A., Sanal, S., & Ismail, A. (2003). Cardiovascular manifestations of substance abuse: Part 1. Cocaine. *Heart Dis, 5,* 187–201.

Gawin, F. H., & Ellinwood, E. H., Jr. (1988). Cocaine and other stimulants: Actions, abuse, and treatment. *N Engl J Med, 318,* 1173–1182.

Gawin, F. H., Riordan, C., & Kleber, H. (1985). Methylphenidate treatment of cocaine abusers without attention-deficit disorder: A negative report. *Am J Drug Alcohol Abuse, 11,* 193–197.

Gay, G. R. (1982). Clinical management of acute and chronic cocaine poisoning. *Ann Emerg Med, 11,* 562–572.

General Accounting Office. (1990). *Methadone maintenance: Some treatment programs are not effective, greater federal oversight needed.* Washington, DC: Author.

Goeders, N. E. (2002). Stress and cocaine addiction. *J Pharmacol Exp Ther, 301*(3), 785–789.

Gold, M. S., Miller, N. S., & Jonas, J. M. (1992). Cocaine (and crack) neurobiology. In J. H. Lowinson, P. Ruiz, & R. B. Millman (Eds.), *Substance abuse: A comprehensive textbook* (2nd ed., pp. 222–235). Baltimore: Williams & Wilkins.

Goldfrank, L. R., & Hoffman, R. S. (1993). The cardiovascular effects of cocaine—update 1992. In H. Sorer (Ed.), *Acute cocaine intoxication: Current methods of treatment* (NIDA Research Monograph No. 123, NIH Publication No. 93-3498, pp. 70–109). Washington, DC: U.S. Government Printing Office.

Goldstein, R. Z., & Volkow, N. D. (2002). Drug addiction and its underlying neurobiological basis: Neuroimaging evidence for the involvement of the frontal cortex. *Am J Psychiatry, 159,* 1642–1652.

Griffin, M. L., Weiss, R. D., Mirin, S. M., & Lange, U. (1989). A comparison of male and female cocaine abusers. *Arch Gen Psychiatry, 46,* 122–126.

Haller, D., Knisely, J., Dawson, K., & Schnoll, S. (1993). Perinatal substance abusers: Psychological and social characteristics. *J Nerv Ment Dis, 181,* 509–513.

Henningfield, J. E., Clayton, R., & Pollin, W. (1990). Involvement of tobacco in alcoholism and illicit drug use. *Br J Addict, 85,* 279–291.

Higgins, S., Budney, A., Bickel, W., & Badger, G. (1994). Participation of significant others in outpatient behavioral treatment predicts greater cocaine abstinence. *Am J Drug Alcohol Abuse, 20,* 47–56.

Higgins, S., Budney, A., Bickel, W., Badger, G., Foerg, F., & Ogden, D. (1995). Outpatient behavioral treatment for cocaine dependence: One-year outcome. *Exp Clin Psychopharmacol, 3,* 205–212.

Higgins, S., Budney, A., Bickel, W., & Foerg, F. (1994). Incentives improve outcome in outpatient behavioral treatment for cocaine dependence. *Arch Gen Psychiatry, 51,* 568–576.

Higgins, S. T., Wong, C. J., Badger, G. J., Ogden, D. E., & Dantona, R. L. (2000). Contingent reinforcement increases cocaine abstinence during outpatient treatment and 1 year of follow-up. *J Consult Clin Psychol, 68,* 64–72.

Hoffman, N. G., Halikas, J. A., Mee-Lee, D., & Weedman, R. D. (1991). *Patient placement criteria for the treatment of psychoactive substance use disorders.* Washington, DC: American Society of Addiction Medicine.

Horner, B., Scheibe, K., & Stine, S. (1996). Cocaine abuse and attention-deficit hyperactivity disorder: Implications of adult symptomatology. *Psychol Addict Behav, 10,* 55–60.

Itkonen, J., Schnoll, S., & Glassroth, J. (1984). Pulmonary dysfunction in free base cocaine users. *Arch Intern Med, 144,* 2195–2197.

Jatlow, P., Hearn, W. L., Elsworth, J. D., Roth, R. H., Bradberry, C. W., & Taylor, J. R. (1991). Cocaethylene inhibits uptake of dopamine and can reach high plasma concentrations following combined cocaine and ethanol use. *NIDA Res Monogr, 105,* 572–573.

Javaid, J. I., Fischman, M. W., Schuster, C. R., Dekirmenjian, H., & Davis, J. M. (1978). Cocaine plasma concentration: Relation to physiological and subjective effects in humans. *Science, 202,* 227–228.

Johanson, C. E., & Schuster, C. R. (1995). Cocaine. In F. L. Bloom & D. J. Kupfer (Eds.), *Psychopharmacology: The fourth generation of progress* (pp. 1685–1697). New York: Raven Press.

Johnston, L. D., O'Malley, P. M., & Bachman, J. G. (2003). *Monitoring the Future national survey results on drug use, 1975–2002. Vol. I: Secondary school students* (NIH Publication No. 03-5375). Bethesda, MD: National Institute on Drug Abuse.

Jones, R. T. (1984). The pharmacology of cocaine. In J. G. Grabowski (Ed.), *Cocaine: Pharmacology, effects and treatment of abuse* (DHHS Publication No. ADM AD4-1325, pp. 34–53). Washington, DC: U.S. Government Printing Office.

Karam, E. G., Yabroudi, P. F., & Melhem, N. M. (2002). Comorbidity of substance abuse and other psychiatric disorders in acute general psychiatric admissions: A study from Lebanon. *Compr Psychiatry, 43,* 463–468.

Karkowski, L. M., Prescott, C. A., & Kendler, K. S. (2000). Multivariate assessment of factors influencing illicit substance use in twins from female–female pairs. *Am J Med Genet, 96,* 665–670.

Kelly, R. F., Sompalli, V., Sattar, P., & Khankari, K. (2003). Increased TIMI frame counts in cocaine users: A case for increased microvascular resistance in the absence of epicardial coronary disease or spasm. *Clin Cardiol, 26,* 319–322.

Kendler, K. S., Jacobson, K. C., Prescott, C. A., & Neale, M. C. (2003). Specificity of genetic and environmental risk factors for use and abuse/dependence of cannabis, cocaine, hallucinogens, sedatives, stimulants, and opiates in male twins. *Am J Psychiatry, 160,* 687–695.

Khantzian, E. J., Gawin, F., Kleber, H. D., & Riordan, C. E. (1984). Methylphenidate treatment of cocaine dependence: A preliminary report. *J Subst Abuse Treat, 1,* 107–112.

Kirby, K. C., Marlowe, D. B., Festinger, D. S., Lamb, R. J., & Platt, J. J. (1998). Schedule of voucher delivery influences initiation of cocaine abstinence. *J Consult Clin Psychol, 66,* 761–767.

Kleinman, P., Miller, A., Millman, R., Woody, G., Todd, T., Kemp, J., & Lipton, D. (1990). Psychopathology among cocaine abusers entering treatment. *J Nerv Ment Dis, 178,* 442–447.

Koob, G. F. (1992). Neurobiological mechanisms in cocaine and opiate dependence. *Res Publications Assoc Res Nerv Ment Dis, 70,* 79–92.

Koob, G. F. (1997, April). Neurochemical explanations for addiction. *Hosp Pract Special Rep,* pp. 12–15.

Kosten, T. R. (1988). *Cocaine treatment: Pharmacotherapies.* Paper presented at the Clinical Applications of Cocaine Research: From Bench to Bedside meeting of the National Institute on Drug Abuse, Rockville, MD.

Kosten, T. R., Rounsaville, B. J., & Kleber, H. D. (1987). A 2.5 year follow-up of cocaine use among treated opioid addicts: Have our treatments helped? *Arch Gen Psychiatry, 44,* 281–284.

Kranzler, H., Satel, S., & Apter, A. (1994). Personality disorders and associated features in cocaine-dependent inpatients. *Compr Psychiatry, 35,* 335–340.

Lambert, N. M., & Hartsough, C. S. (1998). Prospective study of tobacco smoking and substance dependencies among samples of ADHD and non-ADHD participants. *J Learn Disabil, 31,* 533–544.

Laposata, E. A., & Mayo, G. L. (1993). A review of pulmonary pathology and mechanisms associated with inhalation of freebase cocaine ("crack"). *Am J Forensic Med Pathol, 14,* 1–9.

Levin, F. R., Evans, S. M., & Kleber, H. D. (1998). Prevalence of adult attention-deficit hyperactivity disorder among cocaine abusers seeking treatment. *Drug Alcohol Depend, 52,* 15–25.

Lima, M. S., Soares, B. G., Reisser, A. A., & Farrell, M. (2002). Pharmacological treatment of cocaine dependence: A systematic review. *Addiction, 97,* 931–949.

Lombard, J., Levin, I. H., & Weiner, W. J. (1989). [Letter]. *N Engl J Med, 320,* 869.

Lukas, S. E. (1997). *Proceedings of the national consensus meeting on the use, abuse, and sequelae of abuse of methamphetamine with implications for prevention, treatment and research* (DHHS Publication No. SMA 96-8013, pp. 1–37). Washington, DC: U.S. Government Printing Office.

Lysaker, P., Bell, M., Beam-Goulet, J., & Milstein, R. (1994). Relationship of positive and negative symptoms to cocaine abuse in schizophrenia. *J Nerv Ment Dis, 182,* 109–122.

Marlatt, G. A., & Gordon, J. R. (1985). *Relapse prevention: Maintenance strategies in the treatment of addictive behaviors.* New York: Guilford Press.

Marlowe, D., Husband, S., Lamb, R., & Kirby, K. (1995). Psychiatric co-morbidity in cocaine dependence: Diverging trends, Axis II spectrum, and gender differentials. *Am J Addict , 4,* 70–81.

Martino, S., McCance-Katz, E., Workman, J., & Boozang, J. (1995). The development of a dual diagnosis partial hospital program. *Continuum, 2,* 145–165.

McCance-Katz, E. F., Price, L. H., McDougle, C. J., Kosten, T. R., Black, J. E., & Jatlow, P. I. (1993). Concurrent cocaine–ethanol ingestion in humans: Pharmacology, physiology, behavior, and the role of cocaethylene. *Psychopharmacology, 111,* 39–46.

McCarron, M. M., & Wood, J. D. (1983). The cocaine "body packer" syndrome: Diagnosis and treatment. *JAMA, 250,* 1417–1420.

McGonigal, M. D., Cole, J., Schwab, C. W., Kauder, D. R., Rotondo, M. F., & Angood, P. B. (1993). Urban firearm deaths: A five-year perspective. *J Trauma, 35,* 532–536.

Miller, W., & Rollnick, S. (1991). *Motivational interviewing: Preparing people to change addictive behavior.* New York: Guilford Press.

Miner, L. L., & Marley, R. J. (1995). Chromosomal mapping of the psychomotor stimulant effects of cocaine in BXD recombinant inbred mice. *Psychopharmacology, 122,* 209–214.

Mirin, S. M., Weiss, R. D., Griffin, M. L., & Michael, J. L. (1991). Psychopathology in drug abusers and their families. *Compr Psychiatry, 32,* 36–51.

Moore, T., Sorg, J., Miller, L., Key, T., & Resnik, R. (1986). Hemodynamic effects of intravenous cocaine on the pregnant ewe and fetus. *Am J Obstet Gynecol, 155,* 838–888.

Moos, R. H., Mertens, J. R., & Brennan, P. L. (1994). Rates and predictors of four-year readmission among late, middle-aged, and old substance abuse patients. *J Stud Alcohol, 55,* 561–570.

Moos, R. H., & Moos, B. S. (1995). Stay in residential facilities and mental health care as predictors of readmission for with patients with substance use disorders. *Psychiatr Serv, 46,* 66–72.

Muniz, A. E., & Evans, T. (2001). Acute gastrointestinal manifestations associated with use of crack. *Am J Emerg Med, 19,* 61–63.

Najavits, L. M., Gastfriend, D. R., Barber, J. P., Reif, S., Muenz, L. R., Blaine, J., et al. (1998). Cocaine dependence with and without PTSD among subjects in the National Institute on Drug Abuse Collaborative Cocaine Treatment Study. *Am J Psychiatry, 155,* 214–219.

New York State Division of Substance Abuse Services. (1990). *NYS Office of Alcohol and Substance Abuse Services, program statistics* [Data file]. Albany, NY: Author.

Nordahl, T. E., Salo, R., & Leamon, M. (2003). Neuropsychological effects of chronic methamphetamine use on neurotransmitters and cognition: A review. *J Neuropsychiatry Clin Neurosci, 15,* 317–325.

Nurnberg, H. G., Rifkin, A., & Doddi, S. (1993). A systematic assessment of the comorbidity of DSM-III-R personality disorders in alcoholic outpatients. *Compr Psychiatry, 34,* 447–454.

O'Brien, C., Childress, A., Arndt, I., & McLellan, T. (1988). Pharmacologic and behavioral treatments of cocaine dependence: Controlled studies. *J Clin Psychiatry, 49*(Suppl), 17–22.

O'Brien, C., Childress, A., McLellan, T., & Ehrman, R. (1990). Integrating systematic cue exposure with standard treatment in recovering drug dependent patients. *Addict Behav, 15,* 355–365.

Office of the Inspector General, Office of Evaluation and Inspections, and Department of Health and Human Services. (1990). *Crack babies.* Washington, DC: U.S. Government Printing Office.

O'Leary, M. E. (2002). Inhibition of HERG potassium channels by cocaethylene: A metabolite of cocaine and ethanol. *Cardiovasc Res, 53,* 59–67.

Patkar, A. A., Lundy, A., Leone, F. T., Weinstein, S. P., Gottheil, E., & Steinberg, M. (2002). Tobacco and alcohol use and medical symptoms among cocaine dependent patients. *Subst Abuse, 23,* 105–114.

Pristach, C. A., & Smith, C. M. (1990). Medication compliance and substance abuse among schizophrenic patients. *Hosp Commun Psychiatry, 41,* 1345–1348.

Prochaska, J., DiClemente, C., & Norcross, J. (1992). In search of how people change: Applications to addictive behavior. *Am Psychol, 47,* 1102–1114.

Rawson, R. A., Huber, A., Brethen, P., Obert, J., Gulati, V., Shoptaw, S., & Ling, W. (2002). Status of methamphetamine users 2–5 years after outpatient treatment. *J Addict Dis, 21,* 107–119.

Regier, D. A., Farmer, M. E., Rae, D. S., Locke, B. Z., Keith, S. J., Judd, L. L., & Goodwin, F. K. (1990). Comorbidity of mental disorders with alcohol and other drug abuse: Results from the Epidemiologic Catchment Area (ECA) study. *JAMA, 264,* 2511–2518.

Rosenthal, R., Hellerstein, D., Miner, C., & Christian, R. (1994). Positive and negative syndrome typology in schizophrenic patients with psychoactive substance use disorders. *Compr Psychiatry, 35,* 91–98.

Roth, D., Alarcon, F. J., Fernandez, J. A., Preston, R. A., & Bourgoignie, J. J. (1988). Acute rhabdomyolysis associated with cocaine intoxication. *N Engl J Med, 319,* 673–677.

Rounsaville, B. J., Anton, S. F., Carroll, K., Budde, D., Prusoff, B. A., & Gawin, F. (1991). Psychiatric diagnoses of treatment-seeking cocaine abusers. *Arch Gen Psychiatry, 48,* 43–51.

Satel, S. L., & Gawin, F. H. (1989). Migraine-like headache and cocaine use. *JAMA, 261,* 2995–2996.

Schaper, A., Hofmann, R., Ebbecke, M., Desel, H., & Langer, C. (2003). Cocaine–body-packing: Infrequent indication for laparotomy. *Der Chir, 74,* 626–631.

Schindler, C. (1996). Cocaine and cardiovascular toxicity. *Addiction Biology, 1,* 31–47.

Schrank, K. S. (1993). Cocaine-related emergency department presentations. In H. Sorer (Ed.), *Acute cocaine intoxication: Current methods of treatment* (NIDA Research Monograph No. 123, NIH Publication No. 93-3498, pp. 110–128). Washington, DC: U.S. Government Printing Office.

Schuster, C. L., Yu, G., & Bates, A. (1977). Sensitization to cocaine stimulation in mice. *Psychopharmacology, 52,* 185–190.

Schwartz, M. S., Swanson, J. W., & Hannon, M. J. (2003). Detection of illicit substance use among persons with schizophrenia by radioimmunoassay of hair. *Psychiatr Serv, 54,* 891–895.

Seibyl, J., Satel, S., Anthoy, D., & Southwick, S. (1993). Effects of cocaine on hospital course in schizophrenia. *J Nerv Ment Dis, 181,* 31–37.

Seiden, L. S. (1991). Neurotoxicity of methamphetamine: Mechanisms of action and issues related to aging. In M. A. Miller & N. J. Kozel (Eds.), *Methamphetamine abuse: Epidemiologic issues and implications* (NIDA Research Monograph No. 115,

DHHS Publication No. ADM 91-1836, pp. 24–32). Washington, DC: U.S. Government Printing Office.

Seiden, L. S., & Sabol, K. E. (1996). Methamphetamine and methylenedioxymethamphetamine neurotoxicity: Possible mechanisms of cell destruction. In M. D. Majewska (Ed.), *Neurotoxicity and neuropathology associated with cocaine abuse* (NIDA Research Monograph No. 163, NIH Publication No. 96-4019, pp. 251–276). Washington, DC: U.S. Government Printing Office.

Serper, M., Alpert, M., Richardson, N., & Dickson, S. (1995). Clinical effects of recent cocaine use on patients with acute schizophrenia. *Am J Psychiatry, 152,* 1464–1469.

Shaffer, H. J., & Eber, G. B. (2002). Temporal progression of cocaine dependence symptoms in the US National Comorbidity Survey. *Addiction, 97,* 543.

Shoptaw, S., Rawson, R. A., McCann, M. J., & Obert, J. L. (1994). The Matrix model of outpatient stimulant abuse treatment: Evidence of efficacy. *J Addict Dis, 13,* 129–141.

Silverman, K., Higgins, S., Brooner, R., Montoya, I., Cone, E., Schuster, C., & Preston, K. (1996). Sustained cocaine abstinence in methadone maintenance patients through voucher-based reinforcement therapy. *Arch Gen Psychiatry, 53,* 409–415.

Simon, S. L., Domier, C., Carnell, J., Brethen, P., Rawson, R., & Ling, W. (2000). Cognitive impairment in individuals currently using methamphetamine. *Am J Addict, 9*(3), 222–231.

Singer, L. T., Arendt, R., Minnes, S., Farkas, K., Salvator, A., Kirchner, H. L., & Kliegman, R. (2002). Cognitive and motor outcomes of cocaine-exposed infants. *JAMA, 287,* 1952–1960.

Smith, J. E., Koves, T. R., & Co, C. (2003). Brain neurotransmitter turnover rates during rat intravenous cocaine self-administration. *Neuroscience, 117,* 461–475.

Stone, M. H. (1992). Borderline personality disorder: Course of illness. In J. F. Clarkin, E. Marziali, & H. Munroe-Blum (Eds.), *Borderline personality disorder: Clinical and empirical perspectives* (pp. 67–86). New York: Guilford Press.

Stotts, A. L., Schmitz, J. M., Rhoades, H. M., & Grabowski, J. (2001). Motivational interviewing with cocaine-dependent patients: A pilot study. *J Consult Clin Psychol, 69,* 858–862.

Substance Abuse and Mental Health Services Administration. (2001a). *Drug Abuse Warning Network (DAWN)* [Data file]. Rockville, MD: Author.

Substance Abuse and Mental Health Services Administration. (2001b). *National Household Survey* [Data file]. Rockville, MD: Author.

Substance Abuse and Mental Health Services Administration, Office of Applied Studies. (2002). *Treatment Episode Data Set (TEDS): 1992–2000* (National Admissions to Substance Abuse Treatment Services, DASIS Series: S-17, DHHS Publication No. [SMA] 02-3727). Rockville, MD: Author.

Tames, S. M., & Goldenring, J. M. (1986). Madarosis from cocaine use. *N Engl J Med, 314,* 1324.

Tardiff, K., Marzuk, P. M., Leon, A. C., Hirsch, C. S., Stajic, M., Portera, L., & Hartwell, N. (1994). Homicide in New York City: Cocaine use and firearms. *JAMA, 272,* 43–46.

Texter, E. C., Chou, C. C., Merrill, S. L., Laureton, H. C., & Frohlich, E. D. (1964).

Direct effects of vasoactive agents on segmental resistance of the mesenteric and portal circulation: Studies with L-epinephrine, levarterenol, angiotensin, vasopressin, acetylcholine, methacholine, histamine, and serotonin. *J Lab Clin Med*, *64*, 624–633.

Tsuang, M. T., Lyons, M. J., Eisen, S. A., Goldberg, J., True, W., Meyer, J. M., & Eaves, L. J. (1996). Genetic influences on abuse of illicit drugs: A study of 3,297 twin pairs. *Am J Med Genet*, *67*, 473–477.

U.S. Department of Justice, Office of Justice Programs, National Institute of Justice. (2001). *2000 arrestee drug abuse monitoring: Annual report* [Data file]. Washington, DC: Author.

U.S. Department of Justice, Office of Justice Programs, National Institute of Justice. (2003). *National drug threat assessment, 2003* [Data file]. Washington, DC: Author.

Vidaeff, A. C., & Mastrobattista, J. M. (2003). In utero cocaine exposure: A thorny mix of science and mythology. *Am J Perinat*, *20*, 165–172.

Volpe, J. (1992). Effect of cocaine use on the fetus. *N Engl J Med*, *327*, 399–407.

Washton, A. M., Stone, N. S., & Hendrickson, E. C. (1988). Cocaine abuse. In D. M. Donovan & G. A. Marlatt (Eds.), *Assessment of addictive behaviors* (pp. 364–389). New York: Guilford Press.

Weber, J. E., Hollander, J. E., Murphy, S. A., Braunwald, E., & Gibson, C. M. (2003). Quantitative comparison of coronary artery flow and myocardial perfusion in patients with acute myocardial infarction in the presence and absence of recent cocaine use. *J Thromb Thrombolysis*, *14*, 239–245.

Weiss, R. D, Mirin, S. M., Griffin, M. L., Gunderson, J. G., & Hufford, C. (1993). Personality disorders in cocaine dependence. *Compr Psychiatry*, *34*, 145–199.

Weiss, R. D., Pope, H., & Mirin, S. (1985). Treatment of chronic cocaine abuse and attention-deficit disorder, residual type, with magnesium pemoline. *Drug Alcohol Depend*, *15*, 69–72.

Wetti, C. V., Weiss, S. D., Cleary, T. J., & Gyori, E. (1984). Fungal cerebritis from intravenous drug use. *J Forensic Sci*, *29*, 260–268.

Yahne, C. E., Miller, W. R., Irvin-Vitela, L., & Tonigan, J. S. (2002). Magdalena Pilot Project: Motivational outreach to substance abusing women street sex workers. *J Subst Abuse Treatment*, *23*, 49–53.

Ziedonis, D., & Fischer, W. (1996). Motivation-based assessment and treatment of substance abuse in patients with schizophrenia. *Dir Psychiatry*, *16*, 1–7.

Ziedonis, D., Rayford, B., Bryant, B., Kendall, J., & Rounsaville, B. (1994). Psychiatric comorbidity in white and African-American cocaine addicts seeking substance abuse treatment. *Hosp Community Psychiatry*, *45*, 43–49.

CHAPTER 10

Sedatives/Hypnotics
and Benzodiazepines

ROBERT L. DUPONT
CAROLINE M. DUPONT

The sedatives and the hypnotics, especially the benzodiazepines, are widely used in medical practice in the treatment of anxiety, insomnia, epilepsy, and for several other indications (Baldessarini, 2001). The combination of abuse by alcoholics and drug addicts, and the withdrawal symptoms on discontinuation leads to the view that these are "addictive" drugs (DuPont, 2000; Juergens & Cowley, 2003). The pharmacology and the epidemiology of sedatives and hypnotics are reviewed in this chapter, which focuses on the needs of the clinician.

A *sedative* lowers excitement and calms the awake patient, whereas a *hypnotic* produces drowsiness and promotes sleep. The nonbenzodiazepine sedatives generally depress central nervous system (CNS) activity in a continuum, depending on the dose, beginning with calming and extending progressively to sleep, unconsciousness, coma, surgical aesthesia, and, ultimately, to fatal respiratory and cardiovascular depression. Sedatives share this spectrum of effects with many other compounds, including general anesthetic agents, a variety of aliphatic alcohols, and ethyl alcohol. At lower doses, sedatives can cause impaired cognitive and motor functioning (including staggering and slurred speech). Sedation is a side effect of many other medicines, including antihistamines and neuroleptics.

The benzodiazepines resemble the other sedatives, except that they do not produce surgical anesthesia, coma, or death, even at high doses, except when coadministered with other agents that suppress respiration. The benzodiaze-pines can be antagonized by specific agents that do not block the effects of other sedatives. The benzodiazepine antagonists do not produce significant effects in the absence of the benzodiazepines. These properties distinguish the benzodiazepines from the other sedatives and produce a margin of safety that has led to the widespread use of benzodiazepines (Charney, Minie, & Harris, 2001).

The National Comorbidity Survey (NCS) found that 17.2% of the popula-tion had an anxiety disorder in the past 12 months, and 24.9% had a lifetime history of anxiety disorder (DuPont, Dupont, & Rice, 2002; Kessler et al., 1994). These studies establish that the anxiety disorders are the most prevalent class of mental disorders over a 12-month period of time (DuPont, 1995). Using the standard human capital approach to estimate the social costs of illnesses in 1994, the anxiety disorders produced a total social cost of $65 billion (DuPont et al., 2002). Of this total, the cost of all treatments was only $15 billion, whereas $50 billion was due to lost productivity as a result of the often seriously disabling nature of the anxiety disorders. For comparison, using the same meth-odology, the costs of all mental illnesses in 1994 was $204 billion, of which the mood disorders—including depression and bipolar disorders—totaled $42 bil-lion and schizophrenia totaled $45 billion.

The benzodiazepines were introduced in 1960s as comparatively problem-free compared to the barbiturates, which they rapidly replaced. Their popularity reached unprecedented levels in the early 1970s. However, a powerful backlash, labeled the "social issues," emerged, which caused a drop in the use of benzo-diazepines during the 1980s, even though there was a rise in the prevalence of the disorders for which they are used (DuPont, 1986, 1988).

As the benzodiazepines became more controversial, and as various regula-tory approaches were employed to limit their use in medical practice, there was a danger that clinicians would revert to the older and generally more toxic sed-atives and hypnotics, which, in the era of the benzodiazepines, had become unfamiliar (Juergens & Cowley, 2003). Thus, there is more than historical interest in looking at these earlier sedatives, because for some younger medical practitioners, they are new medicines. The use of sedatives and hypnotics for the treatment of anxiety and insomnia in patients with addiction to alcohol and other drugs entails additional risks, especially when benzodiazepines are used (Handelsman, 2002).

For more than three decades, the federal government has tracked the rates of self-reported, nonmedical use of a variety of drugs within the United States, primarily in two surveys—one of high school seniors (Monitoring the Future [MTF]), and the other of Americans 12 years of age and older (National House-hold Survey on Drug Abuse [NHSDA]) (U.S. Department of Health and Human Services, 2001, 2002). The NHSDA separately tracks the use of "tranquilizers" and "sedatives" while the MTF survey tracks "tranquilizers" and "barbiturates." Neither survey identifies "benzodiazepines" specifically. In general, the trends over this extended period of time show a steady rise in nonmedical use, peaking in the late 1970s, followed by a low point in the early 1990s. This was followed by a subsequent upturn in the levels of use that continued into 2001. In 2000, the NHSDA estimated the total number of use Americans, 12 years of age and older, who had used a tranquilizer nonmedically during the prior 30 days as 788,000, down from 950,000 the prior year (U.S. Department of Health and Human Services, 2001). Most of the people who had used a benzodiazepine nonmedically had done so only a few times in their lifetimes. Nonmedical benzodiazepine use, which is different from, and far less common than medical use of the benzodiazepines, is a small but significant part of the overall nonmedical drug problem in the nation.

DISTINGUISHING MEDICAL AND NONMEDICAL USE OF BENZODIAZEPINES

A series of national surveys tracking the medical use of the benzodiazepines showed that their use peaked in 1976 and by the late 1980s had fallen about 25% off that peak rate (DuPont, 1988). A 1979 survey of medical use of the benzodiazepines (near the peak of benzodiazepine use in the United States), showed that 89% of Americans ages 18 years and older had not used a benzodiazepine within the previous 12 months. Of those who had used a benzodiazepine, most (9.5% of all adults) had used the benzodiazepine either less than every day or for less than 12 months, or both, whereas a minority (1.6% of the adult population) had used a benzodiazepine on a daily basis for 12 months or longer. This long-term user group was two-thirds female; 71% were age 50 or older, and most had chronic medical problems, as well as anxiety (DuPont, 1988).

Of those with anxiety disorders in a large community sample, three-fourths were receiving no treatment at all, including not using a benzodiazepine. The 1.6% of the population who are chronic benzodiazepine users can be compared to the 17% of the population suffering from anxiety disorders at any 12-month period. This statistic led many observers to conclude that not only are benzodiazepines not overprescribed but they also may actually be underprescribed, because of the reluctance of both physician and patients to use these medicines (Mellinger & Balter, 1981).

To understand the place of the benzodiazepines in contemporary medical practice, it is important to separate appropriate medical use from inappropriate, nonmedical use. Five characteristics distinguish medical from nonmedical use of all controlled substances, including the benzodiazepines.

1. *Intent.* Is the substance used to treat a diagnosed medical problem, such as anxiety or insomnia, or is it used to get high (or to treat the complications of nonmedical use of other drugs)? Typical medical use of a benzodiazepine or other controlled substance occurs without the use of multiple nonmedical drugs, whereas nonmedical use of the benzodiazepines is usually polydrug abuse. Although alcoholics and drug addicts sometimes use the language of medicine to describe their reasons for using controlled substances nonmedically, "self-administration" or "self-medication" of an intoxicating substance outside the ordinary practice boundaries of medical care is a hallmark of drug abuse (DuPont, 1998).

2. *Effect.* What is the effect of the controlled substance use on the user's life? The only acceptable standard for medical use is that it helps the user live a better life. Typical nonmedical drug use is associated with deterioration in the user's life, even though continued use and denial of the negative consequences of this use are nearly universal.

3. *Control.* Is the substance use controlled only by the user, or does a fully knowledgeable physician share the control of the drug use? Medical drug use is controlled by the physician, as well as the patient, whereas typical nonmedical use is solely controlled by the user.

4. *Legality.* Is the use legal or illegal? Medical use of a controlled substance is legal. Nonmedical drug use of controlled substances, including benzo-diazepines, is illegal.

5. *Pattern.* What is the pattern of the controlled substance use? Typical medical use of controlled substances is similar to the use of penicillin or aspirin, in that it occurs in a medically reasonable pattern to treat an easily recognized health problem other than addiction. Typical use of nonmedical drugs (e.g., alcohol, marijuana, or cocaine), in contrast, takes place at parties or in other social settings. Medical substance use is stable and at a moderate dose level. Nonmedical use of a controlled substance is usually polydrug abuse at high and/or unstable doses (Juergens & Cowley, 2003).

DRUG DEPENDENCE VERSUS PHYSICAL DEPENDENCE

Substance use disorder is a mental disorder defined in the fourth revised edition of the *Diagnostic and Statistical Manual of Mental Disorders* (DSM-IV-TR; American Psychiatric Association, 2000). It includes out-of-control drug use, use outside social and medical sanctions, continued use despite clear evidence of drug-caused problems, and a drug-centered lifestyle. Physical dependence (including withdrawal on discontinuation), in contrast to addiction, is a pharmacological phenomenon in which the user experiences a specific constellation of symptoms for a relatively short period when use of the substance is abruptly discontinued. Physical dependence may, but often does not, accompany substance use disorder (abuse or dependence). The appropriate treatment for addiction, or substance use disorder, is usually long-term, specialized additional treatment followed by prolonged participation in one of the 12-step programs and/or other ongoing support and care. The appropriate treatment for physical dependence, in clear contrast, is gradual dose reduction to permit biological adaptation to lower doses of the dependence-producing substance, leading to zero dosing.

A patient who seeks to continue using a medicine because it is helpful is no more demonstrating "drug-seeking behavior" than is a patient who finds eyeglasses helpful in the treatment of myopia demonstrating "glasses-seeking behavior" if deprived of a corrective lens. Drug abuse and drug dependence are characterized by use despite problems caused by that use (loss of control) and by denial (and dishonesty)—neither of which is seen in appropriate medical treatment (DuPont & Gold, 1995).

Precisely the same confusion of medically trivial physical dependence with serious substance use disorder (addiction) occurs in regard to the use of opiates in the treatment of severe pain. Many patients and many physicians undertreat severe pain, because they are unable to distinguish physical dependence, the benign pharmacological fact of neuroadaptation in medical patients, from the abuse of opiates by drug addicts, a malignant biobehavioral disorder (Savage, 2003).

MEDICAL USE AND ABUSE

The benzodiazepines are among the most widely prescribed psychotropic medicines in the world. The World Health Organization (1988) labeled them "essential drugs" that should be available in all countries for medical purposes. Of the widely used psychotropic drugs, they are the least likely to cause any adverse effects, including serious medical complications and death.

Workplace drug testing is usually limited to identification of marijuana, cocaine, morphine–codeine, amphetamine–methamphetamine, and phencyclidine (PCP). However, benzodiazepines and barbiturates may be added to the test panel. Laboratory positive test results for patients with legitimate prescriptions for benzodiazepines and barbiturates are reported to employers by medical review officers (MROs) as negative, as are other laboratory results that reflect appropriate medical treatment with other controlled substances (MacDonald, DuPont, & Ferguson, 2003).

Several important health concerns about benzodiazepine use that are unrelated to addiction have been expressed, especially about the long-term use of benzodiazepines, including the effects on the brain, the possibility of cerebral atrophy associated with prolonged benzodiazepine use, and other problems, such as memory loss and personality change (American Psychiatric Association Task Force on Benzodiazepine Dependence, Toxicity and Abuse, 1990; Golombok, Moodley, & Lader, 1988). The evidence for these problems is both preliminary and disputed, except for the well-studied acute effect of benzo-diazepines on memory, which has no clinical significance for most patients.

PHARMACOLOGY

In this section, the sedatives and hypnotics are divided for convenience into three groups: barbiturates, "other sedatives and hypnotics," and benzodiaze-pines. We also discuss the newer agents, which are alternatives to the benzo-diazepines.

Barbiturates

Barbital was introduced into medical practice in 1903, and phenobarbital, in 1912. Their rapid success led to the development of over 2,000 derivatives of barbituric acid, with dozens being used in medical practice. The only sedatives to precede the barbiturates were the bromides and chloral hydrate, both of which were in widespread use before the end of the 19th century.

The most commonly used barbiturates today are amobarbital (Amytal), butabarbital (Butisol), mephobarbital (Mebaral), pentobarbital (Nembutal), secobarbital (Seconal), and phenobarbital (Luminal). The first five have an intermediate duration of action, whereas the last, phenobarbital, has a long duration of action. Short-acting barbiturates are used as anesthetics, but not in outpatient medicine.

Barbiturates reversibly suppress the activity of all excitable tissue, with the CNS being particularly sensitive to these effects. Except for the antiepileptic effects of phenobarbital, there is a low therapeutic index for the sedative effects of the barbiturates, with general CNS depression being linked to the desired therapeutic effects. The amount of barbiturates that can cause a fatal overdose is well within the usual size of a single prescription. A common problem with the medical use of the barbiturates for both sedation and hypnosis is the rapid development of tolerance, with a common tendency of medical patients to raise the dose on chronic administration. The barbiturates affect the gamma-aminobutyric acid (GABA) system, producing both a cross-tolerance to other sedating drugs, including alcohol and the benzodiazepines, and a heightened risk of fatal overdose reactions (Charney et al., 2001).

Other Sedatives and Hypnotics

Over the course of the 20th century, several medicines with diverse structures were used as sedatives and hypnotics. In general, the pharmacological properties of these medicines resembled the barbiturates. They produced profound CNS depression, with little or no analgesia. Their therapeutic index was low and their abuse potential was high, similar to the barbiturates. Chloral hydrate (Noctec), ethchlorvynol (Placidyl), ethinamate (Valmid), glutethimide (Doriden), meprobamate (Miltown, Equanil), methyprylon (Noludar), and paraldehyde (Paral) belong in this class of seldom-used medicines that do not have a useful place in contemporary medical practice.

Despite the continued widespread use of antihistamines to treat insomnia, the Food and Drug Administration (FDA), noting the prominent sedative side effects encountered in the administration of antihistamines (including doxylamine, diphenhydramine, and pyrilamine), concluded that the antihistamines are not consistently effective in the treatment of sleep disorders. Tolerance rapidly develops to the sedating effects of these medicines, and the antihistamines can produce paradoxical stimulation. In addition, the antihistamine doses currently approved for the treatment of allergies are inadequate to induce sleep. Antihistamines used to treat sleep disorders can produce daytime sedation because of their relatively long half-lives (Charney et al., 2001).

The use of sedating antidepressants such as Desyrel (trazodone) and Elavil (amitriptyline) to treat insomnia at dose levels lower than are effective for the treatment of depression, such as the use of sedating antihistamines for this indication, is clinically problematic, since these agents may be both less effective and more likely to produce undesirable side effects (especially in producing daytime sedation) than the use of benzodiazepines in this indication (Mendelson et al., 2001).

Benzodiazepines

The benzodiazepines were recognized in animal experiments in the 1950s for their ability to produce "taming" without apparent sedation. Cats, which are extremely sensitive to even small electrical shocks, were obviously sedated when given enough alcohol or barbiturates to prevent anxious avoidance behavior of impending shocks. In contrast, when given benzodiazepines, the cats appeared normal in all of their behavior, except that they did not show the exaggerated anticipatory sensitivity to mild electrical shocks that they showed prior to treatment with benzodiazepines.

Chlordiazepoxide (Librium), the first benzodiazepine used in clinical practice, was introduced in 1961. More than 3,000 additional benzodiazepines have been synthesized, of which about 50 have been used clinically (Baldessarini, 2001). Several of the benzodiazepines, including alprazolam (Xanax), diazepam (Valium), lorazepam (Ativan), and clonazepam (Klonopin) are among not only the most widely prescribed medicines for anxiety but are also the most frequently prescribed medicines worldwide.

The identification of the benzodiazepine receptors in 1977 began the modern era of benzodiazepine research, establishing this class as the best understood of the psychiatric medicines. GABA receptors are membrane-bound proteins divided into three subtypes, GABA-A, GABA-B, and GABA-C receptors. The GABA-A receptors are composed of five subunits that together form the chloride channel, which primarily mediates neuronal excitability (seizures), rapid mood changes, and clinical anxiety, as well as sleep. GABA-B receptors mediate memory, mood, and analgesia. The role of the GABA-C receptors remains unclear. The effects of benzodiazepines are reversed by benzodiazepine antagonists, one of which—flumazenil—is used clinically to reverse rapidly the effects of benzodiazepine overdoses (Charney et al., 2001). The benzodiazepine receptors, part of the GABA system, are found in approximately 30% of CNS synapses and in all species above the level of the shark, demonstrating their fundamental biological importance.

There are pharmacological differences among the individual benzodiazepines that have clinical significance. The differences between the benzodiazepines resemble the differences between the individual medicines in two other major classes of psychotropic medicines: antipsychotics and antidepressants. Although there are many overlapping effects within each class, there are also important differences among the medicines in each class, so that the medicines within a class cannot be used interchangeably. These pharmacological differences among the benzodiazepines include the rapidity of onset (distributional half-life), persistence of active drug and/or metabolite in the body (elimination half-life), major metabolic breakdown pathways (conjugation vs. oxidation), and specific molecular structure (e.g., alprazolam has a unique triazolo ring that may account for some differences in its clinical effects) (Charney et al., 2001). Table 10.1 summarizes these differences for the most widely used benzodiazepines, along with clinically important pharmacological characteristics as they relate to the use and abuse of the benzodiazepines (Chouninard, Lefko-Singh, & Teboul, 1999). Benzodiazepines may produce some clinically relevant effects by mechanisms that do not involve GABA-mediated chloride conductance (Burt & Kamatchi, 1991). The benzodiazepines have only a slight effect on rapid eye movement (REM) sleep, but they do suppress deeper, stage 4 sleep. Although this effect is probably of no clinical significance in most settings, diazepam has been used to prevent "night terrors" that arise in stage 4 sleep.

Speed of Onset

The most important distinction among the benzodiazepines in the substance abuse context is the speed of onset, which determines abuse potential (Griffiths & Werts, 1997). Those benzodiazepines with a slow onset (because they are either slowly absorbed or they must be metabolized to produce an active substance) have a relatively lower abuse potential. Those that rapidly reach peak

TABLE 10.1. Pharmacological Characteristics of Benzodiazepines

Drug	Trade name	Onset of action after oral administration	Rate of metabolism	Metabolized primarily by liver oxidation	Active metabolites	Elimination half-life (hours)	Maximum usual dose (mg/day)
Used primarily to treat anxiety							
Alprazolam	Xanax	Intermediate	Intermediate	Yes	Yes	12–15	4
Chlordiazepoxide hydrochloride	Librium	Intermediate	Long	Yes	Yes	5–30, 10–15	100
Clonazepam[a]	Klonopin	Fast	Long	Yes	No	26–30	2
Clorazepate[a] dipotassium	Tranxene	Fast	Long	Yes	Yes	36–200	60
Diazepam[a,b]	Valium	Fast	Long	Yes	Yes	20–50	40
Halazepam	Paxipam	Intermediate	Long	Yes	Yes	50–100	160
Lorazepam	Ativan	Intermediate	Short	No	No	10–14	6
Oxazepam	Serax	Slow	Short	No	No	5–10	60
Prazepam	Centrax	Slow	Long	Yes	Yes	36–200	60
Used primarily to treat insomnia							
Estazolam	ProSom	Fast	Short	Yes	No	10–24	2
Flurazepam hydrochloride	Dalmane	Intermediate	Long	Yes	Yes	40–100	30
Quazepam	Doral	Fast	Long	Yes	Yes	20–120	30
Temazepam	Restoril	Intermediate	Short	No	Yes	8–12	30
Triazolam	Halcion	Intermediate	Short	Yes	No	2–5	0.25

[a] Approved to treat epilepsy.
[b] Approved as muscle relaxant.

227

brain levels after oral administration are relatively more likely to produce euphoria, and are therefore more likely to be abused by alcoholics and drug addicts. Diazepam has a relatively rapid onset of action and is therefore among the most effective producers of euphoria. In contrast, the more slow-acting benzodiazepines, such as oxazepam (Serax) and prazepam (Centrax), appear to have lower abuse potentials.

Clorazepate and prazepam, with inactive parent compounds, are also less likely to be abused for their euphoric effects because of slower onset of action. Oxazepam and the other slower onset benzodiazepines, like phenobarbital compared to other barbiturates and codeine compared to other opiates, appear to have relatively low abuse potentials.

The relative rapidity of onset of diazepam does not mean that it is more likely than other benzodiazepines to lead to abuse by medical patients who have no addiction history. None of the benzodiazepines, including diazepam, are reinforcing for patients who do not have a history of addiction. On the other hand, the pharmacology of the benzodiazepines suggests that, for patients with a history of addiction to alcohol and other drugs, diazepam may be more likely to be abused than oxazepam, clorazepate, or prazepam (Griffiths & Weerts, 1997).

Some serious students of the pharmacology of benzodiazepines believe that abuse is no more likely for diazepam than for oxazepam (Woods, Katz, & Winger, 1988). Addicts' greater liking for diazepam in some studies, in this view, is the result of the dose: Raise the dose of oxazepam in the double-blind studies, and the liking scores of oxazepam are indistinguishable from those of diazepam. In contrast, other well-respected researchers are convinced that diazepam, lorazepam, and alprazolam have greater abuse potential—not solely because of dosage factors—because of their more rapid absorption and penetration of the blood–brain barrier due to greater lipid solubility (Griffiths & Sannerud, 1987).

Metabolic Pathways

The metabolic pathways of the various benzodiazepines are important clinically, because those benzodiazepines that are metabolized by oxidation in the liver may alter the effects of other drugs. This is illustrated by the "boosting" effect of some benzodiazepines when used by methadone-maintained patients. Although the pharmacology of this effect is not well understood, it appears that simultaneous use of a benzodiazepine (e.g., diazepam or alprazolam) that competes with methadone for oxidative pathways in the liver produces higher peak levels of methadone in the blood (and brain) shortly after methadone is administered. Thus, prior use of some benzodiazepines may enhance brain reward for an hour or so after oral methadone dosages.

Benzodiazepines that have conjugation as the major metabolic pathway are not dependent on liver functioning, so they are less likely to raise methadone plasma levels or to build up plasma levels of the active benzodiazepine in patients who have compromised liver functioning, including alcoholics and the elderly. The benzodiazepines metabolized by conjugation include lorazepam, oxazepam, and temazepam. Thus, because these are less "liked" by methadone-maintained patients and may be better choices for these patients and for patients with compromised liver functioning, a benzodiazepine is to be used.

Oxazepam is both a slow-onset and a conjugated benzodiazepine, making it perhaps the best choice for methadone-maintained patients who are treated with a benzodiazepine. On the other hand, oxazepam has a short elimination half-life, which means it must be taken three or four times a day for continuous therapeutic effects. Oxazepam is no less likely to produce physical dependence (including difficulties on discontinuation) than any other benzodiazepine. Oxazepam is a widely used benzodiazepine in Europe (but not in the United States, where it is commonly abused by drug addicts and alcoholics). Thus, whatever benefit oxazepam may possess for alcoholics and drug addicts compared to other benzodiazepines is relative and not absolute (DuPont, 1988).

Persistence

Persistence of a benzodiazepine (or an active metabolite) in the body is important clinically, because it governs the rapidity of onset of withdrawal symptoms after the last dose for people who have used benzodiazepines for prolonged periods. The benzodiazepines with shorter elimination half-lives are more likely to produce early and pronounced withdrawal symptoms on abrupt discontinuation, whereas those with longer elimination half-lives generally produce more delayed and somewhat attenuated withdrawal symptoms. In general, alprazolam, lorazepam, and oxazepam are more rapidly eliminated than are clorazepate, diazepam, flurazepam, and prazepam. Thus, the benzodiazepines with shorter elimination half-lives are more likely to produce acute withdrawal on abrupt cessation after prolonged use. Clonazepam has a longer elimination half-life than alprazolam or lorazepam, so it is less likely to produce interdose withdrawal symptoms and is more appealing as a withdrawal agent (for the same reason, methadone and phenobarbital are attractive as agents in opiate withdrawal and sedative–hypnotic withdrawal).

When discontinuing treatment with a benzodiazepine abruptly, the speed of onset and the severity of symptoms are greater for benzodiazepines with shorter elimination half-lives (e.g., alprazolam or lorazepam) than for those with a longer half-life (such as clonazepam). However, abrupt discontinuation is not an appropriate medical treatment for benzodiazepine discontinuation after prolonged, everyday use. When short-acting benzodiazepines are withdrawn gradually over several weeks or longer, they do not produce more symptoms of withdrawal than do longer acting benzodiazepines (Sellers et al., 1993).

Although a long half-life may be beneficial in reducing the speed of onset and severity of benzodiazepine withdrawal on abrupt discontinuation, it can be more problematic in other situations. An increase in motor vehicle crash involvement was found in elderly persons using long half-life benzodiazepines, whereas use of shorter half-life benzodiazepines showed no increase in the probability of crashes in elderly persons compared to same-age persons who did not use a benzodiazepine (Hemmelgarn, Suissa, Huang, Boivin, & Pinard, 1997; Wang, Bohn, Glynn, Mogun, & Avom, 2001).

Reinforcement

Three additional aspects of benzodiazepine pharmacology are relevant to the treatment of addicted patients: reinforcement, withdrawal, and tolerance. Reinforcement is the potential for these medicines to be abused or "liked" by alcoholics and drug addicts. In controlled studies, benzodiazepines are not reinforcing or "liked" by either normal or anxious subjects. For example, normal and anxious subjects, given a choice between placebos and benzodiazepines, more often choose the placebo in double-blind acute dose experiments, regardless of the specific benzodiazepine given. In contrast, subjects with a history of addiction in double-blind studies prefer benzodiazepines—especially at high doses—to placebos. Studies have demonstrated that people with a history of addiction show a greater preference for intermediate-acting barbiturates and stimulants, as well as narcotics, than for benzodiazepines. Thus, the benzodiazepines are reinforcing for alcoholics and drug addicts (though not for anxious people or for people who do not have a history of addiction). The benzodiazepines are relatively weak reinforcers compared to opiates, stimulants, and barbiturates among alcoholics and drug addicts.

This research confirms the common clinical observation that benzodiazepines are rarely drugs of choice among addicted people for their euphoric effects (DuPont, 1984, 1988). Although it remains unclear why alcoholics and drug addicts react differently to the benzodiazepines than do normal or anxious subjects, this phenomenon exists with all abused drugs. It is not limited to the benzodiazepines. Normal subjects in double-blind studies do not generally "like" abused drugs, including stimulants, narcotics, and even alcohol. People who are not addicted to alcohol and other drugs do not like the feeling of being intoxicated. Whether addicted people learn to like the intoxicated feeling or whether they have some innate (perhaps genetically determined) difference that explains this characteristic response to alcohol and controlled substances remains an unanswered question of great importance to the prevention of addiction.

When it comes to the outpatient treatment of anxiety in patients with active addiction (e.g., current or recent abuse of alcohol or other drugs), the use of a controlled substance, including benzodiazepines, is generally contraindicated. A number of alternative treatments for anxiety are available, including nonpharmacological treatments, antidepressants, and buspirone (Buspar), a nonsedating antianxiety medicine with no abuse potential. As a general principle, the use of psychotropic medicines, whether controlled (e.g., benzodiazepines) or noncontrolled substances (e.g., antidepressants or antipsychotics), is unlikely to produce a therapeutic benefit for the actively using addicted patient. Stable abstinence is required for these antianxiety medicines to produce therapeutic results.

For patients who have been stable in recovery (including recovering alcoholics) and need treatment for anxiety, it is advisable not to use benzodiazepines, unless the physician can be sure that the patient uses the benzodiazepine only as prescribed and in the absence of any nonmedical drug use, including alcohol use. For many recovering people, successful use of benzodiazepines in the treatment of their anxiety disorders has not threatened their sobriety. We have seen many more patients in recovery who do not want to use any controlled substance and have done well with their anxiety problems, without using a benzodiazepine (Ciraulo et al., 1996; Sattar & Bhatia, 2003).

If a benzodiazepine is to be administered to a recovering person, it may be prudent to use one of the slow-onset medicines (e.g., oxazepam, clorazepate, or prazepam) and to include a family member, as well as the sponsor from a 12-step fellowship in the therapeutic alliance, to help ensure that there is no abuse of the benzodiazepine or any other drug, including alcohol.

Withdrawal

All of the medicines that influence the GABA system show cross-tolerance and similar withdrawal patterns. Because of cross-tolerance within this class of sedatives and hypnotics, an alcoholic or barbiturate addict can be withdrawn under medical supervision using a benzodiazepine. For the same reason, phenobarbital can be used to manage benzodiazepine withdrawal (Wesson, Smith, & Ling, 2003). Compared to other benzodiazepines, however, alprazolam withdrawal may be inadequately covered by substitution. Alprazolam detoxification should include an estimation of daily use and a slow withdrawal over a period of weeks. Clonazepam has been found to be helpful in this condition.

The sedatives/hypnotics withdrawal syndrome, including the potential for withdrawal seizures on abrupt discontinuation, is also a phenomenon of this class of medicines, which argues against abrupt discontinuation of any of these medicines after daily use for more than a few weeks. Cessation of use of the benzodiazepines, along with the other sedatives and hypnotics, can cause withdrawal seizures, because they are potent antiepilepsy drugs that raise the seizure threshold. Medicines that raise the seizure threshold, when abruptly discontinued, produce a rebound drop in the seizure threshold that may cause seizures, even in people who have not previously had an epileptic seizure.

Some recovering people believe that they are more likely to have withdrawal symptoms when they discontinue a benzodiazepine, even if it has been taken within medical guidelines. Research on the topic suggests that this is not the case, but this often contentious issue is best dealt with as an unresolved question in clinical practice.

Tolerance

Tolerance is rapid, and all but complete, to the sedative and to the euphoric effects of the benzodiazepines on repeated administration at a steady dose level for even a few days. This rapidly developing tolerance for both sedation and euphoria/reward is seen clinically when these medicines are used to treat anxiety. Patients often experience sedation or drowsiness when they take their first few benzodiazepine doses, but within a few days of steady dosing, the symptoms of sedation lessen and, for most patients, disappear.

By contrast, tolerance to the antianxiety and antipanic effects of benzodiazepines is nonexistent. Medical patients who are not alcoholics or drug addicts, and who use a benzodiazepine to treat chronic anxiety, obtain substantial beneficial effects at standard, low doses. They do not escalate their benzodiazepine doses beyond common therapeutic levels, even after they have taken benzodiazepines every day for many years.

This distinction between the rapid tolerance to the sedating and the euphoric effects and the absence of tolerance to the antianxiety effects of benzodiazepines is important for the clinician. Patients who use benzodiazepines to get high typically add other substances and escalate their benzodiazepine dose over time. This commonly observed pattern reflects the existence of tolerance to the euphoric effects of benzodiazepines among addicted people. In contrast, typical medical patients using benzodiazepines for their antianxiety effects take them at low and stable doses, without the addition of other drugs, including alcohol.

Some patients who use benzodiazepines daily, even after a long time, do escalate their dose beyond the usually prescribed level, add other drugs (especially alcohol), and/or have a poor clinical response to the benzodiazepine use (inadequate suppression of anxiety). Usually, but not always, these patients have a personal and a family history of addiction to alcohol and other drugs. These same patients sometimes have unusual difficulty in discontinuing their use of benzodiazepines. This group of problems with long-term benzodiazepine use is commonly seen in treatment programs for alcoholics and drug addicts, reinforcing the view in the addiction field that benzodiazepines are ineffective, problem-generating medications, especially after long-term use. Although this pattern of problems exists, it is, in our experience, uncommon in the typical medical or psychiatric practice dealing with anxious patients who do not have a history of addiction. Nevertheless, when it occurs, the best response is discontinuation of benzodiazepine use. For some patients, this requires inpatient treatment.

IDENTIFICATION OF PROBLEMS
AMONG LONG-TERM BENZODIAZEPINE USERS

Physicians frequently encounter patients, or family members of patients, who are concerned about the possible adverse effects of long-term use of a benzodiazepine in the treatment of anxiety or insomnia. In helping to structure the decision making for such a patient, we use the Benzodiazepine Checklist (DuPont, 1986; see Table 10.2). There are four questions to be answered:

1. *Diagnosis.* Is there a current diagnosis that warrants the prolonged use of a prescription medicine? The benzodiazepines are serious medicines that should only be used for serious illnesses.

2. *Medical and nonmedical substance use.* Is the benzodiazepine dose the patient is taking reasonable? Is the clinical response to the benzodiazepine favorable? Is there any use of nonmedical drugs, such as cocaine or marijuana? Is there any excessive use of alcohol (e.g., a total of more than four drinks a week, or more than two drinks a day)? Are other medicines being used that can depress CNS functioning?

3. *Toxic behavior.* Is the patient free of evidence of slurred speech, staggering, accidents, memory loss, or other mental deficits or evidence of sedation?

4. *Family monitor.* Does the family confirm that there is a good clinical response and no adverse reactions to the patient's use of a benzodiazepine? Because people who abuse drugs deny drug-caused problems and often lie to

---

TABLE 10.2 Benzodiazepine Checklist for Long-Term Use

1. *Diagnosis.* Is there a current diagnosis that warrants the prolonged use of a prescription medicine?

2. *Medical and nonmedical substance use.* Is the dose of the benzodiazepine the patient is taking reasonable? Is the clinical response to the benzodiazepine favorable? Is there any use of nonmedical drugs, such as cocaine or marijuana? Is there any excessive use of alcohol (e.g., a total of more than four drinks a week, or more than two drinks a day)? Are there other medicines being used that can depress the functioning of the CNS?

3. *Toxic behavior.* Is the patient free of evidence of slurred speech, staggering, accidents, memory loss, or other mental deficits or evidence of sedation?

4. *Family monitor.* Does the family confirm that there is a good clinical response and no adverse reactions to the patient's use of a benzodiazepine?

Standard for continued benzodiazepine use: a "yes" to all four questions.

their doctors, and because many family members are concerned about long-term benzodiazepine use, we generally ask that a family member come to the office at least once with the patient who is taking a benzodiazepine for a prolonged period. This gives us an opportunity to confirm with the family member, while the patient is present, that benzodiazepine use produces a therapeutic benefit without problems. If there is a problem of toxic behavior or abuse of other drugs, we are more likely to identify it when we speak with the patient's family members; if not, we have an opportunity to educate and reassure both the patient and family members when they are seen together.

Most patients without a history of addiction produce four "yes" answers to these four questions. Even a single "no" answer deserves careful review and may signal the desirability of discontinuation of the benzodiazepine. After completion of the Benzodiazepine Checklist, if there is clear evidence that long-term benzodiazepine use is producing significant benefits and no problems, and if the patient wants to continue using the benzodiazepine (which is, in our experience, a common set of circumstances for chronically anxious patients), then we have no hesitancy in continuing to prescribe a benzodiazepine, even for the patient's lifetime.

On the other hand, many anxious patients, even when they have good responses without problems, want to stop using benzodiazepines. Other patients do not want to stop using a benzodiazepine, but they do show signs of poor clinical response or trouble with the use of a benzodiazepine. In either case, discontinuation is in order, and it is an achievable goal.

Some critics of benzodiazepines, including Stefan Borg and Curtis Carlson of St. Goran's Hospital in Stockholm, Sweden (Allgulander, Borg, & Vikander, 1984), have expressed concerns about the possibility that benzodiazepine use may lead to alcohol problems in patients without a prior history of alcohol abuse, especially in women. The simple advice to a long-term medical user of a benzodiazepine is not to use alcohol, or to use alcohol only occasionally and never more than one or two drinks in 24 hours. Most anxious patients who do not have a prior history of addiction either do not use alcohol at all or use it only in small amounts. The Benzodiazepine Checklist helps the physician, the patient, and the patient's family identify any problems (including alcohol abuse) at early stages, thus facilitating constructive interventions.

LONG-TERM DOSE AND ABUSE

One clinical observation helps the physician identify people who have addiction problems among anxious benzodiazepine users. Most anxious medical users of benzodiazepines have used these medicines at low and stable doses over time, often for many years, with good clinical responses. Dose is a critical and distinguishing variable in long-term benzodiazepine use. People who are addicted to alcohol and other drugs commonly abuse benzodiazepines in high and unstable doses; anxious patients who are not addicted do not. People with active addiction (e.g., who currently use illegal drugs and/or abuse alcohol) seldom report a good clinical response to low and stable doses of benzodiazepines.

We use a simple assessment of dose level: If the patient's typical benzodiazepine dose level is stable at or below one-half the ordinary clinical maximum dose of the prescribed benzodiazepine as recommended in the *Physicians' Desk Reference* (PDR; Medical Economics Data Production, 2003) or in the package insert approved by the FDA for the prescribed benzodiazepine, we call this the "green light" benzodiazepine dose zone. Thus, patients whose daily benzodiazepine dose is stable at or less than 2 mg of alprazolam, 20 mg of diazepam, 5 mg of lorazepam, 4 mg of clonazepam, or 60 mg of oxazepam are in the relatively safe or green-light zone.

The "red light," or danger, zone is above the FDA-approved maximum daily dose (e.g., above 4 mg of alprazolam or 40 mg of diazepam). Except in the treatment of panic, when doses up to two or three times the FDA maximum for chronic anxiety are occasionally needed, it is unusual to see an anxious non-alcohol- or non-drug-abusing patient taking benzodiazepine doses that are this high. Most panic disorder patients, after a few months of treatment, are able to do well (with good panic suppression) in the green light zone, without the physician or the patient making any effort to limit or restrict the benzodiazepine dose level. If vigilance and control are required by the physician to limit the benzodiazepine dose to levels below the maximum recommended doses, this is a poor prognostic sign and a signal that addiction to alcohol and other drugs may be a confounding comorbid disorder.

One common clinical challenge is to see a patient, a family member, or sometimes a physician or therapist who is concerned about "tolerance" and "addiction," because the patient feels compelled to raise the dose of the benzodiazepine over time. In our experience, such worries among patients who lack a personal history of addiction to alcohol or other nonmedical drugs are usually the result of underdosing with the benzodiazepine rather than evidence of addiction. Although some patients with such a presentation are more comfortable taking no medicine at all, most need education about the proper dose of the benzodiazepine. Once the benzodiazepine dose is raised to an ordinary therapeutic level (e.g., well within the green light zone), patients usually feel much better in terms of their symptoms of an anxiety disorder and have no inner pressure to raise the benzodiazepine dose further.

Within the addicted population, several patterns of benzodiazepine abuse have been identified. The most common pattern is the use of a benzodiazepine to reduce the adverse effects of the abuse of other, more preferred drugs. Typical is the suppression of a hangover and other withdrawal phenomena from alcohol use with a benzodiazepine. Patients waking up in the morning after an alcoholic binge may take 10–40 mg or more of diazepam, for example, "just to face the day."

Other common nonmedical patterns are to use benzodiazepines (often alprazolam or lorazepam) concomitantly with stimulants (often cocaine or methamphetamine) to reduce the unpleasant experiences of the stimulant use, and/or to use benzodiazepines (often triazolam [Halcion]) to treat the insomnia that accompanies stimulant abuse.

Benzodiazepines are occasionally used as primary drugs of abuse, in which case they are typically taken orally at high doses. Addicted patients report using doses of 20–100 mg or more of diazepam, or the equivalent doses of other benzodiazepines, for example, at one time. Such high-dose oral use is often repeated several times a day for long periods or on binges. Although, in our experience, such primary benzodiazepine abuse without simultaneous use of other drugs is unusual, it does occur.

Daily use of benzodiazepines, even when there is no dose escalation and no abuse of alcohol or other nonmedical drugs has led to controversy. Clinical experience has shown that even over long periods of daily use, benzodiazepines typically do not lose their efficacy and do not produce significant problems for most patients. An example of this experience was a study of 170 adult patients treated for a variety of sleep disorders continuously with a benzodiazepine for 6 months or longer over a 12-year period. The study found sustained efficacy, with low risk of dose escalation, adverse effects, or abuse (Schenck & Mahowald, 1996).

Discontinuation of Benzodiazepine Use

Discontinuation of sedatives and hypnotics, including the benzodiazepines, can be divided into three categories: (1) long-term low-dose benzodiazepine use, (2) high-dose benzodiazepine abuse and multiple drug abuse, and (3) high-dose abuse of nonbenzodiazepine sedatives and hypnotics (especially intermediate-acting barbiturates). The first group of patients can usually be discontinued on an outpatient basis. Some of the second and even the third group can be treated as outpatients, but most will require inpatient care. Inpatient discontinuation today with managed care is generally reserved for patients who fail at outpatient discontinuation and for those who demonstrate acutely life-threatening loss of control over their drug use. The pharmacological management of inpatient benzodiazepine withdrawal from nontherapeutically high doses of these medicines is covered in standard texts dealing with inpatient detoxification (Wesson et al., 2003).

With respect to withdrawal from benzodiazepines in the context of addiction treatment, the most common problem that addiction treatment professionals experience is that some of their patients who take benzodiazepines also suffer from underlying anxiety disorders and panic attacks. When these patients stop taking a benzodiazepine, they experience a short-term rebound increase in these distressing symptoms. These rebound symptoms, including panic attacks, are difficult for the patients and their physicians to separate from withdrawal symptoms, because they are similar and the time course is also similar, with both types of symptoms occurring at low benzodiazepine doses and peaking during the first or second drug-free week.

There is evidence that most patients who take benzodiazepines at prescribed dose levels can discontinue using them with quite moderate symptoms if the dose reduction is gradual (Busto, Simpkins, & Sellers, 1983; Rickels, Schweizer, Csanalosi, Case, & Chung, 1988). One study found that about half of long-term benzodiazepine users could stop with no withdrawal symptoms (Tyrer, Rutherford, & Huggett, 1981). However, some patients who stop benzodiazepine use, especially after use for many years, do have either prolonged or severe withdrawal symptoms (Noyes, Garvey, Cook, & Perry, 1988). About one in three medical patients with long-term use of a benzodiazepine have clinically significant withdrawal symptoms, even after gradual tapering, and about one in eight patients stopping a benzodiazepine will have prolonged and/or severe symptoms (DuPont, 1988). In any case, discontinuation symptoms (except for abrupt cessation, which can produce seizures and is not indicated) from benzodiazepines are "distressing but not dangerous" (DuPont et al., 1992; Sellers et al., 1993).

There are a number of useful publications on the diagnosis and treatment of chronic anxiety (Davidson, 2003; DuPont, Spencer, & DuPont, 2004; Ross, 1994; Spencer, DuPont, & DuPont, 2004). The benzodiazepines can be used to treat either acute or chronic anxiety, as well as the panic attacks that are commonly associated with anxiety disorders. The benzodiazepines can be used either as needed or every day, and they can be used either alone or with other medicines, most often with antidepressants (Davidson, 1997).

Although all of the benzodiazepines are now off patent, there has been a recent interest in the development of new delivery mechanisms for the two most widely used benzodiazepines (Stahl, 2003). Alprazolam is now available in an extended release formulation, Xanax XR. It has the advantage of slower onset of action, which reduces initial sedation in the hour or two after administration. Slower onset of action also lowers the abuse potential of Xanax XR, since it is the rapid onset of action that triggers the brain reward that addicts seek. This new formulation of alprazolam permits once-a-day, or at most twice-a-day, dosing and reduces the risk of "clock watching," which may be seen with frequent dosing throughout the day. This new formulation of alprazolam may be a significant improvement over the three to four times a day dosing required for the immediate release alprazolam.

Clonazepam has been reformulated for sublingual administration for easy administration without swallowing a pill. This new product is called Klonopin Wafers. In the new formulations of these two benzodiazepines, the manufacturers have moved in opposite directions to maximize two different therapeutic effects. Xanax XR has a slower onset and longer duration of action to smooth the brain level of alprazolam for 24-hour-a-day effectiveness. Sublingual clonazepam has been reformulated to overcome the problems some patients have swallowing pills.

Newer Sedative and Hypnotic Agents

In recent years, a variety of alternatives to the benzodiazepines have become available to treat both anxiety and insomnia. Buspirone (Buspar) has been shown to reduce anxiety in generalized anxiety disorders, but it does not suppress panic attacks, and is not used as a primary treatment of obsessive–compulsive disorder. Buspirone is not abused by alcoholics and drug addicts, and it does not produce withdrawal symptoms on abrupt discontinuation. Like the antidepressants, buspirone requires several weeks of daily dosing to produce antianxiety effects, which are less dramatic from patients' point of view than are the effects produced by the benzodiazepines (Sussman & Stein, 2002).

The antidepressants as a class have been shown to possess antipanic and antianxiety effects opening a new range of uses for these medicines in the treatment of anxiety disorders. The selective serotonin reuptake inhibitors (SSRIs) have emerged as the first-line treatment for many anxiety disorders (Davidson, 2003; DuPont, 1997; Jefferson, 1997). Although the earlier antianxiety and anti-insomnia medicines focused exclusively on the benzodiazepine receptors in the GABA system, the recognition of the importance of serotonin and norepinephrine neurotransmitters in the management of anxiety and insomnia, and the success of buspirone, have stimulated a search for a new generation of antianxiety medicines that are not controlled substances (e.g., they are not abused by alcoholics and drug addicts). Recognition of the withdrawal symptoms associated with abrupt discontinuation of some antidepressants (especially those with shorter half-lives and more anticholinergic properties) have shown that withdrawal is not limited to controlled stubstances (DuPont, 1997).

Two nonbenzodiazepine hypnotic agents have been introduced. Zolpidem (Ambien) and Zaleplon (Sonata) are rapid-onset, short duration of action medicines that act on the benzodiazepine receptors of the GABA system. They have been shown to reduce insomnia. They have largely replaced the benzodiazepines as hypnotic medicines, although they lack the anxiolytic, anticonvulsant, and muscle-relaxant properties of the benzodiazepines (Scharf, Mayleben, Kaffeman, Krall, & Ochs, 1991). Zolpidem and zaleplon are reinforcing to alcoholics and drug addicts, underscoring the fact that the abuse potential of both drugs appears to be similar to that of benzodiazepines. Both medicines impair memory and performance of complex tasks in ways that are similar to the acute effects of benzodiazepines. They do not affect stage 4 sleep, as do the benzodiazepines.

Both zaleplon and zolpidem are effective in relieving sleep-onset insomnia, and both have been approved by the FDA for use up to 7–10 days at a time. Both medicines clinically appear to have sustained hypnotic activity over longer periods of time. Zolpidem has a half-life of about 2 hours, which is consistent with therapeutic activity over a typical 8 hours of sleep. Zaleplon has a 1-hour half-life that offers the possibility of dosing in the middle of the night for broken sleep. For this reason zaleplon is approved for use both at bedtime and in midsleep periods of insomnia.

In recent years, the antiepilepsy medicines, including valproate (Depakote) and gabapentin (Neurontin), have been used as augmenting agents in the treatment of anxiety (Lydiard, 2002).

REFERENCES

Allgulander, C., Borg, S., & Vikander, B. (1984). A 4–6 year follow-up of 50 patients with primary dependence on sedative and hypnotic drugs. *Am J Psychiatry, 141*, 1580–1582.

American Psychiatric Association. (2000). *Diagnostic and statistical manual of mental disorders* (4th text rev. ed.). Washington, DC: Author.

Baldessarini, R. J. (2001). Depression and anxiety disorders. In J. G. Hardman & L. E. Limbird, (Eds.), *Goodman and Gilman's, the pharmacological basis of therapeutics* (10th ed., pp. 447–483). New York: McGraw-Hill.

Burt, D. R., & Kamatchi, G. L. (1991). GABA receptor subtypes: From pharmacology to molecular biology. *FASEB, 5*, 2916–2923.

Busto, U., Simpkins, J., & Sellers, E. M. (1983). Objective determination of benzodiazepine use and abuse in alcoholics. *Br J Addict, 48*, 429–435.

Charney, D. S., Minic, S. J., & Harris, R. A. (2001). Hypnotics and sedatives. In J. G. Hardman & L. E. Limbird, (Eds.), *Goodman and Gilman's, the pharmacological basis of therapeutics* (10th ed., pp. 399–427). New York: McGraw-Hill.

Chouninard, G., Lefko-Singh, K., & Teboul, E. (1999). Metabolism of anxiolytics and hypnotics: Benzodiazepines, buspirone, zopiclone, and zolpidem. *Cell Mol Neurobiol, 19*, 533–552.

Ciraulo, D. A., Sarid-Segal, O., Knapp, C., Ciraulo, A. M., Greenblatt, D. J., & Shader, R. I. (1996). Liability to alprazolam abuse in daughters of alcoholics. *Am J Psychiatry, 153*, 956–958.

Davidson, J. (2003). *The anxiety book*. New York: Penguin/Putnam.

Davidson, J. R. T. (1997). Use of benzodiazepines in panic disorder. *J Clin Psychiatry, 58*(Suppl. 2), 26–31.

DuPont, R. L. (1984). *Getting tough on gateway drugs: A guide for the family*. Washington, DC: American Psychiatric Press.

DuPont, R. L. (1986). *Benzodiazepines: The social issues*. Rockville, MD: Institute for Behavior and Health.

DuPont, R. L. (Ed.). (1988). Abuse of benzodiazepines: The problems and the solutions. *Am J Drug Alcohol Abuse, 14*(Suppl 1), 1–69.

DuPont, R. L. (1995). Anxiety and addiction: A clinical perspective on comorbidity. *Bull Menninger Clin, 59*(Suppl A), A53–A72.

DuPont, R. L. (1997). The pharmacology and drug interactions of the newer antidepressants. *Essential Psychopharmacology, 2,* 7–31.

DuPont, R. L. (1998). Addiction: A new paradigm. *Bull Menninger Clin, 62,* 231–242.

DuPont, R. L. (2000). *The selfish brain: Learning from addiction* (rev. ed.). Center City, MN: Hazelden.

DuPont, R. L., DuPont, C. M., & Rice, D. P. (2002). Economic costs of anxiety disorders. In D. J. Stein & E. Hollander (Eds.), *Textbook of anxiety disorders* (pp. 365–374). Washington, DC: American Psychiatric Press

DuPont R. L., & Gold, M. S. (1995). Withdrawal and reward: implications for detoxification and relapse prevention. *Psychiatr Ann, 25,* 663–668.

DuPont, R. L., Spencer, E. D., & DuPont, C. M. (2004). *The anxiety cure: An eight step program for getting well* (rev. ed.). New York: Wiley.

DuPont, R. L., Swinson, R. P., Ballenger, J. C., Burrows, G. D., Noyes, R., Rubin, R. T., Rifkin, A., & Pecknold, J. C. (1992). Discontinuation effects of alprazolam after long-term treatment of panic-related disorders. *J Clin Psychopharmacol, 12,* 352–354.

Golombok, S., Moodley, P., & Lader, M. (1988). Cognitive impairment in long-term benzodiazepine users. *Psychol Med, 18,* 365–374.

Griffiths, R. R., & Sannerud, C. A. (1987). Abuse of and dependence on benzodiazepines and other anxiolytic/sedative drugs. In H. Meltzer, B. S. Bunney, & J. T. Coyle (Eds.), *Psychopharmacology: The third generation of progress* (pp. 1535–1541). New York: Raven Press.

Griffiths, R. R., & Weerts, E. M. (1994). Benzodiazepine self-administration in humans and laboratory animals: Implications for problems of long-term use and abuse. *Psychopharmacology, 134,* 1–37.

Handelsman, L. (2002). Anxiety in the context of substance abuse. In D. J. Stein & E. Hollander (Eds.), *Textbook of anxiety disorders* (pp. 441–448). Washington, DC: American Psychiatric Press.

Hemmelgarn, B., Suissa, S., Huang, A., Boivin, J.-F., & Pinard, G. (1997). Benzodiazepine use and the risk of motor vehicle crash in the elderly. *JAMA, 278,* 27–31.

Jefferson, J. W. (1997). Antidepressants in panic disorder. *J Clin Psychiatry, 58*(Suppl 2), 20–25.

Juergens, S. M., & Cowley, D.S. (2003). The pharmacology of benzodiazepines and other sedative–hypnotics. In A. W. Graham, T. K. Schultz, M. F. Mayo Smith, & R. K. Ries (Eds.), *Principles of addiction medicine* (3rd ed., pp. 119–139). Chevy Chase, MD: American Society of Addiction Medicine.

Kessler, R. C., McGonagle, K. A., Zhao, S., Nelson, C. B., Hughes, M., Eshleman, S., et al. (1994). Lifetime and 12-month prevalence of *DSM-III-R* psychiatric disorders in the United States: Results from the National Comorbidity Survey. *Arch Gen Psychiatry, 51,* 8–19.

Lydiard, R. B. (2002). Pharmacotherapy for panic disorder. In D. J. Stein & E. Hollander (Eds.), *Textbook of anxiety disorders* (pp. 257–273). Washington, DC: American Psychiatric Press.

MacDonald, D. I., DuPont, R. L., & Ferguson, J. L. (2003). The role of the medical review officer. In A. W. Graham, T. K. Schultz, M. F. Mayo Smith, & R. K. Ries

(Eds.), *Principles of addiction medicine* (3rd ed., pp. 977–985). Chevy Chase, MD: American Society of Addiction Medicine.

Medical Economics Data Production. (2003). *Physicians' desk reference.* Montvale, NJ: Author.

Mellinger, G. D., & Balter, M. B. (1981). Prevalence and patterns of use of psychotherapeutic drugs: Results from a 1979 national survey of American adults. In G. Tognoni, C. Bellantuono, & M. Lader (Eds.), *Epidemiological impact of psycho-tropic drugs* (pp. 117–135). Amsterdam: Elsevier.

Mendelson, W. B., Roth, T., Casella, J., Roehrs, T., Walsh, J., Woods, J. H., et al. (2001). *Report on a conference: The treatment of chronic insomnia: Drug indication, chronic use and abuse liability.* Paper presented at the NCDEU meeting, Phoenix, AZ.

Noyes, R., Garvey, M. J., Cook, B. L., & Perry, P. J. (1988). Benzodiazepine withdrawal: A review of the evidence. *J Clin Psychiatry, 49,* 382–389.

Rickels, K., Schweizer, E., Csanalosi, I., Case, G. W., & Chung, H. (1988). Long-term treatment of anxiety and risk of withdrawal. *Arch Gen Psychiatry, 45,* 444–450.

Ross, J. (1994). *Triumph over fear: A book of help and hope for people with anxiety, panic attacks, and phobias.* New York: Bantam.

Sattar, S. P., & Bhatia, S. (2003). Benzodiazepines for substance abusers. *Curr Psychiatry, l2*(5), 25–34.

Savage, S. R. (2003). Principles of pain management in the addicted patient. In A. W. Graham, T. K. Schultz, M. F. Mayo Smith, & R. K. Ries (Eds.), *Principles of addiction medicine* (3rd ed., pp. 1405–1419). Chevy Chase, MD: American Society of Addiction Medicine.

Scharf, M. B., Mayleben, D. W., Kaffeman, M., Krall, R., & Ochs, R. (1991). Dose response effects of zolpidem in normal geriatric subjects. *J Clin Psychiatry, 52,* 77–83.

Schenck, C. H., & Mahowald, M. W. (1996). Long-term, nightly benzodiazepine treatment of injurious parasomnias and other disorders of disrupted nocturnal sleep in 170 adults. *Am J Med, 100,* 333–337.

Sellers, E. M., Ciraulo, D. A., DuPont, R. L., Griffiths, R. R., Kosten, T. R., Romach, M. K., & Woody, G. E. (1993). Alprazolam and benzodiazepine dependence. *J Clin Psychiatry, 54*(Suppl), 64–74.

Spencer, E. D., DuPont, R. L., & DuPont, C. M. (2004). *The anxiety cure for kids: A guide for parents.* New York: Wiley.

Stahl, S. M. (2003). At long last, long-lasting psychiatric medications: An overview of controlled-released technologies. *J Clin Psychiatry, 64,* 4.

Sussman, N., & Stein, D. J. (2002). Pharmacotherapy for generalized anxiety disorder. In D. J. Stein & E. Hollander (Eds.), *Textbook of anxiety disorders* (pp. 135–141). Washington, DC: American Psychiatric Press.

Tyrer, P., Rutherford, D., & Huggett, D. (1981). Benzodiazepine withdrawal symptoms and propranolol. *Lancet, 1,* 520–522.

U.S. Department of Health and Human Services. (2001, March). *Monitoring the Future—overview of key findings* (NIH Publication No. 02-5105). Rockville, MD: National Institutes of Health, National Institute on Drug Abuse.

U.S. Department of Health and Human Services. (2002). *Results from the 2001 National Household Survey on Drug Abuse* (DHHS Publication No. SMA 02-3758). Rockville, MD: Substance Abuse and Mental Health Services Administration, Office of Applied Studies.

Wang, P. S., Bohn, R. L., Glynn, R. J., Mogun, H., & Avom, J. (2001). Hazardous benzodiazepine regimes in the elderly: Effects of half-life, dosage, and duration on risk of hip fracture. *Am J Psychiatry, 158,* 892–898.

Wesson, D. R., Smith, D. E., & Ling, W. (2003). Pharmacologic interventions for benzodiazepine and other sedative–hypnotic addiction. In A. W. Graham, T. K. Schultz, M. F. Mayo Smith, & R. K. Ries (Eds.), *Principles of addiction medicine* (3rd ed., pp. 721–735). Chevy Chase, MD: American Society of Addiction Medicine.

World Health Organization. (1988). *The use of essential drugs: Third report of the World Health Organization expert committee* (WHO Technical Report Series No. 770). Geneva: Author.

PART IV

SPECIAL POPULATIONS

CHAPTER 11

Polysubstance Use, Abuse, and Dependence

RICHARD N. ROSENTHAL
PETROS LEVOUNIS

DEFINING MULTIPLE SUBSTANCE USE

Diagnostic Approaches

Changes in Diagnostic Criteria from DSM-III to DSM-IV-TR

"Polysubstance dependence" originated in the DSM nomenclature only in 1987, with the introduction of the third revised edition of the *Diagnostic Manual of Mental Disorders* (DSM-III-R; American Psychiatric Association, 1987). Prior to this, in DSM-III (American Psychiatric Association, 1980, p. 179), there was the diagnostic category of "mixed substance abuse," in which criteria for diagnosing substance abuse were met, but either the substances could not be identified or the abuse involved "*so many* substances that the clinician *prefers*" to treat them as a combination rather than define a specific disorder for each substance" (italics added). In addition, in DSM-III, there was an attempt to create clinically meaningful diagnostic categories with respect to dependence on multiple substances, hence the diagnoses "dependence on a combination of opioid and other non-alcoholic substances," an early nod to the high prevalence of use of multiple substances among heroin users, and "dependence on a combination of substances, excluding opioids and alcohol." In parallel with the DSM-III diagnosis for multiple substance abuse, each of these multiple dependence criteria was made only if the substances could not be identified, or the dependence involved *so many* substances that the clinician *preferred* to treat them as a combination rather than define a specific disorder for each substance.

This concept is what underlies the typical, non-DSM use of the term "polysubstance dependence." In DSM-III-R, the concept of polysubstance dependence was formally introduced: The imprecise DSM-III concept of "so many" substances was dropped in favor of a threshold number of substances, and clinician "preference" was eliminated as an option to making such diagnoses. DSM-III-R polysubstance dependence stipulates that the person meets criteria due to repeated use of at least three categories of substances as a group over 6 months, excluding caffeine and nicotine, but does not fulfill dependence criteria for any specific substance (American Psychiatric Association, 1987, p. 185).

In DSM-IV, the concept of polysubstance dependence is more specific (American Psychiatric Association, 1994). However, the DSM-IV versions allow for two different ways to interpret the diagnosis. The first diagnostic concept of polysubstance dependence in DSM-IV is: at least 3 groups of substances repeatedly used by the patient during 12 months that, as a group, meet criteria for dependence, but in which there is no specific drug that independently qualifies for substance dependence. As in all recent versions of the DSM, any substance for which the patient satisfies criteria for dependence should be given that diagnosis independently of other substances used. A second, more exclusive DSM-IV concept of polysubstance dependence is: three or more classes of drugs used by the patient without dependence on any one drug, but the sum of the criteria met for all drugs used is three or more. The definition of "polysubstance dependence" has been clarified somewhat in DSM-IV-TR (American Psychiatric Association, 2000). However, there are still two interpretations possible with the DSM-IV-TR related to polysubstance dependence. One schema focuses on episodes of indiscriminate use of a variety of substances that each meet one criterion, but when added together meet three or more dependence criteria; the other is that full dependence criteria are only met when the drug classes used are grouped together as a whole (First & Pincus, 2002). That stated, as defined by DSM-IV, polysubstance dependence is a relatively rare disorder, and the formal diagnosis is used infrequently by clinicians and researchers (Schuckit et al., 2001).

Clinicians and researchers use the term "polysubstance dependence" more frequently as shorthand for patients for whom the DSM-IV criteria would suggest that the patient fulfills independent dependence criteria for several different substances. Conway, Kane, Ball, Poling, and Rounsaville (2003) call this construct "polysubstance involvement." According to DSM-IV (American Psychiatric Association, 1994, 2000), a patient should have a diagnosis of substance dependence for each substance for which the person meets criteria. Because there is room for misinterpretation between the formal DSM-IV concept of polysubstance dependence and the more frequently used broad concept of use of multiple substances that is also described as "polysubstance dependence," in this chapter we use the convention "multiple substance use disorders" (SUDs) to denote the latter, broad concept, reserving the former for cases in which a formal DSM-based diagnosis has been made. "Multiple SUD" here denotes that the identified subject or sample has two or more formal SUD diagnoses, at least meeting criteria for substance abuse, or meets it by reasonable proxy, such as seeking treatment. "Multiple substance dependence" means that the identified subject or sample meets formal or reasonable proxy criteria for two or more substance dependence disorders.

"Polysubstance Abuse"

Although there was a diagnostic category of "mixed substance abuse" in DSM-III (American Psychiatric Association, 1980, p. 179), there is no diagnosis of polysubstance abuse in DSM-IV-TR (American Psychiatric Association, 2000). There may not be many people who abuse multiple substances over time with clinically significant impact, for whom no one substance is sufficient to make formal abuse criteria. This is because one needs only to satisfy one of the four DSM-IV criteria to pass the threshold for a substance abuse diagnosis related to that particular substance. However, it is conceivable that one could meet a criterion for substance abuse based on use of multiple substances, but not on one in particular. For example, a person could have two arrests for driving under the influence, one for alcohol and the other for cannabis, in the same year.

Descriptive Approaches

Polydrug Use or Polysubstance Use

Most broadly, the literature frequently describes "polydrug use" or "polysubstance use." This nondiagnostic designation generally describes the use of multiple substances rather than framing the use and its effects in clinical terms, which is the intent of diagnosis. As such, polydrug use describes, at minimum, the use of multiple substances, whether licit or illicit. In the treatment research literature, "polydrug use" is often used to describe the lifetime number of drugs regularly used to a threshold SUD, in addition to the index substance (Ball, Carroll, Babor, & Rounsaville, 1995; Feingold, Ball, Kranzler, & Rounsaville, 1996). However, in other than addiction or mental health treatment settings, the expressions "polysubstance use" or "polysubstance abuse" are frequently meant to describe the use by subjects of as few as two substances, such as cocaine and alcohol, alcohol and cannabis, or opiates and cocaine (Ross, Kohler, Grimley, & Bellis, 2003). In a more differentiated conceptualization, the use of multiple substances that cause impairment is frequently described as "polydrug abuse."

   In an effort to further distinguish patterns of use, Grant and Hartford (1990) framed "polydrug use" either as simultaneous, which is the use of multiple drugs at the same occasion, or concurrent, which is the use of different substances on different occasions. Use of different substances is common in patients with alcohol dependence or substance dependence (Caetano & Weisner, 1995), the majority of whom use substances simultaneously (Staines, Magura, Foote, Deluca, & Kosanke, 2001). Longitudinal studies in community samples are able to discriminate between simultaneous and concurrent polydrug use, but a differential impact upon subsequent health outcomes including psychological distress, physical symptoms, and services utilization has not been identified (Earleywine & Newcomb, 1997).

EPIDEMIOLOGY

Readers of the research and clinical addiction literature face a problem in understanding what is meant by terms used to describe multiple SUDs in a specific sample population. These terms are variously given as "polysubstance abuse," "polydrug abuse," "polyaddiction," and "multiple-drug dependence." As stated earlier, "polysubstance abuse" in a narrow DSMs-IV sense, is relatively unlikely to occur, especially in clinical settings, where patients are likely to meet criteria for several SUD diagnoses. On the other hand, the terms "polysubstance abuse" and "polydrug abuse" are frequently used by clinicians and researchers as descriptors of multiple drug use in populations of patients who have an index diagnosis of substance dependence, such as opioid dependence, and who meet at least DSM substance abuse criteria for the other substances.

The use of differing phraseology to describe use of multiple drugs is not limited to the domain of mental health, and addiction clinicians and researchers. Cause of death statements from medical examiners and coroners often use terms such as "polydrug toxicity," "polypharmacy," "multiple drug poisoning," and "polypharmaceutical overdose" to describe multiple-drug-induced deaths (Cone et al., 2003).

Population-Based Studies

When considered in community samples, the presence of an SUD diagnosis elevates lifetime risks of additional SUD diagnoses (Regier et al., 1990). This is true with most classes of abused drugs. For example, the risk for a nonalcohol SUD is elevated among both males and females with alcohol dependence. In the National Comorbidity Survey (NCS), more than 40% of individuals with a DSM-III-R alcohol dependence had, excluding nicotine dependence, co-occurring drug abuse or dependence (Kessler et al., 1997). Between 13 and 18% of those with alcohol abuse will also have a co-occurring lifetime drug use disorder (NCS; Kessler et al., 1997). Lifetime drug use disorder was also present in 21.5% of subjects (odds ratio [OR] = 7.1) with an alcohol use disorder identified in the Epidemiologic Catchment Area survey (ECA; Regier et al., 1990). In addition, among individuals with a nonalcohol substance use disorder in the ECA study, 47.3% also had a lifetime alcohol use disorder. Excluding nicotine dependence, which was not surveyed in the ECA, individuals with cocaine abuse/dependence have the strongest risk (84.8%; OR = 36.3) of any group with an SUD for an additional alcohol use disorder (Regier et al., 1990). In the ECA, the associated use disorder for barbiturates, opiates, amphetamines, and hallucinogens demonstrates an OR for an additional lifetime alcohol use disorder of 10.0 or more (Regier et al., 1990).

However, if one tries to understand the temporal relationship between classes of substances used, lifetime diagnoses do not easily allow for the attribution that the use of multiple substances was temporally coemergent. Therefore, using this threshold to determine multiple-substance abuse may lower its specificity, thus overestimating its prevalence. Past-year prevalence rates are more likely than lifetime rates to provide higher specificity for identifying persons with concurrent multiple-substance use in a subpopulation identified as having two or more SUDs. Unfortunately, few national surveys have presented past-year data on substance use comorbidity. However, data from the 11th, 12th, and 13th National Household Surveys on Drug Abuse (NHSDA; n = 87,915) offer an important source of epidemiological data on drug-related symptoms of dependence, using criteria that can be used to approximate DSM-IV current SUDs (Kandel, Chen, Warner, Kessler, & Grant, 1997).

Adolescents

Adolescent substance users are a subgroup who have been identified as high risk for concurrent polysubstance use, and with that, progression to hazardous use, abuse, or dependence (Brook, Brook, Zhang, Cohen, & Whiteman, 2002). Compared with older age groups, younger users in treatment settings are more likely to report polydrug use (Substance Abuse and Mental Health Services Administration [SAMHSA], 2003b). The NHSDA oversamples subjects who are from 12 to 34 years old, offering community substance use data on adolescents who are not typically covered in other national surveys (Kandel et al., 1997). Although males overall are more likely than females to use or be dependent upon alcohol, cannabis, or cocaine, Kandel and colleagues (1997), using NHSDA data to determine abuse and dependence by proxy, demonstrated that these gender differences for rates of use and of dependence rates among users are largely attenuated among adolescents. Adolescent girls who use alcohol or illicit drugs are at higher risk for dependence than adolescent boys, and among female users of alcohol, cannabis, or cocaine, the rates of dependence are the highest in adolescents compared with older age groups (Kandel et al., 1997).

Clinical Samples

In treatment samples, multiple SUDs are common but typically underdiagnosed (Ananth, Vandeater, Kamal, & Brodsky, 1989; Rosenthal, Hellerstein, & Miner, 1992). In general, the risk for comorbid substance use and other mental disorder diagnoses is increased when comparing clinical to community samples, and the highest rates of comorbid mental disorders–SUDs are typically found in institutional populations, including psychiatric units, substance abuse programs, and jails and prisons (Hien, Zimberg, Weisman, First, & Ackerman, 1997; Jordan, Schlenger, Fairbank, & Caddell, 1996; Kokkevi & Stefanis, 1995; Regier et al., 1990). This is due in part to the selection bias that those most likely admitted to treatment programs are people with impairment due to their drug use. Because of higher severity, they are at higher risk for an additional substance use diagnosis than other drug users.

Comorbidity of various substance use and other mental disorders tends to cluster among certain subsets of the general population, such that more than half of the lifetime alcohol, drug, and mental disorders diagnoses can be found among about 14% of the population (Kessler et al., 1994). In any year, almost 59% of the community sample with an alcohol, drug, or other mental (ADM) disorder meet criteria for three or more lifetime ADM disorders (Kessler et al., 1994). Therefore, compared to the community, treatment settings that aggregate those with SUDs are also most likely to cohort people at the highest risk for multiple SUDs. This is borne out in large-scale family genetics studies. For example, in the Collaborative Study on the Genetics of Alcoholism (COGA), among 1,212 subjects with definite alcohol dependence, recruited from addiction treatment centers, 62% had an additional diagnosis of cannabis and/or cocaine dependence (Bierut et al., 1998).

Treatment Episode Data Set (TEDS) data over the period 1992–2001 consistently revealed that about half of treatment admissions have reported multiple SUDs (SAMHSA, 2003b). This means that in addition to the index substance for which the patient was admitted to treatment, a substantial portion of patients are also abusing other substances. The SAMHSA-sponsored National Survey of Substance Abuse Treatment Services (NSSATS) demonstrated that of the 1,123,239 people receiving treatment in 13,720 responding facilities in 2002, 48% were being treated for abuse or dependence on both alcohol and at least one other substance (SAMHSA, 2003a). Thirty-one percent were in treatment for drug use disorders only, while the remaining 21% were in treatment for alcohol use disorders only. Similarly, data from the 2001 TEDS revealed that 54% of all persons admitted to substance abuse treatment reported multiple substance use, and approximately 42% of all admissions reported problems with both alcohol and drugs (SAMHSA, 2003b). Alcohol and opiates were reported more often as primary substances than as secondary substances (TEDS; SAMHSA, 2003b). The most commonly reported secondary substances were alcohol, marijuana/hashish, and cocaine.

Multiple Substance Use Disorders

The increased risk of comorbidity among treatment-seeking populations over that of the general population has clinical implications for the outcome of treatment (Rosenthal & Westreich, 1999). Patients with multiple SUDs have greater difficulty achieving remission in intensive addiction treatment (Ritsher, Moos, & Finney, 2002). In addition, a history of multiple substance use predicts relapse to drugs in addiction treatment follow-up studies (Walton, Blow, & Booth, 2000). Among patients in treatment for SUDs in a 2-year follow-up study by Walton and colleagues (2000), subjects ($n = 241$) self-reported their current primary substances of choice. Forty-one percent indicated alcohol as the sole drug of abuse. Among the 59.1% who were polysubstance users, the drugs of choice were alcohol, 79.1%; cocaine, 72.7%; marijuana, 48.2%; opiates, 16.5%; sedatives, 13.7%; stimulants, 8.6%; heroin, 9.4%; and hallucinogens, 5.0%.

Nicotine and Multiple Substance Use Disorders

Nicotine dependence has not been traditionally thought of in the context of treating drug abuse problems, even among clinicians trained in addiction treatment. Consequently, when multiple SUDs are discussed, they usually do not include whether the person referred to is a habitual smoker. Nonetheless, over 90% of patients in methadone maintenance treatment are current tobacco smokers, a reasonable proxy for nicotine dependence (Clemmey, Brooner, Chutuape, Kidorf, & Stitzer, 1997). Similarly, 90% of patients in alcoholism inpatient treatment are current smokers (Beatty, Blanco, Hames, & Nixon, 1997). Thus, even among patients identified as having only one current SUD, these individuals are, in fact, multiply drug dependent.

Multiple Substance Use among Alcoholics

The concurrent abuse of alcohol and drugs is a significant problem. Alcohol and drug use disorders frequently overlap, and there are high rates of non-alcohol SUDs among patients in treatment for alcohol use disorders (Beatty et al., 1997). In the 2001 TEDS sample, 72% of all persons admitted to treatment reported alcohol as a primary or secondary substance; 22% of addiction treatment admissions reported primary drug abuse with secondary alcohol abuse, and 20% reported primary alcohol abuse with secondary drug abuse (SAMHSA, 2003b).

Multiple Substance Use among Injecting Heroin Users

Injection drug use is highly correlated with use of multiple substances. Injecting heroin users frequently use multiple drugs in addition to nicotine, such as alcohol, benzodiazepines, cannabis, and amphetamines, and there do not appear to be differences between treatment and nontreatment samples with regard to the number of either lifetime or current dependence diagnoses (Darke & Ross, 1997; Dinwiddie, Cottler, Compton, & Abdallah, 1996; Kidorf, Brooner, King, Chutuape, & Stitzer, 1996). Darke and Ross (1997) recruited a nonrandom sample of 222 Australian heroin injectors, half of whom were in methadone treatment, and found that they had used a mean of 5.3 different classes of substances in the prior 6 months, and 40% had three or more current DSM-III-R dependence diagnoses. Injecting drugs increases the risk for comorbid substance dependence. Dinwiddie and colleagues (1996) found elevated lifetime rates of alcohol, amphetamine, sedative/hypnotic opiate and hallucinogen dependence among injecting drug users (IDUs) compared to non-IDUs with a substantial drug use history.

Severity of psychopathology also appears to be highly associated with multiple substance use. Compared to users of cocaine alone, compulsive simultaneous users of cocaine and heroin ("speedball") have higher Minnesota Multiphasic Personality Inventory (MMPI) scores on depression and trait anxiety, with more severe psychopathology (Malow, West, Corrigan, Pena, & Lott, 1992). With frequent use of this combination, cocaine abusers who are using opiates to reduce the jitters and "crash" of intravenous cocaine use likely increase the risk of heroin dependence in this population (Levin, Foltin, & Fischman, 1996).

Darke and Ross (1997) demonstrated in a sample of Australian heroin injectors that heroin use is correlated strongly with not only multiple substance use but also comorbid psychiatric disorders. Among IDUs, the extent and severity of non-substance-related psychopathology is a strong and linear predictor of the extent of multiple substance dependence. The prevalence of current mood and/or anxiety disorders was about 55%, with 25% having both a current mood and anxiety disorder—in each case, clearly greater than prevalence in the general population (Darke & Ross, 1997; Kessler et al., 1994). Darke and Ross also found a significant positive correlation between the number of lifetime drug dependence diagnoses and the number of lifetime comorbid psychiatric diagnoses in IDUs, and a similar positive correlation ($p < .001$) for current disorders. Although a causal attribution cannot be made, the onset of the mood or anxiety disorder preceded the onset of the heroin dependence in 60–80% of cases, suggesting that use of multiple drugs addresses untreated, underlying psychiatric disorders. However, the increased prevalence of multiple substance dependence in persons with more severe psychopathology might also be due to shared genetic vulnerability; attempts to manage mood and anxiety through self-medication; or disturbances in motivation, judgment, and behavior directly due to psychopathology that increase vulnerability to addiction. In addition, it can be argued that multiple drug use can itself result in a broad range of psychiatric sequelae.

Gender Issues

In the general population, significantly more men than women across ethnic groups (white, black, Hispanic) either use or are dependent on alcohol, cannabis, or cocaine (Kandel et al., 1997). However, women who use nicotine are more likely to meet dependence criteria than men (Kandel et al., 1997). In examining gender effects in opioid dependence, in a study of heroin users, there did not appear to be a gender-based difference in risk for dependence on multiple substances, which may be related to the equivalent risk of mental disorders in this subpopulation (Darke & Ross, 1997). In the general population, there are clear gender differences in the risk for anxiety and mood disorders, with the relative risk for females about double that for males (Kessler et al., 1994). However, in multiple-substance-dependent IDUs, there appears to be no difference by gender in either the lifetime prevalence of mood and anxiety disorders or the current prevalence of anxiety disorders. Only the rate of current depressive disorders is significantly elevated for females over males (Darke & Ross, 1997).

PERSONALITY CORRELATES

In community samples, 28.6% of individuals with a current alcohol use disorder have at least one personality disorder, and 47.7% of those with a current drug use disorder have at least one personality disorder (Grant et al., 2004). Furthermore, of individuals with at least one personality disorder, 16.4% had a current alcohol use disorder and 6.5% had a current drug use disorder. Personality disorders are associated with poorer treatment outcome for patients with alcohol dependence and those with drug dependence (Helzer & Pryzbeck, 1988; Rounsaville, Dolinsky, Babor, & Meyer, 1987). In various treatment settings, patients with SUDs screened with standard instruments meet criteria for personality disorders, with 57–73% having at least one personality disorder diagnosis, and 35–50% having at least two personality disorder diagnoses (Kleinman et al., 1990; Kranzler, Satel, & Apter, 1994; Marlowe et al., 1995; Rounsaville et al., 1998; Skinstad & Swain, 2001). Personality disorder diagnoses are associated with an increased risk of multiple substance use in IDUs (Darke, Williamson, Ross, Teesson, & Lynskey, 2004).

Categorical Personality Disorders

The "Cluster B" personality disorders (antisocial, borderline, narcissistic, and histrionic), as described in DSM-IV, demonstrate elevated rates of SUDs (Mors & Sorensen, 1994). Conversely, in patients with SUDs, there is an elevated rate of Cluster B personality disorders, and multiple-substance-dependent patients are more likely to be diagnosed with Cluster B personality disorders than non-multiple-substance-dependent subjects (Skinstad & Swain, 2001). For example, in 370 patients with heterogenous SUDs, Rounsaville and colleagues (1998) found that 57% had an DSM-III-R personality disorder diagnosis, of which 45.7% were Cluster B, including 27% with antisocial personality disorder (ASPD) and 18.4% with borderline personality disorder (BPD).

Antisocial Personality Disorder

The risk of ASPD among drug-dependent individuals in community samples is 29 times that of the general population, and rates of ASPD among IDUs range between 35 and 71% (Darke et al., 2004; Dinwiddie et al., 1996; Regier et al., 1990). ASPD appears to be a risk factor for multiple substance dependence. For example, patients who meet dependence criteria for both cocaine and alcohol have higher psychiatric severity and are more likely to have ASPD than patients with cocaine dependence only (Cunningham, Corrigan, Malow, & Smason, 1993). Among clinical populations, sociopathy among substance abusers is associated with high treatment dropout and poorer treatment outcome (Leal, Ziedonis, & Kosten, 1994; Woody, McLellan, Luborsky, & O'Brien, 1985). Tómasson and Vaglum (2000) followed 100 treatment-seeking alcoholics with ASPD for 28 months in a European study: Forty-seven percent of the cohort had multiple SUDs and more prior admissions, and they were more frequently involved in fights. The route of drug administration also is associated with elevated risk of ASPD. Compared to non-IDUs with a substantial drug use history, rates of ASPD are elevated in IDUs (Dinwiddie et al., 1996). Increased social deviance is a factor that likely increases risk of access to hard drugs. However, the specific contribution of ASPD to SUD risk is less clearly delineated. Recent family genetics studies suggest that familial aggregation of SUD is largely independent of ASPD (Bierut et al., 1998; Merikangas et al., 1998).

Borderline Personality Disorder

Although ASPD has been the personality disorder that is traditionally diagnosed in patients with SUDs and is typically believed to be responsible for the higher risk of self- and other-harmful behaviors in this population, recent evidence suggests that some proportion of the risk for multiple substance use, as well as suicide attempts and psychiatric severity, is associated with BPD (Darke et al., 2004). Trull, Sher, Minks-Brown, Durbin, and Burr (2000) reviewed 26 studies of the comorbidity of BPD and SUD, and found rates of BPD that ranged from 5 to 65%. Much of the variability between studies was due to different instruments used and populations studied. However, the rate across studies was 57.4%; thus, it is clear that the prevalence of BPD is elevated among patients with SUDs (Trull et al., 2000). BPD is present in 18–34% of cocaine abusers in treatment settings and among 46% of injection heroin users in and out of treatment (Darke et al., 2004; Kleinman et al., 1990; Kranzler, Satel, & Apter, 1994; Marlowe et al., 1995). In a recent study of injection heroin users, 46% of the sample met criteria for BPD, including 38% who also met criteria for comorbid ASPD, yet there appeared to be little increased risk for harmful behaviors among IDUs with ASPD compared to those without ASPD (Darke et al., 2004).

Dimensional Approaches

In addition to the increased rates of SUD in persons with categorically defined personality disorders compared to controls, there are personality dimensions that may be predictive of increased risk for SUDs. Moreover, those with multiple SUDs tend to have more severe personality pathology, as measured on dimensional constructs, than users of single substances, independent of drug of choice (McCormick, Dowd, Quirt, & Zegarra, 1998; Pedersen, Clausen, & Lavik, 1989). Multiple-substance-dependent individuals tend to have high levels of two personality characteristics particularly related to behavioral disinhibition—impulsivity and sensation seeking (see review in Conway et al., 2003). Those with multiple substance dependence score lower in measures of behavioral inhibition (constraint) than those who prefer to use alcohol, cocaine, or cannabis singly (Conway, Swendson, Rounsaville, & Merikangas, 2002).

Impulsivity

Impulsivity/disinhibition appears to be a major factor in both SUD and BPD. Though impulsivity is associated with polysubstance use (O'Boyle & Barratt, 1993), and in addition to the risks for polysubstance abuse attributable to BPD, as described earlier, impulsivity appears more highly elevated in comorbid BPD–SUD than with either disorder alone (Kreudelbach, McCormick, Schulz, & Grueneich, 1993; Morgenstern, Langenbucher, Labouvie, & Miller, 1997). As such, impulsivity may explain some of the increased risk in substance users with BPD for polydrug use and its sequelae. In an analysis of the association between personality and substance use in a nonclinical population screened for alcohol or personality disorders, partialling out trait impulsivity significantly reduced the correlation between BPD or ASPD and the risk for SUD, suggesting that at least part of the association between SUD and personality may be due to underlying personality traits such as impulsivity (Casillas & Clark, 2002). On the balance, increased morbidity in polysubstance abusers might also be explained by a constitutional insensitivity to negative feedback from the environment. Multiple SUD subjects' poor performance on the Gambling Task suggests a heightened tendency to continue reinforced behavior in the context of increasingly negative consequences (Grant, Contoreggi, & London, 2000).

Novelty Seeking

A related personality trait that has been consistently linked with the vulnerability to development of SUD is novelty seeking or sensation seeking. Among children, those with higher sensation seeking are more likely to declare an intention to use alcohol and to have symptoms of substance abuse as adults

(Cloninger, Sigvardsson, & Bohman, 1988; Webb, Baer, & McKelvey, 1995). Generally, persons with SUD exhibit higher levels of this trait compared to those without SUD, whether they are alcoholics or abusers of other substances (Conway et al., 2002). Moreover, users of multiple substances tend to have even higher levels of sensation seeking, such that the greater the involvement in multiple substance dependence, the greater the behavioral disinhibition (Conway et al., 2003; Pedersen et al., 1989). Conversely, the high sensation seekers among cocaine-dependent persons are more likely to have multiple SUD (Ball, Carroll, & Rounsaville, 1994). Conway and colleagues (2003) demonstrated that the number of lifetime substance dependence diagnoses among 325 individuals in addiction treatment was positively and linearly associated with broad psychological measures of behavioral disinhibition. Compared to patients who were dependent on one substance, those who were dependent on two or more substances had higher scores on several different instruments used to rate behavioral undercontrol. All other things being equal (e.g., access, economic status), the more disinhibited a person with a vulnerability to substance dependence, the more likely the thresholds for contact with multiple drugs will be breached, and the vulnerability linked to use of multiple drugs.

Other Characteristics

Multiple-substance-dependent patients in treatment report lower mean levels of self-efficacy and higher mean levels of temptation regarding substance use in comparison to alcohol-only-dependent patients (Edens & Willoughby, 1999). In addition to the increased impulsivity and sensation seeking compared to non-multiple-drug SUD patients, multiple SUD patients score higher on all measures of hostility and aggression (McCormick & Smith, 1995).

Typologic Approaches

Another important development in elucidating the relationship between patterns of substance use, and both categorical and dimensional approaches to measuring personality is the recognition of characteristic patterns, typically grouped into two broad categories among substance abusers, designated Types A and B (Ball, Kranzler, Tennen, Poling, & Rounsaville, 1998). Earlier classification systems in reference to alcoholism had a similar typology, variously referred to as Types 1 and 2 (Cloninger, 1987), which developed out of measures in family genetic studies, or Types A and B (Babor et al., 1992), developed through cluster analyses of a somewhat broader set of patient characteristics. Feingold and colleagues (1996), using a schema analogous to that of Babor and colleagues (1992), replicated the A-B classification in 521 subjects chosen from the community, inpatient, and outpatient drug treatment programs, or outpatient psychiatric treatment programs. Subjects were grouped by presence of alcohol, cocaine, marijuana, or opiate abuse or dependence. The authors found a consistent 60:40 ratio of Type A to Type B for each of the drug groups, suggesting clusters of personality characteristics that are independent of drug of choice. Similarly, in 370 patients attending treatment for alcoholism, cocaine, or opiate dependence, Ball and colleagues (1998) replicated the A-B classification and also found a 60:40 Type A to Type B ratio. Type A substance abusers had less multiple drug use, as well as an older age of onset, fewer years of heavy use, less family history of substance abuse, less impulsivity, and less severe substance abuse. Type B substance abusers tended to be more severe than type A abusers, scoring higher on the personality dimensions of neuroticism, novelty seeking, and harm avoidance. They also had a higher prevalence of multiple substance abuse, an earlier age of onset, more childhood psychiatric symptoms, higher incidence of all Cluster B personality disorders, and more frequent family history of substance abuse (Ball et al., 1998). The Type B profile is quite common in methadone patients, in whom there is a greater prevalence of ASPD than in the general population (Brooner, King, Kidorf, Schmidt, & Bigelow, 1997; Rounsaville et al., 1991).

Compared to drug abusers who are categorized as Type A, Type B is predictive of having multiple SUDs. This is an important refinement in the assessment of drug abusers; since multiple SUD does not occur in non-substance-abusing populations, this distinction gives some predictive power in the target subpopulation of those with SUD. As described earlier, ASPD in persons with SUD is predictive of multiple SUDs, IDU, and higher severity, and an earlier study found that ASPD was one of the best predictors of Type B membership among cocaine abusers (Ball et al., 1995). However, Ball and colleagues (1998) found that the basis for Type A and Type B distinctions in personality dimensions and disorders among the 370 patients in their study remained much the same when the cluster analysis was controlled for presence of ASPD. The typological distinction is not just of heuristic value—Type B patients have more severe SUDs and relapse more quickly after addiction treatment as compared with Type A patients (Babor et al., 1992; Ball et al., 1995). In addition, the more frequent family history of SUD and early onset in Type B patients is consistent with a stronger genetic component compared with late-onset Type A patients.

GENETIC AND FAMILY STUDIES

Vulnerability to substance abuse has general genetic, familial, and nonfamilial environmental factors, as well as factors that appear to be specific to a particular class of substances. A family history of substance abuse is one of the strongest risk factors for development of a SUD (Merikangas et al., 1998). Studies have demonstrated that there are genetic influences on the risk for substance abuse (Tsuang et al., 1996) and that, at least among men, abusing one category of drug is associated with a marked increase in the probability of abusing other classes of drugs (Tsuang et al., 1998). One of the strongest predictors for presence of an SUD is the presence of another SUD (Bierut et al., 1998).

Much of the evidence for the heritability of the general and specific vulnerability for SUD is taken from studies of familial aggregation. Bierut and colleagues (1998) compared siblings of probands with alcohol dependence and those of a control group for the presence of lifetime SUDs. Siblings of alcoholic probands were not only more likely to have a lifetime alcohol use disorder, but they also had an increased risk of cannabis, cocaine, and nicotine dependence. Fifty percent of the alcohol-dependent siblings of alcohol-dependent probands had an additional diagnosis of cannabis and/or cocaine dependence. What is compelling with respect to understanding the risk for multiple substance dependence is that the siblings of cannabis-dependent probands had an increased risk of cannabis dependence, siblings of cocaine-dependent probands had an increased risk for cocaine dependence, and siblings of habitual smokers were at higher risk for nicotine dependence (Bierut et al., 1998). In another study, Tsuang and colleagues (1998) demonstrated that there is a general drug abuse vulnerability factor with genetic, family, and nonfamily environmental components that is shared across all drugs of abuse, in addition to genetic factors that appear to be unique for most classes of drug abuse. So although there appear to be nongenetic general and specific factors for familial transmission of vulnerability to SUDs, multiple SUDs among probands render increased vulnerability to multiple SUDs in relatives, at least through both drug-specific and common genetic factors.

NEUROPSYCHOLOGICAL IMPACT OF MULTIPLE SUBSTANCE USE DISORDERS

As compared with non-polysubstance-using drug abusers, those with multiple SUDs demonstrate the greatest degree of chronic neuropsychological impairment and recover the least function with long-term abstinence (Beatty et al., 1997; Medina, Shear, Schafer, Armstrong, & Dyer, 2003). This may be due in part to the increased cumulative exposure of the brain to drugs and alcohol: Multiple substance users tend to use as much of a particular substance (e.g., alcohol or cocaine) as those who use only alcohol or cocaine (Selby & Azrin, 1998). Selby and Azrin (1998) conducted a comprehensive neuropsychological battery with 355 prison inmates classified by DSM-IV criteria into four groups: those with alcohol use disorders, cocaine use disorders, multiple SUDs, and no history of SUD. The multiple SUDs and the alcohol groups demonstrated significant impairment on most measures compared to the cocaine or no-drug groups, but the multiple SUDs group performed worse than the cocaine alone, alcohol alone or no SUD groups on measures of short-term memory, long-term memory, and visual motor ability. Beatty and colleagues (1997) found analogous results in their neuropsychological evaluation of spatial cognition in multiple SUD and non-multiple-SUD inpatient alcoholics who had at least 3 weeks of sobriety. Multiple SUD patients had significant impairment of geographical knowledge requiring place localization, over and above the impairment on all other measures of visuospatial perception, construction, learning, and memory that all of the alcoholics had compared to controls. After 3 weeks of sobriety, alcoholics with multiple SUD compared to alcoholics without multiple SUD also demonstrate greater memory deficits in tests of recall (Bondi, Drake, & Grant, 1998). The heavy cocaine users among the alcoholics had the worst deficits, suggestive of subcortical dysfunction due to small vessel infarcts. Subjects with multiple SUDs also demonstrated impaired decision making through poor performance on the Gambling Task compared to non-drug-using controls (suggesting dysfunction of the ventromedial prefrontal cortex [Bechara, 1999; Grant et al., 2000]).

Given the neuropsychological effects of multiple SUDs, it is important to recognize that the baseline cognitive function also has a role in vulnerability to multiple SUDs. Premorbid intellectual functioning is a predictor of drug use: Compared to matched non-drug-using controls, multiple substance users were demonstrated to have lower fourth-grade Iowa Test composite and individual scores on Vocabulary, Reading, Language, Work–Study Skills, and Mathematics tests (Block, Erwin, & Ghoneim, 2002)

SPECIAL POPULATIONS

Opioid Dependence and Opioid Maintenance Treatment

Polydrug use is the norm among heroin users. In a study of 329 primary heroin users by Darke and Hall (1995), the most prevalent drugs used during the preceding 6 months were tobacco (94%), cannabis (84%), alcohol (78%), benzodiazepines (64%), amphetamines (42%), cocaine (24%), and hallucinogens (22%); the mean number of drug classes used was 5.2. However, it appears that as they grow older, illicit drug users reduce their range of drugs: Age is inversely correlated in IDUs with the number of current dependence diagnoses, and young males who are not in treatment, and who inject amphetamines, are at higher risk for polysubstance use (Darke & Hall, 1995; Darke & Ross, 1997).

Cocaine Use

The use of cocaine by patients in methadone or buprenorphine maintenance treatment programs has been reported to be as high as 73% in a sample of 1038 newly admitted patients in 15 methadone clinics in New York City (Magura, Kang, Nwakeze, & Demsky, 1998). Contrary to popular belief, the simultaneous use of intravenous heroin and cocaine ("speedball") does not result in a novel set of experiences, nor does it reinforce the effects of either drug when used alone, especially when cocaine and heroin are used in high doses. Cocaine, however, has been shown to alleviate some symptoms of opioid withdrawal, and as such may be used in a self-medicating pattern, as mentioned earlier (Leri, Bruneau, & Stewart, 2003).

Cannabis

Cannabis use among patients in methadone treatment programs has recently been investigated in an attempt to answer the practical question of whether cannabinoid-positive urine toxicology examinations predict poor treatment outcome. Both a recent Israeli study (Weizman, Gelkopf, Melamed, Adelson, & Bleich, 2004) and a review of three U.S. studies (Epstein & Preston, 2003) suggest that cannabis use is not a risk factor for treatment outcome of methadone-maintained outpatients. The authors concluded that cannabinoid-positive urines do not need to be a major focus of clinical attention.

Overdose

In examining both fatal and nonfatal heroin overdoses, the majority of cases involve simultaneous use of alcohol, benzodiazepines, and tricyclic antidepressants (TCAs), such that the toxicology of heroin overdose is probably best described as "polydrug toxicity" (Darke & Hall, 2003; Darke & Zador, 1996). In fatal heroin overdoses, alcohol has been used more than 50% of the time (Darke & Hall, 2003). The mechanism of action for the overdose appears to be the synergistic effect of the various depressants on the central nervous system, leading to respiratory collapse. This is further collaborated by autopsy findings of an inverse relationship between alcohol and morphine blood concentrations; in the presence of alcohol, lower levels of morphine are sufficient to result in death (Darke & Hall, 2003). In a study by Darke and Ross (2000) in Sydney, Australia, both fatal and nonfatal heroin overdoses were linked to concomitant use of TCAs but not selective serotonin reuptake inhibitors (SSRIs), despite the fact that heroin users in Australia predominantly use SSRIs instead of TCAs.

Adolescents, Club Drugs, and the Rave Scene

A recent review of the literature revealed that club drug use [MDMA (3,4-methylenedioxymethamphetamine), ketamine, and GHB (gamma-hydroxybutyric acid)] has reached epidemic proportions and is particularly problematic among adolescents with psychiatric illness, including mood and anxiety disorders, as well as attention-deficit/hyperactivity disorder. Although club drugs originally got their name from nightclubs and raves, adolescents and young adults now use club drugs in both club and nonclub settings (Rosenthal & Solhkhah, in press). Overall, studies of typical MDMA users reveal high rates of multiple drug use (Parrott, Milani, Parmar, & Turner, 2001; Parrott, Sisk, & Turner, 2000; Rodgers, 2000; Schifano, Di Furia, Forza, Minicuci, & Bricolo, 1998). Among treatment seekers, heavy MDMA use is associated with increased psychopathology (Parrott et al., 2000; Schifano et al., 1998). In addition to use of alcohol and cannabis, the heavier the MDMA use, the more likely is the co-use of stimulants and hallucinogens (Scholey et al., 2004). MDMA as a sole drug of abuse is an uncommon phenomenon; thus, it is a reasonable proxy for abuse of multiple substances (Rodgers, 2000).

Raves are large, all-night dance parties, where people come together to use club drugs and "feel like a closely knit family" in what is sometimes called "marching to the beat of Ecstasy." Raves started in England in the early 1980s and have since spread throughout the United States, Europe, South America, and Australia in major urban centers and on college campuses. Adolescents and young adults are particularly drawn to raves, where they feel free to hug, laugh, talk, scream, and dance to "techno" or "house" music under laser lights and the effects of drugs, primarily MDMA (Cohen, 1998). Rave participants often describe looking for a "trance-induced" state or "euphoric transcendence," while smiling, touching, and loving each other in a completely nonviolent setting (Tyler, 1995). Interestingly, a recent study from the Netherlands found a negative association between substance dependence and violent offending (but not criminal recidivism) among a sample of incarcerated male Dutch adolescents (Vreugdenhil, Van Den Brink, Wouters, & Doreleijers, 2003).

Heroin use has been rising among adolescents and young adults, possibly because heroin is now so pure that people can easily sniff or smoke it. An extensive review of descriptive studies of young heroin users revealed, in a pattern similar to that of adult heroin users, substantial multiple substance use and psychiatric comorbidity (Hopfer, Khuri, Crowley, & Hooks, 2002). The same authors also reviewed different treatments of adolescents who use heroin, including therapeutic communities and methadone maintenance, and found that length of time in treatment, regardless of modality, was the best predictor of patient outcome (Hopfer et al., 2002).

Club Drugs and the Circuit Scene

Circuit parties are large-scale dance events, primarily for gay men, where use of multiple drugs is prevalent. Participants often travel from all over the country, and sometimes overseas, to attend these large gatherings that bring together several thousand gay men. MDMA, ketamine, GHB, cocaine, methamphetamine and alcohol are the most frequently used substances. Recent studies by Mansergh and colleagues (2001), Mattison, Ross, Wolfson, Franklin, and San Diego HIV Neurobehavioral Research Center Group (2001), and Lee, Galanter, Dermatis, and McDowell (2003) indicate high rates of simultaneous drug use at circuit parties; the average number of substances ingested by responders on the day of the circuit party studied by Lee and colleagues was 2.4, with a range of 0 to 7. Most people report that using drugs during a circuit party enhances the dancing experience, relieves inhibitions, and improves sex. Others describe multiple substance use as self-medication for depressed mood, anxiety, social isolation, or stress associated with living with HIV disease or AIDS. Some participants report a synergistic effect between drugs, as in the case of the MDMA and ketamine combination; some users believe that it results in a more intense "high," while others feel that ketamine prolongs the effect of MDMA.

Multiple Substance Use and HIV Risk

Multiple substance use at circuit parties has recently become a great concern in the gay community, in the context of the crystal methamphetamine epidemic and the rising incidence of HIV transmission among young gay men in large urban environments. A study of 428 young gay and bisexual men under the San Francisco Young Men's Health Study (Greenwood et al., 2001) found polydrug users to be more likely to be HIV seropositive (OR = 2.05) or of unknown HIV status (OR = 2.78). The common link between HIV seropositivity and multiple substance use has not been demonstrated, but given the preceding discussion, it is reasonable to suspect that an important personality factor may be involved, such as behavioral dyscontrol in the form of impulsivity or sensation seeking. When disinhibiting drugs such as alcohol and GHB are taken concert, a person who has high trait impulsivity is even more likely to engage in risky behavior. For example, Cook and colleagues (2001) identified gay men recently infected with syphilis in Liverpool, United Kingdom, and found that 61% had used GHB as an aphrodisiac in the context of unprotected sex.

The association of multiple substance use and HIV raises medical concerns both in terms of HIV transmission and HIV treatment. Sexual disinhibition and increased risk of HIV transmission have been correlated to substance use, and particularly to stimulants, not only in the gay community but also in a variety of other settings (Levounis, Galanter, Dermatis, Hamowy, & De Leon, 2002). These findings support the hypothesis that multiple substance use may directly result in increased rates of unsafe sex and HIV seroconversion. In terms of HIV treatment, club drugs such as MDMA and GHB interact with protease inhibitors, resulting in dangerously high levels of the club drugs (Harrington, Woodward, Hoofon, & Horn, 1999). Furthermore, patients often fail to adhere to complicated HIV pharmacological regimens during intoxication with or withdrawal from a variety of different drugs of abuse (Lee et al., 2003).

TREATMENT CONSIDERATIONS

At its simplest, treatment of patients with chronic multiple SUDs requires a focus upon each disorder separately, in addition to providing patients with a coherent overall rationale and approach to addiction treatment. Although multiple SUDs have a net negative impact on treatment outcome, Abellanas and McLellan (1993) have shown that patients with multiple SUDs report generally similar motivation for change across drugs of abuse, meaning that their desire to modify their substance use remains consistent across substances. An additional issue is the specific impact of other substance use upon recovery for a particular SUD. Treatment is thus best constructed with a bottom-up approach, using evidence-based approaches where available (Rosenthal, 2004), rather than assuming that optimal treatment should be largely psychotherapeutic or pharmacotherapeutic. For example, there is a clear evidence base for the use of methadone as an agonist therapy for stabilization of opioid dependence (Ciraulo, 2003). However, there is not good evidence that an adequate dose of methadone for treating opioid dependence will suffice in treating cocaine abuse or dependence. Since there is no approved pharmacotherapy for cocaine use disorders at present, the optimal therapy should come from the behavioral treatments, which also have an evidence base. As such, the approach to treating patients with opioid dependence and cocaine dependence should have both pharmacotherapeutic and psychotherapeutic components.

In the acute setting, multiple SUDs present the treatment team with significant challenges. Given a patient's complicated history of recent and chronic use of multiple substances, the clinician in the emergency room or detoxification unit often struggles to make treatment priorities out of a constellation of signs and symptoms that may be the result of intoxication or withdrawal from a number of substances. Given the frequent occurrence of multiple substance use diagnoses (particularly between alcohol and other drugs), any attempt to attribute observed findings associated with comorbid substance use to a single substance, or class of substances, is often difficult, if not impossible. Intoxication from stimulants may result in psychotic symptoms, but so does withdrawal from sedatives. Lethargy is not only a classic sign of opioid intoxication but also a consequence of stimulant withdrawal. A patient who currently uses both benzodiazepines and crystal methamphetamine, and presents with seizures, may be either acutely intoxicated with methamphetamine or suffering from severe benzodiazepine withdrawal, or both. Furthermore, the serious psychosocial complications of multiple SUDs add significantly to the difficulty in treating the already confusing biological manifestations of the illness. As in the case of relapse prevention, the successful management of acute multiple substance use relies primarily upon identification and treatment of each intoxication and withdrawal syndrome separately. For example, patients with serious withdrawal from heroin and alcohol typically require both opioid agonists (e.g., methadone or buprenophine) and benzodiazepines (e.g., chlordiazapoxide or lorazepam), with particular attention to potential synergistic effects between the two classes of medications.

REFERENCES

Abellanas, L., & McLellan, A. T. (1993). "Stage of change" by drug problem in concurrent opioid, cocaine, and cigarette users. *J Psychoactive Drugs, 25,* 307–313.

Ananth, J., Vandeater, S., Kamal, M., & Brodsky, A. (1989). Missed diagnosis of substance abuse in psychiatric patients. *Hosp Community Psychiatry, 40,* 297–299.

American Psychiatric Association. (1980). *Diagnostic and statistical manual of mental disorders* (3rd ed.). Washington, DC: Author.

American Psychiatric Association. (1987). *Diagnostic and statistical manual of mental disorders* (3rd ed., rev.). Washington, DC: Author.

American Psychiatric Association. (1994). *Diagnostic and statistical manual of mental disorders* (4th ed.). Washington, DC: Author.

American Psychiatric Association. (2000). *Diagnostic and statistical manual of mental disorders* (4th ed., text rev.). Washington, DC: Author.

Babor, T. F., Hofmann, M., DelBoca, F. K., Hesselbrock, V., Meyer, R. E, Dolinsky, Z. S., & Rounsaville, B. (1992). Types of alcoholics: I. Evidence for an empirically derived typology based on indicators of vulnerability and severity. *Arch Gen Psychiatry, 49,* 599–608.

Ball, S. A., Carroll, K. M., Babor, T. F., & Rounsaville, B. J. (1995). Subtypes of cocaine abusers: Support for a Type A–Type B distinction. *J Consult Clin Psychol, 63,* 115–124.

Ball, S. A., Carroll, K. M., & Rounsaville, B. J. (1994). Sensation seeking, substance abuse, and psychopathology in treatment-seeking and community cocaine abusers. *J Consult Clin Psychol, 62,* 1053–1057.

Ball, S. A., Kranzler, H. R., Tennen, H., Poling, J. C., & Rounsaville, B. J. (1998). Personality disorder and dimension differences between Type A and type B substance abusers. *J Pers Disord, 12,* 1–12.

Beatty, W. W., Blanco, C. R., Hames, K. A., & Nixon, S. J. (1997). Spatial cognition in alcoholics: Influence of concurrent abuse of other drugs. *Drug Alcohol Depend, 44,* 167–174.

Bechara, A. (1999). Different contributions of the human amygdala and ventromedial prefrontal cortex to decision-making. *J Neurosci, 19,* 5473–5481.

Bierut, L. J., Dinwidie, S. H., Begleiter, H., Crowe, R. R., Hesselbrock, V., Nurnberger, J. I., et al. (1998). Familial transmission of substance dependence: Alcohol, marijuana, cocaine and habitual smoking. *Arch Gen Psychiatry, 55,* 982–988.

Block, R. I., Erwin, W. J., & Ghoneim, M. M. (2002). Chronic drug use and cognitive impairments. *Pharmacol Biochem Behav, 73,* 491–504.

Bondi, M. W., Drake, A. I., & Grant, I. (1998). Verbal learning and memory in alcohol abusers and polysubstance abusers with concurrent alcohol abuse. *J Int Neuropsychol Soc, 4,* 319–328.

Brook, D. W., Brook, J. S., Zhang, C., Cohen, P., & Whiteman, M. (2002). Drug use and the risk of major depressive disorder, alcohol dependence, and substance use disorders. *Arch Gen Psychiatry, 59*, 1039–1044.

Brooner, R. K., King, V. L., Kidorf, M., Schmidt, C. W., & Bigelow, G. E. (1997). Psychiatric and substance use comorbidity among treatment seeking opioid abusers. *Arch Gen Psychiatry, 54*, 71–80.

Caetano, R., & Weisner, C. (1995). The association between DSM-III-R alcohol dependence, psychological distress and drug use. *Addiction, 90*, 351–359.

Casillas, A., & Clark, L. A. (2002). Dependency, impulsivity, and self-harm: Traits hypothesized to underlie the association between cluster B personality and substance use disorders. *J Personal Disord, 16*, 424–436.

Ciraulo, D. A. (2003). Outcome predictors in substance use disorders. *Psychiatr Clin N Am, 26*, 381–409.

Clemmey, P., Brooner, R., Chutuape, M. A., Kidorf, M., & Stitzer, M. (1997). Smoking habits and attitudes in a methadone maintenance treatment population. *Drug Alcohol Depend, 44*, 123–132.

Cloninger, C. R. (1987). A systematic method for clinical description and classification of personality variants. *Arch Gen Psychiatry, 44*, 573–588.

Cloninger, C. R., Sigvardsson, S., & Bohman, M., (1988). Childhood personality predicts alcohol abuse in young adults. *Alcohol Clin Exp Res, 12*, 494–505.

Cohen, R. S. (1998). *The Love Drug: Marching to the beat of Ecstasy.* Binghamton, NY: Haworth Medical Press.

Cone, E. J., Fant, R. V., Rohay, J. M., Caplan, Y. H., Ballina, M., Reder, R. F., et al. (2003). Oxycodone involvement in drug abuse deaths: A DAWN-based classification scheme applied to an oxycodone postmortem database containing over 1000 cases. *J Anal Toxicol, 27*, 57–67.

Conway, K. P., Kane, R. J., Ball, S. A., Poling, J. C., & Rounsaville, B. J. (2003). Personality, substance of choice, and polysubstance involvement among substance dependent patients. *Drug Alcohol Depend, 71*, 65–75.

Conway, K. P., Swendson, J. D., Rounsaville, B. J., & Merikangas, K. R. (2002). Personality, drug of choice, and comorbid psychopathology among substance abusers. *Drug Alcohol Depend, 65*, 225–234.

Cook, P. A., Clark, P., Bellis, M. A., Ashton, J. R., Syed, Q., Hoskins, A., et al. (2001). Re-emerging syphilis in the UK: A behavioral analysis of infected individuals. *Commun Dis Public Health, 4*, 253–258.

Cunningham, S. C., Corrigan, S. A., Malow, R. M., & Smason, I. H. (1993). Psychopathology in inpatients dependent on cocaine or alcohol and cocaine. *Psychol Addict Behav, 7*, 246–250.

Darke, S., & Hall, W. (1995). Levels and correlates of polydrug use among heroin users and regular amphetamine users. *Drug Alcohol Depend, 39*, 231–235.

Darke, S., & Hall, W. (2003). Heroin overdose: Research and evidence-based intervention. *J Urban Health, 80*, 189–200.

Darke, S., & Ross, J. (1997). Polydrug dependence and psychiatric comorbidity among heroin injectors. *Drug Alcohol Depend, 48*, 135–141.

Darke, S., & Ross, J. (2000). The use of antidepressants among injecting drug users in Sydney, Australia. *Addiction, 95*, 407–417.

Darke, S., Williamson, A., Ross, J., Teesson, M., & Lynskey, M. (2004). Borderline personality disorder, antisocial personality disorder and risk-taking among heroin users: Findings from the Australian Treatment Outcome Study (ATOS). *Drug Alcohol Depend*, 74, 77–83.

Darke, S., & Zador, D. (1996). Fatal heroin overdose: A review. *Addiction*, 91, 1765–1772.

Dinwiddie, S. H., Cottler, L., Compton, W., & Abdallah, A. B. (1996). Psychopathology and HIV risk among injection drug users in and out of treatment. *Drug Alcohol Depend*, 43, 1–11.

Earleywine, M., & Newcomb, M. D. (1997). Concurrent versus simultaneous polydrug use: Prevalence, correlates, discriminant validity and prospective effects on health outcomes. *Exp Clin Pharm*, 5, 353–364.

Edens, J. F., & Willoughby, F. W. (1999). Motivational profiles of polysubstance-dependent patients: Do they differ from alcohol-dependent patients? *Addict Behav*, 24, 195–206.

Epstein, D. H., & Preston, K. L. (2003). Does cannabis use predict poor outcome for heroin-dependent patients on maintenance treatment?: Past findings and more evidence against. *Addiction*, 98, 269–279.

Feingold, A., Ball, S. A., Kranzler, H. R., & Rounsaville, B. J. (1996). Generalizability of the type A/type B distinction across different psychoactive substances. *Am J. Drug Alcohol Abuse*, 22, 449–462.

First, M. B., & Pincus, H. A. (2002). The DSM-IV text revision: Rationale and potential impact on clinical practice. *Psychiatr Serv*, 53, 288–292.

Grant, B., & Hartford, T. (1990). Concurrent and simultaneous use of alcohol with sedatives and tranquilizers: Results of a national survey. *J Subst Abuse*, 2, 1–14.

Grant, B. F., Stinson, F. S., Dawson, D. A., Chou, S. P., Ruan, W. J., & Pickering, R. P. (2004). Co-occurrence of 12-month alcohol and drug use disorders and personality disorders in the United States: Results from the National Epidemiologic Survey on Alcohol and Related Conditions. *Arch Gen Psychiatry*, 61, 361–368.

Grant, S., Contoreggi, C., & London, E. D. (2000). Drug abusers show impaired performance in a laboratory test of decision making. *Neuropsychologia*, 38, 1180–1187.

Greenwood, G. L., White, E. W., Page-Shafer, K., Bein, E., Osmond, D. H., Paul, J., & Stall, R. D. (2001). Correlates of heavy substance use among young gay and bisexual men: The San Francisco Young Men's Health Study. *Drug Alcohol Depend*, 61, 105–112.

Harrington, R. D., Woodward, J. A., Hooton, T. M., & Horn, J. R. (1999). Life-threatening interactions between HIV-1 protease inhibitors and the illicit drugs MDMA and gamma-hydroxybutyrate. *Arch Intern Med*, 159, 2221–2224.

Helzer, J. E., & Pryzbeck, T. R. (1988). The co-occurrence of alcoholism with other psychiatric disorders in the general population and its impact on treatment. *J Stud Alcohol*, 49, 219–224.

Hien, D., Zimberg, S., Weisman, S., First, M., & Ackerman, S. (1997). Dual diagnosis subtypes in urban substance abuse and mental health clinics. *Psychiatr Serv*, 48, 1058–1063.

Hopfer, C. J., Khuri, E., Crowley, T. J., & Hooks, S. (2002). Adolescent heroin use: A review of the descriptive and treatment literature. *J Subst Abuse Treat*, 23, 231–237.

Jordan, B. K., Schlenger, W. E., Fairbank, J. A., & Caddell, J. M. (1996). Prevalence of psychiatric disorders among incarcerated women: II. Convicted felons entering prison. *Arch Gen Psychiatry, 53*, 513–519.

Kandel, D., Chen, K., Warner, L. A., Kessler, R. C., & Grant, B. (1997). Prevalence and demographic correlates of symptoms of last year dependence on alcohol, nicotine, marijuana and cocaine in the U.S. population. *Drug Alcohol Depend, 44*, 11–29.

Kessler, R. C., Crum, R. M., Warner, L. A., Nelson, C. B., Schulenberg, J., & Anthony, J. C. (1997). Lifetime co-occurrence of DSM-III-R alcohol abuse and dependence with other psychiatric disorders in the National Comorbidity Study. *Arch Gen Psychiatry, 54*, 313–321.

Kessler, R. C., McGonagle, K. A., Zhao, S., Nelson, C. B., Hughes, M., Eshelman, S., et al. (1994). Lifetime and 12-month prevalence of DSM-III-R psychiatric disorders in the United States: Results from the National Comorbidity Study. *Arch Gen Psychiatry, 51*, 8–19.

Kidorf, M., Brooner, R. K., King, V. L., Chutuape, M. A., & Stitzer, M. L. (1996). Concurrent validity of cocaine and sedative dependence diagnoses in opioid-dependent outpatients. *Drug Alcohol Depend, 42*, 117–123.

Kleinman, P. H., Miller, A. B., Millman, R. B., Woody, G. E., Todd, T., Kemp, J., & Lipton, D. S. (1990). Psychopathology among cocaine abusers entering treatment. *J Nerv Ment Dis, 178*, 442–447.

Kokkevi, A., & Stefanis, C. (1995) Drug abuse and psychiatric comorbidity. *Compr Psychiatry, 36*, 329–333.

Kranzler, H. R., Satel, S., & Apter, A. (1994). Personality disorder and associated features in cocaine-dependent inpatients. *Compr Psychiatry, 35*, 335–340.

Kruedelbach, N., McCormick, R. A., Schulz, S. C., & Grueneich, R. (1993). Impulsivity, coping styles, and triggers for craving in substance abusers with borderline personality disorder. *J Personal Disord, 7*, 214–222.

Leal, J., Ziedonis, D., & Kosten, T. (1994). Antisocial personality disorder as a prognostic factor for pharmacotherapy of cocaine dependence. *Drug Alcohol Depend, 35*, 31–35.

Lee, S. J., Galanter, M., Dermatis H., & McDowell D. (2003). Circuit parties and patterns of drug use in a subset of gay men. *J Addict Dis, 22*, 47–60.

Leri, F., Bruneau, J., & Stewart, J. (2003). Understanding polydrug use: Review of heroin and cocaine co-use. *Addiction, 98*, 7–22.

Levin, F. R., Foltin, R. W., & Fischman, M. W. (1996). Pattern of cocaine use in methadone-maintained individuals applying for research studies. *J Addict Dis, 15*, 97–106.

Levounis, P., Galanter, M., Dermatis, H., Hamowy, A., & De Leon, G. (2003). Correlates of HIV transmission risk factors and considerations for interventions in homeless, chemically addicted and mentally ill patients. *J Addict Dis, 21*, 61–72.

Magura, S., Kang, S. Y., Nwakeze, P. C., & Demsky, S. (1998). Temporal patterns of heroin and cocaine use among methadone patients. *Subst Use Misuse, 33*, 2441–2467.

Malow, R. M., West, J. A., Corrigan, S. A., Pena, J. M., & Lott, W. C. (1992). Cocaine and speedball users: differences in psychopathology. *J Subst Abuse Treatment, 9*, 287–292.

Mansergh, G., Colfax, G. N., Marks, G., Rader, M., Guzman, R., & Buchbinder, S.

(2001). The Circuit Party Men's Health Survey: Findings and implications for gay and bisexual men. *Am J Public Health, 91*, 953–958.

Marlowe, D. B., Husband, S. D., Lamb, R. J., Kirby, K. C., Iguchi, M. Y., & Platt, J. J. (1995). Psychiatric comorbidity in cocaine dependence: Diverging trends, Axis II spectrum and gender differentials. *Am J Addict, 4*, 70–81.

Mattison, A. M., Ross, M. W., Wolfson, T., Franklin, D., & San Diego HIV Neurobehavioral Research Center Group. (2001). Circuit party attendance, club drug use, and unsafe sex in gay men. *J Subst Abuse, 31*, 119–126.

McCormick, R. A., Dowd, E. R., Quirt, S., & Zegarra, J. H. (1998). The relationship of NEO-PI performance to coping styles, patterns of use, and triggers for use among substance abusers. *Addict Behav, 23*, 497–507.

McCormick, R. A., & Smith, M. (1995). Aggression and hostility in substance abusers: The relationship to abuse patterns, coping style, and relapse triggers. *Addict Behav, 20*, 555–562.

Medina, K. L., Shear, P. K., Schafer, J., Armstrong, T. G., & Dyer, P. (2004). Cognitive functioning and length of abstinence in polysubstance dependent men. *Arch Clin Neuropsychol, 19*, 245–258.

Merikangas, K. R., Stolar, M., Stevens, D. E., Goulet, J., Preisig, M. A., Fenton, B., et al. (1998). Familial transmission of substance use disorders. *Arch Gen Psychiatry, 55*, 973–979.

Morgenstern, J., Langenbucher, J., Labouvie, E., & Miller, K. J. (1997). The comorbidity of alcoholism and personality disorders in a clinical population: Prevalence rates and relation to alcohol typology variables. *J Abnorm Psychol, 106*, 74–84.

Mors, O., & Sorensen, L. V. (1994). Incidence and comorbidity of personality disorders among first ever admitted psychiatric patients. *Eur Psychiatry, 9*, 175–184.

O'Boyle, M., & Barratt, E. S. (1993). Impulsivity and DSM-III-R personality disorders. *Pers Individ Dif, 14*, 609–611.

Parrott, A. C., Milani, R., Parmar, R., & Turner, J. J. D. (2001). Ecstasy polydrug users and other recreational drug users in Britain and Italy: Psychiatric symptoms and psychobiological problems. *Psychopharmacology, 159*, 77–82.

Parrott, A. C., Sisk, E., & Turner, J. (2000). Psychobiological problems in heavy "Ecstasy" (MDMA) polydrug users. *Drug Alcohol Depend, 60*, 105–110.

Pedersen, W., Clausen, S. E., & Lavik, N. J. (1989). Patterns of drug use and sensation seeking among adolescents in Norway. *Acta Psychiatr Scand, 39*, 386–390.

Regier, D. A., Farmer, M. E., Rae, D. S., Locke, B. Z., Keith, S. J., Judd, L. L., & Goodwin, F. K. (1990). Comorbidity of mental disorder with alcohol and other drug abuse: Results from the Epidemiologic Catchment Area (ECA) study. *JAMA, 264*, 2511–2518.

Ritsher, J. B., Moos, R. H., & Finney, J. W. (2002). Relationship of treatment orientation and continuing care to remission among substance abuse patients. *Psychiatr Serv, 53*(5), 595–601.

Rodgers, J. (2000). Cognitive performance amongst recreational users of "Ecstasy." *Psychopharmacology, 151*, 19–24.

Rosenthal, R. N. (2004). Concepts of evidence based practice. In A. R. Roberts & K. R. Yeager (Eds.), *Evidence-based practice manual: Research and outcome measures in health and human services* (pp. 20–29). New York: Oxford University Press.

Rosenthal, R. N., Hellerstein, D. J., & Miner, C. R. (1992). Integrated services for treatment of schizophrenic substance abusers: Demographics, symptoms, and substance abuse patterns. *Psychiatr Q, 63*, 3–26.

Rosenthal, R. N., & Solhkhah, R. (in press). Neurobiologic and clinical properties of the "club drugs." In H. R. Kranzler & D. A. Ciraulo (Eds.), *Clinical manual of addiction psychopharmacology*. Arlington, VA, American Psychiatric Press.

Rosenthal, R. N., & Westreich, L. (1999). Treatment of persons with dual diagnoses of substance use disorder and other psychological problems. In B. S. McCrady & E. E. Epstein (Eds.), *Addictions: A comprehensive guidebook* (pp. 439–476). New York: Oxford University Press.

Ross, L., Kohler, C. L., Grimley, D. M., & Bellis, J. (2003). Intention to use condoms among three low-income, urban African American subgroups: Cocaine users, noncocaine drug users, and non-drug users. *J Urban Health, 80*(1), 147–160.

Rounsaville, B. J., Dolinsky, Z. S., Babor, T. F., & Meyer, R. E. (1987). Psychopathology as a predictor of treatment outcome in alcoholism. *Arch Gen Psychiatry, 44*, 505–513.

Rounsaville, B. J., Kosten, T. R., Weissman, M. M., Prusoff, B., Pauls, D., Anton, S. F., & Merikangas, K. (1991). Psychiatric disorders in relatives of probands with opiate addiction. *Arch Gen Psychiatry, 48*, 33–42.

Rounsaville, B. J., Kranzler, H. R., Ball, S., Tennen, H., Poling, J., & Triffleman, E. (1998). Personality disorders in substance abusers: Relation to substance use. *J Nerv Ment Dis, 186*, 87–95.

Schifano, F., Di Furia, L., Forza, G., Minicuci, N., & Bricolo, R. (1998). MDMA ("Ecstasy") consumption in the context of polydrug abuse: A report on 150 patients. *Drug Alcohol Depend, 52*, 85–90.

Scholey, A. B., Parrott, A. C., Buchanan, T., Heffernan, T. M., Ling, J., & Rodgers, J. (2004). Increased intensity of ecstasy and polydrug usage in the more experienced recreational ecstasy/MDMA users: A WWW study. *Addict Behav, 29*, 743–752.

Schuckit, M. A., Danko, G. P., Raimo, E. B., Smith, T. L., Eng, M. Y., Carpenter, K. K., & Hesselbrock, V. M. (2001). A preliminary evaluation of the potential usefulness of the diagnoses of polysubstance dependence. *J Stud Alcohol, 62*, 54–61.

Selby, M. J., & Azrin, R. L. (1998). Neuropsychological functioning in drug abusers. *Drug Alcohol Depend, 50*, 39–45.

Skinstad, A. H., & Swain, A. (2001). Comorbidity in a clinical sample of substance abusers. *Am J Drug Alcohol Abuse, 27*, 45–64.

Staines, G. L., Magura, S., Foote, J., Deluca, A., & Kosanke, N. (2001). Polysubstance use among alcoholics. *J Addict Dis, 20*, 53–69.

Substance Abuse and Mental Health Services Administration, Office of Applied Studies. (2003a). National Survey of Substance Abuse Treatment Services (N-SSATS): 2002 [Data on Substance Abuse Treatment Facilities, DASIS Series: S-19, DHHS Publication No. (SMA) 03-3777]. Rockville, MD: U.S. Dept. of Health and Human Services.

Substance Abuse and Mental Health Services Administration, Office of Applied Studies. (2003b). Treatment Episode Data Set (TEDS): 1992–2001 [National Admissions to Substance Abuse Treatment Services, DASIS Series: S-20, DHHS Publication No. (SMA) 03-3778]. Rockville, MD: U.S. Dept. of Health and Human Services.

Tómasson, K., & Vaglum, P. (2000). Antisocial addicts: The importance of additional Axis I disorders for the 28-month outcome. *Eur Psychiatry, 15,* 443–449.

Trull, T. J., Sher, K. J., Minks-Brown, C., Durbin, J., & Burr, R. (2000). Borderline personality disorder and substance use disorders: A review and integration. *Clin Psychol Rev, 20,* 235–253.

Tsuang, M. T., Lyons, M. J., Eisen, S. A., Goldberg, J., True, W., Lin, N., et al. (1996). Genetic influences on DSM-III-R drug abuse and dependence: A study of 3,372 twin pairs. *Am J Med Genet, 67,* 473–477.

Tsuang, M. T., Lyons, M. J., Meyer, J. M., Doyle, T., Eisen, S. A., Goldberg, J., et al. (1998). Co-occurrence of abuse of different drugs in men: The role of drug-specific and shared vulnerabilities. *Arch Gen Psychiatry, 55,* 967–972.

Tyler, A. (1995). *Street drugs.* London, UK: Hodder & Stoughton.

Vreugdenhil, C., Van Den Brink, W., Wouters, L. F., & Doreleijers, T. A. (2003). Substance use, substance use disorders, and comorbidity patterns in a representative sample of incarcerated male Dutch adolescents. *J Nerv Ment Dis, 191,* 372–378.

Walton, M. A., Blow F. C., & Booth, B. M. (2000). A comparison of substance abuse patients' and counselors' perceptions of relapse risk: Relationship to actual relapse. *J Subst Abuse Treatment, 19,* 161–169.

Webb, J. A., Baer, P. E., & McKelvey, R. S. (1995). Development of a risk profile for intentions to use alcohol among fifth and sixth graders. *J Am Acad Child Adolesc Psychiatry, 34,* 772–778.

Weizman, T., Gelkopf, M., Melamed, Y., Adelson, M., & Bleich, A. (2004). Cannabis abuse is not a risk factor for treatment outcome in methadone maintenance treatment: A 1-year prospective study in an Israeli clinic. *Aust NZJ Psychiatry, 38,* 42–46.

Woody, G. E., McLellan, A. T., Luborsky, L., & O'Brien, C. P. (1985). Sociopathy and psychotherapy outcome. *Arch Gen Psychiatry, 42,* 1081–1086.

CHAPTER 12

Co-Occurring Substance Use Disorders and Other Psychiatric Disorders

ALISA B. BUSCH
ROGER D. WEISS
LISA M. NAJAVITS

Determining better ways to identify and treat individuals with co-occurring substance use disorders (SUDs) and other psychiatric disorders has become increasingly important from clinical, research, and policy perspectives. Several observations have driven this imperative: (1) Co-occurring SUDs with other psychiatric disorders are prevalent (Kessler et al., 1996; Regier et al., 1990) and associated with worse clinical and functional outcomes than either SUDs or other psychiatric disorders alone (Mueller et al., 1994; Ritsher, McKellar, Finney, Otilingam, & Moos, 2002); (2) many people with these co-occurring disorders do not receive adequate treatment (Substance Abuse and Mental Health Service Administration, 2002); and (3) compared to psychiatric patients without co-occurring SUDs, patients with a dual diagnosis tend to use more costly treatments, such as emergency and hospital care (Dickey & Azeni, 1996; Mark, 2003). Together, these observations have led to the development of specific new treatments designed or adapted for this population—although this research is at an early stage.

Within SUD populations, multiple substance use disorders are common (Kessler et al., 1997; Regier et al., 1990). While these individuals can also be considered "dually diagnosed," this chapter focuses exclusively on patients who have an SUD plus a (non-SUD) co-occurring Axis I or II psychiatric disorder.

Additionally, non-SUD Axis I and II psychiatric disorders are here referred to simply as "psychiatric disorders" to distinguish them from substance use disorders.

In this chapter, we review psychosocial and psychopharmacological treatments for dual-diagnosis populations. While increasing methodological rigor is being employed in many of these studies, this research is still at an early stage. Thus, some of the available evidence is from pilot or noncontrolled trials. When evidence from blinded and/or controlled trials is not available for a particular treatment, we review the level of evidence that is available.

EPIDEMIOLOGY

Studies in SUD and psychiatric treatment-seeking populations (McLellan & Druley, 1977; Ross, Glaser, & Germanson, 1988; Rounsaville et al., 1991) have suggested high prevalence rates of co-occurring SUDs and psychiatric disorders. However, treatment-seeking samples may not be representative of community populations, since they tend to have higher rates of comorbidity and may have more severe manifestations of the disorder for which they are seeking treatment. Thus, epidemiological studies of prevalence rates in community populations are important in assessing the true comorbidity prevalence rate.

The two largest U.S. psychiatric epidemiological studies to date, the Epidemiologic Catchment Area (ECA) study (Regier et al., 1990) and the more recent National Comorbidity Survey (NCS; Kessler et al., 1996) demonstrate that co-occurring SUDs and psychiatric disorders are prevalent in community populations. Methodological advancements of the NCS included an expanded scope of the community sample (e.g., the ECA sampled from within five U.S. communities, whereas the NCS sampled nationally representative households), and an advanced version of the *Diagnostic and Statistical Manual of Mental Disorders* (i.e., DSM-III-R [American Psychiatric Association, 1987]). Also, while both studies surveyed most of the more common psychiatric disorders, the ECA did not include posttraumatic stress disorder (PTSD), whereas the NCS did. Neither epidemiological survey included Axis II disorders other than antisocial personality disorder (ASPD). Despite these limitations and differences between the two studies, their results were often qualitatively similar, although the magnitude of their estimates differed somewhat at times. Among persons with psychiatric disorders, the ECA estimated that 30% had a co-occurring SUD. The prevalence varied by diagnosis, however; co-occurring SUDs were most common in individuals with ASPD, followed by those with bipolar I disorder. In SUD populations, the ECA and the NCS estimated that over half will experience Axis I or II psychiatric disorders in their lifetime. These lifetime estimates do not merely reflect rare or historical periods in an individual's history; the 12-month comorbidity prevalence rate of these disorders was also quite high. For example, the NCS estimated that over 33% of those with bipolar disorder would experience an SUD within 12 months, followed by nearly 20% of those with major depression and 15% of those with an anxiety disorder.

THE ASSOCIATION BETWEEN DUAL DIAGNOSIS AND TREATMENT OUTCOME

In both SUD and psychiatric treatment-seeking populations, dually diagnosed patients typically experience worse outcomes than their "singly diagnosed" peers (Ritsher et al., 2002; Schaar & Oejehagen, 2001). However, there are specific populations in which the evidence regarding this is mixed, such as the severely and persistently mentally ill (SPMI) (Farris et al., 2003; Gonzalez & Rosenheck, 2002) and ASPD populations (Cacciola, Alterman, Rutherford, & Snider, 1995; Kranzler, Del Boca, & Rounsaville, 1996). The effect of other psychiatric disorders on SUD outcomes may vary by SUD type. For example, co-occurring major depression appears to predict worse alcohol outcomes (Brown et al., 1998; Greenfield et al., 1998), while there is less evidence for its predicting worse cocaine outcomes (McKay et al., 2002; Rohsenow, Monti, Martin, Michalec, & Abrams, 2002).

There is also evidence (albeit somewhat inconsistent) that gender may play a role in mediating the effect of co-occurring psychiatric disorders on SUD outcome. Major depression in men has been associated with worse SUD outcome (Compton, Cottler, Jacobs, Ben-Abdallah, & Spitznagel, 2003; Rounsaville, Dolinsky, Babor, & Meyer, 1987), although this is not a consistent finding (Kranzler et al., 1996; Powell et al., 1992). In contrast, some studies suggest that female gender has been associated with similar or better SUD outcomes among patients with co-occurring psychiatric disorders (Compton et al., 2003; Rounsaville et al., 1987), except for phobia, which was associated in one study with worse SUD outcome in women (Compton et al., 2003). Finally, ASPD in men has been associated with worse outcomes (Compton et al., 2003; Kranzler et al., 1996); although, the evidence in women has been mixed (Compton et al., 2003; Rounsaville et al., 1987).

THE RELATIONSHIP BETWEEN SUBSTANCE ABUSE AND PSYCHOPATHOLOGY

While determining which disorder is primary in dually diagnosed populations can be useful in clinical research, it may provide little benefit in the clinical management of these patients. Patients with two disorders typically require treatment for both; the exception is patients who present with temporary psychiatric symptoms caused by the substance use or its withdrawal.

Meyer (1986) suggests considering six possible ways in which substance use and other psychopathology may be related:

1. *Psychopathology may be a risk factor for SUDs.* As described previously, studies of patient and community samples have shown that the risk of having a co-occurring SUD is elevated in persons with psychiatric disorders. For example, dopaminergic dysfunction in patients with schizophrenia has been hypothesized to increase their risk of SUDs—particularly cocaine use disorders (Green et al., 1999; Smelson, Losonczy, Kilker, et al., 2002). Another theory, widely known as the "self-medication hypothesis" (Khantzian, 1989, 1997), suggests that psychopathology leads patients to use substances in an attempt to decrease unwanted psychiatric symptoms. For example, a patient with insomnia due to PTSD nightmares may use alcohol or marijuana to induce sleep. Although research has not found direct connections between particular psychopathological symptoms and specific substances (rather, patients tend to misuse a wide variety of substances to "treat" a range of symptoms), the general principle is an important one. It is discussed in more detail in the next section.

2. *Psychiatric disorders and co-occurring SUDs may serve to modify the course of each other in terms of symptomatology, rapidity of onset, and response to treatment.* Also described earlier, there is considerable evidence that comorbidity is associated with worse outcomes. Additionally, there is evidence that patients with schizophrenia and co-occurring SUDs do not respond as well as those without SUDs to similar doses of first-generation antipsychotic medications (Bowers et al., 1990).

3. *Psychiatric symptoms may result from chronic intoxication.* Drug and alcohol use can result in a variety of psychiatric symptoms, such as depression, anxiety, euphoria, psychosis, and dissociative states. Most such symptoms disappear, however, within hours (e.g., cocaine-induced paranoia) (Satel, Southwick, & Gawin, 1991) to weeks (e.g., alcohol-induced anxiety or depression) (Brown, Irwin, & Schuckit, 1991; Brown & Schuckit, 1988).

4. *Long-term substance use can lead to psychiatric disorders that may not remit.* Alcohol-induced long-term cognitive changes, such as those seen in alcohol-induced persisting dementia, exemplify one way in which chronic use of a substance can create enduring change.

5. *Substance abuse and psychopathological symptoms may be meaningfully linked.* Some individuals may use alcohol or drugs in ways that enhance their psychiatric symptoms. For example, patients with ASPD may use alcohol or cocaine, seeking disinhibition and aggression, and patients with bipolar disorder may use cocaine or other stimulants to augment a euphoric mood (Weiss, 1986l; Weiss et al., 1988).

6. *The SUD and psychiatric disorder are unrelated.* The presence of two disorders within an individual does not imply a causal link. For example, both alcohol dependence and depressive disorders are common in the general population; many people with both disorders are not depressed because they drink, nor do they drink because they are depressed. Brunette, Mueser, Xie, and Drake (1997) studied the relationship between severity of substance abuse and severity of schizophrenic symptoms in patients dually diagnosed with both disorders, and found weak relationships and no consistent patterns of relationships between the two sets of symptoms.

The "Self-Medication Hypothesis"

One potential explanation for the increased prevalence rate of co-occurring SUDs among patients with psychiatric disorders has been the "self-medication hypothesis" (Khantzian, 1985, 1997), which postulates that certain drugs may be particularly reinforcing because of particular patients' specific psychopathology.

Two fundamental assumptions underlie this hypothesis: first, that substances are abused to relieve psychological pain, not just to create euphoria; and second, that there is specificity between patients' "drug of choice" preference and the specific intolerable emotions or symptoms that they are attempting to alleviate. For example, patients with social anxiety may be drawn to alcohol to decrease their symptoms, while patients who are prone to violence and anger outbursts may prefer the calming effects of opioids to the potentially disinhibiting effects of alcohol.

A major criticism of the self-medication hypothesis has been its heavy reliance on anecdotal data from patients in psychotherapy and the relative paucity of empirical studies testing it (Aharonovich, Nguyen, & Nunes, 2001). Additionally, intoxicants may produce very different effects acutely compared to the effects of chronic administration. Studies of individuals with heroin (Meyer & Mirin, 1979), cocaine (Post, Kotin, & Goodwin, 1974), and alcohol (Mendelson & Mello, 1966) use disorders have observed a dichotomy between the acute effects of these drugs in producing euphoria or tension relief and the chronic or high-dose effects in producing dysphoria. Several researchers have sought to test empirically the self-medication hypothesis in larger samples. The results have tended not to support the specificity of using a particular addictive substance to alleviate specific psychopathology or mood states (Aharonovich et al., 2001; Weiss, 1992a). However, while not necessarily a validation of the theory that patients use addictive substances to alleviate certain mood states, there is evidence that treating a co-occurring psychiatric disorder (Cornelius et al., 1997; Greenfield et al., 1998) and remission of its symptoms (Hasin, Tsai, Endicott, & Mueller, 1996) can improve SUD outcomes.

Other Theories

Weiss (1992b) suggests three additional mechanisms by which psychopathology can make an individual more vulnerable to SUDs.

1. *Psychopathology may interfere with an individual's judgment or ability to appreciate consequences.* Individuals with psychiatric disorders may be more vulnerable to SUDs, because impaired judgment is often present in many psychiatric syndromes and can interfere with the ability or willingness to understand or change one's behavior. For example, severely depressed patients may have insight regarding the destructive effect of their drinking but may continue to drink due to the pessimism about the possibility and value of change that is part of their depressive disorder. Similarly, the recklessness, irritability, and grandiosity of patients who are manic or hypomanic may interfere with their capacity to appreciate the harmful nature of their substance use.

2. *Psychopathology may accelerate the process of substance dependence by leading to more dysphoria during either chronic use or early abstinence.* It is possible that patients with underlying psychopathology may experience more dysphoria from chronic substance use or more severe withdrawal symptoms when discontinuing drugs or alcohol. Although this potential mechanism has received little study, there is some evidence that cocaine abusers with major depression compared to cocaine abusers without depression may report more severe mood symptoms during abstinence (Gawin & Kleber, 1986).

3. *Psychopathology may reinforce the social context of drug use.* Some patients with severe psychiatric illness may be drawn to a drug-using subculture, because they feel it facilitates socialization or a new peer group. For example, some patients with schizophrenia have described using substances to socialize or be accepted by peers, even though substances increased the risk of psychosis (Drake, Osher, & Wallach, 1989; Spencer, Castle, & Michie, 2002).

Thus, multiple possible motivations and causes contribute to the initiation and maintenance of problematic alcohol and drug use in patients with psychiatric disorders.

DIAGNOSING PSYCHIATRIC DISORDERS IN PATIENTS WITH SUBSTANCE USE DISORDERS

The task of determining whether a patient is suffering from a substance-induced disorder or an independent psychiatric disorder can be complicated. Substances of abuse can cause a wide range of psychiatric symptoms. Clinicians evaluating such patients need to determine whether the disturbance is independent of substance use or related to intoxication or withdrawal. For example, when examining a patient who has a long history of alcohol dependence and depressive symptoms, it can be difficult to determine whether the depressive symptoms result from the direct pharmacological effects of alcohol, the many losses experienced as a result of the alcohol use, feelings of discouragement about the inability to stop drinking, or an independent mood disorder. Other etiologies, such as metabolic disturbances, head trauma, and personality disorders, must also be considered in the differential diagnosis of depressive symptoms in alcohol-dependent patients (Jaffe & Ciraulo, 1986).

Given these considerations, one could ideally establish diagnostic rules to assist in determining whether a psychiatric syndrome is due to substance use or represents a separate and independent disorder. For example, some clinicians may establish a rule that a patient must be abstinent from alcohol and drugs for at least 4 weeks before they can make a diagnosis. Unfortunately, one does not always have the luxury of observing such lengthy abstinent periods (either by historical report or in the present) to assess this. In such circumstances, guidelines, as opposed to strict rules, can be helpful. For example, several studies have indicated that for alcoholics with major depression, treating the depression can have a positive impact on drinking (Cornelius et al., 1997; Greenfield et al., 1998). Thus, while DSM-IV-TR (American Psychiatric Association, 2000) criteria for substance-induced mood disorder suggest at least 4 weeks of observation during abstinence before a clinician can diagnose an independent psychiatric disorder, it also recommends that clinicians should diagnose an independent disorder if the symptoms are qualitatively or quantitatively not what one would expect, given the amount and duration of the substance use. Certain disorders, such as eating disorders and PTSD, can be diagnosed readily, even in the context of substance use or withdrawal, since their symptoms do not closely resemble substance-related syndromes. Indeed, for a diagnosis such as PTSD, which tends to be underdiagnosed in SUD patients, the greater danger is to delay diagnosis; waiting for a period of abstinence may prevent needed treatment for the co-occurring disorder (Najavits, 2004).

Finally, clinicians should consider whether the patient's symptoms are what would be expected upon discontinuation of the abused substance. If there is considerable overlap between the observed symptoms and what one would expect from the drug discontinuation syndrome, then the clinician should wait until either (1) the symptoms resolve, or (2) the symptoms no longer are consistent with what one would expect from drug cessation (i.e., the syndrome one would expect to see after 1 week vs. 1 month of alcohol abstinence). Alternatively, if there is little overlap between the symptoms observed and the expected abstinence syndrome (e.g., bulimia nervosa in an opioid-dependent patient), then the diagnosis can be made without waiting.

DIAGNOSING SUBSTANCE USE DISORDERS AMONG PATIENTS SEEKING TREATMENT FOR PSYCHIATRIC DISORDERS

Co-occurring SUDs are often overlooked in patients seeking treatment for psychiatric disorders. The first step in the accurate diagnosis of SUDs is to systematically ask the patient about the presence of substance use. Structured clinical assessments have been demonstrated to improve detection of SUDs compared to routine assessment in outpatient SPMI (Breakey, Calabrese, Rosenblatt, & Crum, 1998) and inpatient (Albanese, Bartel, Bruno, Morgenbesser, & Schatzberg, 1994) populations; they have also outperformed urine toxicology testing (Albanese et al., 1994). Unfortunately, the increasing acuity of patients on inpatient units and the demanding time constraints of outpatient psychiatric practice (Woodward, Fortgang, Sullivan-Trainor, Stojanov, & Mirin, 1991) may pose challenges to the systematic assessment of SUDs. In one outpatient study, adding the 4-item CAGE (Cut Down, Annoyed, Guilty, Eye-Opener; Ewing, 1984) questionnaire improved the sensitivity of detecting SUDs from 62% to 97% in an SPMI population (Breakey et al., 1998). However, self-report alone, without urine toxicology, can also lead to underdetection of substance use (Claassen et al., 1997; Shaner et al., 1993).

Finally, contingencies play an important role in patients' willingness to self-report substance use. If patients are repeatedly encouraged to be honest in their self-reports, and if they are told (and more importantly, if they believe) that there will be no negative consequences of reporting use (e.g., being discharged from a treatment program or reported to a probation officer or employer), then they are more likely to be forthcoming in reporting their use. If, however, they are concerned that there will be negative consequences, then they are less likely to do so. Thus, self-reports of substance use in an emergency room, where a patient is unlikely to know the clinician and will probably not believe (whether it is true or not) that there will be no negative consequences for disclosing use, are likely to be suspect. However, in an outpatient treatment setting, where a patient has an opportunity to build a relationship with a clinician or treatment team, and perhaps sees other patients self-disclosing and benefiting from that disclosure, self-reports are likely to be more valid (Weiss, 1998).

TREATMENT OF DUALLY DIAGNOSED PATIENTS

A Heterogeneous Population

Since "dually diagnosed" patients comprise a heterogeneous population, it follows that their treatment should perhaps reflect that heterogeneity (Weiss, Mirin, & Frances, 1992); a "one size fits all" approach therefore will likely not be optimal. However, providing group treatments tailored to patients with some degree of diagnostic homogeneity (e.g., patients with bipolar disorder and SUDs) can be a difficult strategy to implement if one is unable to recruit a large enough clinical population for these groups. Similarly, even within diagnostically homogeneous groups, considerable heterogeneity in illness severity and functioning may still exist. Ries, Sloan, and Miller (1997) have suggested a conceptual approach that divides dually diagnosed patients into four major subgroups, according to the severity (i.e., major or minor) of each disorder. Although this is a somewhat crude way to classify patients, it may be helpful in developing an outpatient group treatment program for dually diagnosed patients.

An additional consideration is that not all patients are similar in terms of insight regarding their SUD, nor are they similarly ready to address it. Thus, patients who are undecided whether or not to address their substance use may do better in a group focused on resolving that issue, as opposed to a group in which all participants are actively engaged in treatment and making lifestyle changes to support sobriety. We know of no studies, however, that have tested this idea empirically. It is possible, for example, that having a mix of patient severity levels in one group allows patients the opportunity to learn from those further along in their recovery. This is a central principle of Alcoholics Anonymous (AA), and appears to have strong anecdotal support. Treatments that focus on particular dual diagnoses (e.g., bipolar SUD patients) also have not been directly compared to more general thematic groups (e.g., dual diagnosis groups that are more general, encompassing a wide variety of diagnoses). Thus, it remains an empirical question how the known heterogeneity of such patients should best be addressed within the realistic constraints of specific clinical settings.

Sequential, Parallel, and Integrated Treatment Models

There are three major models in which dually diagnosed patients are treated: sequential, parallel, and integrated treatment. Each is discussed below.

In *sequential treatment*, the more acute condition is treated first, followed by the less acute co-occurring disorder. The same staff may treat both disorders, or the less acute disorder may be treated after transfer to a different program or facility. For example, a manic patient with a cocaine use disorder needs mood stabilization before initiating substance abuse treatment. Conversely, a patient with major depression and alcohol withdrawal delirium is not in a position to discuss treatment adherence to antidepressant medication. Instead, this issue is best addressed when the patient is more stable. Although sequential treatment has the advantage of providing an increased level of attention to the more acute disorder, a typical disadvantage of this model is that patients are often transferred to a different treatment team to address the less acute disorder, and the interrelationship between the two disorders may never be adequately addressed.

In *parallel treatment*, both disorders are treated simultaneously, but not by the same treatment team. For example, a patient may receive treatment for an SUD in an addiction treatment program and for a psychiatric disorder in a mental health clinic. Typically, staff members of each program are very well-versed in their own area of expertise, but not in the other. However, major cross-training efforts on dual diagnosis have improved this situation in the past decade. The different treatment programs may also have different treatment philosophies, which may be confusing to the patient (Mueser, Bellack, & Blanchard, 1992; Ridgely, Goldman, & Willenbring, 1990). For example, in substance abuse treatment programs, clinicians may attribute psychiatric symptoms (e.g., depression and anxiety) to substance use; when a patient attempts to obtain relief, they may view this as "drug-seeking" behavior. Alternatively, staff in psychiatric programs may tend to minimize the importance of substance use and not stress its potential negative consequences.

Unfortunately, patients treated in parallel or sequential programs often receive different experiences based on the treatment settings they enter. The two different programs may provide patients with different feedback on the relationship between their substance use and psychological symptoms. Patients in these situations are then left to attempt to integrate these sometimes disparate approaches themselves. In these circumstances, patients may be accused of "manipulating" and "splitting staff" when they present information obtained in one program that is contradictory to the other.

In *integrated treatment*, the management of both disorders occurs in one treatment setting, and the same clinicians, or team of clinicians, manage both illnesses. Integrated treatment has received increasing interest of researchers and clinicians, fostered by the belief that it is more effective than the other treatment models described earlier.

INTEGRATED PSYCHOSOCIAL TREATMENTS FOR DUALLY DIAGNOSED PATIENTS

Integrated psychosocial treatments have been developed for diverse patient populations with co-occurring SUDs and psychiatric disorders. Here, we review the scope of psychiatric patient populations for which treatments have been developed, followed by a review of specific treatment modalities. While this literature has advanced overall in terms of randomized study designs and manualized treatments, it remains hampered by the limited number of studies and small sample sizes. Thus, while these treatments appear promising, further study is needed.

Severely and Persistently Mentally Ill Populations

Several investigators have examined integrated treatments for SPMI adults. Effectiveness trials by Drake and colleagues have obtained more success in decreasing substance use (Drake et al., 1998; McHugo, Drake, Teague, & Xie, 1999) and hospitalization (McHugo et al., 1999) than in diminishing psychiatric symptoms (Drake, Yovetich, Bebout, Harris, & McHugo, 1998; Drake et al., 1998) or improving functional status or quality of life (Drake et al., 1997). However, these interventions did not compare patients randomized to different treatments. Rather, treatment clinics were assigned to administer one intervention versus another. A recent review of the prospective, controlled trials of integrated treatment programs for SPMI dually diagnosed individuals (Jeffery, Ley, McLaren, & Siegfried, 2003) concluded that methodological flaws precluded determining whether one particular integrated treatment model is more effective than another, or whether integrated treatment in general is superior to nonintegrated treatment for this population. Despite this, much enthusiasm remains for integrated treatment in SPMI populations (Drake et al., 2001). Of note, a recent trial not included in the review approached integrating treatment for dually diagnosed SPMI patients from a different psychosocial treatment perspective and found positive results. Rather than integrating treatment from the perspective of intensive case management and/or housing (as in the studies discussed earlier), patient and caregiver dyads were randomized to routine care versus additional integrated treatment that included motivational interviewing, cognitive-behavioral therapy (CBT), and a family or caregiver intervention for dual-diagnosis patients with schizophrenia. The intervention was associated with improvements in general functioning, psychotic symptoms, and SUD outcomes (Barrowclough et al., 2001). Thus, this field continues to evolve and develop creative new treatments that are being tested with increasing methodological rigor.

Other Psychiatric Populations

In non-SPMI populations, integrated treatment models have also been developed for other patient subpopulations with psychiatric disorders and SUDs such as bipolar disorder (Weiss et al., 2000), personality disorders (Ball, 1998; Linehan et al., 2002), and anxiety disorders such as PTSD (Brady, Dansky, Back, Foa, & Carroll, 2001; Najavits, Weiss, Shaw, & Muenz, 1998), obsessive–compulsive disorder (Fals-Stewart & Schafer, 1992), and social phobia (Randall, Thomas, & Thevos, 2001). With the exception of social phobia, for which integrated CBT for social phobia and alcohol use disorders has yielded worse anxiety and drinking outcomes compared to group CBT geared toward alcohol relapse prevention alone (Randall et al., 2001), preliminary evidence suggests that these new treatments are generating some positive results.

Specific Treatment Modalities

Psychosocial treatments with the potential for broad applicability across several dual-diagnosis populations have also been developed. With the exception of cognitive therapy, most originated in the addiction literature but have demonstrated some efficacy in treating both disorders when adapted specifically for dually diagnosed populations. Below, we briefly describe several of the more common psychosocial interventions studied in populations with co-occurring SUDs and psychiatric disorders.

Cognitive-behavioral therapy (CBT), developed by Beck, Rush, Shaw, and Emery (1979), has been adapted for the treatment of substance abuse (Beck, Wright, Newman, & Liese, 1993). When adapted to specific dually diagnosed populations (e.g., PTSD), additional techniques include the identification of cognitive distortions associated with both disorders (e.g., getting high now as a "reward" for having been deprived in the past), identifying meanings of substance use in the context of PTSD (e.g., as revenge against an abuser), and teaching new coping skills (e.g., setting boundaries) (Najavits et al., 1996).

Relapse prevention therapy (RPT), developed by Marlatt and Gordon (1985), is a form of CBT that focuses on understanding the process of relapse in order to prevent it. RPT can be used as an adjunctive therapy or as a treatment in and of itself. When modified to address dually diagnosed individuals, preventing relapse from both disorders is emphasized. For example, RPT modified for patients with co-occurring bipolar disorder and SUDs (Weiss, Najavits, & Greenfield, 1999; Weiss et al., 2000) teaches patients about triggers for both substance use and bipolar disorder (e.g., erratic sleep behaviors, associating with the wrong people, nonadherence to one's medication regimen).

Motivational interviewing (MI), developed by Miller and Rollnick (1991, 2002), utilizes theory derived from several psychotherapeutic models: systems, client-centered, cognitive-behavioral, and social psychology. MI is also called motivational enhancement, because it is often a brief treatment conducted in as few as two sessions, sometimes aimed at helping the patient accept other psychotherapy (e.g., CBT). Guidelines for modifying MI in dually diagnosed patients with psychotic disorders have been published (Carey et al., 2001; Martino et al., 2002). Recent randomized pilot trials of MI in diverse dually diagnosed populations suggest that it may improve the likelihood of making the transition to outpatient treatment (Swanson, Pantalon, & Cohen, 1999), improve SUD outcomes (Graeber et al., 2003), and decrease psychiatric hospitalization (Daley & Zuckoff, 1998).

The transtheoretical *stages-of-change model* (Prochaska, DiClemente, & Norcross, 1992, 1994) describes a sequential process of five stages of change in recovery for patients with SUDs: precontemplation, contemplation, preparation, action, and maintenance. Osher and Kofoed (1989) have articulated a model similar to stages of change for dually diagnosed patients with severe psychiatric disorders. Adaptations to the stages-of-change model for SPMI dual-diagnosis populations have also been developed, and some have been empirically tested for reliability and validity (Carey, Carey, Maisto, & Purnine, 2002; Velasquez, Carbonari, & DiClemente, 1999) with promising results (Carey et al., 2002; Ziedonis & Trudeau, 1997). Pilot work of a family intervention adapted from the stages-of-change model for this population has also shown promise (Mueser & Fox, 2002).

Twelve-step drug counseling derives directly from the principles of AA and has been adapted for use by professional alcohol and drug counselors (a necessary adaptation, since AA was designed as a self-help group not led by professionals). Two types of treatment emphasize these principles: individual drug counseling (Mercer & Woody, 1999) and 12-step facilitation (TSF) (Nowinski, Baker, & Carroll, 1995). TSF is used by all of the studies described below. Several trials have compared outcomes of dually diagnosed patients treated with TSF groups with outcomes among those treated with various other psychosocial treatments (i.e., CBT, RPT, dialectical behavioral therapy [DBT], or behavioral skills group) (Brooks & Penn, 2003; Fisher & Bentley, 1996; Jerrell & Ridgely, 1995; Linehan, 1993; Linehan et al., 2002; McKay et al., 2002; Ouimette, Gima, Moos, & Finney, 1999). Among them, only one found improved SUD outcomes in TSF versus the comparison integrated treatment (Brooks & Penn, 2003). However, in that study, the TSF group also experienced worsening health and employment status, and psychiatric hospitalization, compared to the group of patients receiving integrated treatment.

Contingency management (CM) interventions reinforce behavior that meets specific, clearly defined, and observable goals (Petry, 2000) such as abstinence (Higgins et al., 1994), medication adherence (Liebson, Tommasello, & Bigelow, 1978), therapy attendance (Helmus, Rhodes, Haber, & Downey, 2001), or completion of treatment goals (Petry, Martin, Cooney, & Kranzler, 2000). Recent empirical evaluations using CM as an adjunctive treatment in dually diagnosed populations suggest that it may offer some benefit in attendance, but its impact on SUD outcomes has been mixed (Helmus, Saules, Schoener, & Roll, 2003; Sigmon, Steingard, Badger, Anthony, & Higgins, 2000).

SELF-HELP GROUPS
AND DUALLY DIAGNOSED INDIVIDUALS

As in other substance-using populations (Miller, Ninonuevo, Klamen, Hoffmann, & Smith, 1997; Ritsher et al., 2002), self-help group attendance has been associated with improved substance use outcomes in dually diagnosed populations (Brooks & Penn, 2003; Ritsher et al., 2002). Whether this is a reflection of self-help groups' improving outcomes directly or a self-selection bias (i.e., patients attending self-help groups may be more likely to remain abstinent because they are more motivated) is unclear.

Despite the fact that self-help groups are both free of charge and geographically accessible (Kurtz, 1997), many dually diagnosed patients do not attend these meetings (Noordsy, Schwab, Fox, & Drake, 1996). Some clinicians may be reluctant to recommend self-help groups to dually diagnosed patients because of concerns that self-help group members might express negative attitudes toward psychotropic medication (Humphreys, 1997). However, recent research indicates that, while this sometimes occurs (Noordsy et al., 1996), it is not prevalent (Meissen, Powell, Wituk, Girrens, & Arteaga, 1999). Moreover, official AA literature states that psychiatric medication, when legitimately prescribed, is appropriate (Alcoholics Anonymous, 1984). When educating patients about the interaction between psychiatric symptoms, drug and alcohol use, and medications, clinicians should inform patients that while some self-help group members may criticize the use of medications, this contradicts official AA policy.

Clinicians may also be concerned that these groups only focus on SUDs (Humphreys, 1997) and may therefore not be as helpful to patients who are struggling with other psychiatric disorders. Recent research suggests that some patients and AA contacts (i.e., persons listed in the AA directories as experienced members) agree (Meissen et al., 1999; Noordsy et al., 1996). However, by encouraging patients to focus on obtaining what AA and similar groups offer, and not expecting AA to provide services outside of its stated mission, clinicians can help dually diagnosed patients to take advantage of these groups.

To address some of these concerns, several dual-focus self-help groups have emerged for participants with co-occurring SUDs and psychiatric disorders (e.g., Double Trouble in Recovery, Dual Recovery Anonymous, and Dual Disorders Anonymous) (Magura et al., 2003). Similar to the literature on self-help groups in the SUD population, positive associations have been found between attendance at dual-focus self-help groups and abstinence (Magura et al., 2003) as well as psychiatric/quality-of-life (Magura, Laudet, Mahmood, Rosenblum, & Knight, 2002) outcomes. Again, whether this is a result of self-selection bias regarding the characteristics of patients who attend these meetings or not is unclear. It is important to consider that the literature on dual-focus self-help groups is an emerging one and is even slimmer than the literature on integrated psychosocial treatments. Further study is needed before conclusions regarding their effectiveness can be drawn.

General Treatment Themes for Dually Diagnosed Patients

Because of the limitations of the empirical literature described earlier regarding psychosocial treatments, it may be helpful to draw on general recommendations provided by various writers on this subject (Bellack & DiClemente, 1999; Carey, 1995; Drake et al., 2001; Drake & Mueser, 2000; Najavits et al., 1996; Rounsaville & Carroll, 1997; Ziedonis, Williams, Corrigan, & Smelsen, 2000). Although treatment modalities differ, some common themes can help guide clinicians who must decide how to intervene with their patients. The suggestions are as follows:

- Be empathic and provide support for the difficulty of living with two disorders, but also provide limit setting.
- Assist patients in setting a goal to stop drug or alcohol use. Explore patients' perceptions of the relationship between their substance use and their psychiatric disorders. As part of this process, also explore the longer term relationship between the two (e.g., an individual may report drinking to reduce social anxiety and feel initially better, but then may feel worse the following day) and discuss the advantages of a drug-free life.
- Educate patients and their family members about the symptoms of both disorders and the causal connections between them.
- Monitor symptoms of both disorders (including the use of biological measures such as urine screens for substance use when indicated).
- Monitor adherence to medications, since nonadherence is a significant risk for relapse.
- To improve functioning and foster the rewards of abstinence, assist patients in developing social, relationship, or vocational skills.
- Attend to patient safety, including attention to human immunodeficiency virus (HIV) and suicidal ideation (both of which have been found to be increased in dually diagnosed patients [Mahler, 1995; Weiss & Hufford, 1999]).
- Have available resources to refer patients to self-help groups for each disorder.
- Discuss with patients what to do and whom to call in case of emergency.
- Provide positive reinforcement for improvements, however small, in each disorder.
- For patients who have had significant periods of recovery, acknowledge these successes and, in a positive way, ask them how they accomplished it. Doing so reminds patients of prior successes and can mitigate the feelings of hopelessness and discouragement that often accompany relapse.
- Take a relapse history to help identify triggers to relapse (e.g., discontinuing medications or treatment, engaging in high-risk behaviors such as socializing where alcohol is present).
- Expect occasional breaks in treatment attendance, and engage in active outreach.

PHARMACOTHERAPY FOR DUALLY DIAGNOSED PATIENTS

During the past decade, the literature regarding when to prescribe pharmaco-therapy for dually diagnosed patients has changed considerably. Previous consensus in the field reflected reluctance to prescribe psychotropic medications in these populations. However, this consensus was based on earlier, method-ologically flawed studies. For example, older studies examining the use of antidepressants in alcoholics often did not use standardized methods to assess the depressed population, had inadequate dosing or duration of antidepres-sants, and sometimes measured mood or drinking outcomes, but not both (Ciraulo & Jaffe, 1981). More recent studies have demonstrated that phar-macotherapy can improve outcomes for the psychiatric disorder and some-times for the SUD as well (Greenfield et al., 1998; Schubiner et al., 2002). Still, it is important also to incorporate psychosocial treatments directed at improving substance use outcomes when treating dually diagnosed patients. The literature on treatments for specific psychiatric disorders is reviewed below.

Major Depression

Nunes and Levin (2004) performed a meta-analysis of antidepressant medica-tion efficacy for the treatment of co-occurring depression and SUD. The results indicated that in this patient population, the efficacy of antidepressants is com-parable to that seen in patients with depression alone. Studies that required at least 1 week of abstinence before treating the depression yielded larger effect sizes and lower placebo response, suggesting that requiring even at least 1 week of abstinence before initiating medication treatment can successfully screen out transient depressive symptoms. Also, studies that exhibited better depression outcomes as a result of antidepressants also showed decreased quantity of sub-stance use. However, rates of sustained abstinence or SUD remission were low across studies, highlighting the importance of treatment directed at the SUD as well when treating these patients.

Bipolar Disorder

Although face validity would suggest that stabilizing mania or hypomania in patients with bipolar disorder would improve impulse control and judgment, and therefore lead to decreases in substance use, the literature is thin regarding the efficacy of mood stabilizing medications on bipolar and SUD outcomes. An open pilot trial by Gawin and Kleber (1984) suggested that lithium may be effective in reducing cocaine use in patients with cyclothymia and cocaine abuse. However, an open trial of lithium in patients with bipolar spectrum dis-orders and cocaine abuse (Nunes, McGrath, Wager, & Quitkin, 1990) demonstrated little efficacy in mood or cocaine outcome measures. An open label trial with valproate in patients with bipolar disorder and SUD (Brady, Sonne, Anton, & Ballenger, 1995) resulted in improvement in mood and substance use measures. Additionally, open-label trials of lamotrigine (Brown, Nejtek, Perantie, Orsulak, & Bobadilla, 2003) and quetiapine (Brown, Nejtek, Perantie, & Bobadilla, 2002) in patients with bipolar disorder and cocaine dependence suggest that these medications may be associated with improved mood symptoms and cocaine craving, although not with significant reductions in cocaine use. Since there have been no double-blind, placebo-controlled studies assessing the efficacy of mood stabilizers or antipsychotic medications in adults with bipolar disorder and SUDs, the results of these open trials can be seen as preliminary at best. However a double-blind, placebo-controlled, 6-week trial of lithium in adolescents with bipolar disorder and substance dependence (Geller et al., 1998) found lithium to be efficacious for outcomes in both disorders.

Schizophrenia

Unfortunately, the literature on the pharmacological treatment of patients with schizophrenia and SUDs is limited to retrospective or open-label prospective studies, some of which lack a comparison group. For example, an open trial of desipramine added to antipsychotic treatment in an integrated dual-diagnosis relapse prevention program has shown promise in reducing cocaine use and improving psychiatric symptoms (Ziedonis, Richardson, Lee, Petrakis, & Kosten, 1992). Additionally, preliminary reports suggest that there may be a potential benefit of second-generation antipsychotic medications such as clozapine (Buckley, Thompson, Way, & Meltzer, 1994; Drake et al., 2000; Zimmet, Strous, Burgess, Kohnstamm, & Green, 2000), olanzapine (Littrell, Petty, Hilligoss, Peabody, & Johnson, 2001), and risperidone (Smelson, Losonczy, Davis, et al., 2002) in improving substance use outcomes in populations with co-occurring schizophrenia. Clozapine has been hypothesized to be uniquely beneficial: Its unique pharmacological receptor activity may correct underlying reward system deficits of patients with schizophrenia and SUDs (Green, Zimmet, Strous, & Schildkraut, 1999; LeDuc & Mittleman, 1995). Additionally, when administered in low doses (50 mg or less) to normal volunteers, clozapine has been shown to attenuate the subjective high and rush associated with cocaine, as well as its pressor effect (Farren et al., 2000).

Despite these encouraging findings, there is evidence from normal study volunteers that low-dose clozapine may increase cocaine blood levels and cause near-syncope (Farren et al., 2000). However, to our knowledge, there are no case reports or studies documenting clinically significant syncopal episodes in patients with schizophrenia and stimulant use disorders who are prescribed clozapine. Thus, while the introduction of second-generation antipsychotics are encouraging in their potential to improve SUD outcomes in this dually diagnosed population, well-designed controlled trials are needed to establish safety, tolerability, and efficacy in this population.

Anxiety Disorders

The use of benzodiazepines in populations with SUDs and co-occurring psychiatric disorders is controversial. This issue has been explored almost exclusively in populations with anxiety and alcohol use disorders. The prevalence of benzodiazepine use among patients with alcohol use disorders is greater than in the general population but comparable to psychiatric disorder populations (Ciraulo, Sands, & Shader, 1988). Clinicians are often understandably concerned that prescribing benzodiazepines to these patients may lead to either a worsening of the alcohol use disorder, the development of a benzodiazepine use disorder, or potentiation of the benzodiazepine effect when combined with alcohol. Preliminary evidence from case reports (Adinoff, 1992) and a prospective naturalistic study (Mueller, Goldenberg, Gordon, Keller, & Warshaw, 1996) suggests that there may be a carefully selected subpopulation of patients with co-occurring alcohol use and anxiety disorders for whom long-term prescription of benzodiazepine may not affect sobriety or result in benzodiazepine misuse. However, it may not improve outcomes either. For example, a retrospective naturalistic study of veterans with PTSD and SUD found that physicians were less likely to prescribe benzodiazepines for those with SUD (Kosten, Fontana, Sernyak, & Rosenheck, 2000). While those with prescribed benzodiazepines did not have worse outcomes, chronic benzodiazepine treatment (independent of a co-occurring SUD) did not improve anxiety or social functioning in these patients either. Similarly, Brunette, Noordsey, Xie, and Drake (2003) followed SPMI patients with SUDs annually for 6 years and found that the rate of benzodiazepine prescribing was high (up to 63%) but not associated with differences in substance use remission, hospitalization, or, interestingly, reductions in anxiety or depression. Also, unsurprisingly, patients prescribed benzodiazepines were more likely to abuse them than those who were not. While controlled trials are needed to explore these issues more fully, the findings from these reports add further to concerns that the long-term use of benzodiazepines in these populations perhaps offers the risk of abuse or dependence without great potential for clinical benefit.

Another pharmacological alternative in this population is buspirone, which does not have abuse potential. Thus far, there have been three double-blind, placebo-controlled studies of buspirone in patients with alcohol dependence and anxiety—generalized anxiety disorder (GAD) (Tollefson, Montague-Clouse, & Tollefson, 1992), GAD and "other nonpanic anxiety" (Malcolm et al., 1992), or "anxious alcoholics" (Kranzler et al., 1994). Two of the studies found buspirone to be associated with improvements in anxiety and alcohol use outcomes (Kranzler et al., 1994; Tollefson et al., 1992). Although there have been concerns that buspirone's antianxiety effect is more limited in patients with a prior history of benzodiazepine use (Schweizer, Rickels, & Lucki, 1986), a pooled analysis of eight placebo-controlled randomized trials of patients with GAD (DeMartinis, Rynn, Rickels, & Mandos, 2000) found that patients with either remote (defined as at least 1 month duration) or no prior benzodiazepine treatment experienced improved anxiolysis, fewer adverse events, and clinical improvement similar to that with benzodiazepines compared to patients with recent benzodiazepine treatment. Thus, patients who have not received benzodiazepines for at least 1 month may benefit from buspirone.

Attention-Deficit/Hyperactivity Disorder

Although stimulants have been the most extensively studied treatment for adult attention-deficit/hyperactivity disorder (ADHD) (Levin, Evans, & Kleber, 1999), there are concerns that they may worsen the course of the SUDs or be subject to abuse themselves in dually diagnosed populations (Gawin, Riordan, & Kleber, 1985). At the same time, it has also been observed that a childhood history of ADHD worsens outcomes for cocaine dependence (Carroll & Rounsaville, 1993). Therefore, improving a patient's difficulties with inattention and hyperactivity may have beneficial effects on substance abuse as well (Levin et al., 1999). Consistent with this, prospective studies of children who received stimulant treatment for ADHD indicate that stimulants have a protective effect against future development of SUDs as an adult (Wilens, 2001).

Although not as well-studied as stimulants, nonstimulant medications that lack abuse potential are possible alternatives in the treatment of ADHD. In adult populations, only bupropion (Wilens et al., 2002), desipramine (Wilens et al., 1996), and atomoxetine (Michelson et al., 2003) have undergone double-blind, placebo-controlled study and demonstrated effectiveness in the treatment of hyperactivity and inattention. However, none of these trials included patients with active SUDs. To our knowledge, the only published trials of antidepressants as treatment for ADHD in populations with a current co-occurring SUD are a single-blind trial of bupropion for adult ADHD and cocaine abuse (Levin, Evans, McDowell, Brooks, & Nunes, 2002), and an open-label study of venlafaxine in patients with ADHD and alcohol use disorder (Upadhyaya, Brady, Sethuraman, Sonne, & Malcolm, 2001). Both showed improvements in hyperactivity and inattention, as well as improved substance use outcomes. However, these results need to be replicated in larger, more rigorous studies.

Clinical trials of methylphenidate in adults with ADHD and a history of cocaine use disorders have also shown promising results. Both open-label trials of long-acting methylphenidate (Castaneda et al., 2000; Levin, Evans, McDowell, & Kleber, 1998) and a double-blind, placebo-controlled study of regular methylphenidate (Schubiner et al., 2002) in adults with ADHD and cocaine dependence have all been consistent in that ADHD symptoms improved, and no escalation of the stimulant dose was observed. However, while the open trial by Levin and colleagues (1998) indicated reductions in cocaine craving and use, Schubiner and colleagues (2002) found no evidence of improved cocaine outcomes in their double-blind, placebo-controlled trial. Pemoline is a stimulant thought to have lower abuse potential than methylphenidate. However, there are no controlled trials of pemoline in this population, and its increased risk of hepatotoxicity, while small, makes its safety in this population unclear (Levin, Evans, & Kleber, 1999). Despite limited evidence that stimulants may be safely used in this population to treat ADHD without worsening SUD outcomes (and perhaps improving them), their use in these patients remains controversial.

What to Do When the Pharmacological Treatment for the Co-Occurring Psychiatric Disorder Has Abuse Potential

As evidenced in numerous studies, treating a co-occurring psychiatric disorder can often have positive outcomes in both reducing substance use and helping the specific psychiatric disorder for which it is prescribed. However, what if the pharmacological treatment has the potential to worsen or create a new SUD? This dilemma is often considered in treating patients who suffer with SUDs and co-occurring anxiety disorders or ADHD, when clinicians ask themselves, "Is it safe to prescribe stimulants/benzodiazepines for this patient?"

Pharmacotherapies that do not have abuse potential should be considered first-line treatments before prescribing stimulants or benzodiazepines in these populations (Ciraulo & Nace, 2000; Levin et al., 1999), and it is important that patients receive adequate trials (i.e., dose and duration) of these medications before they are abandoned. Psychosocial treatments with demonstrated efficacy should also be tried before prescribing an abusable medication. For example, CBT has demonstrated efficacy for anxiety disorders (Beck et al., 1993) and should be explored before prescribing a benzodiazepine. If these first-line treatments fail to improve the anxiety or ADHD symptoms adequately, then the following guidelines are suggested when prescribing stimulants or benzodiazepines in these patient populations (Ciraulo & Nace, 2000; Levin et al., 1999):

- *Select preparations that limit the potential for abuse.* Medications with longer half-lives or sustained-release preparations have lower abuse potential and are therefore preferable in these populations. Select as low a dose as possible. For benzodiazepines, avoid as-needed-basis prescribing in lieu of a fixed dosing schedule. Limit the number of pills given with each prescription, and keep a log of the pills prescribed. Frequent patient contact can help the clinician assess whether the medication is helpful, as well as whether it is being overused.
- *Use objective measures to document improvements.* For example, using a

standardized assessment such as the Adult Behavior Checklist (Murphy & Barkley, 1996) or the Beck Anxiety Inventory (Beck, Epstein, Brown, & Steer, 1988) can help document improvements (or lack thereof).

- *Monitor substance use.* Patients should be asked about alcohol and drug use, and other sources of information (urine screens, collateral information from family members) should be strongly considered.
- *Enlist family members in supporting and monitoring the patient.* Verify the efficacy and appropriate use of the medication with family members.
- *Patients should safeguard medications.* While the patient may not abuse the medication, family members may.
- *Monitor prescriptions.* Keep careful track of the number of pills you prescribe, and beware of warning signs of abuse, such as premature requests for refills or "lost prescriptions." These usually indicate overuse of the medication.

Pharmacotherapy Targeting Substance Dependence in Dually Diagnosed Populations

Although pharmacotherapies aimed specifically at decreasing alcohol or drug use (e.g., naltrexone, disulfiram) can be efficacious in improving SUD outcomes in non-dually-diagnosed populations, the literature on the use of these medications in dually diagnosed populations is quite thin. Concerns that disulfiram may cause or exacerbate psychosis (Mueser, Noordsy, Fox, & Wolfe, 2003) have contributed to a reluctance to prescribe it in patients with SPMI (Kingsbury & Salzman, 1990). While there have been no controlled studies of disulfiram in populations with alcohol dependence and SPMI, there have been a few published case reports (Brenner, Karper, & Krystal, 1994) and case series (Kofoed, Kania, Walsh, & Atkinson, 1986; Mueser et al., 2003) describing its tolerability and potential benefit for improving alcohol outcomes and hospitalization rates for those who remain in treatment. Additionally, there is preliminary evidence that naltrexone may improve drinking outcomes in patients with alcohol dependence and schizophrenia (Batki et al., 2002) or major depression (Salloum et al., 1998). The benefit or tolerability of naltrexone in patients with bipolar disorder and alcohol disorders is less clear, based on one case report (Sonne & Brady, 2000).

INTEGRATION OF PSYCHOTHERAPY AND PHARMACOTHERAPY FOR DUALLY DIAGNOSED PATIENTS

Integrated psychosocial treatments are increasingly accepted and provided to patients as more and varied evidence accrues regarding their benefits. However, there continue to be few trials that integrate novel psychosocial treatments with novel pharmacotherapies. Instead, most treatments either focus on new pharmacological or new psychosocial interventions. Despite this, more recent research has emphasized the importance of integrating pharmacological and psychotherapeutic treatment options.

FUTURE DIRECTIONS

In the approximately 20 years since researchers and clinicians in the mental health and addictions fields first noted the high prevalence rate of comorbidity and poorer outcomes in dually diagnosed populations, important strides have been made in further understanding the epidemiology and sequelae of these disorders, as well as the critical need to develop specific treatments for these populations. Significant progress has been made in developing new treatments, testing them with increasing methodological rigor, and developing optimal treatment methods for these often poorly served patient populations. In the next decade, we are hopeful that this continued research effort will translate into improved treatment methods and outcomes in these patients.

ACKNOWLEDGMENTS

This work was supported by Grant Nos. K02 DA00326 (Dr. Weiss), R01 DA015968 (Drs. Busch and Weiss), U10 DA015831 (Drs. Busch, Weiss, and Najavits), and K02 DA00400 (Dr. Najavits) from the National Institute on Drug Abuse.

REFERENCES

Adinoff, B. (1992). Long-term therapy with benzodiazepines despite alcohol dependence disorder. *Am J Addict, 1*(4), 288–293.

Aharonovich, E., Nguyen, H. T., & Nunes, E. V. (2001). Anger and depressive states among treatment-seeking drug abusers: Testing the psychopharmacological specificity hypothesis. *Am J Addict, 10*(4), 327–334.

Albanese, M. J., Bartel, R. L., Bruno, R. F., Morgenbesser, M. W., & Schatzberg, A. F. (1994). Comparison of measures used to determine substance abuse in an inpatient psychiatric population. *Am J Psychiatry, 151*(7), 1077–1078.

Alcoholics Anonymous. (1984). *The AA member: Medications and other drugs* [Brochure]. New York: Alcoholics Anonymous World Services.

American Psychiatric Association. (1987). *Diagnostic and statistical manual of mental disorders* (3rd ed., rev.). Washington, DC: Author.

American Psychiatric Association. (2000). *Diagnostic and statistical manual of mental disorders* (4th ed.). Washington, DC: Author.

Ball, S. A. (1998). Manualized treatment for substance abusers with personality disorders: Dual focus schema therapy. *Addict Behav, 23*(6), 883–891.

Barrowclough, C., Haddock, G., Tarrier, N., Lewis, S. W., Moring, J., O'Brien, R., et al. (2001). Randomized controlled trial of motivational interviewing, cognitive behavior therapy, and family intervention for patients with comorbid schizophrenia and substance use disorders. *Am J Psychiatry, 158*(10), 1706–1713.

Batki, S. L., Dimmock, J., Cornell, M., Wade, M., Carey, K. B., & Maisto, S. A. (2002). *Directly observed naltrexone treatment of alcohol dependence in schizophrenia: Preliminary analysis.* San Francisco: Research Society on Alcoholism.

Beck, A. T., Epstein, N., Brown, G., & Steer, R. A. (1988). An inventory for measuring clinical anxiety—psychometric properties. *J Consult Clin Psychol, 56,* 893–898.

Beck, A. T., Rush, A. J., Shaw, B. F., & Emery, G. (1979). *Cognitive therapy of depression.* New York: Guilford Press.

Beck, A. T., Wright, F. D., Newman, C. F., & Liese, B. S. (1993). *Cognitive therapy of substance abuse.* New York: Guilford Press.

Bellack, A. S., & DiClemente, C. (1999). Treating substance abuse among patients with schizophrenia. *Psychiatr Serv, 50*(1), 75–80.

Bowers, M. B., Mazure, C. M., Nelson, J. C., & Jatlow, P. I. (1990) Psychotogenic drug use and neuroleptic response. *Schizophr Bull, 16*(1), 81–85.

Brady, K. T., Dansky, B. S., Back, S. E., Foa, E. B., & Carroll, K. M. (2001). Exposure therapy in the treatment of PTSD among cocaine-dependent individuals: Preliminary findings. *J Subst Abuse Treat, 21*(1), 47–54.

Brady, K. T., Sonne, S. C., Anton, R., & Ballenger, J. C. (1995). Valproate in the treatment of acute bipolar affective episodes complicated by substance abuse: A pilot study. *J Clin Psychiatry, 56*(3), 118–121.

Breakey, W. R., Calabrese, L., Rosenblatt, A., & Crum, R. M. (1998). Detecting alcohol use disorders in the severely mentally ill. *Community Ment Health J, 34*(2), 165–174.

Brenner, L. M., Karper, L. P., & Krystal, J. H. (1994). Short-term use of disulfiram with clozapine. *J Clin Psychopharmacol, 14*(3), 213–215.

Brooks, A. J., & Penn, P. E. (2003). Comparing treatments for dual diagnosis: Twelve-step and self-management and recovery training. *Am J Drug Alcohol Abuse, 29*(2), 359–383.

Brown, E. S., Nejtek, V. A., Perantie, D. C., & Bobadilla, L. (2002). Quetiapine in bipolar disorder and cocaine dependence. *Bipolar Disord, 4*(6), 406–411.

Brown, E. S., Nejtek, V. A., Perantie, D. C., Orsulak, P. J., & Bobadilla, L. (2003). Lamotrigine in patients with bipolar disorder and cocaine dependence. *J Clin Psychiatry, 64*(2), 197–201.

Brown, R. A., Monti, P. M., Myers, M. G., Martin, R. A., Rivinus, T., Dubreuil, M. E., & Rohsenow, D. J. (1998). Depression among cocaine abusers in treatment: Relation to cocaine and alcohol use and treatment outcome. *Am J Psychiatry, 155*(2), 220–225.

Brown, S. A., Irwin, M., & Schuckit, M. A. (1991). Changes in anxiety among abstinent male alcoholics. *J Stud Alcohol, 52*(1), 55–61.

Brown, S. A., & Schuckit, M. A. (1988). Changes in depression among abstinent alcoholics. *J Stud Alcohol, 49*(5), 412–417.

Brunette, M. F., Mueser, K. T., Xie, H., & Drake, R. E. (1997). Relationships between symptoms of schizophrenia and substance abuse. *J Nerv Ment Dis, 185*(1), 13–20.

Brunette, M. F., Noordsey, D. L., Xie, H., & Drake, R. E. (2003). Benzodiazepine use and abuse among patients with severe mental illness and co-occurring substance use disorders. *Psychiatr Serv*, *54*(10), 1395–1401.

Buckley, P., Thompson, P., Way, L., & Meltzer, H. Y. (1994). Substance abuse among patients with treatment-resistant schizophrenia: Characteristics and implications for clozapine therapy. *Am J Psychiatry*, *151*(3), 385–389.

Cacciola, J. S., Alterman, A. I., Rutherford, M. J., & Snider, E. C. (1995). Treatment response of antisocial substance abusers. *J Nerv Ment Dis*, *183*, 166–171.

Carey, K. B. (1995). Treatment of substance use disorders and schizophrenia. In A. F. Lehman & L. B. Dixon (Eds.), *Double jeopardy: Chronic mental illness and substance use disorders* (pp. 85–108). Chur, Switzerland: Harwood.

Carey, K. B., Carey, M. P., Maisto, S. A., & Purnine, D. M. (2002). The feasibility of enhancing psychiatric outpatients' readiness to change their substance use. *Psychiatr Serv*, *53*(5), 602–608.

Carey, K. B., Purnine, D. M., Maisto, S. A., & Carey, M. P. (2001). Enhancing readiness-to-change substance abuse in persons with schizophrenia: A four-session motivation-based intervention. *Behav Modif*, *25*(3), 331–384.

Carroll, K. M., & Rounsaville, B. J. (1993). History and significance of childhood attention deficit disorder in treament-seeking cocaine abusers. *Compr Psychiatry*, *34*, 75–86.

Castaneda, R., Levy, R., Hardy, M., & Trujillo, M. (2000). Long-acting stimulants for the treatment of attention-deficit disorder in cocaine-dependent adults. *Psychiatr Serv*, *51*, 169–171.

Ciraulo, D. A., & Jaffe, J. H. (1981). Tricyclic antidepressants in the treatment of depression associated with alcoholism. *J Clin Pharmacol*, *1*, 146–150.

Ciraulo, D. A., & Nace, E. P. (2000). Benzodiazepine treatment of anxiety or insomnia in substance abuse patients. *Am J Addict*, *9*(4), 276–284.

Ciraulo, D. A., Sands, B. F., & Shader, R. I. (1988). Critical review of the liability of benzodiazepine abuse among alcoholics. *Am J Psychiatry*, *145*(12), 1501–1506.

Claassen, C. A., Gilfillan, S., Orsulak, P., Carmody, T. J., Battaglia, J., & Rush, A. J. (1997). Substance use among patients with a psychotic disorder in a psychiatric emergency room. *Psychiatr Serv*, *48*(3), 353–358.

Compton, W. M., Cottler, L. B., Jacobs, J. L., Ben-Abdallah, A., & Spitznagel, E. L. (2003). The role of psychiatric disorders in predicting drug dependence treatment outcomes. *Am J Psychiatry*, *160*(5), 890–895.

Cornelius, J. R., Salloum, I. M., Ehler, J. G., Jarrett, P. J., Cornelius, M. D., Perel, J. M., et al. (1997). Fluoxetine in depressed alcoholics: A double-blind, placebo-controlled trial. *Arch Gen Psychiatry*, *54*(8), 700–705.

Daley, D. C., & Zuckoff, A. (1998). Improving compliance with the initial outpatient session among discharged inpatient dual diagnosis clients. *Soc Work*, *43*, 470–473.

DeMartinis, N., Rynn, M., Rickels, K., & Mandos, L. (2000). Prior benzodiazepine use and buspirone response in the treatment of generalized anxiety disorder. *J Clin Psychiatry*, *61*(2), 91–94.

Dickey, B., & Azeni, H. (1996). Persons with dual diagnoses of substance abuse and major mental illness: Their excess costs of psychiatric care. *Am J Public Health*, *86*(7), 973–977.

Drake, R. E., Essock, S. M., Shaner, A., Carey, K. B., Minkoff, K., Kola, L., et al. (2001).

Implementing dual diagnosis services for clients with severe mental illness. *Psychiatr Serv, 52*(4), 469–476.

Drake, R. E., McHugo, G. J., Clark, R. E., Teague, G. B., Xie, H., Miles, K., & Ackerson, T. H. (1998). Assertive community treatment for patients with co-occurring severe mental illness and substance use disorder: A clinical trial. *Am J Orthopsychiatry, 68,* 201–215.

Drake, R. E., & Mueser, K. T. (2000). Psychosocial approaches to dual diagnosis. *Schizophr Bull, 26,* 105–118.

Drake, R. E., Osher, F. C., & Wallach, M. A. (1989). Alcohol use and abuse in schizophrenia: A prospective community study. *J Nerv Ment Dis, 177,* 408–414.

Drake, R. E., Xie, H., McHugo, G. J., & Green, A. I. (2000). The effects of clozapine on alcohol and drug use disorders among patients with schizophrenia. *Schizophr Bull, 26,* 441–449.

Drake, R. E., Yovetich, N. A., Bebout, R. R., Harris, M., & McHugo, G. J. (1997). Integrated treatment for dually diagnosed homeless adults. *J Nerv Ment Dis, 185,* 298–305.

Ewing, J. A. (1984). Detecting alcoholism: The CAGE questionnaire. *JAMA, 252,* 1905–1907.

Fals-Stewart, W., & Schafer, J. (1992). The treatment of substance abusers diagnosed with obsessive–compulsive disorder: An outcome study. *J Subst Abuse Treat, 9,* 365–370.

Farren, C. K., Hameedi, F. A., Rosen, M. A., Woods, S., Jatlow, P., & Kosten, T. R. (2000). Significant interaction between clozapine and cocaine in cocaine addicts. *Drug Alcohol Depend, 59,* 153–163.

Farris, C., Brems, C., Johnson, M. E., Well, R., Burns, R., & Kletti, N. (2003). A comparison of schizophrenic patients with or without coexisting substance use disorder. *Psychiatr Q, 74,* 205–222.

Fisher, M. S., & Bentley, K. J. (1996). Two group therapy models for clients with a dual diagnosis of substance abuse and personality disorder. *Psychiatr Serv, 47,* 1244–1250.

Gawin, F., & Kleber, H. D. (1986). Abstinence symptomatology and psychiatric diagnoses in cocaine abusers: Clinical observations. *Arch Gen Psychiatry, 43,* 107–113.

Gawin, F., Riordan, C., & Kleber, H. (1985). Methylphenidate treatment of cocaine abusers without attention deficit disorder: A negative report. *Am J Drug Alcohol Abuse, 11,* 193–297.

Gawin, F. H., & Kleber, H. D. (1984). Cocaine abuse treatment: Open pilot trial with desipramine and lithium carbonate. *Arch Gen Psychiatry, 41,* 903–909.

Geller, B., Cooper, T. B., Sun, K., Zimerman, B., Frazier, J., Williams, M., & Heath, J. (1998). Double-blind and placebo-controlled study of lithium for adolescent bipolar disorders with secondary substance dependency. *J Am Acad Child Adolesc Psychiatry, 37,* 171–178.

Gonzalez, G., & Rosenheck, R. A. (2002). Outcomes and service use among homeless persons with serious mental illness and substance abuse. *Psychiatr Serv, 53,* 437–446.

Graeber, D. A., Moyers, T. B., Griffith, G., Guajardo, E., & Tonigan, S. (2003). A pilot study comparing motivational interviewing and an educational intervention in patients with schizophrenia and alcohol use disorders. *Community Ment Health J,* *39,* 189–202.

Green, A. I., Zimmet, S. V., Strous, R. D., & Schildkraut, J. J. (1999). Clozapine for comorbid substance use disorder and schizophrenia: Do patients with schizophrenia have a reward-deficiency syndrome that can be ameliorated by clozapine? *Harv Rev Psychiatry,* *6,* 287–296.

Greenfield, S. F., Weiss, R. D., Muenz, L. R., Vagge, L. M., Kelly, J. F., Bello, L. R., & Michael, J. (1998). The effect of depression on return to drinking: A prospective study. *Arch Gen Psychiatry,* *55,* 259–265.

Hasin, D. S., Tsai, W.-Y., Endicott, J., & Mueller, T. I. (1996). The effects of major depression on alcoholism: Five-year course. *Am J Addict,* *5,* 144–155.

Helmus, T. C., Rhodes, G., Haber, M., & Downey, K. K. (2001). Reinforcement of counseling attendance utilizing a high and low magnitude of reinforcement in a 22-day detoxifcation program. *Drug Alcohol Depend,* *63*(Suppl 1), 65.

Helmus, T. C., Saules, K. K., Schoener, E. P., & Roll, J. M. (2003). Reinforcement of counseling attendance and alcohol abstinence in a community-based dual-diagnosis treatment program: A feasibility study. *Psychol Addict Behav,* *17,* 249–251.

Higgins, S. T., Budney, A. J., Bickel, W. K., Foerg, F. E., Donham, R., & Badger, G. J. (1994). Incentives improve outcome in outpatient behavioral treatment of cocaine dependence. *Arch Gen Psychiatry,* *51,* 568–576.

Humphreys, K. (1997). Clinicians' referral and matching of substance abuse patients to self-help groups after treatment. *Psychiatr Serv,* *48,* 1445–1449.

Jaffe, J. H., & Ciraulo, D. A. (1986). Alcoholism and depression. In R. E. Meyer (Ed.), *Psychopathology and addictive disorders* (pp. 293–320). New York: Guilford Press.

Jeffery, D. P., Ley, A., McLaren, S., & Siegfried, N. (2004). Psychosocial treatment programmes for people with both severe mental illness and substance misuse. *Cochrane Database Syst Rev,* *4.*

Jerrell, J. M., & Ridgely, M. S. (1995). Comparative effectiveness of three approaches to serving people with severe mental illness and substance abuse disorders. *J Nerv Ment Dis,* *183,* 566–576.

Kessler, R. C., Crum, R. M., Warner, L. A., Nelson, C. B., Schulenberg, J., & Anthony, J. C. (1997). Lifetime co-occurrence of DSM-III-R alcohol abuse and dependence with other psychiatric disorders in the National Comorbidity Survey. *Arch Gen Psychiatry,* *54,* 313–321.

Kessler, R. C., Nelson, C. B., McGonagle, K. A., Edlund, M. J., Frank, R. G., & Leaf, P. J. (1996). The epidemiology of co-occurring addictive and mental disorders: Implications for prevention and service utilization. *Am J Orthopsychiatry,* *66,* 17–31.

Khantzian, E. J. (1985). The self-medication hypothesis of addictive disorders: focus on heroin and cocaine dependence. *Am J Psychiatry,* *142,* 1259–1264.

Khantzian, E. J. (1989). Addiction: Self-destruction or self-repair? *J Subst Abuse Treat,* *6*(2), 75.

Khantzian, E. J. (1997). The self-medication hypothesis of substance use disorders: A reconsideration and recent applications. *Harv Rev Psychiatry,* *4,* 231–244.

Kingsbury, S. J., & Salzman, C. (1990). Disulfiram in the treatment of alcoholic patients with schizophrenia. *Hosp Commun Psychiatry,* *41,* 133–134.

Kofoed, L., Kania, J., Walsh, T., & Atkinson, R. M. (1986). Outpatient treatment of patients with substance abuse and coexisting psychiatric disorders. *Am J Psychiatry, 143*, 867–872.

Kosten, T. R., Fontana, A., Sernyak, M. J., & Rosenheck, R. (2000). Benzodiazepine use in posttraumatic stress disorder among veterans with substance abuse. *J Nerv Ment Dis, 188*, 454–459.

Kranzler, H. R., Burleson, J. A., Del Boca, F. K., Babor, T. F., Korner, P., Brown, J., & Bohn, M. J. (1994). Buspirone treatment of anxious alcoholics: A placebo-controlled trial. *Arch Gen Psychiatry, 51*, 720–731.

Kranzler, H. R., Del Boca, F. K., & Rounsaville, B. J. (1996). Comorbid psychiatric diagnosis predicts three-year outcomes in alcoholics: A posttreatment natural history study. *J Stud Alcohol, 57*, 619–626.

Kurtz, L. F. (1997). *Self-help and support groups: A handbook for practitioners.* Thousand Oaks, CA: Sage.

LeDuc, P., & Mittleman, G. (1995). Schizophrenia and psychostimulant abuse: A review and re-analysis of clinical evidence. *Psychopharmacology, 121*, 407–427.

Levin, F. R., Evans, S. M., & Kleber, H. D. (1999). Practical guidelines for the treatment of substance abusers with adult attention-deficit hyperactivity disorder. *Psychiatr Serv, 50*, 1001–1003.

Levin, F. R., Evans, S. M., McDowell, D. M., Brooks, D. M., & Nunes, E. (2002). Bupropion treatment for cocaine abuse and adult attention-deficit/hyperactivity disorder. *J Addict Dis, 21*, 1–16.

Levin, F. R., Evans, S. M., McDowell, D. M., & Kleber, H. D. (1998). Methylphenidate treatment for cocaine abusers with adult attention-deficit/hyperactivity disorder: A pilot study. *J Clin Psychiatry, 59*, 300–305.

Liebson, I. A., Tommasello, A., & Bigelow, G. E. (1978). A behavioral treatment of alcoholic methadone patients. *Ann Intern Med, 89*, 342–344.

Linehan, M. M. (1993). Dialectical behavior therapy for treatment of borderline personality disorder: Implications for the treatment of substance abuse. In L. S. Onken, J. D. Blaine, & J. J. Boren (Eds.), *Behavioral treatments for drug abuse and dependence* (NIDA Research Monograph No. 137, DHHS Publication No. 93-3684, pp. 201–216). Washington, DC: U.S. Government Printing Office.

Linehan, M. M., Dimeff, L. A., Reynolds, S. K., Comtois, K. A., Welch, S. S., Heagerty, P., & Kivlahan, D. R. (2002). Dialectal behavior therapy versus comprehensive validation therapy plus 12-step for the treatment of opioid dependent women meeting criteria for borderline personality disorder. *Drug Alcohol Depend, 67*, 13–26.

Littrell, K. H., Petty, R. G., Hilligoss, N. M., Peabody, C. D., & Johnson, C. G. (2001). Olanzapine treatment for patients with schizophrenia and substance abuse. *J Subst Abuse Treat, 21*, 217–221.

Magura, S., Laudet, A. B., Mahmood, D., Rosenblum, A., & Knight, E. (2002). Adherence to medication regimens and participation in dual-focus self-help groups. *Psychiatr Serv, 53*, 310–316.

Magura, S., Laudet, A. B., Mahmood, D., Rosenblum, A., Vogel, H. S., & Knight, E. L. (2003). Role of self-help processes in achieving abstinence among dually diagnosed persons. *Addict Behav, 28*, 399–413.

Mahler, J. (1995). HIV, substance use, and chronic mental illness. In A. F. Lehman & L. B. Dixon (Eds.), *Double jeopardy: Chronic mental illness and substance use disorders* (pp. 159–175). Chur, Switzerland: Harwood.

Malcolm, R., Anton, R. F., Randall, C. L., Johnston, A., Brady, K., & Thevos, A. (1992). A placebo-controlled trial of buspirone in anxious inpatient alcoholics. *Alcohol Clin Exp Res, 16,* 1007–10013.

Mark, T. L. (2003). The costs of treating persons with depression and alcoholism compared with depression alone. *Psychiatr Serv, 54,* 1095–1097.

Marlatt, G. A., & Gordon, G. R. (1985). *Relapse prevention: Maintenance strategies in the treatment of addictive behaviors.* New York: Guilford Press.

Martino, S., Carroll, K., Kostas, D., Perkins, J., & Rounsaville, B. (2002). Dual diagnosis motivational interviewing: A modification of motivational interviewing for substance-abusing patients with psychotic disorders. *J Subst Abuse Treat, 23,* 297–308.

McHugo, G. J., Drake, R. E., Teague, G. B., & Xie, H. (1999). Fidelity to assertive community treatment and client outcomes in New Hampshire Dual Disorders study. *Psychiatr Serv, 50,* 818–824.

McKay, J. R., Pettinati, H. M., Morrison, R., Feeley, M., Mulvaney, F. D., & Gallop, R. (2002). Relation of depression diagnoses to 2-year outcomes in cocaine-dependent patients in a randomized continuing care study. *Psychol Addict Behav, 16,* 225–235.

McLellan, A. T., & Druley, K. A. (1977). Non-random relation between drugs of abuse and psychiatric diagnosis. *J Psychiatr Res, 13,* 179–184.

Meissen, G., Powell, T. J., Wituk, S. A., Girrens, K., & Arteaga, S. A. (1999). Attitudes of AA contact persons toward group participation by persons with a mental illness. *Psychiatr Serv, 50,* 1079–1081.

Mendelson, J. H., & Mello, N. K. (1966). Experimental analysis of drinking behavior of chronic alcoholics. *Ann NY Acad Sci, 133,* 828–845.

Mercer, D. E., & Woody, G. E. (1999). *An individual drug counseling approach to treat cocaine addiction: The collaborative cocaine treatment study model* (Therapy Manuals for Drug Abuse No. 3). Rockville, MD: U.S. Department of Health and Human Services, National Institute on Drug Abuse.

Meyer, R. E. (1986). How to understand the relationship between psychopathology and addictive disorders: Another example of the chicken and the egg. In R. E. Meyer (Ed.), *Psychopathology and addictive disorders* (pp. 3–16). New York: Guilford Press.

Meyer, R. E., & Mirin, S. M. (1979). *The heroin stimulus: Implications for a theory of addiction.* New York: Plenum Press.

Michelson, D., Adler, L., Spencer, T., Reimherr, F. W., West, S. A., Allen, A. J., et al. (2003). Atomoxetine in adults with ADHD: Two randomized, placebo-controlled studies. *Biol Psychiatry, 53,* 112–120.

Miller, N. S., Ninonuevo, F. G., Klamen, G. L., Hoffmann, N. G., & Smith, D. E. (1997). Integration of treatment and posttreatment variables in predicting results of abstinence-based outpatient treatment after one year. *J Psychoactive Drugs, 29,* 239–248.

Miller, W. R., & Rollnick, S. (1991). *Motivational interviewing: Preparing people to change addictive behavior.* New York: Guilford Press.

Miller, W. R., & Rollnick, S. (2002). *Motivational interviewing: Preparing people for change* (2nd ed.). New York: Guilford Press.

Mueller, T. I., Goldenberg, I. M., Gordon, A. L., Keller, M. B., & Warshaw, M. G. (1996). Benzodiazepine use in anxiety disordered patients with and without a history of alcoholism. *J Clin Psychiatry, 57,* 83–89.

Mueller, T. I., Lavori, P. W., Keller, M. B., Swartz, A., Warshaw, M. G., Hasin, D., et al. (1994). Prognostic effect of the variable course of alcoholism on the 10-year course of depression. *Am J Psychiatry, 151,* 701–706.

Mueser, K. T., Bellack, A. S., & Blanchard, J. J. (1992). Comorbidity of schizophrenia and substance abuse: Implications for treatment. *J Consult Clin Psychol, 60,* 845–856.

Mueser, K. T., & Fox, L. (2002). A family intervention program for dual disorders. *Community Ment Health J, 38,* 253–270.

Mueser, K. T., Noordsy, D. L., Fox, L., & Wolfe, R. (2003). Disulfiram treatment for alcoholism in severe mental illness. *Am J Addict, 12,* 242–252.

Murphy, K. R., & Barkley, R. A. (1996). Prevalence of DSM-IV symptoms of ADHD in adult licensed drivers. *J Atten Disord, 1,* 147–161.

Najavits, L. M. (2004). Assessment of trauma, PTSD, and substance use disorder: A practical guide. In J. P. Wilson & T. Keane (Eds.), *Assessing psychological trauma and PTSD* (pp. 466–491). New York: Guilford Press.

Najavits, L. M., Weiss, R. D., & Liese, B. S. (1996). Group cognitive-behavioral therapy for women with PTSD and substance use disorder. *J Subst Abuse Treat, 13,* 13–22.

Najavits, L. M., Weiss, R. D., Shaw, S. R., & Muenz, L. R. (1998). "Seeking safety": Outcome of a new cognitive-behavioral psychotherapy for women with posttraumatic stress disorder and substance dependence. *J Trauma Stress, 11,* 437–456.

Noordsy, D. L., Schwab, B., Fox, L., & Drake, R. E. (1996). The role of self-help programs in the rehabilitation of persons with severe mental illness and substance use disorders. *Community Ment Health J, 32,* 71–81.

Nowinski, J., Baker, S., & Carroll, K. (1995). *Twelve step facilitation therapy manual: A clinical research guide for therapists treating individuals with alcohol abuse and dependence* (Vol. 1). Rockville, MD: National Institute on Alcohol Abuse and Alcoholism.

Nunes, E. V., & Levin, F. R. (2004). Treatment of depression in patients with alcohol or other drug dependence: A meta-analysis. *JAMA, 291,* 1887–1896.

Nunes, E. V., McGrath, P. J., Wager, S., & Quitkin, F. M. (1990). Lithium treatment for cocaine abusers with bipolar spectrum disorders. *Am J Psychiatry, 147,* 655–657.

Osher, F. C., & Kofoed, L. (1989). Treatment of patients with psychiatric and psychoactive substance use disorders. *Psychiatr Serv, 40,* 1025–1030.

Ouimette, P. C., Gima, K., Moos, R. H., & Finney, J. W. (1999). A comparative evaluation of substance abuse treatment. IV: The effect of comorbid psychiatric diagnoses on amount of treatment, continuing care, and 1-year outcomes. *Alcohol Clin Exp Res, 23,* 552–557.

Petry, N. M. (2000). A comprehensive guide to the application of contingency management procedures in clinical settings. *Drug Alcohol Depend, 58,* 9–25.

Petry, N. M., Martin, B., Cooney, J. L., & Kranzler, H. R. (2000). Give them prizes, and they will come: Contingency management for treatment of alcohol dependence. *J Consult Clin Psychol, 68,* 250–257.

Post, R. M., Kotin, J., & Goodwin, F. K. (1974). The effects of cocaine on depressed patients. *Am J Psychiatry, 131,* 511–517.

Powell, B. J., Penick, E. C., Nickel, E. J., Liskow, B. I., Riesenmy, K. D., Campion, S. L., & Brown, E. F. (1992). Outcomes of co-morbid alcoholic men: A 1-year follow-up. *Alcohol Clin Exp Res, 16,* 131–138.

Prochaska, J. O., DiClemente, C., & Norcross, J. C. (1992). In search of how people change: Applications to addictive behaviors. *Am Psychol, 47,* 1102–1114.

Prochaska, J. O., Norcross, J. C., & DiClemente, C. C. (1994). *Changing for good.* New York: Morrow.

Randall, C. L., Thomas, S., & Thevos, A. K. (2001). Concurrent alcoholism and social anxiety disorder: A first step toward developing effective treatments. *Alcohol Clin Exp Res, 25,* 210–220.

Regier, D. A., Farmer, M. E., Rae, D. S., Locke, B. Z., Keith, S. J., Judd, L. L., & Goodwin, F. K. (1990). Comorbidity of mental disorders with alcohol and other drug abuse: Results from the Epidemiologic Catchment Area (ECA) study. *JAMA, 264,* 2511–2518.

Ridgely, S., Goldman, H. H., & Willenbring, M. (1990). Barriers to the care of persons with dual diagnoses: Organizational and financing issues. *Schizophr Bull, 16,* 123–132.

Ries, R. K., Sloan, K., & Miller, N. (1997). Dual diagnosis: concept, diagnosis, and treatment. In D. Dunner (Ed.), *Current psychiatric therapy* (pp. 173–180). Philadelphia: Saunders.

Ritsher, J. B., McKellar, J. D., Finney, J. W., Otilingam, P. G., & Moos, R. H. (2002). Psychiatric comorbidity, continuing care and mutual help as predictors of five-year remission from substance use disorders. *J Stud Alcohol, 63,* 709–715.

Rohsenow, D. J., Monti, P. M., Martin, R. A., Michalec, E., & Abrams, D. B. (2002). Brief coping skills treatment for cocaine abuse: 12-month substance use outcomes. *J Consult Clin Psychol, 68,* 515–520.

Ross, H. E., Glaser, F. B., & Germanson, T. (1988). The prevalence of psychiatric disorders in patients with alcohol and other drug problems. *Arch Gen Psychiatry, 45,* 1023–1031.

Rousanville, B. J., Anton, S. F., Carroll, K., Budde, D., Prusoff, B. A., & Gawin, F. (1991). Psychiatric diagnosis of treatment-seeking cocaine abusers. *Arch Gen Psychiatry, 48,* 43–51.

Rounsaville, B. J., & Carroll, K. M. (1997). Individual psychotherapy for drug abusers. In J. H. Lowinson, P. Ruiz, R. B. Millman, & J. G. Langrod (Eds.), *Substance abuse: A comprehensive textbook* (pp. 430–439). Baltimore: Williams & Wilkins.

Rounsaville, B. J., Dolinsky, Z. S., Babor, T. F., & Meyer, R. E. (1987). Psychopathology as a predictor of treatment outcome in alcoholics. *Arch Gen Psychiatry, 44,* 505–513.

Salloum, I. M., Cornelius, J. R., Thase, M. E., Daley, D. C., Kirisci, L., & Spotts, C. (1998). Naltrexone utility in depressed alcoholics. *Psychopharmacol Bull, 34,* 111–115.

Satel, S., Southwick, S., & Gawin, F. H. (1991). Clinical features of cocaine-induced paranoia. *Am J Psychiatry, 148,* 495–499.

Schaar, I., & Oejehagen, A. (2001). Severely mentally ill substance abusers: An 18-month follow-up study. *Soc Psychiatry Psychiatr Epidemiol, 36,* 70–78.

Schubiner, H., Saules, K. K., Arfken, C. L., Johanson, C. E., Schuster, C. R., Lockhart, N., et al. (2002). Double-blind placebo-controlled trial of methylphenidate in the treatment of adult ADHD patients with comorbid cocaine dependence. *Exp Clin Psychopharmacol, 10*(3), 286–294.

Schweizer, E., Rickels, K., & Lucki, I. (1986). Resistance to the anti-anxiety effect of buspirone in patients with a history of benzodiazepine use. *N Engl J Med, 314*, 719–720.

Shaner, A., Khalsa, M. E., Roberts, L., Wilkins, J., Anglin, D., & Hsieh, S. C. (1993). Unrecognized cocaine use among schizophrenic patients. *Am J Psychiatry, 150*, 758–762.

Sigmon, S. C., Steingard, S., Badger, G. J., Anthony, S. L., & Higgins, S. T. (2000). Contingent reinforcement of marijuana abstinence among individuals with serious mental illness: A feasibility study. *Exp Clin Psychopharmacol, 8*(4), 509–517.

Smelson, D. A., Losonczy, M. F., Davis, C. W., Kaune, M., Williams, J., & Ziedonis, D. (2002). Risperdone decreases craving and relapses in individuals with schizophrenia and cocaine dependence. *Can J Psychiatry, 47*, 671–675.

Smelson, D. A., Losonczy, M. F., Kilker, C., Starosta, A., Kind, J., Williams, J., & Ziedonis, D. (2002). An analysis of cue reactivity among persons with and without schizophrenia who are addicted to cocaine. *Psychiatr Serv, 53*, 1612–1616.

Sonne, S. C., & Brady, K. T. (2000). Naltrexone for individuals with comorbid bipolar disorder and alcohol dependence. *J Clin Psychopharmacol, 20*, 114–115.

Spencer, C., Castle, D., & Michie, P. T. (2002). Motivations that maintain substance use among individuals with psychotic disorders. *Schizophr Bull, 28*, 233–247.

Substance Abuse and Mental Health Services Administration. (2002). *Report to Congress on the prevention and treatment of co-occurring substance abuse disorders and mental disorders*. Washington, DC: Authors.

Swanson, A. J., Pantalon, M. V., & Cohen, K. R. (1999). Motivational interviewing and treatment adherence among psychiatric and dually diagnosed patients. *J Nerv Ment Dis, 187*, 630–635.

Tollefson, G. D., Montague-Clouse, J., & Tollefson, S. L. (1992). Treatment of comorbid generalized anxiety in a recently detoxified alcoholic population with a selective serotonergic drug (buspirone). *J Clin Pharmacol, 12*, 19–26.

Upadhyaya, H. P., Brady, K. T., Sethuraman, G., Sonne, S. C., & Malcolm, R. (2001). Venlafaxine treatment of patients with comorbid alcohol/cocaine abuse and attention-deficit/hyperactivity disorder: A pilot study. *J Clin Psychopharmacol, 21*, 116–117.

Velasquez, M. M., Carbonari, J. P., & DiClemente, C. C. (1999). Psychiatric severity and behavior change in alcoholism: The relation of the transtheoretical model variables to psychiatric distress in dually diagnosed patients. *Addict Behav, 24*, 481–496.

Weiss, R. D. (1986). Psychopathology in chronic cocaine abusers. *Am J Drug Alcohol Abuse, 12*, 17–29.

Weiss, R. D. (1992a). Drug abuse as self-medication for depression: An empirical study. *Am J Drug Alcohol Abuse, 18*, 121–129.

Weiss, R. D. (1992b). The role of psychopathology in the transition from drug use to abuse and dependence. In M. Glantz & R. Pickens (Eds.), *Vulnerability to drug abuse* (pp. 137–148). Washington, DC: American Psychological Association.

Weiss, R. D. (1998). Validity of substance use self-reports in dually diagnosed outpatients. *Am J Psychiatry, 155*, 127–128.

Weiss, R. D., Griffin, M. L., Greenfield, S. F., Najavits, L. M., Wyner, D., Soto, J. A., & Hennen, J. A. (2000). Group therapy for patients with bipolar disorder and substance dependence: Results of a pilot study. *J Clin Psychiatry, 61,* 361–367.

Weiss, R. D., & Hufford, M. R. (1999). Substance abuse and suicide. In D. Jacobs (Ed.), *Harvard Medical School guide to assessment and intervention in suicide* (pp. 300–310). New York: Simon & Schuster.

Weiss, R. D., Mirin, S. M., & Frances, R. J. (1992). The myth of the typical dual diagnosis patient. *Hosp Community Psychiatry, 43,* 107–108.

Weiss, R. D., Najavits, L. M., & Greenfield, S. F. (1999). A relapse prevention group for patients with bipolar and substance use disorders. *J Subst Abuse Treat, 16,* 47–54.

Weiss, R. D., Najavits, L. M., Greenfield, S. F., Soto, J. A., Shaw, S. R., & Wyner, D. (1988). Psychopathology in cocaine abusers: Changing trends. *J Nerv Ment Dis, 176,* 719–725.

Wilens, T. E. (2001, Fall). Does the medicating of ADHD increase or decrease the risk for later substance abuse? An evaluation of the literature [Insert]. *Am Assoc Addict Psychiatry News,* pp. 1–4.

Wilens, T. E., Biederman, J., Prince, J., Spencer, T. J., Faraone, S. V., Warburton, R., et al. (1996). Six-week, double-blind, placebo-controlled study of desipramine for adult attention deficit hyperactivity disorder. *Am J Psychiatry, 153,* 1147–1153.

Wilens, T. E., Spencer, T. J., Biederman, J., Girard, K., Doyle, R., Prince, J., et al. (2002). A controlled clinical trial of bupropion for attention deficit hyperactivity disorder in adults. *Am J Psychiatry, 158,* 282–288.

Woodward, B., Fortgang, J., Sullivan-Trainor, M., Stojanov, H., & Mirin, S. M. (1991). Underdiagnosis of alcohol dependence in psychiatric inpatients. *Am J Drug Alcohol Abuse, 17,* 373–388.

Ziedonis, D., Richardson, T., Lee, E., Petrakis, I., & Kosten, T. (1992). Adjunctive desipramine in the treatment of cocaine abusing schizophrenics. *Psychopharmacol Bull, 28,* 309–314.

Ziedonis, D., & Trudeau, K. (1997). Motivation to quit using substances among individuals with schizophrenia: Implications for a motivation-based treatment model. *Schizophr Bull, 23,* 229–238.

Ziedonis, D., Williams, J., Corrigan, P., & Smelsen, D. A. (2000). Management of substance abuse in schizophrenia. *Psychiatr Ann, 30,* 67–75.

Zimmet, S. V., Strous, R. D., Burgess, E. S., Kohnstamm, S., & Green, A. I. (2000). Effect of clozapine on substance use in patients with schizophrenia and schizoaffective disorder: A retrospective study. *J Clin Psychopharmacol, 20,* 94–98.

CHAPTER 13

Pathological Gambling
and Other "Behavioral" Addictions

JON E. GRANT
MARC N. POTENZA

Several disorders, particularly those formally categorized in the fourth edition of the *Diagnostic and Statistical Manual of Mental Disorders* (DSM-IV-TR) as impulse control disorders (ICDs) not elsewhere classified, have been described as "behavioral" addictions (American Psychiatric Association, 2000). The ICDs include pathological gambling (PG), kleptomania, intermittent explosive disorder, trichotillomania, and pyromania, and diagnostic criteria for compulsive computer use, compulsive sexual behavior, and compulsive buying (CB) have been proposed. Although there exists some controversy regarding the most precise categorization of these disorders, mounting evidence supports phenomenological, clinical, epidemiological, and biological links between behavioral and drug addictions. As such, it seems increasingly important that individuals involved in the prevention and treatment of substance use disorders (SUDs) have a current understanding of ICDs and the potential for future research findings to guide prevention and treatment efforts for addictions in general.

PG represents the most thoroughly investigated ICD; consequently, this chapter largely focuses on PG, the relationship of PG to SUDs, and current treatment options for PG. We will also review two other ICDs (kleptomania and CB) that, despite having been less studied than other psychiatric disorders, have been receiving increasing attention from clinicians and researchers.

CORE FEATURES OF BEHAVIORAL AND DRUG ADDICTIONS

Behavioral and drug addictions share common core qualities: (1) repetitive or compulsive engagement in a behavior despite adverse consequences; (2) diminished control over the problematic behavior; (3) an appetitive urge or craving state prior to engagement in the problematic behavior; and (4) a hedonic quality during the performance of the problematic behavior. These features have led to a description of ICDs as "addictions without the drug."

Clinical similarities between ICDs and SUDs are best reflected in the diagnostic criteria for PG. Criteria for PG (Table 13.1) share common features with those for SUDs (American Psychiatric Association, 2000), including aspects of tolerance, withdrawal, repeated unsuccessful attempts to cut back or stop, and impairment in major areas of life functioning (Blanco, Moreyra, Nunes, Saiz-Ruiz, & Ibanez, 2001). Epidemiological data also support a relationship between PG and SUDs, with high rates of co-occurrence in each direction (Potenza, Fiellin, Heninger, Rounsaville, & Mazure, 2002). Phenomenological

---

TABLE 13.1. Diagnostic Criteria for Pathological Gambling

A. Persistent and recurrent maladaptive gambling behavior as indicated by five (or more) of the following:

(1) is preoccupied with gambling (e.g., preoccupied with reliving past gambling experiences, handicapping or planning the next venture, or thinking of ways to get money with which to gamble)

(2) needs to gamble with increasing amounts of money in order to achieve the desired excitement

(3) has repeated unsuccessful efforts to control, cut back, or stop gambling

(4) is restless or irritable when attempting to cut down or stop gambling

(5) gambles as a way of escaping from problems or of relieving a dysphoric mood (e.g., feelings of helplessness, guilt, anxiety, depression)

(6) after losing money gambling, often returns another day to get even ("chasing" one's losses)

(7) lies to family members, therapist, or others to conceal the extent of involvement with gambling

(8) has committed illegal acts such as forgery, fraud, theft, or embezzlement to finance gambling

(9) has jeopardized or lost a significant relationship, job, or educational or career opportunity because of gambling

(10) relies on others to provide money to relieve a desperate financial situation caused by gambling

B. The gambling behavior is not better accounted for by a Manic Episode

---

Note From American Psychiatric Association (2000, p. 674). Copyright 2000 by the American Psychiatric Association. Reprinted by permission.

data further support a relationship between behavioral and drug addictions: For example, high rates of PG and SUDs have been reported during adolescence and young adulthood (Chambers & Potenza, 2003); the telescoping phenomenon (reflecting the rapid rate of progression from initial to problematic behavioral engagement in women as compared with men) initially described for alcoholism has been applied to PG (Potenza et al., 2001); and similar typologies to those defining groups with alcoholism have been proposed for PG (Lesieur, 2000; Potenza, Steinberg, McLaughlin, Rounsaville, & O'Malley, 2000). Emerging biological data, such as those identifying common genetic contributions to alcohol use and gambling disorders (Slutske et al., 2000) and common brain activity changes underlying gambling urges and cocaine cravings (Potenza et al., 2002), provide further support for a shared relationship between PG and SUDs.

OTHER MODELS FOR IMPULSE CONTROL DISORDERS

Although much data from diverse sources support a close relationship between PG and SUDs, other non-mutually-exclusive proposed models for ICDs include categorizations as obsessive–compulsive spectrum (Potenza & Hollander, 2002) and affective spectrum (McElroy et al., 1996) disorders. The range of medication classes (serotonin reuptake inhibitors [SRIs], mood stabilizers, opioid antagonists) investigated in the treatment of ICDs reflects the different categorizations.

Conceptualization of ICDs within an obsessive–compulsive spectrum is based on common features of repetitive thoughts and behaviors (Potenza & Hollander, 2002). Although clinical aspects, such as ritualistic behaviors, are shared between obsessive–compulsive disorder (OCD) and ICDs, other aspects seem different (e.g., the ego-syntonic nature of gambling in PG and the ego-dystonic nature of compulsions in OCD). Although some evidence support high rates of co-occurring OCD and ICDs (McElroy, Hudson, Pope, Keck, & Aizley, 1992), multiple studies do not report an association (Grant & Kim, 2001, 2002a; Potenza et al., 2002). Personality features of individuals with ICDs (impulsive, reward and sensation seeking) differ from those with OCD (harm avoidant) (Kim & Grant, 2001). Biological differences also exist; for example, whereas increased activity in corticobasal ganglionic–thalamic circuitry has been described during symptom provocation studies of OCD, relatively decreased activity in these brain regions was observed in cue elicitation studies in PG (Potenza et al., 2003). Family history and large-scale epidemiological studies have also not demonstrated associations between PG and OCD (Potenza et al., 2002). Thus, there is less evidence linking PG to OCD than to SUDs.

The association of ICDs with mood disorders has led to their grouping as an affective spectrum disorder (McElroy et al., 1996). Many people with ICDs report that the pleasurable yet problematic behaviors alleviate negative emotional states. Because the behaviors are risky and self-destructive, the question has been raised whether ICDs reflect subclinical mania or cyclothymia. The elevated rates of co-occurrence between ICDs and depression, and bipolar disorder support their inclusion within an affective spectrum, as do early reports of treatment response to SRIs, mood stabilizers, and electroconvulsive therapy (McElroy, Hudson, Pope, Keck, &White, 1991; McElroy et al., 1996). However, as has been suggested with SUDs, depression in ICDs may be distinct from primary or uncomplicated depression; for example, depression in ICDs may represent a response to shame and embarrassment (Grant & Kim, 2002a). In addition, rates of co-occurrence of ICDs and bipolar disorder may not be as high as initially thought (Grant & Kim, 2001, 2002a), and the response to SRIs not as robust as initially anticipated (McElroy et al., 1991). Nonetheless, brain imaging studies have found common regional brain activity differences distinguishing bipolar subjects from controls, and PG subjects from controls, during a cognitive task involving attention and response inhibition (Potenza et al., 2003). For these reasons, the relationship between ICDs and mood disorders requires clarification, particularly because appropriate classification has implications for treatment development.

EPIDEMIOLOGY

Arguably the best data on the prevalence of ICDs exist for PG. A recent meta-analysis of 120 published studies and a national prevalence study estimate that the lifetime prevalence of serious gambling (meeting DSM criteria for PG) among adults ranges from 0.9 to 1.6% (National Opinion Research Center, 1999; Shaffer, Hall, Vander Bilt, 1999), with past-year rates for adults ranging from 0.6 to 1.1% (National Opinion Research Center, 1999; Shaffer & Hall, 1996).

Rates of problem gambling, a less severe form of disordered gambling than PG, not presently defined in the DSM, have been estimated at an additional 3–5% of the general adult population. As with SUDs, higher rates of problem gambling and PG have been reported in males, particularly during adolescence and young adulthood.

Although the precise prevalence of kleptomania remains unknown, a preliminary estimate of 0.6% has been reported (Goldman, 1991). Furthermore, there is emerging evidence that kleptomania may be more common than initially thought (Grant, Potenza, Levine, & Kim, in press). Estimates of the lifetime prevalence of compulsive buying have ranged from 1.1 to 5.9% (Christenson et al., 1994; McElroy, Keck, Pope, Smith, & Strakowski, 1994).

ETIOLOGY

A growing body of literature implicates multiple neurotransmitter systems (e.g., serotonergic, dopaminergic, noradrenergic, opioidergic), as well as familial and inherited factors, in the pathophysiology of ICDs (Potenza & Hollander, 2002).

The most consistent findings involve the serotonin (5-hydroxyindole or 5-HT) system, believed to underlie impulse control (Potenza & Hollander, 2002). Evidence for serotonergic involvement in ICDs comes in part from studies of platelet monoamine oxidase B (MAO-B) activity, which correlates with cerebrospinal fluid (CSF) levels of 5-hydroxyindoleacetic acid (5-HIAA, a metabolite of 5-HT) and is considered a peripheral marker of 5-HT function (Potenza & Hollander, 2002). Low CSF 5-HIAA levels have been found to correlate with high levels of impulsivity and sensation seeking (Potenza & Hollander, 2002). Pharmacological challenge studies that measure hormonal response after administration of serotonergic drugs also provide evidence for serotonergic dysfunction in ICDs (Potenza & Hollander, 2002).

Dopaminergic systems influencing rewarding and reinforcing behaviors have also been implicated in ICDs. "Reward deficiency syndrome," a hypothesized hypodopaminergic state involving multiple genes and environmental stimuli that puts an individual at high risk for multiple addictive, impulsive, and compulsive behaviors, is one proposed mechanism (Blum et al., 2000). Alterations in dopaminergic pathways have been proposed as underlying the seeking of rewards (gambling, drugs) that trigger the release of dopamine and produce feelings of pleasure (Blum et al., 2000).

Noradrenergic systems, believed to underlie arousal, excitement, and sensation seeking, have been implicated in impulsive behaviors (Potenza & Hollander, 2002). Anticipation of or engagement in seemingly impulsive behaviors can activate the autonomic nervous system. Correlations between scores on the extroversion scale of the Eysenck Personality Questionnaire and markers of noradrenergic functioning (e.g., CSF or plasma 3-methoxy-4-hydroxyphenylglycol [MHPG] levels, urinary outputs of norepinephrine and its major metabolites) suggest a disturbance in central noradrenergic system functioning in PG (Roy, De Jong, & Linnoila, 1989).

The mu opioid system is believed to underlie urge regulation through the processing of reward, pleasure, and pain, at least in part via modulation of dopamine neurons in mesolimbic pathway through gamma-aminobutyric acid (GABA) interneurons (Potenza & Hollander, 2002). Opioidergic involvement in ICDs comes from studies of naltrexone, a mu opioid receptor antagonist with efficacy in reducing the urges in ICDs (Grant & Kim, 2002b; Kim, Grant, Adson, & Shin, 2001).

PATHOLOGICAL GAMBLING

Clinical Characteristics

PG shares many features with SUDS. Gambling usually begins in childhood or adolescence, with males tending to start at an earlier age (Chambers & Potenza, 2003; Grant & Kim, 2001). Higher rates of PG are observed in men, with a telescoping phenomenon observed in females (Potenza, Steinberg, et al., 2001). PG has been described as a chronic, relapsing condition (Potenza, Kosten, & Rounsaville, 2001). High rates of PG in adolescents and young adults suggest a similar natural history to that observed with SUDs (Chambers & Potenza, 2003).

Other gender-related differences in PG have been described. Female as compared with male pathological gamblers tend to have problems with non-strategic forms of gambling, such as slot machines and bingo, whereas men are more likely than women to have problems with strategic forms, such as sports and card gambling (Potenza, Steinberg, et al., 2001). As is the case of SUDS and specific substances, the extent to which problems with specific forms of gambling might relate to prevention and treatment efforts requires further investigation. Both female and male gamblers report that advertisements are a common trigger of their urges to gamble, although females are more likely to report that feeling bored or lonely may also trigger their urges to gambling (Grant & Kim, 2001; Ladd & Petry, 2002).

As with SUDs, financial and marital problems are common (Grant & Kim, 2001) and often include illegal behaviors, such as stealing, embezzlement, and writing bad checks (Grant & Kim, 2001; Potenza et al., 2000). Cognitive features have also been reported as common between PG and SUDs; for example, both groups have been found to have high rates of temporal discounting of rewards and to perform disadvantageously on decision-making tasks (Bechara, 2003).

Co-Occurring Disorders

Studies consistently find that patients with PG have high rates of lifetime mood (60–76%), anxiety (16–40%), and personality (87%) disorders, particularly antisocial personality disorder (Black & Moyer, 1998; Crockford & el-Guebaly, 1998). Elevated rates of CB, compulsive sexual behavior, and intermittent explosive disorder have also been found (Black & Moyer, 1998).

High rates of co-occurrence have been reported for SUDs (including nicotine dependence) and PG, with the highest odds ratios generally observed between gambling and alcohol use disorders (Cunningham-Williams, Cottler, Compton, & Spitznagel, 1998; Welte, Barnes, Wieczorek, Tidwell, & Parker, 2001). A Canadian epidemiological survey estimated that the relative risk for an alcohol use disorder is increased 3.8-fold when disordered gambling is present (Grant, Kushner, & Kim, 2002), and odds ratios ranging from 3.3 to 23.1 have been reported between PG and alcohol abuse/dependence in U.S. population-based studies (Cunningham-Williams et al., 1998; Welte et al., 2001).

Treatment

Given the high rates of placebo response often observed in treatment trials of PG, the treatment section focuses on findings from double-blind, placebo-controlled trials (see Table 13.2).

Antidepressants

SRIs are the most well-studied pharmacotherapy for PG. In a double-blind study with one subject, 125 mg/day of clomipramine resulted in significant improvement. The patient sustained improvement for 28 weeks on a dose of 175 mg/day (Grant, Kim, & Potenza, 2003). Fluvoxamine has demonstrated mixed results in two placebo-controlled, double-blind studies, with one 16-week crossover study supporting its efficacy at an average dose of 207 mg/day (Hollander et al., 2000), and a second 6-month parallel-arm study with high rates of dropout finding no significant difference in response to active or placebo drug (Blanco, Petkova, Ibanez, & Saiz-Ruiz, 2002).

Paroxetine at doses between 20 and 60 mg/day (average end-of-study dose = 52 mg/day) has been shown in a short-term, parallel-arm, placebo-controlled, double-blind study to be well-tolerated and efficacious in the treatment of PG (Kim, Grant, Adson, Shin, & Zaninelli, 2002). However, a 16-week multicenter study of paroxetine did not find a statistically significant difference between active drug and placebo, perhaps in part due to the high placebo response rate (48% to placebo, 59% to active drug) (Grant, Kim, Potenza, et al., 2003). A similarly high placebo response rate was seen in a recent study using sertraline (Saiz-Ruiz et al., 2005).

Opioid Antagonists

Given their ability to modulate dopaminergic transmission in the mesolimbic pathway, mu opioid receptor antagonists have been investigated in the treatment of PG. Initially, open-label treatment suggested the efficacy of naltrexone, an FDA-approved treatment for alcohol dependence, in reducing the intensity of urges to gamble, gambling thoughts, and gambling behavior when

TABLE 13.2. Double-Blind, Placebo-Controlled Pharmacotherapy Trials for Impulse Control Disorders

Disorder	Reference	Treatment	Duration	Sample size	Mean daily dose (± SD)	Outcome
Pathological gambling	Hollander et al. (2000)	*Fluvoxamine* (Luvox)	Crossover 16 weeks with a 1-week placebo lead-in	15 enrolled, 10 completers	195 mg (± 50)	Fluvoxamine superior to placebo on CGI and PG-YBOCS
Pathological gambling	Potenza & Hollander (2002)	Olanzapine (Zyprexa)	7 weeks	23 Video Poker gamblers enrolled, 21 completers	10 mg (± 0)	No significant difference found between olanzapine and placebo-treated groups
Pathological gambling	Kim et al. (2001)	Naltrexone (ReVia)	12 weeks with 1-week placebo lead-in	89 enrolled, 45 completers	188 mg (± 96)	Naltrexone group significantly improved compared with placebo on CGI and G-SAS
Pathological gambling	Hollander et al. (2005)	Lithium carbonate SR (Lithobid SR)	10 weeks	40 bipolar-spectrum patients enrolled, 29 completers	1,170 mg (± 221)	Lithium group significantly improved compared with placebo on CGI, PG-YBOCS, and CARS-M
Pathological gambling	Blanco et al. (2002)	Fluvoxamine (Luvox)	6 months	32 enrolled, 13 completers	200 mg	Fluvoxamine not statistically significant from placebo except in young males

Disorder	Study	Medication	Design	N	Dose	Outcome
Pathological gambling	Kim et al. (2002)	Paroxetine (Paxil)	8 weeks with 1-week placebo lead-in	53 enrolled, 41 completers	51.7 mg (± 13.1)	Paroxetine group significantly improved compared to placebo on CGI
Pathological gambling	Grant et al. (2003)	Paroxetine (Paxil)	16 weeks	76 enrolled, 45 completers	50 mg (± 8.3)	Paroxetine and placebo groups with comparable improvement on all measures
Pathological gambling	Saiz-Ruiz et al. (2005)	Sertraline (Zoloft)	6 months	66 enrolled, 37 completers	95 mg	Sertraline and placebo groups with comparable improvement to CCPGQ
Compulsive buying	Black et al. (2000)	Fluvoxamine (Luvox)	9 weeks with 1-week placebo lead-in	23 enrolled, 18 completers	220 mg	Fluvoxamine and placebo groups with comparable improvement on YBOCS-SV and CGI
Compulsive buying	Ninan et al. (2000)	Fluvoxamine (Luvox)	13 weeks	37 enrolled, 23 completers	215 mg (± 76.5)	Fluvoxamine and placebo groups with comparable improvement on YBOCS-CB, CGI, and GAF
Compulsive buying	Koran et al. (2003)	Citalopram (Celexa)	7-week open-label followed by 9 weeks randomized	24 enrolled, 15 randomized	42.1 mg (± 15.3)	Citalopram group significantly improved compared to placebo on YBOCS-SV and CGI

Note. PG-YBOCS, Yale–Brown Obsessive Compulsive Scale Modified for Pathological Gambling; YBOCS-SV, Yale–Brown Obsessive Compulsive Scale—Shopping Version; YBOCS-CB, Yale–Brown Obsessive Compulsive Scale Modified for Compulsive Buying; CGI, Clinical Global Impression scale; G-SAS, Gambling Symptom Assessment Scale; GAF, Global Assessment of Functioning; CARS-M, Clinician-Administered Rating Scale for Mania; CCPGQ, Criteria for Control of Pathological Gambling Questionnaire.

receiving high dose (range = 50–250 mg/day; mean dose of 157 mg/day) (Grant, Kim, & Potenza, 2003). A larger double-blind study using a mean naltrexone dose of 188 mg/day confirmed these earlier findings (Kim, Grant, Adson, & Shin, 2001). In particular, individuals reporting higher intensity gambling urges responded preferentially to treatment (Kim et al., 2001).

Mood Stabilizers

A recent double-blind study found sustained-release lithium carbonate superior to placebo in 29 bipolar-spectrum pathological gamblers over 10 weeks (Hollander, Pallanti, & Baldini-Rossi, 2005). Bipolar spectrum disorders were defined as including DSM-IV diagnoses of bipolar II disorder, bipolar disorder not otherwise specified (NOS), and cyclothymia, and mood swings that occurred at times unrelated to gambling urges/behavior.

Atypical Antipsychotics

Atypical antipsychotics have been explored as augmenting agents in the treatment of nonpsychotic disorders and behaviors, including OCD. Olanzapine was not found to be superior to placebo in the treatment of video poker pathological gamblers (Potenza & Hollander, 2002). A case report described symptom improvement following the initiation of olanzapine at 10 mg/day in the treatment of a woman with PG and schizophrenia (Grant, Kim, & Potenza, 2003). Further systematic investigation of the potential of atypical antipsychotics, particularly in treating individuals with co-occurring psychotic disorders and PG, seems indicated.

Psychotherapy

Multiple behavioral treatments have been investigated (Petry & Roll, 2001). Cognitive therapy focuses on changing the patient's beliefs regarding perceived control over randomly determined events. Case reports have demonstrated success with cognitive therapy (Petry & Roll, 2001), and further support is derived from two randomized trials. In the first, individual cognitive therapy resulted in reduced gambling frequency and increased perceived self-control over gambling when compared with a wait-list control group (Sylvain, Ladouceur, & Boisvert, 1997). A second trial that included relapse prevention also produced improvement in gambling symptoms compared to a wait-list group (Ladouceur et al., 2001).

Cognitive-behavioral therapy has also been used to treat pathological gambling, including one published randomized trial (Echeburua, Baez, & Fernandez-Montalvo, 1996). In this study, four groups were compared: (1) individual stimulus control and *in vivo* exposure with response prevention, (2) group cognitive restructuring, (3) a combination of 1 and 2, and (4) a wait-list control. At 12 months, rates of abstinence or minimal gambling were higher in the individual treatment (69%) compared with group cognitive restructuring (38%) and the combined treatment (38%). An independent controlled trial, based on cognitive behavioral therapies used in the treatment of SUDs and including relapse prevention strategies, is currently underway, with initial results suggesting the efficacy of manually driven cognitive-behavioral therapy (Petry & Roll, 2001).

Brief interventions in the form of workbooks have also been studied. One study assigned gamblers to a workbook alone (which included cognitive-behavioral and motivational enhancement techniques) or to the workbook in addition to one clinician interview (Dickerson, Hinchy, & England, 1990). Both groups reported significant reductions in gambling at a 6-month follow-up. Similarly, a separate study assigned gamblers to a workbook, a workbook plus a telephone motivational enhancement intervention, or a wait list. Compared to gamblers using the workbook alone, those assigned to the motivational intervention and workbook reduced gambling throughout a 2-year follow-up period (Hodgins, Currie, & el-Guebaly, 2001).

Two studies have also tested aversion therapy and imaginal desensitization in randomized designs. In the first study, both treatments resulted in improvement in a small sample of patients (McConaghy, Armstrong, Blaszczynski, & Allcock, 1983). In the second study, 120 pathological gamblers were randomly assigned to aversion therapy, imaginal desensitization, *in vivo* desensitization, or imaginal relaxation. Participants receiving imaginal desensitization reported better outcomes at 1-month and up to 9 years later (McConaghy, Blaszczynski, & Frankova, 1991).

KLEPTOMANIA

Kleptomania (stealing madness) was formally designated a psychiatric disorder in DSM-III, and the core features include (1) a recurrent failure to resist an impulse to steal unneeded objects; (2) an increasing sense of tension before committing the theft; (3) an experience of pleasure, gratification or release at the time of committing the theft; and (4) stealing that is not performed out of anger, vengeance, or due to psychosis (American Psychiatric Association, 2000).

Clinical Characteristics

Kleptomania usually appears first during late adolescence or early adulthood (Goldman, 1991). The course is generally chronic, with waxing and waning of symptoms. Women are twice as likely as men to suffer from kleptomania (Grant & Kim, 2002a).

Like individuals with SUDs, most with kleptomania try unsuccessfully to stop. In one study, all participants reported increased urges to steal when trying to stop (Grant & Kim, 2002a). The diminished ability to stop often leads to feelings of shame and guilt, reported in most (77.3%) subjects (Grant & Kim, 2002a). Of married subjects, less than half had disclosed their behavior to their spouses due to shame and guilt (Grant & Kim, 2002a).

Although people with kleptomania often steal various items from multiple places, the majority steal from stores. In one study, 68.2% of patients reported that the value of stolen items had increased over time (Grant & Kim, 2002a), a finding suggestive of tolerance. Patients may keep, hoard, discard, give as gifts, or return stolen items (McElroy et al., 1991). Many (64–87%) have been apprehended at some time due to their behavior (McElroy et al., 1991), and 15–23% report having been jailed (Grant & Kim, 2002a). Although the majority of the patients who were apprehended reported that their urges to steal were diminished after the apprehension, their symptom remission generally lasted only for a few days or weeks (McElroy et al., 1991). Together, these findings demonstrate a continued engagement in the problematic behavior despite adverse consequences, a core feature of addiction.

Co-Occurring Disorders and Family History

High rates of other psychiatric disorders have been found in patients with kleptomania. Rates of lifetime comorbid affective disorders range from 59% (Grant & Kim, 2002a) to 100% (McElroy et al., 1991). The rate of comorbid bipolar disorder has been reported as ranging from 9% (Grant & Kim, 2002a) to 60% (McElroy et al., 1991). Studies have also found high lifetime rates of comorbid anxiety disorders (60–80%; McElroy et al., 1991, 1992), ICDs (20–46%; Grant, 2003), SUDs (23–50%; Grant & Kim, 2002a; McElroy et al., 1991), and eating disorders (60%; McElroy et al., 1991).

Individuals with kleptomania are more likely to have a first-degree relative with a psychiatric disorder compared to nonaffected controls (Grant, 2003), In addition, high rates of mood (20–35%) and substance use disorders (15–20%) have been observed in first-degree relatives of patients with kleptomania (McElroy et al., 1991).

Treatment

Pharmacotherapy

Only case reports, two small case series, and one open-label study of pharmacotherapy have been performed for kleptomania. Given the high placebo response rates observed in the treatment of ICDs, findings from these studies should be interpreted cautiously. Various medications have been studied in case reports or case series, and several have been found effective: fluoxetine, nortriptyline, trazodone, clonazepam, valproate, lithium, fluvoxamine, paroxetine, and topiramate (Grant & Kim, 2002b; McElroy et al., 1991).

The only formal trial of medication for kleptomania involved 10 subjects in a 12-week, open-label study of naltrexone. A mean dose of 145 mg/day resulted in a significant decline in the intensity of urges to steal, stealing thoughts, and stealing behavior (Grant & Kim, 2002b).

Psychotherapy

Although multiple types of psychotherapies have been described in the treatment of kleptomania, no controlled trials exist in the literature. Treatments described in case reports as demonstrating success include psychoanalytic, insight-oriented, and behavioral therapies (Goldman, 1991; McElroy et al., 1991). Because no controlled trials of therapy for kleptomania have been published, the efficacies of these interventions are difficult to evaluate.

COMPULSIVE BUYING

Originally termed "oniomania" by Kraeplin and Bleuler, CB has been described for over 100 years (Christenson et al., 1994). Although not specifically recognized in the DSM-IV-TR, the following CB diagnostic criteria have been proposed: (1) maladaptive preoccupation with or engagement in buying (evidenced by frequent preoccupation with or irresistible impulses to buy, frequent buying of items that are not needed or not affordable, or shopping for longer periods of time than intended); (2) preoccupations or the buying lead to significant distress or impairment; and (3) the buying does not occur exclusively during hypomanic or manic episodes (McElroy et al., 1994).

Clinical Characteristics

As with other ICDs and SUDs, the onset of CB appears to occur during late adolescence or early adulthood, although the full disorder may take several years to develop (Christenson et al., 1994). Unlike most SUDs, CB shows a female preponderance, ranging from 80–92% in clinical samples (Christenson et al., 1994; McElroy et al., 1994; Schlosser, Black, Repertinger, & Freet, 1994).

CB is characterized by repetitive urges to shop that are most often unprovoked but may be triggered by being in stores. These urges may worsen during times of stress, emotional difficulties, or boredom. Urges are generally intrusive, and most patients attempt to resist them, although usually unsuccessfully. Buying often results in large debts, marital or family disruption, and legal consequences (Christenson et al., 1994). Although the behavior is pleasurable and momentarily relieves the urges to shop, guilt, shame, and embarrassment generally follow buying episodes.

A positive interaction with salespeople is often described as a motivating factor in CB. The items bought vary considerably, and can include clothing, jewelry, books, and auto parts. Most items are not used or removed from the packaging, and many are given away, returned, or hoarded (Christenson et al., 1994).

Co-Occurring Disorders and Family History

Rates of co-occurring mood disorders range from 28 to 95% (Christenson et al., 1994; McElroy et al., 1994; Schlosser et al., 1994), with the mood disorder often preceding the compulsive buying by at least 1 year (Christenson et al., 1994). Lifetime histories of anxiety (41–80%), substance use (30–46%), eating (17–35%%), and impulse control (21–40%) disorders are fairly common (Christenson et al., 1994; McElroy et al., 1994; Schlosser et al., 1994). In addition, patients with CB frequently report first-degree relatives with SUDs (25%), mood disorders (20%), or CB (10%) (Black, Repertinger, Gaffney, & Gabel, 1998).

Treatment

Pharmacotherapy

The effectiveness of pharmacotherapies in treating CB is beginning to be systematically investigated (see Table 13.2). Case reports and open-label studies have suggested that the following agents may be beneficial: nortriptyline, fluoxetine, buproprion, lithium, clomipramine, naltrexone, fluvoxamine, citalopram, and valproate (Black, Monahan, & Gabel, 1997; Koran, Bullock, Hartston, Elliott, & D'Andrea, 2002; McElroy et al., 1994).

In the first of two double-blind fluvoxamine studies, 37 subjects were treated for 13 weeks. Only 9 of 20 patients assigned to medication were responders (mean dose of 215 mg/day), and this rate did not differ significantly from that in the placebo group (8 of 17 were responders) (Ninan et al., 2000). In the second double-blind study, Black, Gabel, Hansen, and Schlosser (2000) treated 23 patients for 9 weeks, following a 1-week placebo lead-in phase. Using a mean dose of 200 mg/day, no differences in response rates were observed between the groups treated with active and placebo drug.

A double-blind study using citalopram, however, suggests the efficacy of selective SRIs in treating CB. Seven weeks of open-label treatment was followed by randomization of responders to medication or placebo for another 9 weeks. Patients taking active citalopram demonstrated statistically significant decreases in terms of the frequency of shopping, as well as the intensity of thoughts and urges concerning shopping (Koran, Chuong, Bullock, & Smith, 2003).

Psychotherapy

There are no formal studies of psychotherapy for CB. Several case reports suggest that possible effective psychotherapeutic interventions might include exposure and response prevention, and supportive or insight-oriented psychotherapy (McElroy et al., 1994).

CONCLUSIONS

Behavioral addictions, such as the ICDs, have historically received relatively little attention from clinicians and researchers. As such, our understanding of the basic features of these disorders is relatively primitive. Future research investigating ICDs and their relationship to SUDs holds significant promise in advancing prevention and treatment strategies for addiction in general.

REFERENCES

American Psychiatric Association. (2000). *Diagnostic and statistical manual of mental disorders* (4th ed., text rev.). Washington, DC: Author.

Bechara, A. (2003). Risky business: emotion, decision-making, and addiction. *J Gambl Stud, 19,* 23–51.

Black, D. W., Gabel, J., Hansen, J., & Schlosser, S. (2000). A double-blind comparison of fluvoxamine versus placebo in the treatment of compulsive buying disorder. *Ann Clin Psychiatry, 12,* 205–211.

Black, D. W., Monahan, P., & Gabel, J. (1997). Fluvoxamine in the treatment of compulsive buying. *J Clin Psychiatry, 58,* 159–163.

Black, D. W., & Moyer, T. M. (1998). Clinical features and psychiatric comorbidity of subjects with pathological gambling behavior. *Psychiatr Serv, 49,* 1434–1439.

Black, D. W., Repertinger, S., Gaffney, G. R., & Gabel, J. (1998). Family history and psychiatric comorbidity in persons with compulsive buying: Preliminary findings. *Am J Psychiatry, 155,* 960–963.

Blanco, C., Moreyra, P., Nunes, E. V., Saiz-Ruiz, J., & Ibanez, A. (2001). Pathological gambling: Addiction or compulsion? *Semin Clin Neuropsychiatry, 6,* 167–176.

Blanco, C., Petkova, E., Ibanez, A., & Saiz-Ruiz, J. (2002). A pilot placebo-controlled study of fluvoxamine for pathological gambling. *Ann Clin Psychiatry, 14,* 9–15.

Blum, K., Braverman, E. R., Holder, J. M., Lubar, J. F., Monastra, V. J., Miller, D., et al. (2000). Reward deficiency syndrome: A biogenetic model for the diagnosis and treatment of impulsive, addictive, and compulsive behaviors. *J Psychoactive Drugs, 32*(Suppl 1), 1–68.

Chambers, R. A., & Potenza, M. N. (2003). Neurodevelopment, impulsivity, and adolescent gambling. *J Gambl Stud, 19*, 53–84.

Christenson, G. A., Faber, R. J., de Zwaan, M., Raymond, N. C., Specker, S. M., Ekern, M. D., et al. (1994). Compulsive buying: Descriptive characteristics and psychiatric comorbidity. *J Clin Psychiatry, 55*, 5–11.

Crockford, D. N., & el-Guebaly, N. (1998). Psychiatric comorbidity in pathological gambling: A critical review. *Can J Psychiatry, 43*, 43–50.

Cunningham-Williams, R. M., Cottler, L. B., Compton W. M. III, & Spitznagel, E. L. (1998). Taking chances: Problem gamblers and mental health disorders—results from the St. Louis Epidemiologic Catchment Area study. *Am J Public Health, 88*, 1093–1096.

Dickerson, M., Hinchy, J., & England, L. S. (1990). Minimal treatments and problem gamblers: A preliminary investigation. *J Gambl Stud, 6*, 87–102.

Echeburua, E., Baez, C., & Fernandez-Montalvo, J. (1996). Comparative effectiveness of three therapeutic modalities in psychological treatment of pathological gambling: Long term outcome. *Behav and Cogn Psychother, 24*, 51–72.

Goldman, M. J. (1991). Kleptomania: Making sense of the nonsensical. *Am J Psychiatry, 148*, 986–996.

Grant, J. E. (2003). Family history and psychiatric comorbidity in persons with kleptomania. *Compr Psychiatry, 44*, 437–441.

Grant, J. E., & Kim, S. W. (2001). Demographic and clinical features of 131 adult pathological gamblers. *J Clin Psychiatry, 62*, 957–962.

Grant, J. E., & Kim, S. W. (2002a). Clinical characteristics and associated psychopathology of 22 patients with kleptomania. *Compr Psychiatry, 43*, 378–384.

Grant, J. E., & Kim, S. W. (2002b). Kleptomania: Emerging therapies target mood, impulsive behavior. *Curr Psychiatry, 1*, 45–49.

Grant, J. E., Kim, S. W., & Potenza, M. N. (2003). Advances in the pharmacological treatment of pathological gambling. *J Gambl Stud, 19*, 85–109.

Grant, J. E., Kim, S. W., Potenza, M. N., Blanco, C., Ibanez, A., Stevens, L. C., et al. (2003). Paroxetine treatment of pathological gambling: A multi-center randomized controlled trial. *Int Clin Psychopharmacol, 18*, 243–249.

Grant, J. E., Kushner, M. G., & Kim, S. W. (2002). Pathological gambling and alcohol use disorder. *Alcohol Res Health, 26*, 143–150.

Grant, J. E., Potenza, M. N., Levine, L., & Kim, D. (in press). Prevalence of impulse control disorders in adult psychiatric inpatients. *Am J Psychiatry*.

Hodgins, D. C., Currie, S. R., & el-Guebaly, N. (2001). Motivational enhancement and self-help treatments for problem gambling. *J Consult Clin Psychol, 69*, 50–57.

Hollander, E., DeCaria, C. M., Finkell, J. N., Begaz, T., Wong, C. M., & Cartwright, C. (2000). A randomized double-blind fluvoxamine/placebo crossover trial in pathological gambling. *Biol Psychiatry, 47*, 813–817.

Hollander, E., Pallanti, S., & Baldini-Rossi, N. (2005). Does sustained-release lithium reduce impulsive gambling and affective instability versus placebo in pathological gamblers with bipolar spectrum disorders? *Am J Psychiatry, 162*, 137–145.

Kim, S. W., & Grant, J. E. (2001). Personality dimensions in pathological gambling disorder and obsessive–compulsive disorder. *Psychiatry Res, 104*, 205–212.

Kim, S. W., Grant, J. E., Adson, D. E., & Shin, Y. C. (2001). Double-blind naltrexone and placebo comparison study in the treatment of pathological gambling. *Biol Psychiatry, 49,* 914–921.

Kim, S. W., Grant, J. E., Adson, D. E., Shin, Y. C., & Zaninelli, R. M. (2002). A double-blind placebo-controlled study of the efficacy and safety of paroxetine in the treatment of pathological gambling. *J Clin Psychiatry, 63,* 501–507.

Koran, L. M., Bullock, K. D., Hartston, H. J., Elliott, M. A., & D'Andrea, V. (2002). Citalopram treatment of compulsive shopping: An open-label study. *J Clin Psychiatry, 63,* 704–708.

Koran, L. M., Chuong, H. W., Bullock, K. D., & Smith, S. C. (2003). Citalopram for compulsive shopping disorder: An open-label study followed by double-blind discontinuation. *J Clin Psychiatry, 64,* 793–798.

Ladd, G. T., & Petry, N. M. (2002). Gender differences among pathological gamblers seeking treatment. *Exp Clin Psychopharmacol, 10,* 302–309.

Ladouceur, R., Sylvain, C., Boutin, C., Lachine, S., Doucette, C., Leland, J., & Jacques, C. (2001). Cognitive treatment of pathological gambling. *J Nerv Ment Dis, 189,* 774–780.

Lesieur, H. R. (2000). Commentary: types, lotteries, and substance abuse among problem gamblers. *J Am Acad Psychiatry Law, 28,* 404–407.

McConaghy, N., Armstrong, M. S., Blaszczynski, A., & Allcock, C. (1983). Controlled comparison of aversive therapy and imaginal desensitization in compulsive gambling. *Br J Psychiatry, 142,* 366–372.

McConaghy, N., Blaszczynski, A., & Frankova, A. (1991). Comparison of imaginal desensitization with other behavioral treatments of pathological gambling: A two to nine year follow-up. *Br J Psychiatry, 159,* 390–393.

McElroy, S. L., Hudson, J. I., Pope, H. G., Keck, P. E., & Aizley, H. G. (1992). The DSM-III-R impulse control disorders not elsewhere classified: Clinical characteristics and relationship to other psychiatric disorders. *Am J Psychiatry, 149,* 318–327.

McElroy, S. L., Keck, P. E., Pope, H. G., Smith, J. M. R., & Strakowski, S. M. (1994). Compulsive buying: A report of 20 cases. *J Clin Psychiatry, 55,* 242–248.

McElroy, S. L., Pope, H. G., Hudson, J. I., Keck, P. E., & White, K. L. (1991). Kleptomania: A report of 20 cases. *Am J Psychiatry, 148,* 652–657.

McElroy, S. L., Pope, H. G., Jr., Keck, P. E., Hudson, J. I., Phillips, K. A., & Strakowski, S. M. (1996). Are impulse-control disorders related to bipolar disorder? *Compr Psychiatry, 37,* 229–240.

National Opinion Research Center. (1999). *Overview of the national survey and community database research on gambling behavior: Report to the National Gambling Impact Study Commission.* Chicago: Author.

Ninan, P. T., McElroy, S. L., Kane, C. P., Knight, B. T., Castor, L. S., Rose, S. E., et al. (2000). Placebo-controlled study of fluvoxamine in the treatment of patients with compulsive buying. *J Clin Psychopharmacol, 20,* 362–366.

Petry, N. M., & Roll, J. M. (2001). A behavioral approach to understanding and treating pathological gambling. *Semin Clin Neuropsychiatry, 6,* 177–183.

Potenza, M. N., Fiellin, D. A., Heninger, G. A., Rounsaville, B. J., & Mazure, C. M. (2002). Gambling: An addictive behavior with health and primary care implications. *J Gen Intern Med, 17,* 721–732.

Potenza, M. N., & Hollander, E. (2002). Pathological gambling and impulse control disorders. In J. T. Coyle, C. Nemeroff, D. Charney, & K. L. Davis (Eds.), *Neuropsychopharmacology: The 5th generation of progress* (pp. 1725–1741). Baltimore: Lippincott/Williams & Wilkins.

Potenza, M. N., Kosten, T. R., & Rounsaville, B. J. (2001). Pathological gambling. *JAMA, 286,* 141–144.

Potenza, M. N., Leung, H. C., Blumberg, H. P., Peterson, B. S., Fulbright, R. K., Lacadie, C. M., et al. (2003). An fMRI Stroop study of ventromedial prefrontal cortical function in pathological gamblers. *Am J Psychiatry, 160,* 1990–1994.

Potenza, M. N., Steinberg, M. A., McLaughlin, S. D., Rounsaville, B. J., & O'Malley, S. S. (2000). Illegal behaviors in problem gambling: Analysis of data from a gambling helpline. *J Am Acad Psychiatry Law, 28,* 389–403.

Potenza, M. N., Steinberg, M. A., McLaughlin, S. D., Wu, R., Rounsaville, B., & O'Malley, S. S. (2001). Gender-related differences in the characteristics of problem gamblers using a gambling helpline. *Am J Psychiatry, 158,* 1500–1505.

Potenza, M. N., Steinberg, M. A., Skudlarski, P., Fulbright, R. K., Lacadie, C. M., Wilber, M. K., et al. (2003). Gambling urges in pathological gamblers: An fMRI study. *Arch Gen Psychiatry, 60,* 828–836.

Roy, A., De Jong, J., & Linnoila, M. (1989). Extraversion in pathological gamblers: Correlates with indexes of noradrenergic function. *Arch Gen Psychiatry, 46,* 679–681.

Saiz-Ruiz, J., Blanco, C., Ibanez, A., Masramon, X., Gomez, M. M., Madrigal, M., et al. (2005). Sertraline treatment of pathological gambling. *J Clin Psychiatry, 66,* 28–33.

Schlosser, S., Black, D. W., Repertinger, S., & Freet, D. (1994). Compulsive buying: Demography, phenomenology, and comorbidity in 46 subjects. *Gen Hosp Psychiatry, 16,* 205–212.

Shaffer, H. J., & Hall, M. N. (1996). Estimating the prevalence of adolescent gambling disorders: A quantitative synthesis and guide toward standard gambling nomenclature. *J Gambl Stud, 12,* 193–214.

Shaffer, H. J., Hall, M. N., & Vander Bilt, J. (1999). Estimating the prevalence of disordered gambling behavior in the United States and Canada: A research synthesis. *Am J Public Health, 89,* 1369–1376.

Slutske, W. S., Eisen, S., True, W. R., Lyons, M. J., Goldberg, J., & Tsuang, M. (2000). Common genetic vulnerability for pathological gambling and alcohol dependence in men. *Arch Gen Psychiatry, 57,* 666–673.

Sylvain, C., Ladouceur, R., & Boisvert, J. M. (1997). Cognitive and behavioral treatment of pathological gambling: A controlled study. *J Consult Clin Psychol, 65,* 727–732.

Welte, J., Barnes, G., Wieczorek, W., Tidwell, M. C., & Parker, J. (2001). Alcohol and gambling pathology among U.S. adults: Prevalence, demographic patterns and comorbidity. *J Stud Alcohol, 62,* 706–712.

CHAPTER 14

Substance Abuse
in Minority Populations

JOHN FRANKLIN
MARYLINN MARKARIAN

This chapter highlights issues in the treatment of addictive disorders in African Americans, Hispanic Americans, Asian Americans, and Native Americans. Cultural competency of caregivers in treatment programs is vital but is often lacking (Westermeyer, 1995). Substantial knowledge gaps still exist in minority substance abuse, and continued research in this area is needed. The growing ethnic diversity of the United States makes the significance of these issues even greater. According to the 2000 census, African Americans make up 12.2% of the population, Hispanics 11.8%, Asian Americans/Pacific Islanders 3.9%, Native Americans 0.7%, and whites 71.4% (U.S. Bureau of the Census, 2002). The fastest growing ethnic groups are Hispanics and Asian Americans. It is estimated by the year 2060, the U.S. non-Hispanic white population will be a minority. This chapter reviews selected data on addictive disorders in minority populations.

Divisions along ethnic lines can be complicated by variations in country of origin, religious and spiritual orientation, and political and economic conditions. These differences may influence the clinical presentation and therapeutic needs of the patient. Other variables include socioeconomic status, educational level, occupational stability, dwelling situation, marital status, family of origin, and age.

Thus, a middle-class African American woman with a college degree and stable employment, dwelling in a reasonably safe neighborhood, may share a daily world outlook toward the future more similar to that of a European American woman of a similar background than to a single, unemployed African American mother dwelling in an inner city. Their experiences within ethnic groups can be vastly different. There are scant data about differences in biological vulnerability for substance abuse between ethnic groups (Berrettini & Persico, 1996; Chan, McBride, Thomasson, Ykenny, & Crabb, 1994; Goldman et al., 1993), but new, yet unconfirmed biological findings are presented later in this chapter. This chapter highlights socioeconomic issues in substance abuse treatment for minorities.

Ethnic differences among women have received attention in the literature. In terms of alcohol, African American families produce more abstainers than do European and Hispanic American families. African American women may express more conservative drinking norms (Herd, 1997). African American women have rates of heavy drinking comparable to European American rates; however, they report fewer social and personal problems related to drinking. African American women may be more insulated from alcohol-related social problems by their families, communities, and churches. A larger proportion of African American women, however, experience alcohol-related health problems than do European American cohorts (Herd, 1989). One study of African American and Native American pregnant women shows African American women using higher quantities of malt liquor (higher alcohol content) (Graves & Kaskutas, 2001). African American women exhibit higher rates of fetal alcohol syndrome. These findings may be attributed to issues such as nutrition and access to health care. Concurrent illicit drug use may also be a contributing factor. In 1998, the percentage of African American women using illicit drugs during the preceding month, compared to European American cohorts, was 8.1 versus 7.6% in whites (Substance Abuse and Mental Health Services Administration, 2000). There are higher rates of cocaine use in African American and Hispanic women compared to Asian or Hispanic women.

Hispanic American women are more likely than European American women to abstain, though there is a one-sided convergence with increasing acculturation. For example, in one study, 75% of Mexican immigrant women abstained from alcohol, whereas 38% of third-generation Mexican American women were abstainers (Gilbert, 1991). Younger American-born Hispanic women are more likely to report moderate to heavy drinking than their immigrant cohorts. Mexican American women who use substances suffer significantly higher lifetime rates of physical and sexual assault (Lown & Vega, 2001). A substantially higher percentage of Native American/Alaskan Native women drink compared to whites, blacks, or Hispanics.

African American women in treatment often have myriad needs: employment, child care, and treatment for victimization and psychiatric symptoms. Personal losses, such as death of loved ones, separation, and loss of child custody, have a profound impact on drug use in African American women (Roberts, 1999). Women in substance abuse treatment are oversampled in terms of sexual abuse. In a study of 1,272 randomly selected women in a jail predominant for women of color, 8% had a comorbidity of severe mental disorder and substance abuse (Abram, Teplin, & McClelland, 2003). Life stress has been found to be a strong correlate of crack cocaine use in African American women (Boyd, Hill, Holmes, & Purnell, 1998), as is gang affiliation in women (Harper & Robinson, 1999). Child care has traditionally been a major obstacle to substance abuse treatment, but especially for minorities, although this is not unique to ethnic minorities. Financial restriction is a fundamental barrier to treatment for women, with added hardship for more women belonging to ethnic/minority groups.

Supportive networks are important to substance abuse recovery, irrespective of child care needs. A strong focus on the development of supports is indicated in the treatment of addicted women. Isolation among addicted women occurs for multiple reasons, including feelings of shame, guilt, and depression, and minority women may experience a double stigma. Creative social networks should be a strong focus of recovery for addicted minority women. It may be necessary to utilize extended family, as well as supports outside the family who serve as positive maternal figures. Respect for family systems is especially important in treating Hispanic women (Ruiz, Langrod, & Alksne, 1981).

AFRICAN AMERICANS

Heavy alcohol use by white men peaks in the 20s, then declines. Based on 1-month prevalence data, African American teens ages 12–17, compared to white teens of similar age, drink heavily less often, 0.7% versus 3.4%. However, by the age of 26, heavy use of alcohol is similar, 7.8% in blacks versus 7.1% in whites. Heavy use among black men is relatively low in the early years, peaks in middle age, then declines (Herd, 1990). One hypothesis of the etiology is that issues of racism and limited opportunities become more evident as African Americans mature into adulthood. The factors involved in the later onset of heavy alcohol use in African Americans and the subsequent rise in alcohol use need further research.

Diagnostic screening instruments for substance abuse in African Americans have been shown to be valid (Duncan, Duncan, & Strycker, 2002). In a large inpatient sample, African Americans were found to have later onset of use but earlier onset of alcohol-related problems (Hesselbrock, Hesselbrock, Segal, Schuckit, & Bucholz, 2003). In addition, the prevalence of alcohol-related problems in black men showed significant differences in psychosocial distress compared to that of white men (Herd, 1994). The greatest differences between the groups were found in scores for loss of control, symptomatic drinking, binge drinking, health problems, and problems with friends and relatives. Blacks and whites had similar drinking patterns, as measured by frequency and maximum amounts consumed. Black men were significantly less permissive in attitudes toward alcohol use in particular situations, such as driving a car or spending time with small children in a parental role. Further analyses showed that the higher rates of alcohol-related problems were not fully accounted for by social and demographic differences between black and white men.

An earlier study by Herd (1990), reporting on data from a 1984 national survey, showed similar findings of greater alcohol-related problems among black men than among white men in the past year. The exception was drunk driving, in which white men scored higher. Black men scored higher on symptoms of physical dependence and health problems. Here, the rates of frequent heavy drinking were lower, not higher, for black men. Limited financial resources and access to health care likely also contributed to the higher prevalence of alcohol-related health problems in black men. African Americans may be at higher risk for hepatic damage and cirrhosis from drinking (Singh & Hoyert, 2000; Stewart, 2002). Herd (1994) suggested that this finding may represent a longer duration of heavy use, as opposed to more discrete phases of heavy alcohol use seen in some white men. The body, it is hypothesized, is less resilient to alcohol toxicity at older ages.

Jones-Webb, Hsiao, and Hannan (1995) found that lower socioeconomic class seems to have a more profound influence on alcohol-related problems for black men than for white men, as did other researchers (Barr, Farrell, Barnes, & Welte, 1993; Herd, 1994; Jones, 1989). Black men of lower socioeconomic status may experience more overt forms of discrimination and may be more likely to reside in communities in which there is more police surveillance. Group norms may be predictive of problematic alcohol use in African Americans (Jones-Webb, Snowden, Herd, Short, & Hannan, 1997). Greater ethnic identity may be protective against problematic drinking (Herd & Grube, 1996). Lower neighborhood cohesion has been associated with adolescent drug and alcohol problems.

Polymorphism of the ADH2*3 alcohol dehydrogenase metabolic enzyme may play a role in alcohol expectations in African Americans (Ehlers, Carr, Betancourt, & Montane-Jaime, 2003). Lower P3 amplitudes during event-related potentials have also been reported in alcoholic African Americans (Ehlers et al., 2003). The association of alcohol use and hypertension may be particularly problematic in African American men (Russell, Cooper, Frone, & Peirce, 1999). The association between hypertension and illicit drug use has also been reported (Kim, Dennison, Hill, Bone, & Levine, 2000). Ziedonis, Rayford, Bryant, and Rounsaville (1994) have reported on differential rates of lifetime psychiatric comorbidity in black and white cocaine addicts, with whites having significantly higher rates of lifetime depression, alcohol dependence, and attention deficit and conduct disorder. African Americans often exhibit significant general coping skills but fewer treatment resources compared to whites (Conigliaro et al., 2000; Walton, Blow, & Booth, 2001). There is some evidence that substance abuse in whites may be associated with greater underlying psychopathology, whereas African Americans may have greater social and environmental factors (Roberts, 1999). Early initiation of sexual activity may be predictive of later substance abuse in African Americans (Stanton et al., 2002).

Historically, a greater proportion of African Americans abstain from illicit drug use than do whites. This difference is especially pronounced in the 12–25 age groups. However, public databases such as the Client Data Acquisition Process and Drug Abuse Warning Network (DAWN) suggest that African Americans and Hispanics are overrepresented in categories of heroin and cocaine use. Since the 1980s, we have seen up-and-down patterns of perceived harm among high school students. However, data still show a higher overall prevalence of illicit drug use in blacks: 8.2% in blacks versus 6.1% in whites (Substance Abuse and Mental Health Services Administration, 2000). Higher rates of marijuana and cocaine use account for the difference. In the 1998 National Household Survey on Drug Abuse (NHSDA), African Americans had higher prevalence of marijuana (5 vs. 6.6%) and cocaine (0.7 vs. 1.3%) (Substance Abuse and Mental Health Services Administration, 2000). The gap between white and black adolescents' marijuana use has disappeared. African Americans have higher rates of marijuana use by age 20 (Brown, Flory, Lynam, Leukefeld, & Clayton, 2004; Reardon & Buka, 2002). Also emerging from epidemiology studies is a somewhat higher concentration of heroin use among blacks as compared to whites. The NHSDA (Substance Abuse and Mental Health Services Administration, 2000) shows that past-month use of any illicit drug is higher for whites between the ages of 12 and 25, and higher for African Americans age 26 and up. Asian/Pacific Islanders show the lowest rates of past-month use across all age groups.

As with alcohol, illicit drug use appears to take a greater toll on African Americans' health, as measured by emergency department data. African Americans are overrepresented, as a percentage of the population, in emergency room (ER) visits. Whites represent 57.5% of ER visits compared to 21.4% by African Americans (DAWN, 2004; National Institute on Drug Abuse, 2003). Although DAWN data are derived from large cities where African American populations are proportionally high, this is still an overrepresentation of ER visits for drug abuse. African Americans are more likely than whites to be treated and released rather than hospitalized. The 1998 NHSDA showed cocaine is the primary drug leading to the ER visits for African Americans. African Americans are also overrepresented in medical examiners' morbidity data. They account for 30% of drug-related deaths, while making up 23% of the population of the cities surveyed in DAWN. Cocaine is the most frequent cause of death, 56.7%, followed by heroin and morphine. Much of the information about hard core drug use comes from similar data derived from public facilities. These data may seriously underestimate the number of persons who obtain alternative treatment for medical and psychosocial problems.

Literature reviewed by Brown, Alterman, Rutherford, Cacciola, and Zaballero (1993) suggest that correlates of heroin abuse may be educational impairment, poor employment history, history of legal problems, including incarceration, and possibly psychiatric problems. A national sample of by Kandel and Davies (1991) showed that early sexual intercourse was associated with elevated lifetime cocaine use among all ethnic groups; and that a correlate to cocaine use was daily marijuana use (defined by use at least 20 times in the last 30 days).

Low rates of condom use among cocaine, marijuana, and alcohol abusers may be contributing to an HIV epidemic among African Americans (Kingree & Betz, 2003; Timpson, Williams, Bowen, & Keel, 2003). Cocaine use, in particular, may contribute to intracerebral bleeding, renal failure, chest pain, and myocardial infarctions in African Americans (Oureshi et al., 2001). In addition, the severity of asthma exacerbation seems to be worse in African American urban settings (Rome, Lippmann, Dalsey, Taggart, & Pomerantz, 2000). Several groups are also studying strategies to decrease cigarette smoking in African Americans (Ahluwalia, Harris, Catley, Okuyemi, & Mayo, 2002; Benowitz, 2002; Okuyemi, Ahluwalia, Richter, Mayo, & Resnicow, 2001).

A coarse reading of this literature might imply that some intrinsic nature within the ethnic groups accounts for the differences. Lillie-Blanton, Anthony, and Schuster (1993) conducted a study in which they regrouped participants according to neighborhood rather than race or ethnicity. They held constant social and environmental risk factors that likely influence the racial comparisons and applied this design to the apparent differences in crack cocaine use among whites, Hispanics, and African Americans. This interesting analysis revealed that the odds ratios did not vary significantly among the ethnic groups. Being African American did not place individuals at higher risk for crack use. Though this analysis does not refute the epidemiological findings of the study, it does suggest that the apparent differences may be more a product of social conditions, including availability of drugs, than are issues intrinsic to ethnicity. Drug trafficking, often concentrated in minority neighborhoods, is a risk factor for use (Li, Feigelman, Stanton, Galbraith, & Huang, 1998).

Among African American and European Americans, there may be different mu receptor polymorphisms (Crowley et al., 2003). However, strong evidence has yet established that these gene findings are associated with actual drug use (Kranzler, Gelernter, O'Malley, Hernandez-Avila, & Kaufman, 1998). One report found no association between particular dopamine receptor alleles and cocaine dependence in African Americans (Gelernter, Kranzler, & Satel, 1999). Negative findings have also been reported for the association between serotonin transporter polymorphisms and aggression in African American cocaine dependence (Patkar et al., 2002).

It is well-known that as a result of the "war on drugs" and other pressures, African Americans arrested for drug-related charges are overrepresented in prisons and jails. Inequalities in sentencing factors may indicate subtle racism. For example, the differential sentencing for crack cocaine use, which is more prevalent in black communities, and powder cocaine has been a matter of national debate.

Access to treatment is still a problem for African Americans (Zule, Lam, & Wechsberg, 2003). Some argue that prevention and treatment of substance abuse and HIV in African American communities must recognize and address institutional racism, sociopolitical exploitation, patterns drug of distribution, limited employment opportunities, and historical African American coping strategies (Adimora et al., 2001; Agar & Reisinger, 2002; Bowser & Bilal, 2001). Increasing gainful employment is a particularly powerful intervention (Petry, 2003). Poverty in black neighborhoods compared to white neighborhoods may have a greater impact on alcohol-related problems. Many in the African American community stress the issues of self-help and community empowerment to combat divisive elements leading to drug and alcohol use. As a result, network therapy may have a particular role in more distressed communities. In a large Veterans Administration residential study, African Americans had similar rates of program participation to whites but tended to do better in aftercare programs with greater African American staff presence (Rosenheck & Seibyl, 1998). Another study, using data from the National Collaborative Study, found that social and peer relationship problems predicted 18.8% of the variance for future substance use in an urban adolescent population (Friedman & Glassman, 2002). School dropout rates have been associated with injection drug use in African Americans; dropout rates should be targeted for intervention (Obot & Anthony, 2000; Obot, Hubbard, & Anthony, 1999).

Problackness and awareness of racial oppression have been associated with negative substance use attitudes (Gary & Berry, 1985). Strong ethnic identity may protect against substance abuse and should be incorporated in treatment programs, especially for adolescents (Brook, Balka, Brook, Win, & Gursen, 1998, Longshore, 1999). However, one study reported high levels of cultural identity to be positively associated with heavy drug use (James, Kim, & Armijo, 2000). Culturally sensitive interventions have been shown to enhance getting people into treatment and improving outcomes (Dushay, Singer, Weeks, Rohena, & Gruber, 2001; Longshore, Grills, & Annon, 1999). There is no question that standard treatment approaches highlighted in the rest of this book can readily be applied to all ethnic groups. Standard cognitive-behavioral treatments have been shown to be as effective for African Americans as for whites (Milligan, Nich, & Carroll, 2004).

Misdiagnosis of psychiatric comorbidities in African Americans can limit treatment effectiveness (Baker & Bell, 1999). There is an association between substance abuse and suicide in black men but it may be less robust than that in white men (Garlow, 2002; Kaslow et al., 2000). The core features of loss of control and compulsivity that make a drug abuser or alcoholic are not dissimilar between ethnic groups. However, as we continue to tailor treatment to individuals, racial and cultural factors have to be addressed.

Should programs in primarily African American communities be especially designed to promote cultural sensitivity? In some sense this goes on naturally. The feel, look, and language of an Alcohol Anonymous (AA) meeting in an African American community is different from that in a white self-help group. AA had its beginnings in the Oxford movement and was initially white and middle class. However, given that the church and spiritual dimensions of black life are an integral aspect of black culture, it is not surprising that AA has been successfully transplanted to the black community. There have been attempts to develop and describe culturally sensitive mental health facilities (Deitch & Solit, 1993; Rowe & Grills, 1993). These attempts often are trapped in a quagmire of definitions of culture, race, and what is crucial to a culturally relevant program. Culturally relevant programs might promote positive racial and cultural identity, enhance self-esteem, increase self-determination, and appreciate traditional African American values. Afrocentric values stress relationships, verbal fluidity, emotional expressiveness, and spirituality. A study of substance abuse programs, using the National Drug Abuse Treatment System Survey, suggests that culturally competent treatment is holistic and emphasizes employment, spiritual strength, and physical health (Howard, 2003a). Programs that hire staff that mirror patients' ethnic background may minimize racial bias. In addition, possessing knowledge of African American history and culture is a component of a culturally competent program (Howard, 2003b).

Research questions related to primary hypotheses that especially address ethnic concerns are needed. There may be dimensions to an all-black treatment program that go beyond variables currently thought to be important. Ethnic biological differences, if any exist, of African Americans need further work. Differences in health outcome and possibly medication responses need further consideration. The issue of matching or nonmatching of therapist or patient along racial and ethnic dimensions has been a subject of considerable discussion in mental health and has a role in the substance abuse field. Matching of racial and cultural attributes between therapist and client may enhance empathy or in some cases result in therapist overidentification with the client. Empathy and respect of others' cultural norms are an essential components to any discussion of cultural sensitivity.

HISPANIC AMERICANS

Hispanics comprise a heterogeneous group, including Mexican Americans, Puerto Ricans, Cuban Americans, and others. As with other ethnic groups, a greater number of Hispanic men drink alcohol and use drugs than do Hispanic women. Mexican American men are more likely to abstain than other Hispanic men. However, they drink more heavily and report more alcohol-related problems. Puerto Rican men have the highest prevalence of illicit drug use, 10% versus 5% of Mexican Americans (Substance Abuse and Mental Health Services Administration, 2000). White Hispanic men have high rates of cirrhosis, especially among Mexican Americans (Stinson, Grant, & Dufour, 2001). Self-reported rates of drinking and driving are highest in Hispanics and whites (Caetano & Clark, 2000). In New York City, cocaine- and opiate-positive urine analysis in victims of firearms deaths are highest in Latino men (Galea et al., 2003). Also, Latinos and African Americans have higher rate of overdose deaths. Cuban men had fewer abstainers, a smaller proportion of heavy drinkers, and fewer alcohol-related problems. Drinking increases with education and income for both sexes (Caetano, 1989).

According to the 1995 NHSDA, for all age groups except 12–17 years, Hispanics had the fewest members in the "ever used any illicit drug" category as compared to whites and African Americans. Data derived from the NHSDA (1996–1997) reported that Hispanics are more likely to binge drink and use drugs more heavily. Caetano and Medina-Mora (1990) compared the drinking patterns of Mexican Americans and Mexicans living in Mexico. A more permissive attitude about alcohol use was associated with acculturation. Alcohol use increased with acculturation in both Mexican men and woman. However, Mexican Americans reported fewer alcohol-related problems than did Mexican men living in Mexico. For Mexican women born in the United States, abstention rates steadily decreased and rates of infrequent drinking steadily increased with acculturation. This pattern is not seen in Mexican-born women living in the United States (Caetano & Medina-Mora, 1990). Similarly, in South Florida, U.S.-born Hispanic young adults have increased rates of substance abuse and mental health problems compared to Hispanic immigrants. Inhalant use is reported to be high among Hispanic youth in southwestern border states. Polymorphism of the alcohol dehydrogenase 2 gene and P450 2E1 has been reported to contribute to development of alcoholism in Mexican American men (Konishi et al., 2003).

Among people of need, Hispanics and African Americans compared to whites have greater unmet need for alcohol and drug abuse treatment. Hispanics receive active treatment 22.4% of the time, and African American 25% of the time, versus whites at 37% (Wells, Klap, Koike, & Sherbourne, 2001). Language can be the most concrete barrier to adequate treatment for Hispanics in communities without adequate Spanish-speaking facilities. However, cultural sensitivity is not guaranteed by just speaking the language. In the state of Massachusetts, Latinos are one-third less likely to enter residential treatment (Lundgren, Amodeo, Ferguson, & Davis, 2001). For example, Spanish-speaking male staff must be able to treat female clients with respect and be sensitive to sexual, family, and child-rearing issues. A number of authors (e.g., Szapocznik

& Fein, 1995) identify family issues as being perhaps the most important component of addiction treatment of the Hispanic client.

Gfroerer and De La Rosa (1993) found that parents' attitudes and use of drugs, licit or illicit, played an important role in the drug use behavior of 12- to 17-year-old Hispanic youth. Parents need to be informed clearly and honestly about their influence. Also, the role of family should be well understood by treatment staff. Each family member has a function within the family. If properly educated, the family members can each provide support, using their already established role. Some of the traditional roles, according to Ruiz and colleagues (1981), are the elderly, esteemed for their wisdom, the father for his authority, the mother for her devotion, and the children for their future promise. Denial of alcoholism may be extensive in Hispanic fathers who drink only on the weekend and fulfill work obligations. Szapocznik and Fein (1995) included the cultural tradition of interdependence with extended family made up of uncles, aunts, cousins, and lifelong friends. Basically, the functional family does include any person who has day-to-day contact with and a role in the family. The family is an important resource and must be integrated into the treatment.

ASIAN AMERICANS

People of Asian heritage make up nearly 3.9% of the U.S. population according to U.S. Bureau of the Census (2002): Chinese Americans (the largest group, 24%), Filipinos (20%), Asian Indians (12%), Koreans (12%), Japanese (12%), and Vietnamese (9%). Other countries of Asian immigration include Mongolia, Pakistan, Nepal, Bangladesh, Burma, Thailand, Cambodia, Malaysia, Singapore, and others. Many languages, cultures, and political systems are represented. Most of the world's major religions are represented, including Buddhism, Hinduism, Judaism, Christianity, and Islam. These religions have varying views regarding alcohol use. Alcohol use is prohibited in the Moslem teachings. Hinduism and Buddhism suggest avoidance of alcohol and other mind-altering substances. The Judeo-Christian perspective is more lenient and incorporates alcohol use into some religious ceremonies. These views affect the way the society, the family, and the problem drinker deal with the concept and acceptance of alcoholism. Acceptance and availability of treatment for individuals also have an impact.

The well-described "flushing" reaction seen in some Asian people has been linked to variations of aldehyde dehydrogenase isoenzymes. The reaction occurs because of a limited ability to degrade acetaldehyde to acetic acid. The toxic acetaldehyde is responsible for the flushing, headache, nausea, and other symptoms of alcohol use estimated to occur in 47–85% of Asians (National Institute on Alcohol and Alcoholism, 2000). This was thought to explain the lower rates of alcohol abuse among Asians. However, studies have shown that sociocultural factors play a substantial role in alcohol use (Johnson & Nagoski, 1990; Newlin, 1989).

Some major databases on alcoholism in ethnic minority populations do not include information on Asian Americans. The Epidemiologic Catchment Area (ECA) study placed Asian Americans in the "other" category. Two national studies do survey Asians as a specific category: DAWN and the NHSDA (Substance Abuse and Mental Health Administration, 2000). The percentage of past-month use among Asians/Pacific Islanders is 2.8%, the lowest among the major ethnic groups. The 1-month prevalence for Native Hawaiians and other Pacific Islanders is 6.2%, versus 2.7% for Asians. However, the Korean subgroup of Asians has a 6.9% prevalence rate, similar to that of African Americans. The available research literature is mostly community based or pertains to a specific subgroup within the Asian American community, such as students. Given these limitations, a number of studies show that there is significant variation in drinking patterns among the different Asian groups. There is some evidence that rates of heavy drinking are higher for Filipino Americans (29%) and Japanese Americans (28.9%), followed by Korean Americans (25.8%) and Chinese Americans (14.2%) (Kitano & Chi, 1989). The breakdown by sex found heavy drinking in 11.7% of Japanese women, 3.5% of Filipino women, and 0.8% of Korean women, whereas Chinese women registered near zero. In a large inpatient sample, Alaskan Native men and women had earlier onsets of alcohol dependence (Hesselbrock et al., 2003). Interestingly, there is a Japanese AA-like organization called the All Nippon Sobriety Association (Gomberg, 2003).

Potential treatment problems in the Asian American community begin with the lack of acceptance of alcoholism and drug addictions as treatable illnesses. Ja and Aoki (1993) write about the typical chain of events in the life of an intact Asian family when substance abuse begins to appear. Often, substance abuse problems are ignored or denied, with the hope that they will disappear. Also, the family will make efforts to conceal it from the community to avoid embarrassment and shame. Prevention or early treatment is unlikely in this family and community dynamic. When denial is overwhelming, the family breaks down and may resort to shaming and other attempts at punishment. The family may also turn to extended family members and elders, basically moving gradually outward from nuclear family to external community. There is a deep sense of failure on the part of the family by the time members resort to outside professional help. It is not uncommon at this point to have family members completely turn over the alcoholic or addict and resist participation themselves. The client is often still in denial and resistant to treatment, until an alliance with staff is facilitated.

Treatment barriers begin with ignorance of the actual extent of drug and alcohol problems in the Asian American community. Asians are thought of by many as model immigrants. The 1960s brought a large wave of educated, skilled

Asian professionals. Migration since the 1970s has resulted in people with less education, and fewer language and work skills immigrating to the United States (Varma & Siris, 1996). Many of them entered as refugees from war-ravaged countries. Poverty, overcrowded domiciles, discrimination, and other social problems are present in the lives of Asian Americans; however, documentation of these problems is sparse. This notion of "model" immigrant may be hurting the Asian American community from outside and within. It also lends itself to the denial within the community and amplifies the elements of shame and embarrassment felt by the family.

Better documentation of the extent of drug and alcohol abuse in the Asian American population would, ideally, enhance the funding for culturally sensitive education and treatment. Education at the community level is needed to foster awareness and acceptance, and assist in prevention. Treatment programs that target Asian Americans might consider the insular and private style of the Asian American family. Also essential is recognition of the dominance of the family and community over the psychological and social needs of the individual. Acceptance of these differences would decrease conflict between the families and treatment providers. This show of respect for their values might facilitate the families' participation in the treatment. A treatment goal for all individuals should be reintegration back into their family and community, if at all possible.

NATIVE AMERICANS

More than 200 Native American tribes have a differential use of illicit substances. Studies show that Native American/Alaskan Native youth have twice the prevalence of cigarette, alcohol, marijuana, and cocaine use as that of Hispanics, blacks, or whites. Alcohol abuse is recognized as a significant problem among Native Americans (Shalala, Trujillo, Nolan, & D'Angelo, 1996). The CAGE questionnaire, however, has not been particularly useful among Native Americans (Saremi et al., 2001). Conduct disorder has been found to be a significant risk factor for alcohol dependence in Navajo Indians (Kunitz et al., 1999). In the past, arrest rates secondary to alcohol use for Native Americans were reported to be 12 times the national average (Stewart, 1964). In a Michigan Monitoring the Future study, Native American adolescents had the highest levels of tobacco, alcohol, and illicit drug use (Wallace et al., 2002). Native American/Alaskan Native youth may also participate in more risky behaviors (Frank & Lester, 2002). Although the alcohol mortality rate for Native Americans was three to four times the national average, evidence indicates that there has been a decrease in mortality since 1969 (Burns, 1995). This drop seems to be in concert with the doubling of alcohol treatment services by the Indian

Health Service in the 1980s. Primary case settings may be important for detecting substance use (Shore, Manson, & Buchwald, 2002).

Illicit drug use among Native Americans is less clear, because the data available are poor. Furthermore, the use of hallucinogens has an important role in some Native American religious rituals. The heterogeneity of Native American cultures is plainly evident and further discourages simplistic discussions of Indian culture. The "firewater" myth states that alcohol introduced to Native Americans by white settlers produced exaggerated biological effects in such persons. Garcia-Andrade, Wall, and Ehlers (1997), however, found less subjective intoxication among nonalcoholic Mission Indian men with greater Native American heritage. The same researchers implicate alcohol expectancy and metabolism rates as possible differential effects among members of this tribe (Garcia-Andrade et al., 1997; Wall, Garcia-Andrade, Thomasson, Cole, & Ehlers, 1996).

Native Americans share a belief in the unity and sacredness of all nature. Individual or ethnic groups may be more or less familiar with their own culture. Confrontational approaches, successful in many Anglo programs, cause Native Americans to shy away. Risk factors for alcohol and drug use in Native Americans parallel many of the same issues of other disenfranchised groups. Attempts at assimilation of Native American culture, in the context of isolation from mainstream opportunities, have contributed to further cultural stress. The recent increase in Indian-owned casinos has offered monetary opportunities, but also the possibilities of increased gambling and substance abuse. The breakdown of Native American culture, a factor that allowed alcohol to take a foothold, has been reversing in recent years. Self-determination and a return to traditional spiritual and healing beliefs have helped springboard alternative indigenous models of alcohol and drug recovery.

REFERENCES

Abram, K. M., Teplin, L. A., & McClelland, G. M. (2003). Comorbidity of severe psychiatric disorders and substance use disorders among women in jail. *Am J Psychiatry, 160*(5), 1007–1010.

Adimora, A. A., Schoenbach, V. J., Martinson, F. E., Donaldson, K. H., Fullilove, R. E., & Aral, S. O. (2001). Social context of sexual relationships among rural African Americans. *Sex Transm Dis, 28*(2), 69–76.

Agar, M., & Reisinger, H. S. (2002). A heroin epidemic at the intersection of histories: The 1960s epidemic among African Americans in Baltimore. *Medical Anthropol, 21*(2), 115–156.

Ahluwalia, J., Harris, K. J., Catley, D., Okuyemi, K. S., & Mayo, M. S. (2002). Sustained-release bupropion for smoking cessation in African Americans: A randomized controlled trail. *JAMA, 288*(4), 468–474.

Baker, F. M., & Bell, C. C. (1999). Issues in the psychiatric treatment of African Americans. *Psychiatr Serv, 50*(3), 362–368.

Barr, K. E. M., Farrell, M. P., Barnes, G. M., & Welte, J. W. (1993). Race, class and gender differences in substance abuse: Evidence of a middle-class/under-class polarization among black males. *Social Problems, 403,* 314–327.

Berrettini, W. H., & Persico, A. M. (1996). Dopamine D2 receptor gene polymorphisms and vulnerability to substance abuse in African Americans. *Biol Psychiatry, 40,* 144–147.

Bowser, B. P., & Bilal, R. (2001). Drug treatment effectiveness: African-American culture in recovery. *J Psychoactive Drugs, 33*(4), 391–402.

Boyd, C., Guthrie, B., Pohl, J., Whitmarsh, J., & Henderson, D. (1998). African American women who smoke crack cocaine: Sexual trauma and the mother–daughter relationship. *J Psychoactive Drugs, 26*(3), 243–247.

Boyd, C. J., Hill, E., Holmes, C., & Purnell, R. (1998). Putting drug use in context: Lifelines of African-American women who smoke crack. *J Subst Abuse Treat, 15*(3), 235–249.

Brook, J. S., Balka, E. B., Brook, D. W., Win, P. T., & Gursen, M. D. (1998). Drug use among African Americans: Ethnic identity as a protective factor. *Psychol Rep, 83*(3 Pt. 2), 1427–1446.

Brown, L. S., Jr., Alterman, A. I., Rutherford, M. J., Cacciola, J. S., & Zaballero, A. R. (1993). Addiction Severity Index scores of four racial/ethnic and gender groups of methadone maintenance patients. *J Subst Abuse, 5*(3), 269–279.

Brown, T. L., Flory, K., Lynam, D. R., Leukefeld, C., & Clayton, R. R. (2004). Comparing the developmental trajectories of marijuana use of African-American and Caucasian adolescents: Patterns, antecedents, and consequences. *Exp Clin Psychopharmacol, 12*(1), 47–56.

Burns, T. R. (1995). How does IHS relate administratively to the high alcoholism mortality rate? *Am Indian Alsk Native Ment Health Res, 6*(3), 31–45.

Caetano, R. (1989). Drinking patterns and alcohol problems in a national sample of U.S. Hispanics. In D. L. Spiegler, D. A. Tate, S. S. Aitken, & C. M. Christian (Eds.), *Alcohol use among U.S. ethnic minorities: Proceedings of a conference on the epidemiology of alcohol use and abuse among ethnic minority groups* (NIAAA Research Monograph No. 18, DHHS Publication No. ADM 89-1435, pp. 147–162). Washington, DC: U.S. Government Printing Office.

Caetano, R., & Clark, C. L. (2000). Hispanics, blacks and whites driving under the influence of alcohol: Results from the 1995 National Alcohol Survey. *Accid Anal Prev, 32*(1), 57–64.

Caetano, R., & Medina-Mora, M. E. (1990, June). Reasons and attitudes toward drinking and abstaining: A comparison of Mexicans and Mexican-Americans. In *Epidemiologic trends in drug use: Community epidemiology work group proceedings* (pp. 173–191). Rockville, MD: National Institute of Drug Abuse.

Chan, R. J., McBride, A. W., Thomasson, H. R., Ykenney, A., & Crabb, D. W. (1994). Allele frequencies of the preproenkephalin A (PENK) gene CA repeat in Asians, African-Americans, and Caucasians: Lack of evidence for different allele frequencies in alcoholics. *Alcohol Clin Exp Res, 18*(3), 533–535.

Conigliaro, J., Maisto, S. A., McNeil, M., Kraemer, K., Kelley, M. E., Conigliaro, R., & O'Connor, M. (2000). Does race make a different among primary care patients with alcohol problems who agree to enroll in a study of brief interventions? *Am J Addict*, 9(4), 321–330.

Crowley, J. J., Oslin, D. W., Patkar, A. A., Gottheil, E., DeMaria, P. A. Jr., O'Brien, C. P., et al. (2003). A genetic association study of the mu opioid receptor and severe opioid dependence. *Psychiatr Genet*, 13(3), 169–173.

Deitch, D., & Solit, R. (1993). International training for drug abuse treatment and the issue of cultural relevance. *J Psychoactive Drugs*, 25(1), 87–95.

Drug Abuse Warning Network (DAWN). (2004). *Mortality data from DAWN, 2002.* (DAWN Series D-25, DHHS Publication No. [SMA] 04-3875). Rockville, MD. *http://dawninfo.samhsa.gov/old_dawn/pubs_94_02/mepbus/default.asp*

Duncan, S. C., Duncan, T. E., & Strycker, L. A. (2002). A multilevel analysis of neighborhood context and youth alcohol and drug problems. *Prev Sci*, 3(2), 125–133.

Dushay, R. A., Singer, M., Weeks, M. R., Rohena, L., & Gruber, R. (20010. Lowering HIV risk among ethnic minority drug users: Comparing culturally targeted intervention to a standard intervention. *Am J Drug Alcohol Abuse*, 27(3), 501–524.

Ehlers, C. L., Carr, L., Betancourt, M., & Montane-Jaime, K. (2003). Association of the ADH2*3 allele with greater alcohol expectancies in African-American young adults. *J Stud Alcohol*, 64(2), 176–181.

Frank, M. L., & Lester, D. (2002). Self-destructive behaviors in American Indian and Alaska Native high school youth. *Am Indian Alsk Native Ment Health Res*, 10(3), 24–32.

Friedman, A. S., & Glassman, K. (2002). Family risk factors versus peer risk factors for drug abuse: A longitudinal study of an African-American urban community sample. *J Subst Abuse Treat*, 18(3), 267–275.

Galea, S., Ahern, J., Tardiff, K., Leon, A., Coffin, P. O., Derrk, K., & Vlahov, D. (2003). Racial/ethnic disparities in overdose mortality trends in New York City, 1990–1998. *J Urban Health*, 80(2), 201–211.

Garcia-Andrade, C., Wall, T. L., & Ehlers, C. L. (1997, July). The firewater myth and response to alcohol in mission Indians. *Am J Psychiatry*, 154(7), 983–988.

Garlow, S. J. (2002). Age, gender and ethnicity differences in patterns of cocatin and ethanol use preceding suicide. *Am J Psychiatry*, 159(4), 615–619.

Gary, L., & Berry, G. (1985). Predicting attitudes toward substance use in a black community. *Community Ment Health J*, 21, 45–51.

Gelernter, J., Kranzler, H., & Satel, S. L. (1999). No association between D$_2$ dopamine receptr (DRD2) alleles or haplotypes and cocaine dependence or severity of cocaine dependence in European- and African-Americans. *Biol Psychiatry*, 45(3), 340–345.

Gfroerer, J., & De La Rosa, M. (1993). Protective and risk factors associated with drug use among Hispanic youth. *J Addict Dis*, 12(2), 87–107.

Gilbert, M. J. (1991). Acculturation and changes in drinking patterns among Mexican-American women. *Alcohol Health Res World*, 15(3), 234–238.

Goldman, D., Brown, G. L., Albaugh, B., Robin, R., Goodson, S. , Trunzo, M., et al. (1993). DRD2 dopamine receptor genotype, linkage disequilibrium, and alcoholism in American Indians and other populations. *Alcohol Clin Exp Res*, 17(2), 199–204.

Gomberg, E. S. (2003). Treatment for alcohol-related problems: Special populations: Research opportunities. *Recent Dev Alcohol*, 16, 313–333.

Graves, K., & Kaskutas, L. A. (2001). Beverage choice among Native-American and African-American urban women. *Alcohol Clin Exp Res*, 26(2), 218–222.

Harper, G. W., & Robinson, W. L. (1999). Pathways to risk among inner-city African-American adolescent females: The influence of gang membership. *Am J Community Psychol*, 27(3), 383–404.

Herd, D. (1989). The epidemiology of drinking patterns and alcohol-related problems among U.S. blacks. In D. Spiegler, D. Tate, D. S. Aitkens, & C. Christian (Eds.), *Alcohol use among U. S. ethnic minorities* (NIAAA Research Monograph No. 18, DHHS Publication No. ADM 89-1435, pp. 3–50). Washington, DC: U.S. Government Printing Office.

Herd, D. (1990). Subgroup differences in drinking patterns among black and white men: Results from a national survey. *J Stud Alcohol*, 51(3), 221–232.

Herd, D. (1994). Predicting drinking problems among black and white men: Results from a national survey. *J Stud Alcohol*, 55, 61–71.

Herd, D. (1997). Sex ratios of drinking patterns and problems among blacks and whites: Results from a national survey. *J Stud Alcohol*, 58(1), 75–82.

Hesselbrock, M. N., Hesselbrock, V. M., Segal, B., Schuckit, M. A., & Bucholz, K. (2003). Ethnicity and psychiatric comorbidity among alcohol-dependent persons who receive inpatient treatment: African Americans, Alaska Natives, Caucasians and Hispanics. *Alcohol Clin Exp Res*, 27(8), 1368–1373.

Howard, D. L. (2003a). Are the treatment goals of culturally competent outpatient substance abuse treatment units congruent with their client profile? *J Subst Abuse Treat*, 24(2), 103–113.

Howard, D. L. (2003b). Culturally competent treatment of African-American clients among a national sample of outpatient substance abuse treatment units. *J Subst Abuse Treat*, 24(2), 89–102.

Ja, D., & Aoki, B. (1993). Substance abuse treatment: Cultural barriers in the Asian-American community. *J Psychoactive Drugs*, 25(1), 61–71.

James, W. H., Kim, G. K., & Armijo, E. (2000). The influence of ethnic identity on drug use among ethnic minority adolescents. *J Drug Educ*, 30(3), 265–280.

Johnson, R. C., & Nagoski, C. T. (1990). Asians, Asian-Americans, and alcohol. *J Psychoactive Drugs*, 22(1), 45–52.

Jones, R. J. (1989). *The socio-economic context of alcohol use and depression: Results from a national survey of black and white adults.* Paper presented at the 15th annual Ketil Bruun Alcohol Epidemiology Symposium, Maastricht, The Netherlands.

Jones-Webb, R., Hsiao, C., & Hannan, P. (1995). Relationships between socioeconomic status and drinking problems among black and white men. *Alcohol Clin Exp Res*, 19(3), 623–627.

Jones-Webb, R., Snowden, L., Herd, D., Short, B., & Hannan, P. (19970. Alcohol-related problems among black, Hispanic and white men: The contribution of neighborhood poverty. *J Study Alcohol*, 58(5), 539–545.

Kaslow, N., Thompson, M., Meadows, L., Chance, S., Puett, R., Hollins, L., et al. (2000). Risk factors for suicide attempts among African-American women. *Depress Anxiety*, 12(1), 13–20.

Kim, M. T., Dennison, C. R., Hill, M. N., Bone, L. R., & Levine, D. M. (2000). Relationship of alcohol and illicit drug use with high blood pressure care and control among urban hypertensive black men. *Ethn Dis*, 10(2), 175–183.

Kingree, J. B., & Betz, H. (2003). Risky sexual behavior in relation to marijuana and alcohol use among African-American, male adolescent detainees and their female partners. *Drug Alcohol Depend, 72*(2), 197–203.

Kitano, H. H. L., & Chi, I. (1989). Asian Americans and alcohol: The Chinese, Japanese, Koreans, and Filipinos in Los Angeles. In D. Spiegler, D. Tate, S. Aitkens, & C. Christian (Eds.), *Alcohol use among U.S. ethnic minorities* (NIAAA Research Monograph No. 18, DHHS Publication No. ADM 89-1435, pp. 373–382). Washington, DC: U.S. Government Printing Office.

Konishi, T., Calvillo, M., Leng, A. S., Feng, J., Lee, T., Lee, H., et al. (2003). The ADH3*2 and CYP2E1 c2 alleles increase the risk of alcoholism in Mexican-American men. *Exp Mol Pathol, 74*(2), 183–189.

Kranzler, H. R., Gelernter, J., O'Malley, S., Hernandez-Avila, C. A., & Kaufman, D. (1998). Association of alcohol or other drug dependence with alleles of the mu opioid receptor gene (OPRM1). *Alcohol Clin Exp Res, 22*(6), 1356–1359.

Kunitz, S. J., Gabriel, K. R., Levy, J. E., Henderson, E., Lampert, K., McCloskey, J., et al. (1999). Alcohol dependence and conduct disorder among Navajo Indians. *J Stud Alcohol, 60*(2), 159–167.

Li, X., Feigelman, S., Stanton, B., Galbraith, J., & Huang, W. (1998). Drug trafficking and drug use among urban African-American adolescents: A casual analysis. *J Adolesc Health, 23*(5), 280–288.

Lillie-Blanton, M., Anthony, J., & Schuster, C. R. (1993). Probing the meaning of racial/ethnic group comparisons in crack cocaine smoking. *JAMA, 296*(8), 993–997.

Longshore, D. (1999). Help-seeking by African-American drug users: A prospective analysis. *Addict Behav, 24*(5), 683–686.

Longshore, D., Grills, C., & Annon, K. (1999). Effects of a culturally congruent intervention on cognitive factors related to drug-use recovery. *Subst Use Misuse, 34*(9), 1223–1241.

Lown, A. E., & Vega, W. A. (2001). Alcohol abuse and dependence among Mexican-American women who report violence. *Alcohol Clin Exp Res, 25*(10), 1479–1486.

Lundgren, L. M., Amodeo, M., Ferguson, F., & Davis, K. (2001). Racial and ethnic differences in drug treatment entry of injection drug users in Massachusetts. *J Subst Abuse Treat, 21*, 145–153.

Milligan, C. O., Nich, C., & Carroll, K. M. (2004). Ethnic differences in substance abuse treatment retention, compliance, and outcome from two clinical trials. *Psychiatr Serv, 55*(2), 167–173.

National Institute on Alcohol Abuse and Alcoholism. (2000, June). *10th Special Report to the U.S. Congress on Alcohol and Health*. Rockville, MD: Author.

Newlin, D. B. (1989). The skin-flushing response: Autonomic, self-report and conditioned responses to repeated administrations of alcohol in Asian men. *J Abnorm Psychol, 98*, 421–425.

Obot, I. S., & Anthony, J. C. (2000). School dropout and injecting drug use in a national sample of white, non-Hispanic American adults. *J Drug Educ, 30*(2), 145–155.

Obot, I. S., Hubbard, S., & Anthony, J. C. (1999). Level of education and injecting drug use among African Americans. *Drug Alcohol Depend, 55*(1–2), 177–182.

Okuyemi, K. S., Ahluwalia, J. S., Richter, K. P., Mayo, M. S., & Resnicow, K. (2001).

Differences among African-American light, moderate and heavy smokers. *Nicotine Tob Res, 3*(1), 45–50.

Patkar, A. A., Berrettini, W. H., Hoehe, M., Thornton, C. C., Gottheil, E., Hill, K., & Weinstein, S. P. (2002). Serotonin transporter polymorphisms and measures of impulsivity, aggression and sensation-seeking among African-American cocaine-dependent individuals. *Psychiatry Res, 110*(2), 103–115.

Petry, N. M. (2003). A comparison of African-American and non-Hispanic Caucasian cocaine-abusing outpatients. *Drug Alcohol Depend, 69*(1), 43–49.

Qureshi, A. I., Mohammad, Y., Suri, M. F., Bramimah, J., Janardhan, V., Guterman, L. R., et al. (2001). Cocaine use and hypertension are major risk for intracerebral hemorrhage in young African Americans. *Ethn Dis, 11*(2), 311–319.

Reardon, S. F., & Buka, S. L. (2002). Differences in onset and persistence of substance abuse and dependence among whites, blacks and Hispanics. *Public Health Rep, 117*(Suppl 1), S51–S59.

Roberts, C. A. (1999). Drug use among inner-city African-American drug users: The process of managing loss. *Qual Health Res, 9*(5), 620–638.

Rome, L. A., Lippmann, M. L., Dalsey, W. C., Taggart, P., & Pomerantz, S. (2000). Prevalence of cocaine use and its impact on asthma exacerbation in an urban population. *Chest, 117*(5), 1324–1329.

Rosenheck, R., & Seibyl, C. L. (1998). Participation and outcome in a residential treatment and work therapy program for addictive disorders: The effects of race. *Am J Psychiatry, 155*(8), 1029–1034.

Rowe, D., & Grills, C. (1993). African-centered drug treatment: An alternative conceptual paradigm for drug counseling with African-American clients. *J Psychoactive Drugs, 25*(1), 21–33.

Ruiz, P., Langrod, J., & Alksne, L. (1981). Rehabilitation of the Puerto Rican addict: A cultural perspective. *Int J Addict, 16*(5), 841–847.

Russell, M., Cooper, M. L., Frone, M. R., & Peirce, R. S. (1999). A longitudinal study of stress, alcohol and blood pressure in community-based samples of blacks and non-blacks. *Alcohol Res Health, 23*(4), 299–306.

Saremi, A., Hanson, R. L., Williams, D. E., Roumain, J., Robin, R. W., Long, J. C., et al. (2001). Validity of the CAGE questionnaire in an American Indian population. *J Stud Alcohol, 62*(3), 294–300.

Shore, J., Manson, S. M., & Buchwald, D. (2002). Screening for alcohol abuse among urban Native Americans in a primary care setting. *Psychiatr Serv, 53*, 757–760.

Singh, G. K., & Hoyert, D. L. (2000). Social epidemiology of chronic liver disease and cirrhosis mortality in the United States, 1935–1997: Trends and differentials by ethnicity, socioeconomic status and alcohol consumption. *Hum Biol, 72*(5), 801–820.

Stanton, B., Li, X., Pack, R., Cottrell, L., Harris, C., & Burns, J. M. (2002). Longitudinal influence of perceptions of peer and parental factors on African-American adolescent risk involvement. *J Urban Health, 79*(4), 536–548.

Stewart, O. (1964). Questions regarding American Indian criminality. *Human Organ, 23*, 61–66.

Stewart, S. H. (2002). Racial and ethnic differences in alcohol-associated aspartate aminotransferase and gamma-glutamyltransferase elevation. *Arch Intern Med, 162*(19), 2236–2239.

Stinson, F. S., Grant, B. F., & Dufour, M. C. (2001). The critical dimension of ethnicity in liver cirrhosis mortality statistics. *Alcohol Clin Exp Res*, 25(8), 1181–1187.

Substance Abuse and Mental Health Services Administration. (2000). *National Household Survey on Drug Abuse: Population estimates* (DHHS Publication No. BK0355). Washington, DC: U.S. Government Printing Office.

Szapocznik, J., & Fein, S. (1995). *Issues in preventing alcohol and other drug abuse among Hispanic/Latino families* (CSAP Cultural Competence Series 2, DHHS Publication No. SMA 95-3034). Washington, DC: U.S. Government Printing Office.

Timpson, S. C., Williams, M. L., Bowen, A. M., & Keel, K. B. (2003). Condom use behaviors in HIV-infected African American crack cocaine users. *Substance Abuse*, 24(4), 211–220.

U.S. Bureau of the Census. (2002). *Current population reports*. Washington, DC: U.S. Government Printing Office.

Varma, S., & Siris, S. (1996). Alcohol abuse in Asian Americans. *Am J Addict*, 5(2), 136–143.

Wall, T. L., Garcia-Andrade, C., Thomasson, H. R., Cole, M., & Ehlers, C. L. (1996). Alcohol elimination in Native American Mission Indians: An investigation of interindividual variation. *Alcohol Clin Exp Res*, 20(7), 1159–1164.

Wallace, J. M., Jr., Bachman, J. G., O'Malley, P. M., Johnston, L. D., Schulenberg, J. E., & Cooper, S. M. (2002). Tobacco, alcohol, and illict drug use: Racial and ethnic differences among U.S. high school seniors, 1976–2000. *Public Health Rep*, 117(Suppl 1), S67–S75.

Walton, M. A., Blow, F. C., & Booth, B. M. (2001). Diversity in relapse prevention needs: Gender and race comparisons among substance abuse treatment patients. *Am J Drug Alcohol Abuse*, 27(2), 225–240.

Wells, K., Klap, R., Koike, A., & Sherbourne, C. (2001). Ethnic disparities in unmet need for alcoholism, drug abuse and mental health care. *Am J Psychiatry*, 158(12), 2027–2032.

Westermeyer, J. (1995). Cultural aspects of substance abuse and alcoholism: Assessment and management. *Psychiatr Clin North Am*, 18(3), 589–605.

Ziedonis, D., Rayford, B., Bryant, K. J., & Rounsaville, B. (1994). Psychiatric comorbidity in white and African-American cocaine addicts seeking substance abuse treatment. *Hosp Community Psychiatry*, 45(1), 43–49.

Zule, W. A., Lam, W. K., & Wechsberg, W. M. (2003). Treatment readiness among out-of-treatment African-American crack users. *J Psychoactive Drugs*, 35(4), 503–510.

CHAPTER 15

Addictions in the Workplace

AVRAM H. MACK
JEFFREY P. KAHN
RICHARD J. FRANCES

Clinicians are frequently asked to address addictions in the workplace, including prevention, treatment, assessment of performance, benefit structure, disability, and risk management. Anyone involved with these topics must recognize issues of importance to the organization, the individual, the public safety, and the relevant laws and ethics (Kahn & Langlieb, 2002). And, as in any situation in which the clinician is a third party, privacy, confidentiality, and other ethical considerations must be appropriately addressed. This chapter serves as an introduction to this complex task. We begin by exploring the problems posed by substance use, abuse, and dependence in the workplace, the laws that govern the organizations roles, and the issues faced by psychiatrists involved in these situations; we then describe aspects of management of the problems and, finally, address a number of specific occupations in which particular issues are important. Chapter 4 in this volume, on drug testing, covers its use in the workplace and highlights these issues as related to sports and professional athletes.

THE PROBLEM: EXTENT AND CAUSES

The use of illicit or addictive substances in the workplace can have devastating effects, including accidents, injuries, disability, lateness/absenteeism, theft, reduced performance, and reduced morale. By 1998, the societal cost of drug abuse was $143.4 billion, with lost productivity accounting for around $100 billion of that amount (Office of National Drug Control Policy, 2001). It is projected that the cost to business of alcohol abuse is $185 billion, with lost productivity accounting for 70% of that amount (National Institute on Alcohol Abuse and Alcoholism, 2001). Beyond lost productivity, however, are other costs, including liability for workplace accidents due to intoxication or the association with violence (see Chapter 16 on forensic addiction psychiatry, this volume). The Substance Abuse and Mental Health Services Administration (SAMSHA) has published findings from recent National Household Survey on Drug Abuse (NHSDA) studies on the extent of use and institutional policies (Office of Applied Studies, 1999). Since any type of worker at any level of hierarchy can cause an accident or be violent, it is important to consider every case individually and to take each case seriously.

The nature of the use, abuse, and dependence of both alcohol and illicit substances in the workplace is generally similar to that out of the workplace. Many different substances are used by individuals with many different psychological backgrounds and in different places in the organizational hierarchy, before, during, or after business hours. Individuals who use or abuse certain performance-enhancing substances include military pilots, musicians, artists, and athletes. A 1997 study of workplace alcohol use on a national level found that 7.6% of full-time employees were heavy drinkers (five or more drinks on 5 or more days in the month prior to the survey) and a third of those also were using illicit drugs (Office of Applied Studies, 1999).

Why should the leadership of an organization care about occupational substance use? In addition to compassion, quality of productivity, and quality of work environment, there are many other compelling reasons why attention should be given to the matter: the potential for worker's compensation claims, the potential for violence, and legal liability. A significant relationship between use of alcohol and the likelihood of a claim of injury was demonstrated in one prospective study of municipal railways operators (Raglans et al., 2002). Both violence and sexual harassment in the workplace are associated with substance abuse. Besides prevention of loss and liability, various legal foundations guide the way in which organization leaders seek and manage workers with substance use disorders (SUDs). The 1970 Occupational Safety and Health Act, the 1988 Drug-Free Workplace Act, the 1990 Americans with Disabilities Act (Westreich, 2002), and the Family and Medical Leave Act all established legal guidelines for addressing and treating substance use at the workplace. On the other hand, the Contract with America Advancement Act of 1996 removed addictions from coverage under Social Security. It is always advisable to ask an attorney to provide the applicable statutes before providing an opinion. Furthermore, since drug–alcohol testing has been frequently challenged, all organizations should seek specific guidance on current and local standards for enforcement of testing.

Organizational Contributions to Substance Misuse

From the organization's perspective, the paramount issue is how or why substance use has transgressed into the workplace. The consultant's function is to address the areas upon which to focus, including organizational permissiveness, work stress, culture and attitude, and the worker's preemployment understanding of tolerated behavior.

Permissiveness

Each workplace has its own personality, and its own view of substance use. Some are militantly antidrug, while others are relatively *laissez-faire*. When top leadership may be impaired or in denial, the whole organization may be affected. Fads, outbreaks, and epidemics of drug use in organizations can also occur.

Culture and Attitude

This includes both the culture created by the organizational setup and the unofficial practices of those in the organization (e.g., chewing tobacco among baseball players). In terms of institutional structure, one study compared the organization of two groups of employees in the United States: one organized in a typical manner, the other based on Japanese principles. The latter group had fewer problems (Ames, Grube, & Moore, 2000).

Work Stress

A lack of specificity has impeded the creation of workplace stress reduction programs that would diminish the putative stress–addiction relationship (Roman & Blum, 2002). Studies that have measured "burnout" have failed to link "burnout" with alcohol abuse or use. However, alcohol use has been associated with less-specific measures of occupational stress (Crum, Muntaner, Waton, & Anthony, 1995).

Diagnosis, Case Findings, and Recognition

An important role for the organization and for the consultant is detecting cases of substance abuse in the work setting. This function must be handled with finesse on many levels, including, among others, the company structure, reporting, confidentiality rules, and the requirement of periodical medical evaluations. The first opportunity to identify problem substance use is before the individual becomes an employee: the preemployment screen. Human resources/

benefits officers should be trained to recognize the importance of physical, historical, or social signals of misuse, and this should, with a low threshold of suspicion, lead to further inquiry, including, for example, direct questioning, professional evaluation, or request for records of prior treatment.

Once the individual is an employee, sources include physical findings (e.g., stench of cannabis, bottles of alcohol, change in work performance, reports from others; ideally, confidential or anonymously), violence or legal problems, or the development of associated medical problems. The extent to which the dependent or abusing worker spends most of his or her time thinking about (obtaining, concealing, using) the drug leaves less time for work or anything else. Many addicts in the workplace are able to conceal their drug use for years! Supervisors should be trained to spot problems, and workers should also be provided education for self-diagnosis.

A tenet of addiction is continued use despite adverse consequences. Denial of a problem is a challenge, and confrontation is often part of the intervention. The first steps to recovery are recognition of a problem and agreeing to a need for help. The addict is unwilling (earlier in the course of addiction) or unable (in the later stages) to stop use. Sadly, the employer who says "Get help or you're fired" often has more leverage than family or friends.

Loss of control is an important criterion for addiction, and one of the more confusing aspects for employers to comprehend. Over time, untreated drug use progresses from social and recreational use to more problematic heavy use, and finally to out-of-control addiction. In order to understand the loss of control, addiction must be presented to third parties as a progressive, not static, illness. Of course, denial of this progression is characteristic: It is difficult to accept the eventual loss of control. The addict at first minimizes the damage, then blames others as justification for continued abuse, which may be followed by rationalizing his or her behavior.

In this progression, the first step toward successful treatment of alcohol or drug addiction in the workplace is the direct confrontation of denial. The employer or partners often have more leverage and more emotional neutrality than a family member. The supervisor does not make a diagnosis but does recommend an evaluation by a professional. The substance abuser is usually unwilling to seek help on his or her own, and must be made to see the adverse consequences of not stopping drug use (e.g., loss of job, divorce). The employee is given the choice of treatment or termination, and the usual result is a referral to an Employee Assistance Program (EAP).

Diagnosing Specific Substances in the Workplace

It is important to remember that each drug may have a different course in the workplace, and relapse depends very much on the drug being used.

Stimulants and Cocaine

Dependence or abuse of stimulants and cocaine is difficult to detect in the workplace; they produce no odor and no hangovers. Users are often workers who were once industrious but now have difficulty concentrating and staying alert. Physical signs of cocaine or stimulant abuse do become apparent. Frequent unexplained absences, lateness, inability to sit still, and excessive trips to the restroom, along with paranoia, irritability, and hypomanic symptoms, should lead the employer to suspect stimulant, especially cocaine, abuse. Crashing, depression, and abuse of sedatives are also signs.

Marijuana

The marijuana-dependent individual who smokes daily will have deficits in vocational, social, and psychological functioning. Common findings include inability to concentrate, difficulty with judgement and fine motor coordination, memory impairment, and social withdrawal. Lethargy, depression, and a loss of goal-directed behavior are common. In the workplace, the results can be dangerous to the individual user, coworkers, and the general public, depending on the occupation of the user.

Opiates and Opioids

Both legal and illicit opiates and opioids are major problems in the workplace. The heroin addict is frequently absent and late. He or she is prone to accidents because of heroin intoxication (lethargy, somnolence, difficulty concentrating, impaired motor coordination and judgment) or withdrawal. Injuries resulting in disability and theft or embezzlement to support the dependence are common. The abuse of legally prescribed opiates has increasingly been portrayed in the lay press. Regular use of these substances leads to a high level of tolerance and to a withdrawal syndrome identical to that of heroin. Use of "hard drugs," such as heroin or opiates, has stigmatized many individuals in the past. For those who are motivated to quit, compassion and support in the workplace can make a big difference in successful abstinence from this class of substance, and persons maintained on methadone or buprenorphine are frequently able to work well.

Sedatives/Hypnotics

As is the case with the prescription opioids, employees become adept at concealing their dependence on these medications. Intoxication can be dangerous if the employee is required to drive, operate equipment, or perform complex tasks. Cases of acute stress disorder and posttraumatic stress disorder (PTSD) drastically increased on Wall Street after the September 11, 2001, terrorist attacks. Disasters, terrorism, and war pose additional workplace stress, and concomitant increases in abuse of these substances will likely occur with them.

TREATMENT AND INTERVENTIONS

Addiction psychiatrists may be called upon for preemployment screening, fitness-for-work evaluations, crisis situations, case management, treatment, or to review organizational policy regarding substances. Before any contact with a patient, the addiction psychiatrist working in the occupational setting must have a clear sense of his or her duty. Interactions between a clinician/consultant and an employee/patient are complicated by the various roles inherent in the setup. At the least, the patient must be made aware of policy regarding confidentiality and the physician's dual agency. One SAMHSA-sponsored group demonstrated the utility of such an approach when enacted by an EAP (Lapham, McMillan, & Gregory, 2003).

Preemployment Screening

Preemployment screening to identify various potential problems, including substance abuse, may produce referrals for evaluation. In addition, it is helpful to educate employers about how to screen and when to refer. Those who perform these screens need to have a low threshold for referral. Important information can be gleaned from reference letters, a history of arrests, the admission of medical problems, or the applicant's physical appearance. Special attention should be paid not only to use but also to use in the workplace.

Once all the information has been gathered, the question is what to do with it. There are two important questions for the consultant: (1) Is the behavior a treatable condition, and (2) has it affected occupational function in the past? With these questions in mind, the psychiatrist may come to a recommendation, especially when considering the type of work being sought. It would be foolhardy to reject every single potential employee simply because he or she has misused a substance. Hiring talented persons in stable recovery makes good business sense.

Problem Organizations

For the organization that has sought the consultant's advice, there is an assumption that change is sought: that a problem has been identified. The consultant must gather a bird's-eye view of the organization, from the demographics of the employer to the proximity of the work location to areas high in drug trafficking. One should even determine the type of beverages served at company functions. There may be a need to discuss perceptions of permissiveness and of the actual written or unwritten consequences of legal or illicit substance use during work hours.

Is some cases an organization may choose to become a "drug-free work-place." The implications of this go beyond psychiatric consultation and require legal advice. The Drug Enforcement Agency (2004) has provided a guideline for implementing this standard.

Random Drug Testing

Preemployment and periodic mandatory, random urine testing for illicit drugs has become a controversial topic in recent years. The main argument in favor of mandatory urine testing is deterrence of illicit drug use, both at work and at home. Random testing is mandated by federal regulations for the transportation industry, for example. Those who are opposed to mandatory urine testing say that it is a violation of constitutional rights to privacy. And even with safe-guards, concerns are also raised about reporting errors and potential breaches of confidentiality. An employee's right to privacy must be balanced with society's best interests. As mentioned earlier, any testing program needs to be developed in concert with legal consultation.

The third party must be reminded that urine tests do not distinguish drug use from drug abuse or dependence. This can only be done with a comprehensive medical and psychiatric history, and physical examination. At best, laboratory tests are adjunctive and provide diagnostic confirmation. It is accepted in the treatment community that urine testing is a useful adjunct in the treatment of the drug-dependent individual, but not all drug users are abusers.

Nonrandom Testing

There are a number of situations in which testing is done on a nonrandom basis, including when there is reasonable suspicion, after an accident or violence, or as a part of a posttreatment follow-up. Employees seem to favor tests following accidents (Howland, Mangione, Lee, Bell, & Levine, 1996).

Brief Interventions

After an assessment has been made, brief interventions are sometimes the requisite next step. It can be immensely helpful to have the individual's family be a part of the intervention. The family is the mediator between the individual and his or her culture, and the family environment is where attitudes toward drugs are first learned.

The Employee Assistance Program Model

When available, it is ideal to place the employee's "case" within the EAP. The overall approach of the EAP is to identify and treat the drug-abusing employee and to help the employee maintain his or her career and productivity, rather than to fire him or her. EAPs provide both primary and secondary prevention. They make job-based evaluations and referrals, and some also provide substance abuse treatment, thus increasing job retention and lowering complications. EAPs are valuable for workers in that they provide a nonthreatening place to obtain alcohol and drug abuse information and counseling, as well as early diagnosis and treatment. In some companies, up to 40% of the employees use EAPs; approximately 17% of these are for substance abuse. Approximately 30,000 EAP programs exist in the United States. They have been in decline recently as managed care has grown. Employers are generally in favor of the EAP system, since they feel that, in the long run, it is more cost-effective to treat employees than to fire them and retrain new ones. Seeing recovering alcoholics and drug abusers return to work happier and more productive is also helpful for company morale. Insurance companies are generally in favor of EAPs, since successful substance abuse treatment has been shown to reduce overall medical costs. Company EAPs vary in demeanor, from stern to forgiving, and also from a moral to a medical model (which most EAPs encourage).

By definition, EAPs are in a difficult position. They are the advocate of the employee, yet at the same time must protect the interests of the employer. And although patient confidentially must be preserved in all types of mental health treatment, in order for the EAP to be effective, there must be some degree of communication with the employee's supervisor, union, or personnel office. It is important that the guidelines for communication of this type be clear at the very beginning of treatment. In most programs, the employer communicates with the EAP regarding job performance, and the EAP provides the employer with periodic progress reports, without divulging confidential information. The "success rate" of the EAP has been cited to be 70% (Blum, Martin, & Roman, 1992), although outcome measures require further refinement.

More often than not, participation is voluntary, though for some employees referral is an alternative to a job action. It is best for the EAP to be proactive about its roles (Lapham et al., 2003). Education about the EAP is essential, and a clearly written policy indicating that drug use will not be tolerated is helpful as well. EAPs can also train both employees and supervisors. Supervisors should be trained to (1) understand their role in implementation of the policy, (2) observe and document job performance problems, (3) confront employees who are unsatisfactory in job performance, (4) understand the effects of substances in the workplace, and (5) know how to refer employees with suspected problems to the EAP or other mental health professional. Employees should be taught the dangers of alcohol and drug abuse to themselves and their families; the negative effects of substances on job performance, health, and safety; company policy and consequences of violating it; the functions of the EAP; drug testing policy and confidentiality; and the ways in which they can get help.

There are important limitations to EAPs. First, many executives, upper level managers, and company presidents do not seek treatment for substance abuse through their EAPs. They often prefer off-site treatment programs or clinicians for the following reasons: (1) Their substance abuse may involve an illicit drug rather than alcohol; (2) company morale would suffer if it became known, for example, that the CEO was a cocaine addict; and (3) it is difficult to be treated by someone they employ. Second, the EAP focus on substance abuse can lead to referral to broadly trained clinicians, and less careful attention to other emotional and psychiatric problems. Many of these patients benefit from consultation with an addiction psychiatrist.

SPECIAL POPULATIONS

Each of the many special work populations may differ in terms of types of drugs used, reasons for use (e.g., boredom, exhilaration, etc.), and potential consequences.

Athletes

Athletes are usually young adults whose jobs involve stardom, celebrations, disappointments, access to illicit drugs, large amounts of cash, great physical exertion, and great physiological reserve. Sometimes the athlete may be trying to make the grade in any way possible, or may be little-noticed. Drug misuse may be for enhancement of performance, recreation, pleasure, or self-medication of pain.

A vast number of substances are used by athletes to improve their performance. Many have been discovered and regulated (or banned), many more exist now, and others will surface in the future. These substances are regulated mostly because they affect fair competition or may endanger the user; this sort of use, often diagnosed as other substance use disorder, includes steroids, nutritional supplements, or stimulants or opioids.

Athletes use all kinds of addictive substances recreationally, including cocaine, marijuana, and tobacco. The use of smokeless tobacco is endemic among baseball players (including college and high school players) (Colborn, Cummings, & Michaelek, 1989). Coaches and those concerned about players must be able to make recommendations for treatment regardless of "who" the player is.

Executives and Other VIPs

Some special considerations exist for dealing with substance-abusing executives and leaders, because their impact on other people magnifies the effects of their problems. Moreover, they are often insulated from help by virtue of their position and may feel pressure to appear professional and authoritative. Some executives have always dealt with emotional distress by covering it over, perhaps through self-medication with drugs or alcohol. Similarly, others have relied on the socially lubricating effects of alcohol, or on the short-term performance enhancement of cocaine for their success. Leaders with addictions feel further impelled to avoid advice and help, and can end up feeling quite "lonely at the top." Being at the top of the heap can enable substance use. Executives can make their own schedule in a way that allows for substance use. Some feel that ordinary rules do not apply to them—a feeling that is further compounded by the physical and psychological effects of substance abuse. Among VIPs such as media celebrities, the acquired narcissism that accompanies a successful career can lead to greater difficulty in reaching out for or accepting help.

Employees often feel helpless and demoralized when faced with a distressed and possibly substance-abusing boss. Under these circumstances, employees (and other executives) commonly protect the impaired executive. This can include doing his or her work, ignoring inappropriate instructions, covering up mistakes, and helping to keep the secret. This is sometimes rationalized as "The Devil you know is better than the Devil you don't know."

As a result, management, human resources, and occupational medicine personnel need to be alert to signs of possible substance abuse. This includes visible distress or intoxication, impaired judgment or performance, decreased interpersonal skills, unexplained absences, and more. An ombudsman program offers a discrete and protected channel for employee concerns, as can a confidential occupational medicine department. If a problem is noticed at work, the executive needs to be approached by senior management, human resources, occupational medicine personnel, or an ombudsman. The approach should be discrete and focus on genuine business performance concerns. Occasionally, it is appropriate to involve family members in the process.

It is important that any clinical treatment not treat the executive as a VIP. To do so often results in attempts by the patient to control the treatment, minimize problems, avoid comprehensive psychiatric and medical evaluation and treatment, or avoid Alcoholics Anonymous (AA) or similar programs.

Health Care Workers

Health care workers (HCWs), a diverse group that includes, for example, academic physicians, floor nurses, and laboratory technicians, share a niche in a workplace that combines high stress and sometimes access to addictive substances, or to the hardware needed for their use (e.g., syringes, alcohol swabs). It may be no surprise that they often use substances to cope. This area has received a fair amount of research attention. For physicians, all 50 states have systems for physician health.

Occupational stresses in the health care setting may contribute to substance misuse. One study that viewed the 2002 Washington-area sniper shootings as terrorism found that among employees of a local hospital, with high exposure to trauma, the perception of safety was inversely proportional to the risk of alcohol misuse. Conversely, the use of alcohol was a risk factor for acute stress disorder (odds ratio = 5.1) (Greiger, Fullerton, Ursano, & Reeves, 2003).

Abuse is widespread among both nurses and physicians. Using an anonymous survey, Trinkoff and Storr found (1998) that 32% of nurses admitted to use of substances. For physicians, alcohol use may be common: One study suggested a 12% rate of abuse (Moore, Mead, & Pearson, 1990). Physicians may be among the most resistant to seek help for a real problem (Aach et al., 1992). Physicians also have a high risk factor for addiction. Actually, adults who have grown up in families with addiction have a tendency to choose health care professions. Physicians have higher access to pharmaceutical drugs but are less inclined to use street drugs. In the New York State Physicians' Health Program, 88% of the participants used alcohol or prescription drugs, and only 12% used marihuana or cocaine. Additional risk factors for SUDs in physicians have been postulated to be "pharmacological optimism," intellectual strength, strong will, love of challenges, instrumental use of medications, and a daily need for denial (Mansky, 1999).

As in other professions, there may be a need to tailor treatments for this group. New research has demonstrated that prevention aimed at HCWs can be successful (Lapham, Chang, & Gregory, 2000). Confidentiality is a major concern in the care of HCWs, and many centers are especially adept at caring for HCWs (e.g., Talbott Recovery Program). Physicians may gain help through two mutual-help groups, caduceus groups and International Doctors in Alcoholics Anonymous, which supplement mainstream 12-step programs.

High-Responsibility Workers: Air Traffic Controllers, Machine Operators, Drivers, and Pilots

One of the most difficult issues with regard to working with this population is in considering when and where to speak up about the dangers posed by the worker, especially when the consultant has a dual agency. While a therapeutic alliance is central to treatment, an important role of the addiction psychiatrist is to confront denial and to protect the public (Leeman, Cohen, & Parkas, 2001) whether the setting is occupational or private. Notwithstanding the narrowness of the *Tarasoff* duties, the therapist should remind the patient of the legal liabilities that result from the risky behavior. One should consider referral to another caretaker if the patient refuses to bring his or her dangerous behavior to a halt.

The American Society for Addiction Medicine guidelines (2000) recognize that reporting substance abuse is necessary when there is an "immediate threat to public safety," which might be construed to be anytime a person drives under the influence of alcohol.

For the worker with people's lives in his or her hands, there may be no "safe" level of blood alcohol. One study performed in the United Kingdom demonstrated that despite a lack of sense of sleepiness following a lunch with alcohol, drivers driving at the typical "circadian dip" who were at half the legal alcohol limit nonetheless performed worse on driving and evidenced electroencephalographic (EEG) evidence of alteration (Horne, Reyner, & Barrett, 2003). Alcohol certainly increased preexisting sleepiness in this experimental design. One study demonstrated that substance abuse of all drug classes is higher than expected among construction workers (Hersh, McPherson, & Cook, 2002).

Both governmental and commercial aviation systems have been keenly aware of the problem of alcohol and flying for some time. It is an environment "unforgiving" of mistakes. Little research has been conducted on the issue and policies designed to stop use (Cook, 1997). Actually, it is in the unregulated, general aviation sphere that most accidents occur today.

Of course, both alcohol and nicotine are legal drugs. There are no guidelines regarding nicotine at all. Changes in regulations about use of tobacco may have potentially created a situation in which pilots may go through nicotine withdrawal during flight (Giannakoulas, Katramados, Melas, Diamantopoulos, & Chimonas, 2003).

Individuals with Access to Weapons: Police and the Military

Akin to HCWs, police and military workers may be at high risk of causing harm when intoxicated, in that they have access to lethal weapons such as firearms. There are countless anecdotes about suicides and murders done by policemen while intoxicated. The full impact on veterans of the war on terrorism and those who have fought in Afghanistan and Iraq is not clear and will emerge over the years to come. Those who learn to kill during war may be more prone to substance use, violence, and posttraumatic stress disorder, with signs of these apparent in the workplace.

During the Vietnam War, a large number of American servicemen and women were abusers of drugs, ranging from heroin to marijuana. This phenomenon was partially explained by the prevailing culture, availability of drugs in the war theater, antipathy for the war, and stresses of the war experience. Strangely, the addiction to heroin did not generally continue once the users returned to the United States, which reinforced the concept that addiction can be halted. Since that period, the U.S. military has been highly attentive to drug abuse among its ranks.

Performance-enhancing drugs may be more prevalent in the armed forces than recreational drugs. There is anecdotal evidence that military pilots are increasingly being asked to use sedatives for sleep and stimulants during the period of their missions. Unfortunately, soldiers leaving the military get little help with the transition to civil life.

We advocate that supervisors have an extremely low threshold for addressing such problems when they arise. Any institutionalized tendency to minimize such dangers should be addressed as well. Amnesty programs or anonymous reporting may help. Military medical services often are organized to care for large numbers of individuals, and some bases have begun programs for surveillance of individuals who are at risk, or who demonstrate "drug-seeking behaviors" (Lewis & Gaule, 1999). Unfortunately, the military does not provide much treatment for drug abusers and tends to process them out of the military.

CONCLUSION

The practice of addiction psychiatry in occupational settings can be complex, but it also may produce important assistance to organizations. Ideally, further research will be publicized and made more generalized.

REFERENCES

Aach, R. D., Girard, D. E., Humphrey, H., McCue, J. D., Reuben, D. B., Smith, J. W., et al. (1992). Alcohol and other substance abuse and impairment among physicians in residency training. *Ann Int Med, 116,* 245–254.

American Society of Addiction Medicine. (2000). Public policy statement on reporting of patient information related to fitness for driving or other potentially dangerous activities. *J Addict Dis, 19,* 125–127.

Ames, G. M., Grube, J. W., & Moore, R. S. (2000). Social control and workplace drinking norms: a comparison of two drinking cultures. *J Stud Alcohol, 61,* 203–219.

Blum, T. C., Martin, J. K., & Roman, P. M. (1992). A research note of EAP prevalence, components, and utilization. *J Employee Assist Res, 1,* 209–229.

Colborn, J. W., Cummings, K. M., & Michaelek, A. M. (1989). Correlates of adolescent's use of smokeless tobacco. *Health Ed Q, 16,* 91–100.

Cook, C. C. H. (1997). Alcohol policy and aviation safety. *Addiction, 97,* 793–804.

Crum, R., Muntaner, C., Waton, W., & Anthony, J. (1995). Occupational stress and the risk of alcohol abuse and dependence. *Alcohol Clin Exp Res, 19,* 647–655.

Drug Enforcement Agency. (2004). *Guidelines for a drug-free workforce.* Retrieved on July 11, 2004, from *www.usdoj.gov/dea/demand/dfmanual/index.html*

Giannakoulas, G., Katramados, A., Melas, N., Diamantopoulos, I., & Chimonas, E.

(2003). Acute effects of nicotine withdrawal syndrome in pilots during flight. *Aviat Space Environ Med, 74,* 247–251.

Greiger, T. A., Fullerton, C. S., Ursano, R. J., & Reeves, J. J. (2003). Acute stress disorder, alcohol use, and perception of safety among hospital staff after the sniper attacks. *Psychiatr Serv, 54,* 1383–1387.

Hersh, R. K., McPherson, T. L., & Cook, R. F. (2002). Substance use in the construction industry: A comparison of assessment methods. *Subst Use Misuse, 37,* 1331–1358.

Horne, J. A., Reyner, L. A., & Barrett, P. R. (2003). Driving impairment due to sleepiness is exacerbated by low alcohol intake. *Occup Environ Med, 60,* 689–692.

Howland, J., Mangione, T. W., Lee, M., Bell, N., & Levine, S. (1996). Employee attitudes toward work-site alcohol testing. *J Occup Environ Med, 38,* 1041–1046.

Kahn, J., & Langlieb, A. (2002). Mental health and productivity in the workplace. San Francisco: Jossey-Bass.

Lapham, S., Chang, G., & Gregory, C. (2000). Substance abuse intervention for health care workers: A preliminary report. *J Behav Health Serv Res, 27,* 131–143.

Lapham, S. C., McMillan, G., & Gregory, C. (2003). Impact of an alcohol misuse intervention for health care workers: 2. Employee Assistance Programme utilization, on the job injuries, job loss, and health services utilization. *Alcohol Alcohol, 38,* 183–188.

Leeman, C. P., Cohen, M. A., & Parkas, V. (2001). Should a psychiatrist report a bus drivers' alcohol and drug abuse?: An ethical dilemma. *Gen Hosp Psychiatry, 23,* 333–336.

Lewis, P., & Gaule, D. (1999). Dealing with drug-seeking patients: The Tripler Army Medical Center experience. *Milif Med, 164,* 838–840.

Mansky, P. A. (1999). Issues in the recovery of physicians from addictive illnesses. *Psychiatr Q, 70,* 107–122.

Moore, R. D., Mead, L., & Pearson, T. A. (1990). Youthful precursors of alcohol abuse in physicians. *Am J Med, 88,* 332–336.

National Institute on Alcohol Abuse and Alcoholism. (2001, January). *Alcohol Alert 51.* Retrieved on December 20, 2004, from *www.niaaa.nih.gov/publications/aa51.htm*

Office of Applied Studies. (1999). *Worker drug use and workplace policies and programs: results from the 1994 and 1997 NHSDA* (SAMHSA). Rockville, MD: Author.

Office of National Drug Control Policy. (2001). *The economic costs of drug abuse in the United States, 1992–1998* (Publication No. NCJ-190636). Washington, DC: Executive Office of the President.

Raglans, D., Krause, N., Greiner, B. A., Holman, B. L., Fisher, J. M., & Cunradi, C. B. (2002). Alcohol consumption and incidence of workers' compensation claims: A 5-year prospective study of urban transit operators. *Alcohol Clin Exp Res, 26,* 1388–1394.

Roman, P. M., & Blum, T. C. (2002). The workplace and alcohol problem prevention. *Alcohol Res Health, 26,* 49–47.

Trinkoff, A. M., & Storr, C. L. (1998). Substance use among nurses: Differences among specialties. *Am J Public Health, 88,* 581–555.

Westreich, L. (2002). Americans and the Americans with Disabilities Act. *J Am Acad Psychiatry Law, 30,* 355–363.

CHAPTER 16

Addiction and the Law

AVRAM H. MACK
RICHARD J. FRANCES
SHELDON I. MILLER

Legal problems, from violence to accidents to crime, frequently accompany use of substances of abuse and vice versa. Clinicians who deal with addicted patients need a grasp of many forensic psychiatry issues in order to practice with skill and communicate effectively in legal settings. This chapter covers a wide range of issues relative to addiction and the law, including issues in criminal justice system (e.g., not guilty by reason of insanity [NGRI], treatment for parolees or probationers, pleas for sentence reduction, advice to Drug Courts) or other settings, and civil matters such as inpatient and outpatient commitment, child custody, competence, and confidentiality.

It is likely that the addiction psychiatrist will have interactions with the legal system. A significant portion of the growing number of incarcerated Americans suffers from addictions. Conversely, around 20% of patients with addictions have sociopathy and major problems with the law, including offenses such as driving while intoxicated (DWI), drug possession, and prescription forgery. Addiction work among this population may involve clinical care or expert testimony. In each scenario, knowledge of the interface between addiction psychiatry and the law is very important. This chapter is geared for the general psychiatrist or the addiction psychiatrist who needs guidance in consulting as an expert in the intersection of substances and the law, which simultaneously can be interesting, rewarding, anxiety provoking, and hazardous.

PSYCHIATRY AND THE LAW

Any psychiatrist may, willingly or not, become involved in legal issues. The uninitiated must become familiar with general knowledge on the law and psychiatry (Group for the Advancement of Psychiatry, 1991; Gutheil, 1998; Rosner, 2003). Some universals should be stated. First, in the United States, "local rules" matter. Every jurisdiction has its own laws, rules, case law, and administrative regulations under which medicine and psychiatry are practiced, and these should be reviewed by the psychiatrist before addressing the facts.

Second, in the United States, administrative, criminal, and civil cases are set in an adversarial system in which one side is pitted against the other. The adversarial system can create situations in which the expert is attacked by the opposing side, and such attacks have gone as far as complaints to professional or ethical boards, but experts very rarely have been accused of perjury (Binder, 2002). Thus, maintaining a professional stance is vital. The forensic expert is always better served in the position of friend to the Court (as is the case in Drug Courts), rather than to one of the parties.

Third, it is important to be aware that there is an opprobrium against "junk science." The psychiatrist who serves as an expert witness under oath should be prepared for his or her ideas to be questioned, perhaps in great detail and in comparison with the general knowledge of the field. Until recently, the Federal standard was that created by the *Frye* case, otherwise known as the "general acceptance test," but *Daubert v. Merrell Dow* and subsequent cases established a new precedent with which experts should be familiar (Gutheil & Stein, 2000) in order to be ethical and effective.

ADDICTION AND THE LAW

There are areas of psychiatry and addiction testimony that are contested, even if clinically valid and important. Therefore, some guidance into what is said about addictions and substances in court may be useful.

"Addiction": A Courtroom Definition

"Addiction" is a powerful word, and it should not be misused. Its meaning carries biological, behavioral, and social connotations. Among physicians, it has been interchangeable with "substance dependence," and this has been linked to demonstrable alterations in neural activity. However, the medical community also has come to consider food, gambling, and sex as "addictions," and attorneys, clients, and some doctors may wish to apply the suffix "-ism" to any behavior they wish to portray as compulsive or uncontrollable. There has been a backlash to the expanding application of this word and, so far, courts have objected to this expansion; so one should exercise caution in using the term "addiction" when discussing behaviors rather than substances of abuse.

Basics of Diagnosis

In forensic situations, it is essential to utilize diagnostic terms that are accepted by all parties. The legal sphere is not the setting to further academic theories. The addiction psychiatrist must be vigilant about new theories and their premature application, and should inform his or her side of the need to be critical of the assertions of the other side's expert. Notwithstanding current scientific theories, the current classification of mental disorders, the *Diagnostic and Statistical Manual of Mental Disorders* (DSM-IV-TR; American Psychiatric Association, 2000a) is the standard. On the other hand, DSM-IV-TR has an "imperfect fit" with the needs of courts: For example, the court often asks the expert for predictions on the future, or degree of dangerousness, neither of which has a DSM category. In addition, courts and attorneys frequently misunderstand DSM-IV-TR substance use disorder (SUD) diagnoses, which should be clarified.

Assessment

There is no such thing as a "complete psychiatric assessment." All forensic psychiatry assessments must be done with a particular focus and a question in mind. The forensic assessment of a subject for whom substances of abuse are present needs to include a thorough review of all history, including medical, psychiatric, and social function (we discuss correctional setting assessment below). It is acceptable to utilize standardized instruments, especially insofar as these may provide normalized data with which to make comparisons. Collateral sources of data are essential. Laboratory studies may be important, depending on the time setting. Sinha and Easton (1999) have provided a guide for a "Forensic Substance Abuse Evaluation."

ADDICTION AND CRIMINAL LAW

Criminality, Violence, and Substance Abuse

The various substances of abuse all seem to be associated with aggression or violence during intoxication or withdrawal (Hoaken & Stewart, 2003), or with effects on personality when used chronically.

Among the substances, alcohol has been most scrutinized: Independent of crime and incarceration, the relationship between alcohol and aggression (including suicide) has been well documented (Graham et al., 1998) in both epidemiological (Murdoch, Pihl, & Ross, 1990) and "laboratory" (controlled environment) studies (Bushman & Cooper, 1990). The findings of the Epidemiologic Catchment Area (ECA) Study indicated that those who met criteria for antisocial personality disorder were 21 times as likely to develop abuse or dependence on alcohol at some point in their lives (Moeller & Dougherty, 2001). There is a relationship between violence and other substances as well, including nicotine and cannabis. The basis of these relationships is unknown, although theories abound from biological, environmental, to social causes.

In terms of the relationship between substance use and crime, the link is well documented. Seventy percent of those arrested for violent offenses test positive for substances (Sinha & Easton, 1999). The MacArthur study found violence to be greatest among mentally ill persons using substances (Monahan & MacArthur Violence Risk Assessment Study, 2001). In this vein, some have suggested that the decline in violent crimes in the United States in the 1990s was related to changes in the use of alcohol and other drugs (Greenfield & Henneberg, 2001). There is an association between severity of abuse and frequency of criminal acts, especially as abuse becomes dependence.

Associations between certain types of violence and substances also have been studied: Male-to-female domestic violence is associated with substance use. There is evidence suggesting that alcohol precedes or accompanies marital violence, especially among men (Leonard & Quigley, 1999), and especially during pregnancy. Studies have shown that there is an increased risk of child abuse and child neglect when substances are used (Schuck & Widom, 2003). Finally, substances commonly are used by perpetrators of sexual assault. In perhaps 50% of all cases, the perpetrator has used alcohol.

Accidents and injuries are clear consequences of substance use. Clinicians who treat addicted persons may sense a need to report use in order to prevent such events, especially for those whose personal or professional activities may place others at great risk. This is not guided by *Tarasoff* considerations, in which there are intended targets (Felthous, 1993). Our advice is to seek out the laws in one's own state and Federal law. Clinicians may need to make difficult choices and should at least feel free to contact the interested professional or regulatory bodies. Seeking clarification from a judge may be helpful as well, when there is a wish to report in questionable cases (see Chapter 15 on workplace addictions, this volume).

Substances in the Courtroom

In the Anglo-American adversarial criminal justice system, the basic goal of criminal proceedings is to establish responsibility for the illegal event. A major tenet of responsibility is the intention of the actor. A criminal conviction requires the proof of *mens rea* or, "intent" to do the evil act, and it is around this concept that almost all debate and reasoning about substances hinge.

Over time, case law and statutes have almost completely eviscerated intoxication as a defense against responsibility, but substances and their effects still have a place in criminal proceedings in terms of the mitigation of responsibility, when substance use treatment is mandated as an alternative to incarceration, or when the long-term medical or psychiatric effects of substances interfere with the defendant's ability to proceed. This section reviews these areas. The "irresistible impulse" defense, an antiquated and little-used argument, asserts that an impulse to commit the offense could not be resisted by the offender.

There are few situations in which responsibility cannot be assigned to the criminal offender. These include insanity, involuntary intoxication, and being otherwise incompetent (such as being a minor). Voluntary intoxication itself is not an excuse; nor has it been over the past 500 years of Anglo-American law, but it may alter the punishment (Slovenko, 1995). When "specific intent" is required to be convicted of a particular charge (e.g., murder rather than manslaughter for a homicide), voluntary intoxication has been successfully used as a defense—that the perpetrator could not have had the specific intent as required by law. In some states, when accidents occur while a person is intoxicated, the presence or absence of *mens rea* when the substance is first ingested must be assessed when determining intent (Wagenaar & Toomey, 2002).

In general, intoxication can be exculpatory when it occurs via trickery or under duress, in the case of previously unknown susceptibility to an atypical reaction or side effect to a substance or medication. This is described by Myers and Vondruska (1998). In this sort of defense, *mens rea* is negated. However, in some jurisdictions, there are specific guidelines and limitations for an acceptable involuntary intoxication defense (Downs & Billick, 2000).

"Strict liability crimes" are those in which *mens rea* is not required for a conviction. These include driving while intoxicated or driving under the influence (DWI or DUI). In a number of states, maximum sentences are mandated if death results from a driver who was DWI yet there was only a minimal impact from the substance. "Settled insanity" is a situation in which long-term use, which is different from an acute intoxication or toxic psychosis, leads to a chronic injury (Slovenko, 1995).

Diminished capacity, a partial defense allowed in some jurisdictions, is used to reduce the integrity of the *mens rea* partial defense in cases in which *specific intent* is required. If the defense is able to prove the lack of *specific intent*, then guilt could be found for a lesser/other crime that does not have such requirement. This is contrary to the NGRI defense. According to the diminished capacity defense, due to intoxication, whether voluntary or not, the person could not deliberate. The expert must check with the attorney as to which charge is a specific intent crime and what rules apply in which jurisdictions. For example, a person suffering from delirium tremens may strike out at a health care worker he perceives to be a bear coming toward him. Genetic factors should, perhaps, be taken into account in a wise and just sentencing.

"Blackouts" are real phenomena that can occur in the occasional user, as well as in the chronic abuser or the alcohol-dependent person. They can lead to a person being unable to account for hours or days of his or her life. During a blackout, the individual may not be perceived by observers to have any impairment of cognitive or intellectual ability. This does not mean that committed acts were not intended. State-dependent memory may also occur, with return of some learning during intoxication. In some cases in which criminal or civil offenses have been alleged, the defendant who is an abuser of drugs or alcohol may state that he or she is not able to comment upon the act because he or she was in a state of "blackout." The actor's apparent lack of impairment during the actions leads to very different accounts of the action.

ADDICTION AND CIVIL MATTERS

Civil matters are often encumbered by addictions. The topics of civil law range from family matters (e.g., divorce, custody) to administrative proceedings (e.g., medical or pilot's license proceedings), to personal injury, to negligence to wills and estates. As in criminal proceedings, the psychiatrist may be asked to place the substance use in the context of the past behavior or to make predictions about future behavior. We discuss a number of frequently visited topics. Issues relating to the workplace and the Americans with Disabilities Act (ADA) are discussed in Chapter 15, this volume.

Family and Matrimonial Law

In disputes over divorce, custody, guardianship, adoption, or child safety, the substance use of any involved party is commonly at issue. The expert is often asked to comment upon the substance use of parents and effects on the child, with recommendations for custody, visitation, and treatment as a pretense for rights. The presence of an SUD does not mean lack of fitness, but it can be a factor. The fiercely adversarial nature of these proceedings often impedes the formation of a valid picture.

Personal Injury

When an individual who is injured sues another party for damages, the defendant might allege that the plaintiff was intoxicated at the time. Either side might need an addiction psychiatrist to assist or rebuff the claim of intoxication and long-term addiction. Injured parties may also blame the party that provides the substance of abuse. Many cases have exposed the liability of bars, bartenders, and parents of minors (Wagenaar, 2001).

Disability

Claims for disability insurance (whether through the state or a private organization) may be based on a claim of addiction. Each case is decided on its own merits, but addiction psychiatrists are naturally the experts of choice. If the case goes to court, the expert would seem essential. Complex management of addictions in pain cases requires expertise to sort out whether or not return to work is indicated or possible.

Other areas in which an addiction psychiatrist may have special expertise include malpractice cases, either when a patient alleged that a physician made a patient become addicted, or when the physician was impaired by substances. Since workplace actions frequently lead to legal consequences, the addiction psychiatrist is frequently involved in consultation regarding the workplace (Chapter 15, this volume). Sexual harassment cases may be brought in either criminal or civil settings and addictions may be raised as in issue in such cases as well.

ADDICTION AND CORRECTIONAL PSYCHIATRY

The nationwide decline in crime has been associated with a rise in the number of incarcerated Americans, and a great proportion of these individuals have active SUDs or are dually diagnosed. It is important for a psychiatrist to review the issues of correctional psychiatry, so that he or she may be prepared to advise on screening, treatment, and recommendations for release. Basic guidelines have been delineated for correctional facilities both by the American Psychiatric Association Manuscript (American Psychiatric Association, 2000b) and the National Commission on Correctional Health Care (2003).

There are three very different incarceration settings: lockup (upon arrest), jail (following arraignment, during trial, prior to sentencing, or in sentences of up to 1 year), and prison (postsentencing more than 1 year). Psychiatric issues differ greatly among these settings (Weinstein, Kim, Mack, Malavade, & Saraiya, in press). SUDs present different pictures in each setting.

Correctional Center Epidemiology

Substance use and SUDs are essentially epidemic among the incarcerated. Peters, Greenbaum, Edens, Carter, and Ortiz (1998) found that 74% of inmates in the U.S. criminal justice system have a lifetime DSM-IV SUD. Abram and Teplin (1991) found that a large majority of male jail detainees with severe mental disorders had a co-occurring SUD at some point in their lifetime. More than half who had current severe psychiatric disorders had a co-occurring SUD or had used a substance at the time of arrest. These prevalence rates were significantly higher than rates in the general population, and were also higher than rates found in patient populations (Abram & Teplin, 1991). Among women jail detainees in Cook County, 72% with a current severe mental disorder had a co-occurring SUD at some point in their lifetime (Abram, Teplin, & McClelland, 2003). These rates were higher than those found among women in the general population and among male jail detainees. Likewise, the rates of co-occurring mental disorders are elevated among the incarcerated. Peters and Hills estimated in 1993 that between 3 and 11% of all inmates have both substance use and psychiatric diagnoses. This is a population that requires solid assessment for the misuse of substances.

Benefits of Addressing the Problem

The first stage of benefit is in terms of reduction of the aggression of intoxication. Finding and treating intoxication and withdrawal also reduce the potential for morbidity and mortality associated with intoxication (e.g., cocaine) or withdrawal (e.g., alcohol). Proper recognition of SUDs can lead to long-term benefits for the institution: When individuals receive treatment for addiction, research has shown that focused, rehabilitation-oriented treatment can lead to favorable outcomes following incarceration (Gendreau, 1996; Knight, Simpson, & Hiller, 1999), and moreso if aftercare is provided (Griffith, Hiller, Knight, & Simpson, 1999). A number of measures from a process evaluation of a therapeutic community program suggest that the presence of a therapeutic community within a prison is associated with significant advantages for management of the institution, including lower rates of infractions, reduced absenteeism among correctional staff, and virtually no illicit drug use among inmates. Over the longer term, the offender and society benefit, because there is a reduced likelihood of eventual recidivism.

Case Findings

Clearly the cases are present and should be found, but how can they, or should they, be found? This is an area of enormous interest with few answers. From lockups to jails to prisons, the potential types of misuse differ; therefore, so does the value of particular screening approaches and treatment plan choices. A resource for those interacting with juveniles should be available as well (McClelland, Teplin, & Abram, 2004).

New Arrest or Surrender

When an individual enters custody directly from the outside world, any of the drugs of abuse may be present. This "intake" is a most critical time, when the staff must be most careful to look for intoxication, overdose, or active withdrawal from any substance, but especially alcohol, benzodiazepines, or other sedatives. It is common for those who are surrendering to have had a "last hit" before entering incarceration. For long-term users who are not actively intoxicated or in withdrawal, the opportunity to be referred to rehabilitation programs can be missed. Medical screening at intake can likewise be of great importance, because it alone may produce evidence of an SUD. Conversely, a history of an SUD prompts further, specialized medical assessment. These individuals are at high risk for infectious diseases such as human immunodeficiency virus (HIV) and the viral hepatidities, especially hepatitis C (Baillargeon et al., 2003).

Screening instruments and other manner of case finding need to be appropriate for the setting. In general, searching for SUDs among the incarcerated is difficult because of a high degree of antisocial personality style, which includes denial and sometimes the wish not to attend to one's addiction. For this reason, the authority must use instruments or simple assumptions to lead to the case. Instruments such as the Michigan Alcoholism Screening Test (MAST) and the CAGE Questionnaire are helpful in the assessment of alcohol use in the primary care setting but have not been specifically assessed for use among prisoners. It is likely that the single best means of finding cases is through face-to-face clinical evaluations with nonaggressive interviewing styles. Additionally, findings on physical examinations, such as spider angiomata, needle tracks, nasal septum injuries, or autonomic arousal may trigger suspicion. Testing of body fluids or hair is seen as costly and inefficient, since it basically serves to confirm either use in the past days or at some point in the past 3 months. Nonetheless, urine, blood, and hair testing, which all have high rates of sensitivity and specificity for cannabis, opiates, benzodiazepines, and alcohol, can help (see Chapter 4, this volume). Screening for SUDs must also be geared to detect comorbid psychiatric conditions, which are common among the addicted incarcerated population.

Long-Term Incarceration

For those who remain in custody for months or years, another approach is needed. In this setting, there is the opportunity for treatment and possibly rehabilitation. On the other hand, drugs and alcohol also make their way to prisoners. Authorities and clinicians must be ready to address both issues.

There is great variation in the available resources given to long-term treatment of addictions among the incarcerated. Unfortunately, many prison systems do not address addiction in long-term inmates. Or in some systems, addiction is addressed only in the last months of incarceration. On the other hand, other systems have ongoing Alcoholics Anonymous (AA) meetings, education, and group, and even individual, psychotherapies.

Dispositions after Prison

Addiction psychiatrists may work with parole boards to mandate treatment. There may be times when the psychiatrist is asked to comment to a parole board about an inmate who is addicted in prison or beforehand. On discharge, both inmates with SUDs and those with SUDs comorbid with psychiatric conditions are at high risk of relapse, which may affect criminality as well. One Scottish study found that of the increased deaths after release, many were intravenous drug users, especially those with HIV (Bird & Hutchinson, 2003). Some parole boards mandate treatment either using their own authority or by referring parolees to the mandated treatment programs (see below). Such requirements have been accepted in the case of sex offenders but have not been successfully utilized for addictions to this point.

When asked by a court to suggest a treatment plan for the addicted offender, it is best to offer multiple modes of treatment and surveillance. Consider residential, groups, day treatment, medication management, and others. The period of treatment should be a minimum of 1 year. Random screens are best done twice weekly. Attendance at required activities should be required. The clinician should reevaluate the individual on some regular basis.

ALTERNATIVES AND ADJUNCTS TO, AND DIVERSIONS FROM, THE INCARCERATION/JUSTICE SYSTEM

For those with SUDs who have been or will likely become dangerous to themselves or others, various states, counties, and federal government agencies have been developing ways in which to intervene. This includes "diversion" programs (such as drug courts), as well as mandated treatment laws. These institutions may protect the public from violence or accidents, and they may reduce expenditure on incarceration.

"Diversion" refers to institutions, practices, and laws that divert criminal offenders who have a mental disorder or an SUD out of the standard criminal justice system and into alternatives. There are moral and economic rationales for diversion, which may occur at any stage of the justice process, from arrest to sentencing. A review of the many programs can be found in a volume by the Council of State Governments (2002).

Drug courts, one type of diversion, are special courts given the responsibility to handle cases involving substance-abusing offenders through comprehensive supervision, drug testing, treatment services, and immediate sanctions and incentives. These courts mandate treatment, seem to have low recidivism rates, and lead to education, cost savings, and drug-free babies. They have been shown to have good outcomes, to save money, and to reduce criminal recidivism.

States have created laws that can be used to force those with either mental disorders or SUDs into treatment plans. Thomsen Hall and Appelbaum (2002) have commented on the valid legal basis for this approach. In *Robinson v. California*, the U.S. Supreme Court ruled in 1961 that "a state might establish a program of compulsory treatment for those addicted to narcotics. Such a program might require periods of involuntary confinement and penal sanctions might be imposed for failure to comply with established treatment procedures." As of 1997, 31 states and the District of Columbia had statutes specifically allowing involuntary treatment or commitment for dependent individuals. This can be inpatient or outpatient treatment, or partial hospitalization. The criteria and processes for commitment vary by state but usually require a judicial hearing in which the individual's or the community's safety is seen to be endangered by the refusal of the patient to be in treatment. The use of monitored disulfiram administration has been shown to increase compliance (Brewer, 1993).

CONCLUSION

In 1939, Penrose accurately predicted an inverse relationship between the number of individuals in a society who are psychiatrically hospitalized and those with psychiatric disorders who are incarcerated. For patients released from state, municipal, Veterans Administration, and private hospitals, homelessness, comorbid addiction, and incarceration have resulted. In this era of continued hospital deinstitutionalization and increased incarceration, psychiatrists are increasingly essential in forensic, legal, and correctional settings. This will be true so long as long-term institutions for the mentally ill are absent and community resources are inadequate; the next-best alternative will be the implementation and expansion of procedures and practices of diversion from the justice system. Clinicians could have the greatest impact on helping addicted and mentally ill offenders and reducing their placement in the justice system by advocating for effective diversion programs that not only promote proper medical care and maintain liberty rights but also protect the public. Clinicians need also to know how best to use coercion wisely and compassionately as a means to confront denial, engage patients in treatment, and liberate them from the ravages and confinement of their addiction. Working with these addicted patients, who suffer more than most of humanity, can be personally interesting and rewarding.

REFERENCES

Abram, K. M., & Teplin, L. A. (1991). Co-occurring disorders among mentally ill jail detainees: implications for public policy. *Am Psychol, 46*, 1036–1045.

Abram, K. M., Teplin, L. A., & McClelland, G. M. (2003). Comorbidity of severe psychiatric disorders and substance abuse disorders among women in jail. *Am J Psychiatry, 160*, 1007–1010.

American Psychiatric Association. (2000a). *Diagnostic and statistical manual of mental disorders* (4th ed., rev. text). Washington, DC: Author.

American Psychiatric Association. (2000b). *Psychiatric services in jails and prisons* (2nd ed.). Washington, DC: Author.

Baillargeon, J., Wu, H., Kelley, M. J., Grady, J., Linthicum, L., & Dunn, K. (2003). Hepatitis C seroprevalence among newly incarcerated inmates in the Texas correctional system. *Public Health, 117*, 43–48.

Binder, R. L. (2002). Liability for the psychiatrist expert witness. *Am J Psychiatry, 159*, 1819–1825.

Bird, S. M., & Hutchinson, S. J. (2003). Male drugs-related deaths in the fortnight after release from prison: Scotland, 1996–99. *Addiction, 98*, 185–190.

Brewer, C. (1993). Recent developments in disulfiram treatment. *Alcohol Alcohol, 28*, 383–395.

Bushman, B. J., & Cooper, H. M. (1990). Effects of alcohol on human aggression: An integrative research review. *Psychol Bull, 107*, 341–354.

Council of State Governments. (2002). *Criminal Justice/Mental Health Consensus Project.* New York: Author.

Downs, L., & Billick, S. B. (2000). Involuntary intoxication. *J Am Acad Psychiatry Law, 28*, 368–369.

Felthous, A. R. (1993). Substance abuse and the duty to protect. *Bull Am Acad Psychiatry Law, 21*, 419–426.

Gendreau, P. (1996). Offender rehabilitation: What we know and what needs to be done. *Crim Justice Behav, 23*, 144–161.

Graham, K., Leonard, K. E., Room, R., Wild, T. C., Pihl, R. O., Bois, C., & Single, E. (1998). Current directions in research on understanding and preventing intoxicated aggression. *Addiction, 93*, 659–676.

Greenfield, L. A., & Henneberg, M. A. (2001). Victim and offender self-reports of alcohol involvement in crime. *Alcohol Res Health, 25*, 20–31.

Griffith, J. D., Hiller, M. L., Knight, K., & Simpson, D. D. (1999). A cost-effectiveness analysis of in-prison therapeutic community treatment and risk classification. *Prison J, 79*, 352–368.

Group for the Advancement of Psychiatry, Committee on Psychiatry and Law. (1991). The mental health professional and the legal system. *Rep Group Adv Psychiatry, 131*, 1–192.

Gutheil, T. G. (1998). *The psychiatrist in court: A survival guide.* Washington, DC: American Psychiatric Press.

Gutheil, T. G., & Stein, M. D. (2000). Daubert-based gatekeeping and psychiatric/psychologic testimony in court: Review and proposal. *J Psychiatry Law, 28*, 235–251.

Hoaken, P. N. S., & Stewart, S. H. (2003). Drugs of abuse and the elicitation of human aggressive behavior. *Addict Behav, 28*, 1533–1554.

Knight, K., Simpson, D. D., & Hiller, M. L. (1999). Three year reincarceration outcomes for in-prison therapeutic community treatment in Texas. *Prison J, 79*, 337–351.

Leonard, K., & Quigley, B. (1999). Drinking and marital aggression in newlyweds: An event-based analysis of drinking and the occurrence of husband marital aggression. *J Stud Alcohol, 60*, 537–545.

McClelland, G. M., Teplin, L. A., & Abram, K. M. (2004). Detection and prevalence of substance use among juvenile detainees. *Office of Juvenile Justice and Delinquency Prevention Bulletin*. Retrieved July 10, 2004, from *www.ojjdp.ncjrs.org/publications/ PubAbstract.asp?pubi=11680*

Moeller, F. G., & Dougherty, D. M. (2001). Antisocial personality disorder, alcohol, and aggression. *Alcohol Res Health*, 25, 5–11.

Monahan, J., & MacArthur Violence Risk Assessment Study. (2001). *Rethinking risk assessment: The MacArthur study of mental disorder and violence*. Oxford, UK: Oxford University Press.

Murdoch, D., Pihl, R. O., & Ross, D. (1990). Alcohol and crimes of violence: Present issues. *Int J Addict*, 25, 1065–1081.

Myers, W. C., & Vondruska, M. A. (1998). Murder, minors, selective serotonin reuptake inhibitors, and the involuntary intoxication defense. *J Am Acad Psychiatry Law*, 26, 487–496.

National Commission on Correctional Health Care. (2003). *Standards for health services in prisons*. Chicago: Author.

Penrose, L. (1939). Mental disease and crime: Outline of a comparative study of European statistics. *Br J Med Psychol*, 18, 1–15.

Peters, R. H., Greenbaum, P. E., Edens, J. F., Carter, C. R., & Ortiz, M. M. (1998). Prevalence of DSM-IV substance abuse and dependence disorders among prison inmates. *Am J Drug Alcohol Abuse*, 24, 573–587.

Peters, R. H., & Hills, H. A. (1993). Inmates with co-occurring substance abuse and mental health disorders. In H. J. Steadman & J. J. Cocozza (Eds.), *Mental illness in America's prisons* (pp. 159–212). Seattle, WA: National Coalition for the Mentally Ill in the Criminal Justice System.

Rosner, R. (Ed.). (2003). *Textbook of forensic psychiatry* (2nd ed.). New York: Oxford University Press.

Schuck, A. M., & Widom, C. S. (2003). Childhood victimization and alcohol symptoms in women: an examination of protective factors. *J Stud Alcohol*, 64(2), 247–256.

Sinha, R., & Easton, C. (1999). Substance abuse and criminality. *J Am Acad Psychiatry Law*, 27, 513–526.

Slovenko, R. (1995). *Psychiatry and criminal culpability*. New York: Wiley.

Thomsen Hall, K., & Appelbaum, P. (2002). The origins of commitment for substance abuse in the U.S. *J Am Acad Psychiatry Law*, 30, 33–45.

Wagenaar, A. C. (2001). Liability of commercial and social hosts for alcohol-related injuries: A national survey of accountability norms and judgments. *Public Opin Q*, 65, 344–368.

Wagenaar, A. C., & Toomey, T. L. (2002). Effects of minimum drinking age laws: Review and analyses of the literature from 1960 to 2000. *J Stud Alcohol Suppl*, 63(Suppl 14), 206–225.

Weinstein, H., Kim, D., Mack A., Malavade, K., & Saraiya, A. (in press). Correctional psychiatry. In C. Scott (Ed.), *The clinical handbook of correctional psychiatry*. Washington, DC: American Psychiatric Press.

CHAPTER 17

Pain and Addiction

RUSSELL K. PORTENOY
DAVID LUSSIER
KENNETH L. KIRSH
STEVEN D. PASSIK

The complex issues at the interface between pain management and chemical dependence have received increasing attention during the past decade. The most intense focus from the clinical perspective has been on the evolving role for opioid therapy. In an interesting paradox, specialists in addiction usually focus on the role of these drugs as a major cause of abuse, whereas pain specialists focus on their role as essential medications for pain and suffering. Although each discipline, of course, is aware of the problems addressed by the other, the antithetical nature of these perspectives historically has supported a lack of communication between these two groups.

Given the extraordinary prevalence and interactions between pain and chemical dependence, this lack of communication must be challenged. Both chronic pain and substance abuse are highly prevalent problems. Numerous surveys, both domestic and international, have recorded a prevalence rate for chronic pain that is as high as 40% (Verhaak, Kerssens, Dekker, Sorbi, & Bensing, 1998). Suveys of substance abuse in the United States have indicated that 6–10% of the population regularly use illicit drugs, and approximately 33% have sampled one of these drugs at least once (Colliver & Kopstein, 1991; Groerer & Brodsky, 1992; Regier et al., 1984). It is inevitable that clinicians encounter patients with pain who abuse drugs, and the need to address issues that relate to both pain and drug abuse occurs commonly.

The expanding role of opioid therapy in the treatment of chronic pain lends particular urgency to the need for an accurate and dispassionate appraisal of the benefits and risks associated with pain control and chemical dependence. Medical perceptions surrounding opioid therapy have cycled dramatically during the past century (Musto, 1999; Rock, 1977). A more liberal approach to prescribing began during the latter part of the 20th century with worldwide endorsement of opioid therapy for cancer pain. This spurred a more gradual acceptance of the view that opioid therapy may be appropriate for larger numbers of patients with chronic pain. During the past 10 years, this acceptance has advanced throughout the community of pain specialists, driven by favorable experiences with these drugs, incontrovertible evidence of widespread undertreatment of pain, and the reduced stigmatization of opioid drugs. From this perspective, opioid use was encouraged, with relatively little focus on the potential risks associated with abuse, addiction, and diversion. Indeed, for some practitioners, the myth of inevitable addiction was replaced by another myth, based on the misapprehension that chronic pain patients are somehow "immune" to the problems of misuse, abuse, addiction, or diversion (Friedman, 1990).

Pain specialists now have begun to realize that the issues related to chemical dependence are central to the safe and effective use of opioids as analgesics for chronic pain. The emphasis is now on a balanced perspective, in which potential therapeutic benefits are weighed against this risk. With a balanced perspective, the divide between professionals in addiction medicine and pain medicine is narrowing, and a new level of discourse may enhance the ability of each discipline to comprehend clinical phenomena and formulate questions for research.

DEFINITIONS AND PHENOMENOLOGY

Redefining Abuse and Addiction

Both clinical practice and research depend on a valid nomenclature for the phenomena associated with drug abuse and addiction. Unfortunately, this terminology has been problematic historically, and clarification is a necessary first step in advancing the understanding of the relationship between pain and chemical dependence.

Tolerance

Tolerance is a pharmacological property defined by the need for increasing doses of a drug to maintain effects (Dole, 1972; Martin & Jasinski, 1969). It implies that exposure to the drug itself is the "driving force" for the physiological changes that result in declining effects. It may involve one drug effect, any combination of effects, or all effects simultaneously.

Although tolerance is commonly regarded to be a problematic occurrence during opioid therapy, this characterization only applies to analgesic or other potentially positive drug effects. Tolerance to adverse effects, such as respiratory depression, nausea, and sedation, typically occurs rapidly and is a favorable outcome. By opening the "therapeutic window," this type of tolerance improves the risk:benefit ratio and allows dose titration in a manner that optimizes benefit.

In contrast, tolerance to analgesia is not favorable and can potentially lead to several adverse outcomes. Clinicians and patients alike commonly express concerns that tolerance will compromise analgesic therapy by necessitating progressively higher, and ultimately unsustainable, doses. Equally important, the drug-induced decline in the reinforcing effects of these drugs could, in the subpopulation predisposed to addiction, impel dose escalation in an effort to regain these effects, thereby potentially contributing to the development of the compulsive drug use (Wikler, 1980; American Psychiatric Association, 2000).

The concern about declining analgesic effects has not been borne out during an extensive clinical experience with the long-term administration of opioid drugs for the treatment of chronic pain (Nghiemphu & Portenoy, 2000; Portenoy, 1994). Most patients with chronic pain achieve an opioid dose associated with a favorable balance between analgesia and side effects, and remain at this dose for prolonged periods. When the need for dose escalation occurs, there are usually findings consistent with worsening pain (such as progression of a pain-producing lesion), and tolerance cannot be said to be the "driving force" for dose escalation. Interestingly, addicts who receive methadone for maintenance therapy also appear largely unaffected by the development of tolerance to the blocking actions of this drug.

Moreover, a strongly reinforcing effect (a "high") is distinctly uncommon when opioids are administered for pain in the nonaddicted population. The development of tolerance to these effects is now viewed as neither necessary nor sufficient for the development of addiction.

Physical Dependence

Physical dependence is defined solely by the occurrence of an abstinence syndrome following abrupt dose reduction or administration of an antagonist (Dole, 1972; Martin & Jasinski, 1969; Redmond & Krystal, 1984). The dose and duration of treatment required to produce clinically significant physical dependence in humans varies remarkably, and it is prudent to assume that the potential for withdrawal exists after an opioid has been administered repeatedly for only a few days.

There continues to be confusion about the differences between physical dependence and addiction. Physical dependence, like tolerance, has been suggested to be a component of addiction (American Psychiatic Association, 2000); specifically, the desire to avoid withdrawal has been postulated to create behavioral contingencies that reinforce drug-seeking behavior (Wikler, 1980). Although this phenomenon may be important in the subpopulation of individuals predisposed to addiction, it has no relevance for the vast majority of patients who receive opioid therapy for the treatment of acute or chronic pain. Physical dependence does not preclude the uncomplicated discontinuation of opioids during multidisciplinary pain management of nonmalignant pain (Halpern & Robinson, 1985), and opioid therapy is routinely stopped without difficulty in the cancer patients whose pain disappears following effective antineoplastic therapy.

In the clinical setting, therefore, the capacity to experience abstinence should never be labeled "addiction." Unless abstinence is intentionally or unintentionally induced by discontinuation of therapy or administration of an antagonist (including a partial agonist like buprenorphine or an agonist–antagonist opioid), the phenomenon of physical dependence is subclinical and not an issue in practice.

Abuse and Addiction

The definitions of abuse and addiction are complex when potentially abusable drugs are prescribed for specific medical indications (Kirsh, Whitcomb, Donaghy, & Passik, 2002). In the nomenclature of the American Psychiatric Association (2000), substance abuse refers to a maladaptive pattern of drug use associated with some manifest harm to the user or others. A less restrictive definition characterizes drug abuse as any use outside of socially accepted norms (Rinaldi, Steindler, Wilford, & Goodwin, 1998). Although the latter definition raises concerns about cultural sensitivity in labeling abuse, it can be applied more easily to misuse of prescribed analgesics and therefore has greater utility in the clinical setting. For the clinician, the use of any illicit drug, the maladaptive use of alcohol, and the use of prescribed drugs in a manner not intended by the clinician all may be perceived as abuse. If a prescribed regimen is inappropriately used in a manner that is not persistent or extreme, however, the term "misuse" is sometimes applied.

The American Psychiatric Association (2000) uses the term "substance dependence" to refer to addiction and defines this disorder as a maladaptive pattern of drug use associated with harm and, most importantly, characterized by compulsive drug use. Although this definition can be applied broadly to pain patients, it has been criticized because of specific criteria that include tolerance and physical dependence. Other definitions of addiction developed by specialists in addiction medicine (American Psychiatric Association, 2000; Rinaldi et al., 1988; Wikler, 1980; World Health Organization, 1969) have been similarly criticized.

In an effort to bridge the gap between pain specialists and addiction specialists, a working group jointly created by the American Society of Addiction Medicine, the American Pain Society, and the American Academy of Pain Medicine has developed a definition that has now been endorsed by all three professional societies:

> Addiction is a primary, chronic, neurobiologic disease, with genetic, psychosocial, and environmental factors. . . . It is characterized by behaviors that include one or more of the following: impaired control over drug use, compulsive use, continued use despite harm, and craving. (Savage et al., 2003, p. 662)

This definition is a useful starting point for clinicians and future investigators. Studies are needed to characterize each of the criteria empirically and to define the predictive validity of the various behaviors subsumed by each.

Aberrant Drug-Related Behaviors and Their Differential Diagnosis

The diagnosis of addiction is based on the observation of a drug-related phenomenology that meets defined criteria. In the clinical setting, where opioids or other potentially abusable drugs are prescribed for legitimate medical purposes, a broad range of aberrant drug-related behaviors occurs, from those that are relatively mild and limited (e.g., use of a prescribed dose to self-medicate a problem not intended by the clinician, such as insomnia) to those that are profound (e.g., injection of an oral formulation). On the basis of clinical experience, these drug-related behaviors have been divided into those that are more or less egregious and likely to predict addiction (Table 17.1).

The observation that aberrant drug-related behavior varies in severity and may or may not meet criteria for the diagnosis of addiction suggests that drug-related phenomenology in the clinical setting has a differential diagnosis (Table 17.2). Recognition of these potential disorders, which are not mutually exclusive, should guide a careful, ongoing assessment, the goal of which is to establish the nature of the problem for the purpose of treatment planning (Passik, Kirsh, & Portenoy, 2002; Passik & Portenoy, 1998).

The concept of "pseudoaddiction" is included in the differential diagnosis of aberrant drug-related behaviors and is particularly challenging when patients have both pain and comorbid substance use disorders. "Pseudoaddiction" refers to the occurrence of problematic behavior related to desperation associated with unrelieved pain. Paradoxically, the behaviors disappear if access to analgesic medication is increased. Originally described in the cancer population

TABLE 17.1. Aberrant Drug-Related Behaviors

Behaviors more suggestive of an addiction disorder

- Selling prescription drugs
- Prescription forgery
- Stealing or "borrowing" drugs from others
- Injecting oral formulations
- Obtaining prescription drugs from nonmedical sources
- Obtaining drugs from multiple medical sources without informing or despite prohibition
- Concurrent abuse of alcohol or illicit drugs
- Multiple episodes of self-escalation of dose, despite warnings not to do so
- Multiple episodes of prescription "loss"
- Evidence of functional deterioration unexplained by the pain or other comorbidity
- Repeated resistance to changes in therapy despite clear evidence of adverse effects

Behaviors less suggestive of an addiction disorder

- Aggressive complaining about the need for more drug
- Drug hoarding during periods of reduced symptoms
- Requesting specific drugs
- Openly acquiring similar drugs from other medical sources
- Occasional unsanctioned dose escalation
- Unapproved use of the drug to treat another symptom
- Reporting psychic effects not intended by the clinician
- Resistance to a change in therapy associated with "tolerable" adverse effects
- Expression of family concerns

(Weissman & Haddox, 1989), the term is now commonly applied to patients with any type of chronic pain.

Patients with addiction also may develop an increase in drug seeking that is driven by uncontrolled pain. In some cases, this behavior reflects both addiction and pseudoaddiction. If the patient is receiving a prescribed opioid for pain, the diagnosis may only be clarified if medical access to the drug is increased in a structured plan. Should drug-seeking behavior continue in this context, the likelihood that pseudoaddiction predominates is less.

TABLE 17.2. Differential Diagnosis of Aberrant Drug-Related Behavior

- Addiction
- Pseudoaddiction
- Psychiatric disorders
  - Axis I disorders (e.g., depression, anxiety, somatoform)
  - Axis II disorders (e.g., borderline personality, sociopathic personality)
- Encephalopathy (confusion in dose and interval of prescription)
- Criminal intent

Impulsive drug use also may be unrelated to both addiction and pseudo-addiction. Instead, it may reflect the existence of another psychiatric disorder. For example, patients with borderline personality disorder may exhibit aberrant drug taking to express fear and anger, or to improve chronic boredom. Similarly, some patients use opioids to self-medicate symptoms of anxiety or depression, insomnia, or problems of adjustment.

Other causes of problematic drug-related behaviors occur uncommonly in the clinical setting. Occasionally, drugs are misused because of a confusional state. This problem is exemplified by the repetitive use of a hypnotic at night, particularly in the elderly. Rarely, patients engage in criminal behavior, diverting controlled prescription drugs for profit.

Categories of Substance Abusers

The challenge of pain assessment and management in the population with substance abuse presumably varies with many specific characteristics. For example, patients with a history of addiction presumably pose greater concerns as a group than those whose involvement with drugs never reached this level. Similarly, it is likely that patients with a remote history of drug abuse or addiction have a greater potential for responsible drug use than those who are actively abusing (Fultz, 1975; Gonzales & Coyle, 1992; Macaluso, Weinberg, & Foley, 1988). These observations may influence the assessment of risk during therapy and thereby guide therapeutic decision. Studies are badly needed to confirm and clarify the nature of these impressions given their relevance to practice.

Patients who are receiving opioid agonist therapy for opioid addiction, either methadone or buprenorphine maintenance, represent another important subgroup. A recent survey indicated that 37% of methadone patients experience chronic severe pain, and 65% report interference by pain with functioning (sleep, affect, physical activity, and social relationships) (Rosenblum et al., 2003). Two-thirds of those with chronic severe pain had been prescribed an opioid analgesic during the 3 months prior to the survey.

Like those patients who have a remote history of substance abuse, those who are receiving a substitution therapy and have a well-established recovery probably can control a therapeutic opioid regimen, as long as it is carefully monitored and structured. Indeed, it is likely that undertreatment of chronic pain, which may relate to clinician bias, reluctance of patients to seek care, or reduced effectiveness of standard therapy because of opioid tolerance, is a greater risk in this population than the occurrence of iatrogenic relapse. Studies are needed, however, to evaluate the risks and benefits of opioid treatment in this population and the barriers to effective therapy.

The treatment of pain in patients with active drug abuse is particularly challenging. Pain management in this population is complicated by the drug use itself, the adverse physical and psychosocial consequences that result, and common medical and psychiatric comorbidities. The degree of psychopathology may be severe enough that a useful therapeutic alliance is impossible, and both the veracity of the complaints and adherence to prescribed therapies become major problems. Some patients cannot be treated with any potentially abusable drug.

Careful assessment is again critical to appropriate management. The types of drugs abused, the extent of the consequences, and the comorbidities must be clarified. An understanding of the past psychiatric condition of the patient can provide a context for therapeutic decisions. For example, sociopathy is relatively common among a subset of addicts (Hill, Haertzen, & Davis, 1962; Hill, Haertzen, & Glaser, 1960), and information about the occurrence of sociopathic behaviors prior to the diagnosis of chronic pain can inform the decision to treat with potentially abusable drugs. Straightforward questioning about illegal practices may yield surprisingly frank answers, from which an assessment of these behaviors can be made.

Categories of Patients with Pain

Patients with pain can be categorized in several clinically meaningful ways. Some distinctions are particularly relevant to the selection of treatment approaches.

Most patients who require opioid therapy present with acute monophasic pain that may accompany trauma or a procedure and is expected to be self-limited. When severe, the short-term administration of an opioid drug is widely considered to be medically appropriate treatment. Surveys suggest that these pain syndromes are often undertreated (Edwards, 1990; Perry & Heidrich, 1982).

Recurrent acute pains also are extremely prevalent. They include common painful disorders, such as headache and dysmenorrhea, and many diseases associated with periodic flares, including sickle-cell anemia, inflammatory bowel disease, and some arthritides or musculoskeletal disorders. The preferred treatment of these recurrent pains varies with the diagnosis and severity. The use of opioid therapy is conventional practice for some, such as the pain of sickle-cell anemia. The decision to implement a trial should be based on an assessment of pain characteristics and risks, rather than on diagnosis alone.

A third category is chronic pain associated with cancer or other progressive medical disease. Opioid therapy is considered to be the major therapeutic approach for patients with moderate or severe cancer pain (American Pain Society, 2003; Portenoy & Lesage, 1999), and pain associated with advanced medical illness of other types, including pain due to AIDS.

The role of opioid therapy in chronic pain syndromes of other types is less well accepted (see below). These syndromes include numerous disorders associated with nonprogressive organic lesions, such as osteoarthritis and various nerve injuries. They also include many syndromes defined solely by the pattern of pain and associated symptoms, including chronic daily headache syndrome, fibromyalgia, chronic pelvic pain of unknown origin, and many cases of back and neck pain. A small subgroup has pain and disability that is perceived by the clinician to be primarily related to psychopathology. These patients are characterized in psychiatric parlance as having a somatoform disorder (American Psychiatric Association, 2000), usually a pain disorder. More generically, the term "chronic pain syndrome" is often applied, denoting a chronic pain associated with a high level of disability and psychiatric comorbidity. Finally, some patients with chronic pain have no identifiable medical or psychiatric syndrome; these pains are best termed "idiopathic" (Arner & Myerson, 1988).

PAIN ASSESSMENT AND MANAGEMENT

The skills required to treat pain in any patient population include the ability to perform a comprehensive assessment and select a treatment strategy based on the diagnostic formulation. If drug therapy is used for pain, competent management depends on the ability to implement state-of-the-art prescribing principles. For opioid pharmacotherapy, the latter skills must be accompanied by the capacity to perform an assessment of the risks associated with misuse, abuse, addiction and diversion, and the ability to manage these risks over time. These skills are particularly needed in the population of chronic pain patients with a history of substance abuse.

Pain Assessment

Chronic pain is a complex, multidimensional phenomenon. It is commonly associated with other symptoms and disturbances in function. It is best conceptualized as a chronic illness that can be managed but seldom cured. The goals of therapy usually relate to comfort, functional restoration, and improved quality of life.

Given this complexity, comprehensive pain assessment requires history taking that focuses on the pain complaint, its consequences, prior treatments, relevant comorbidities, and other elements in a routine history. The characteristics of the pain include intensity, temporal features, location, quality, and provoking or relieving factors. Intensity should be measured, usually with a verbal rating scale (e.g., "mild," "moderate," "severe") or a numerical scale (e.g., "0–10"). The selection of the specific metric is less important than its regular application over time. Pain quality is assessed by eliciting verbal descriptors, such as "sharp," "burning," "lancinating," or "dull." The temporal pattern includes onset, course (progressive, stable, or fluctuating) and daily pattern.

The history also must characterize the impact of the pain and specifically query both physical and psychosocial functioning. The objective is to understand the role of the pain in the patient's life. Depending on the patient, this may require a discussion about work, social engagements, intimate relationships, interactions with health care providers, or other experiences.

The history of prior treatments for the pain should illuminate both prescribed and nonprescribed therapies. If prescribed drugs have been used, it is important to review the doses and durations of therapy, and to determine whether the lack of effectiveness was related to side effects.

Relevant comorbidities should be explored in both the physical and psychosocial domains. The psychosocial history should seek information on premorbid psychiatric disease, work and education history, current psychological state (particularly anxiety and depression), and premorbid interpersonal problems. A history of substance use is essential and should include information about the prior and present use of both licit (e.g., alcohol, tobacco, over-the-counter and prescription drugs) and illicit drugs.

In patients with a known history of substance abuse, the interviewer must gather detailed information on the specific pattern of addictive behaviors (e.g., drugs, routes, frequency of administration, means of acquisition, means of financing). The perceived relationship between these behaviors and the pain should be clarified.

History, physical examination, and results of diagnostic studies provide the data for a meaningful interpretation of the pain. This interpretation can be viewed from several perspectives. First, an etiology for the pain should be characterized, if possible. This etiology, which is usually reflects some structural pathology, may be a target for primary treatment.

Second, the data may allow labeling of the pain by syndrome. Syndrome identification can be very useful in guiding the selection of the appropriate management plan and indicating prognosis. Appropriate diagnosis of specific pain syndromes is facilitated by the taxonomy of pain developed by the International Association for the Study of Pain (Merskey & Bogduk, 1994).

Third, the information should permit inferences to be drawn about the predominating pathophysiology. Most broadly, pain can be classified as having a pathogenesis that is organic, psychogenic (e.g., somatoform disorder), mixed, or unclassifiable (idiopathic pain). Pain with a predominating organic contribution can be described as either nociceptive or neuropathic (American Psychiatric Association, 2000; Arner & Myerson, 1988; Portenoy, Payne, & Jacobsen, 1999). Although this is a gross simplification of complex biological processes, it has clinical utility and is widely employed. Nociceptive pain is perceived to be consistent with the degree of evident tissue injury, and is therefore conceptualized as being related to the ongoing activation of pain-sensitive primary afferent neurons. Subtypes include somatic pain (related to injured somatic structures, such as bone and joint) and visceral pain (related to injury to visceral structures). Neuropathic pain results from aberrant somatosensory processing in the central or peripheral nervous system and is disproportionate to the extent of evident tissue injury. There are numerous well-defined syndromes, including postherpetic neuralgia, painful neuropathy, poststroke pain, phantom limb pain, and complex regional pain syndrome (reflex sympathetic dystrophy and causalgia).

The distinction between nociceptive and neuropathic pain has clinical relevance. If a pain is nociceptive and the underlying etiology can be eliminated, or isolated from the central nervous system, long-term analgesia is expected. The profound analgesia associated with joint replacement illustrates this observation. In contrast, the diagnosis of a neuropathic pain suggests the use of medications that appear relatively specific for pains of this type (see below).

Management of Chronic Pain

The pain assessment guides the selection of therapies. For the patient with chronic pain, particularly pain associated with disability, a multimodality strategy targeted to both pain and disability may be preferable. There are numerous

---

TABLE 17.3. Therapeutic Strategies for Pain Management

1. Primary therapies directed against the underlying etiology
2. Primary analgesic therapies
   - Pharmacological approaches
     Examples: Nonopioid analgesics
     Adjuvant anaglesics
     Opioid analgesics
   - Rehabilitative approaches
     Examples: Physical/occupational therapy
     Orthoses/prostheses
   - Psychological approaches
     Examples: Cognitive-behavioral therapy
   - Anesthesiological approaches
     Examples: Neural blockade
     Neuraxial infusion
   - Neurostimulatory approaches
     Examples: Transcutaneous electrical nerve stimulation
     Dorsal column stimulation
   - Surgical approaches
     Examples: Cordotomy
   - Complementary and alternative medicine approaches
     Examples: Acupuncture
     Massage
     Neutraceuticals
   - Lifestyle changes
     Examples: Weight loss
     Exercise

approaches that may be combined in such a strategy (Table 17.3). If primary therapy against an identified etiology is possible, and appropriate, this should be considered as symptomatic treatments are offered.

Analgesic Pharmacotherapy

Drugs used to treat chronic pain can be divided in three categories: non-opioid analgesics (acetaminophen and the nonsteroidal anti-inflammatory drugs [NSAIDs]), adjuvant analgesics, and the opioids. Opioid pharmaco-therapy is most relevant for the current discussion.

OPIOID ANALGESICS

Pain specialists now consider long-term opioid therapy to be a major element in the approach to chronic pain, and specialists in pain medicine and in addiction medicine have begun to discuss the role of this approach in patients with histories of drug abuse or addiction. During the past few years, there has been a dramatic increase in the willingness of primary care physicians to consider long-term treatment for selected patients. As a result, overall access to these drugs has risen substantially. Concurrently, indicators of abuse and diversion have also tracked upward. Warnings raised by regulators and law enforcement have begun to increase concerns on the part of prescribers about the possibility of investigation and even sanction for prescribing opioids. This concern has been a constant in the United States for many decades and has been viewed by pain specialists as a significant barrier to appropriate opioid use.

The call for a more balanced approach to the role of opioid drugs derives from this present tension. Whether from the larger perspective of society or health care, or the microperspective of the individual clinician, the appropriate paradigm now emphasizes the need for a more nuanced perspective. This perspective accepts the legitimate role of opioid therapy in the management of appropriate patients with chronic pain (and the likelihood that prescribing needs to be increased to address the problem of undertreated pain) and concurrently recognizes the need to minimize the risk of adverse outcomes associated with chemical dependence. This paradigm now forms the foundation for the management principles that guide opioid therapy (Table 17.4).

Patient Selection. It is no longer appropriate to peremptorily reject the use of opioid drugs solely on the basis of pain syndrome or the psychiatric condition of the patient. Given the existing data and a large clinical experience, the most reasonable posture is to consider a trial of opioid therapy for *any* patient with chronic or frequently recurrent pain of moderate to severe intensity, and then to base the decision to proceed or not on the responses to the following questions:

TABLE 17.4. Proposed Guidelines for the Management of Long-Term Opioid Therapy

1. Chronic opioid therapy should be considered for any patient with chronic or frequently recurrent pain of moderate to severe intensity, based on the responses to the following questions: (a) What is conventional practice for pain of this type? (b) Are opioids likely to work well? (c) Is the patient at relatively increased risk of side effects by virtue of medical comorbidities or their treatments? (d) Are there other available therapies that might be considered in lieu of an opioid trial, for which there is evidence of the same or better efficacy at no greater risk? (e) Is the patient likely to manage opioid therapy responsibly? (f) Does this patient have a pain problem for which opioid therapy could be administered given the clinician's knowledge and skills; if not, could the patient be managed with the help of a consultant, or should referral be considered?

2. A single clinician should take primary responsibility for treatment. Treatment must be preceded by a comprehensive assessment that includes a detailed evaluation of current and past drug use. Past medical records should be obtained, and if needed, other health care providers, family, and pharmacies should be contacted to assess prior drug-taking behavior.

3. Patients should give informed consent before the start of therapy and the consent discussion should be documented in the medical record. This discussion should cover the issue of addiction, potential for cognitive impairment and other side effects, and the goals of the therapy.

4. Based on the assessment, clarify expectations regarding risk of problematic drug-related behavior and structure a treatment approach based on the level of risk. The approach may or may not incorporate actions such as very frequent visits, urine drug screening, required treatment by a mental health care provider or addiction medicine specialist, requirement to participate in ongoing addiction treatment, a written agreement stipulating expectations and consequences for problematic behavior, a requirement to use one pharmacy and do pill counts at visits, treatment with only long-acting drugs, and other strategies. None of these approaches are needed for some patients; others require very tight controls to enhance monitoring and assist the patient in maintaining responsible use.

5. After drug selection, doses should be given on an around-the-clock basis if the pain is continuous; several weeks should be agreed upon as the period of initial dose titration, and although improvement in function should be continually stressed, meaningful partial analgesia should be accepted as the appropriate goal of therapy.

6. Failure to achieve at least partial analgesia at relatively low initial doses in the patient with no substantial prior exposure raises questions about the potential treatability of the pain syndrome with opioids; such an occurrence should lead to reassessment of the pain syndrome.

7. Emphasis should be given to attempts to capitalize on improved analgesia by gains in physical and social function. Opioid therapy should be considered complementary to other analgesic and rehabilitative approaches.

8. Exacerbations of pain may occur and, following a careful assessment, the clinician may decide to increase the stable dose. This change in therapy should be stated clearly for the patient and documented in the medical record. If repeated dose escalation is needed to maintain pain control, the clinician should reevaluate the pain syndrome and the patient.

9. Ongoing monitoring of a range of outcomes is essential. At each contact, assessment should specifically address (a) comfort (degree of analgesia; self-report instruments may be helpful but should not be required); (b) opioid-related side effects; (c) functional status (physical and psychosocial); (d) existence of aberrant drug-related behaviors.

10. Initially, most patients must be seen and assessed at least monthly. If therapy is uneventful and consistently beneficial, monitoring can become less frequent. If, however, monitoring reveals problematic drug-related behavior, this should initiate an evaluation intended to interpret the phenomenon. Treatment for a new diagnosis (e.g., addiction) may be needed, as well as a new strategy for the analgesic drugs. In some cases, tapering and discontinuation of opioid therapy will be necessary. Other patients may appropriately continue therapy within a revised structure for monitoring therapy (see item 4). Consideration should be given to consultation with an addiction medicine specialist.

11. Documentation is essential, and the medical record should specifically address comfort, side effects, functional status, and the occurrence of aberrant behaviors repeatedly during the course of therapy.

1. What is conventional practice for pain of this type?
2. Are there other available therapies that might be considered in lieu of an opioid trial, for which there is a reasonable likelihood of the same or better efficacy at no greater risk?
3. Is the patient at relatively increased risk of side effects by virtue of medical comorbidities or their treatments?
4. Is the patient likely to manage opioid therapy responsibly?
5. Is a trial of opioid therapy in this patient appropriate given the clinician's knowledge and skills; if not, could the patient be managed with the help of a consultant, or should referral be considered?

These questions apply to all patients, irrespective of drug use history. They imply that there is no population for whom opioids are absolutely contraindicated, but that concerns such as the ability to control drug use are central in the decision-making process.

Principles of Prescribing. Guidelines for the selection and administration of opioid drugs derive from knowledge of opioid pharmacology and clinical experience (American Pain Society, 2003; Portenoy & Lesage, 1999; World Health Organization, 1996) and follow a few key principles.

1. *Issues in drug selection.* Opioids can be classified as pure agonists and agonist–antagonist drugs (Table 17.5). In contrast to the pure agonists, the agonist–antagonist opioids, including the mixed agonist–antagonists (e.g., pentazocine, nalbuphine, butorphanol, dezocine) and the partial agonists (e.g., buprenorphine), are characterized clinically by a ceiling effect for analgesia, the capacity to precipitate an abstinence syndrome in patients who are physically dependent on pure agonists, and a lesser degree of "liking" by those with the disease of addiction (Houde, 1979; Hoskin & Hanks, 1991). Some (pentazocine and butorphanol) have an incidence of psychomimetic effects substantially greater than that of the agonist drugs.

With the exception of buprenorphine, which now is also used as agonist therapy for opioid addiction, the agonist–antagonist drugs are not generally considered for chronic pain management. Although these drugs appear to have less abuse potential than the pure agonists and therefore might be selected for longer term use in patients with drug abuse histories, no specific data support the comparative safety and efficacy of this approach, and most pain specialists employ pure agonist drugs even with these patients. Because of the risk of precipitating an abstinence syndrome, agonist–antagonists should not be administered to patients who have developed physical dependence to opioids.

In the United States, the most common approach to the treatment of moderate pain involves the administration of a product combining a nonopioid analgesic (acetaminophen, aspirin, or ibuprofen) and an opioid (hydrocodone, codeine, oxycodone, or propoxyphene). If the maximum daily dose of the nonopioid analgesic is reached without providing adequate pain relief, the patient is considered for a trial of a single entity pure agonist drug. Tramadol is a centrally acting analgesic with a mechanism that is partially opioid and also is commonly tried for moderate pain.

Pure agonist drugs commonly employed for severe pain include morphine, hydromorphone, oxycodone, fentanyl (transdermal formulation), levorphanol, oxymorphone (rectal formulation and oral formulation in development), and methadone. Some clinicians use meperidine in this setting, but this generally should be avoided because of potential toxicity (dysphoria, tremulousness, hyperreflexia, and seizures) related to the accumulation of a metabolite (normeperidine), especially in renally impaired patients (Kaiko et al., 1983).

The modified-release, long-acting drugs now are usually favored for the treatment of chronic pain. These include several morphine formulations, transdermal fentanyl, and an oxycodone formulation. Other modified release drugs, such as oxymorphone, hydromorphone, and buprenorphine, will most likely be available soon. Methadone is long acting by virtue of its half-life; it, too, is often considered in this setting (see below).

There is great individual variation in the response to the different pure agonist drugs, an observation that has justified the use of sequential opioid trials to identify the most favorable drug. This practice is generally known as opioid "rotation" (de Stoutz, Bruera, & Suarez-Almazor, 1995). Initial drug selection is usually influenced by prior experience with opioids, cost, and the preferences of the patient. Morphine has active metabolites that accumulate in patients with renal insufficiency (Peterson, Randall, & Paterson, 1990; Sjogren, 1997) and may be less preferred when renal function is expected to vary. On the basis of extensive clinical observation, transdermal fentanyl may be preferred when opioids are expected to cause severe constipation or other gastrointestinal toxicities. Despite the media awareness of oxycodone abuse, there is no substantive evidence that this drug possesses characteristics that increase its risk relative to others. Nonetheless, if street value is an issue that influences drug selection, drugs that raise concern now include oxycodone, hydrocodone, and hydromorphone.

Methadone is gaining in popularity as a drug for long-term opioid therapy for pain. It is relatively inexpensive, has no active metabolites, and may possess high potency when substituted for another pure mu agonist drug. The latter effect may be related to the d-isomer of the commercially available racemic mixture, which is an antagonist at the N-methyl-D-aspartate (NMDA) receptor (Bruera & Neumann, 1999). Studies of NMDA antagonists suggest that this effect may be associated with an independent analgesic potential, and the ability to partially reverse opioid tolerance (Davis & Inturrisi, 1999).

Enthusiasm for the expanded use of methadone as an analgesic is tempered by several characteristics. Despite its long half-life, and contrary to its daily

TABLE 17.5. Opioid Asnalgesics

	Equianalgesic doses[a]	Half-life (hours)	Peak effect (hours)	Duration of effect (hours)	Comments
			Pure agonists (morphine-like)		
Morphine	10 i.m. 20–60 p.o.[b]	2–3 2–3	0.5–1 1.5–2	3–6 4–7	Standard comparior for opioids. Multiple routes available.
Controlled-release morphine	20–60 p.o.[b]	2–3	3–4	8–12	
Sustained-release morphine	20–60 p.o.[b]	2–3	4–6	24	
Hydromorphone	1.5 i.m. 7.5 p.o.	2–3 2–3	0.5–1 1–2	3–4 3–4	Multiple routes available.
Oxycodone	20–30 p.o.	2–3	1	3–6	Combined with aspirin or acetaminophen for moderate pain; available orally without coanalgesic for severe pain.
Controlled-release oxycodone	20–30	2–3	3–4	8–12	
Oxymorphone	1 i.m. 10 p.r.	— —	0.5–1 1.5–3	3–6 4–6	No oral formulation.
Meperidine	75 i.m. 300 p.o.	2–3 2–3	0.5–1 1–2	3–4 3–6	More CNS excitation than with other opioids. Not preferred for chronic pain due to potential toxicity.
Heroin	5 i.m.	0.5	0.5–1	4–5	Analgesic action due to metabolites, predominantly in morphine; not available in United States.
Levorphanol	2 i.m. 4 p.o.	12–15	0.5–1	3–6	Long half-life; accumulation occurs after starting or increasing dose.
Methadone	10 i.m. 20 p.o.	12– >150	0.5–1.5	4–8	Risk of delayed toxicity due to accumulation; useful to start to start dosing on p.r.n. basis, with close monitoring.
Codeine	130 i.m. 200 p.o.	2–3	1.5–2	3–6	Usually combined with nonopioid.

					Comments
Propoxyphene hydrochloride or napsylate	—	12	1.5–2	3–6	Toxic metabolite accumulates with overdose but not significant at doses used clinically; often combined with nonopioid.
Hydrocodone	—	2–4	0.5–1	3–4	Only available combined with acetaminophen.
Dihydrocodeine		2–4	0.5–1	3–4	Only available combined with acetaminophen or aspirin.
Partial agonists					
Buprenorphine	0.4 i.m. 0.8 s.l.	2–5 2–3	0.5–1 5–6	4–6	Can produce withdrawal in opioid-dependent patients; has ceiling for analgesia; s.l. tablet not available in United States.
Mixed agonist–antagonists					
Pentazocine	60 i.m. 180 p.o.	2–3 2–3	0.5–1 1–2	3–6 3–6	Produces withdrawal in opioid-dependent patients; oral formulation combined with naloxone or nonopioid in the United States; ceiling doses and side-effect profile limits role in chronic pain.
Nalbuphine	10 i.m.	4–6	0.5–1	3–6	Same as pentazocine. No oral formulation. Not preferred for chronic pain.
Butorphanol	2 i.m.	2–3	0.5–1	3–4	Same as nalbuphine.
Dezocine	10 i.m.[c]	1.2–7.4	0.5–1	3–4	Same as nalbuphine.

Note. p.o, orally; i.m., intramuscularly; p.r, rectally; p.r.n., as needed; s.l., sublingually; CNS, central nervous system.

[a] Dose that provides analgesia equivalent to 10 mg i.m. morphine. These ratios are useful guides when switching drugs or routes of administration. When switching drugs, reduce the equianalgesic dose of the new drug by 25–50% to account for incomplete cross-tolerance. The major exception to this is methadone, which appears to manifest a greater degree of incomplete cross-tolerance than other opioids; when switching to methadone, reduce the equianalgesic dose by 75–90%.

[b] Extensive survey data suggest that the relative potency of i.m.:p.o. morphine of 1:6 changes to 1:2–3 with chronic dosing.

[c] Approximate equianalgesic dose suggested from meta-analysis of available comparative studies.

administration in the treatment of opioid addiction, the use of methadone as an analgesic requires multiple doses per day. The long and variable half-life, which ranges from 12 hours to more than 150 hours (Plummer, Gourlay, Cherry, & Cousins, 1988), increases the risk of accumulation during dose titration. Patients who are predisposed to adverse effects due to advanced age or major organ failure require particularly careful monitoring (for a period of more than 1 week) when the dose of methadone is increased. There also have been recent concerns about the potential for methadone to cause a prolonged QT syndrome, and thereby predispose to serious cardiac arrhythmias (Kornick et al., 2003). The data are yet limited, and studies are underway to evaluate this further.

2. *Issues in the selection of a route.* The oral and transdermal routes are preferred for chronic opioid therapy due to their simplicity and acceptability. Chronic parenteral administration, either continuous subcutaneous infusion or continuous intravenous infusion through an indwelling venous access device, is usually considered in selected patients with advanced medical illness. Neuraxial infusion via the epidural or subarachnoid route has achieved a high level of sophistication and is available in developed countries for a small subgroup of chronic pain patients, typically those with intolerable side effects from systemic drugs (Plummer et al., 1991; Smith et al., 2002). The utility of this approach is likely to increase as studies establish the effectiveness of drug combinations and new drugs are approved specifically for intraspinal use.

Alternative routes have also been developed to deliver short-acting opioids for the treatment of breakthrough pain. Oral transmucosal fentanyl citrate is now available and has an onset of effect substantially faster than orally administered drugs (Fine, Marcus, Just De Boer, & Van der Oord, 1991). Other systems, including iontophoretic transdermal, buccal, and intrapulmonary drug delivery, are in development.

3. *Issues in dosing.* The most important step in optimizing opioid therapy is individualization of the dose through a process of dose titration. It is usually more effective to prevent the recurrence of pain than to abort it, and fixed-schedule dosing is preferred when treating continuous or frequently recurrent pain. "As needed" dosing may be useful during the initiation of therapy and is most commonly employed when a short-acting "rescue" opioid is combined with a long-acting drug to treat acute exacerbations of pain (breakthrough pain) (Portenoy et al., 1999). Although the addition of a rescue opioid is conventional practice in the management of cancer pain, it should be viewed as an option that may or may not be appropriate in any specific case. The use of rescue medication may be particularly problematic in those with a history of addictive disease, whose potential for abuse or relapse may be greater with access to a short-acting opioid.

Once an opioid and route of administration are selected, the dose should be increased until adequate analgesia occurs or intolerable and unmanageable adverse effects supervene. The opioid responsiveness of a specific pain syndrome can only be ascertained by dose escalation to limiting adverse effects. The opioid dose is immaterial as long as the patient attains a favorable balance between analgesia and adverse effects.

Although doses typically stabilize for prolonged periods during long-term management, dose escalation is usually required at intervals to maintain analgesia. In patients with progressive medical illness, this dose escalation is usually explained by a worsening of the pain-producing organic lesion (Nghiemphu & Portenoy, 2000; Portenoy, 1994). As observed previously, experience with long-term management of pain suggests that tolerance is rarely the "driving force" for dose escalation in the clinical setting.

Relative potencies have been determined for most pure agonist drugs in single-dose analgesic assays (Table 17.5). Using potency ratios, equianalgesic dose tables have been created that provide guidance when switching drugs or routes of administration (Indelicato & Portenoy, 2002). Due to incomplete cross-tolerance between opioids, which may result in a potency greater than anticipated for the newly initiated drug, a change from one drug to another should always be accompanied by a 25–50% reduction in the calculated equianalgesic dose. The exceptions to this include methadone, which should be reduced by 75–90% when initiated after treatment with another pure agonist drug, and transdermal fentanyl, which should be started at the dose indicated in the package insert (dose reduction already has been built in to these recommendations). The extent to which the equianalgesic dose is reduced by a safety factor can be adjusted up or down depending on the clinical condition of the patient, specifically the severity of the pain, the existence of opioid-related side effects, and the severity of medical comorbidities.

4. *Side effect management.* The management of side effects is an essential part of opioid therapy. By adequately treating side effects, it is often possible to titrate the opioid to a higher dose and thereby increase the responsiveness of the pain. Although respiratory depression fosters the greatest concern, tolerance to this adverse effect develops rapidly, and it is very uncommon if the opioid is titrated according to the accepted dosing guidelines. Constipation is the most frequent side effect encountered with chronic opioid therapy. Patients otherwise predisposed to constipation by virtue of advanced age or medical comorbidity should be considered for a prophylactic bowel regimen when opioid therapy is initiated. Although somnolence and mental clouding is frequent at the start of opioid treatment, these effects usually subside in a few days. In the absence of other medical problems, long-term opioid therapy should be accompanied by clear thinking; the capacity to drive or otherwise function at a high level should be considered goals of the treatment. Occasionally, the analgesic response is satisfactory but therapy is persistently compromised by somnolence or mental clouding. One option in this setting, which generally is accepted by pain specialists, is coadministration of a psychostimulant (such

as methylphenidate, modafinil, or dextroamphetamine) (Bruera, Fainsinger, MacEachern, & Hanson, 1992). Given the potential for stimulant abuse and new side effects, the use of such a drug requires careful assessment of risks versus benefits, and appropriate monitoring if treatment is initiated. Nausea or other gastrointestinal symptoms, such as anorexia or bloating, occur commonly early in therapy and are usually managed with a antiemetic. Because the experience of side effects with one opioid does not predict the occurrence of the same symptoms with another one, opioid rotation is always an option for the treatment of a challenging side effect.

5. *Risk assessment and management.* Extensive experience in the management of cancer pain has suggested that long-term opioid therapy of an older population with no prior history of substance abuse is rarely associated with de novo development of abuse or addiction. Similarly, very large surveys of patients who receive opioids to treat acute pain indicate that this therapy has a very low risk of precipitating addiction. These reassuring experiences, however, do not mean that the long-term administration of opioids to all populations carries a low risk of abuse, addiction, or diversion. Indeed, given the base rates of addiction in the population at large, the reality that neither the prevalence nor the pattern of aberrant drug-related behaviors during pain therapy are known, and the experience of pain specialists who commonly encounter drug abuse in the referred population they treat, it is prudent to perform an assessment of risk in all patients. Based on this assessment, treatment can be structured in a way that facilitates monitoring and assists the patient who needs help in controlling drug use.

The most consistent predictor of misuse and abuse during opioid therapy appears to be a history of substance abuse. Surveys have begun to identify other predictors and develop validated methods for categorizing risk (Adams et al., 2004; Chabal, Erjavec, Jacobson, Mariano, & Chaney, 1997; Coambs & Jarry, 1996; Compton, Darakjian, & Mitto, 1998; Friedman, Li, & Mehrotra, 2003). There is presently no single, well-accepted measure or risk profile. In addition to a history of drug abuse, factors that may raise a "red flag" include a report by the patient about concern related to control of the medication, a family history of drug abuse, a personal or family history of significant psychiatric disease, problematic behaviors with other prescribed drugs, a criminal record, and frequent automobile accidents.

Based on this assessment, the clinician should categorize the patient by degree of perceived risk. Proactive strategies for prescribing should be applied in some combination for those whose risk is perceived to be relatively high (Table 17.4). These strategies may include a written agreement defining the parameters of acceptable behavior; urine drug screening; frequent visits; various rules concerning pill counts, concurrent treatment for addiction or other psychiatric disease, and response to lost prescriptions; no use of short-acting drugs; and similar approaches. For the person who is perceived to be at relatively limited risk, these strategies may be limited (e.g., frequent visits only until the relationship is established). For those perceived to be at high risk, such as the addict only recently in a recovery program, all of the strategies can be required.

These strategies should be explained to the patient as the foundation needed by the clinician to act in the patient's best interest. They are not punitive and should not undermine the therapeutic alliance. Indeed, experience suggests that the patient with addiction and pain often will correctly perceive in this effort that the clinician is willing to undertake a relatively labor-intensive approach in an effort to provide pain relief.

During treatment, monitoring for aberrant drug-related behavior should be undertaken as a routine, similar to the conventional monitoring of efficacy (analgesia), side effects, and potential benefits on function (Table 17.4). In some cases, this monitoring may appropriately be limited to the history; in others, the patient must be required to permit contacts between the clinician and others, such as family, other physicians, a sponsor, or a pharmacist. The occurrence of aberrant drug-related behavior should initiate reevaluation, so that appropriate interpretation of the behavior is possible (discussed earlier). If the decision is made to continue prescribing, the structure of therapy usually should be altered to impose additional controls. These enhance the ability to monitor in the future and may assist the fragile patient in maintaining responsible drug use.

OTHER ANALGESIC DRUGS

Acetaminophen and the NSAIDs. The analgesia provided by nonopioid analgesics is characterized by a ceiling effect, which usually limits the use of these drugs to pain that is usually moderate in severity. In the absence of relative contraindications, however, it is reasonable to undertake trials of these drugs in all types of pain. Based on clinical observations, they are least likely to be helpful in neuropathic pain and are most clearly indicated in pain associated with inflammatory diseases (e.g., rheumatoid arthritis).

Acetaminophen possesses analgesic properties similar to aspirin but is better tolerated and lacks the adverse effects of NSAIDs. The main concern associated with its use is the hepatotoxicity encountered with overdose. The usual maximum daily dose is 4,000 mg. In those with liver disease (e.g., hepatitis C) or chronic alcoholism (Zimmerman & Maddrey, 1995), the risk of hepatotoxicity is greater, and acetaminophen should be used in far lower doses, or avoided altogether.

NSAIDs comprise an extremely diverse group of drugs (Table 17.6), all of which inhibit the enzyme cyclo-oxygenase (COX), thereby reducing the synthesis of prostaglandins. Cyclo-oxygenase is produced in at least two isoforms, COX-1 and COX-2. The "constitutive" isoform COX-1 is involved in physio-

TABLE 17.6. Nonsteroidal Anti-Inflammatory Drugs

Chemical Class	Drug	Recommended starting dose (mg/day orally)[a]	Recommended maximum dose (mg/day orally)
	Nonselective COX inhibitors		
Salicylates	Aspirin	2,600	6,000
	Diflunisal	1,000 × 1	1,500
	Choline magnesium trisalicylate	1,500 × 1, then 1,000	4,000
	Salsalate	1,500 × 1, then 1,000	4,000
Propionic acids	Ibuprofen	1,600	4,200
	Naproxen	500	1,500
	Naproxen sodium	550	1,375
	Fenoprofen	800	3,200
	Ketoprofen	100	300
	Flurbiprofen	100	300
	Oxaprozin	600	1,800
Acetic acids	Indomethacin	75	200
	Tolmetin	600	2,000
	Sulindac	300	400
	Diclofenac	75	200
	Ketorolac	40	40
	Ketorolac (i.m.)	30 (loading)	60
	Etodolac	600	1,200
Oxicams	Piroxicam	20	40
	Meloxicam	7.5	15
Naphthylalkanones	Nabumetone	1,000	2,000
Fenamates	Mefenamic acid	500 × 1	1,000
	Meclofenamic acid	150	400
Pyrazoles	Phenylbutazone	300	400
	Selective COX-2 inhibitors		
	Celecoxib	200	400
	Valdecoxib	20	40

[a] In elderly persons on multiple drugs or those with renal insufficiency, starting dose should be one-half to two-thirds of the recommended starting dose.

logical processes, whereas the "inducible" COX-2 is mostly produced as part of the inflammatory cascade. A higher selectivity for the COX-2 isozyme is therefore desirable in order to achieve higher analgesic and anti-inflammatory activities with fewer adverse effects. The various NSAIDs vary in their COX-2 selectivity. Commercially available drugs with high COX-2 selectivity comprise celecoxib and valdecoxib; at a relatively low dose, meloxicam is also highly selective. The appropriate positioning of the COX-2 selective drugs is still controversial; they are most clearly appropriate in patients who have not tolerated the nonselective COX-1/COX-2 inhibitors and those at increased risk of gastrointestinal complications.

The potential for toxicity during NSAID therapy influences the decision to initiate therapy, the selection of drug, and the approach to dosing and monitoring. The most important toxicities are gastrointestinal, renal, and cardiovascular.

Approximately 10% of patients treated with a nonselective COX-1/COX-2 NSAID experience clinically important gastrointestinal toxicity, and gastric or duodenal ulcers occur in about 2% (Loeb, Ahlquist, & Talley, 1992). The risk of gastrointestinal toxicity is increased with advanced age (older than 60 years old), higher NSAID dose, concomitant administration of a corticosteroid, a history of ulcer disease or previous gastrointestinal complication from NSAIDs, and possibly by heavy alcohol or cigarette consumption (Hernandez-Diaz & Rodriguez, 2000; Loeb et al., 1992). The risk of ulcer can be reduced but not eliminated (Mamdani et al., 2002) by use of the selective COX-2 inhibitors or by concurrent administration of gastroprotective therapy, including a proton pump inhibitor (e.g., omeprazole), misoprostol (a prostaglandin analogue), or a H2 blocker (La Corte, Caselli, Castellino, Bajocchi, & Trotta, 1999).

Renal function depends on both COX-1 and COX-2 isoforms; consequently, any NSAID can cause serious renal toxicity, including acute renal failure and hyperkalemia. NSAIDs should be used with caution in those with renal disease, and all patients should have regular monitoring of renal function. The nonselective COX-1/COX-2 NSAIDs can cause a bleeding diathesis by interfering with platelet activity; this potential toxicity does not occur with the COX-2 selective agents. Symptomatic coronary artery disease during treatment with the selective COX-2 drug, rofecoxib, recently led to the withdrawal of this drug from the U.S. market. At the present time, this problem is not believed to be a class effect. Patients at risk for atherothrombotic disease who are treated with a COX-2 selective drug should also receive aspirin therapy.

Adjuvant Analgesics. Adjuvant analgesics are drug that have primary indications other than pain but can be analgesic in some pain conditions (Lussier & Portenoy, 2003). This category is extremely diverse, representing numerous drugs in many classes (Table 17.7). Some of these drugs have analgesic properties in several pain syndromes and are therefore referred as "multipurpose

TABLE 17.7 Adjuvant Analgesics

Indication	Drug class	Examples
Multipurpose analgesics	Antidepressants	
	Tricyclic antidepressants	Amitriptyline, doxepin, nortriptyline, desipramine
	SSRIs	Paroxetine, citalopram
	SNRI	Venlafaxine, duloxetine
	Others	Bupropion, trazodone, maprotiline
	Alpha^2-adrenergic agonists	Clonidine, tizanidine
	Corticosteroids	Dexamethasone, prednisone
Adjuvants for neuropathic pain	Anticonvulsants	Gabapentin, lamotrigine, pregabalin oxcarbazepine, topiramate, levetiracetam, zonisamide, carbamazepine, phenytoin, valproate
	Local anesthetics	Lidocaine, mexiletine
	N-Methyl-D-aspartate blockers	Ketamine, dextromethorphan, amantadine
	Sympatholytics	Prazosin, phentolamine, phenoxybenzamine, beta blockers
	Topical agents	Local anesthetics, capsaicin, NSAIDs
	Miscellaneous	Baclofen, calcitonin
Adjuvants for musculoskeletal pain	"Muscle relaxants"	Orphenadrine, carisoprodol, methocarbamol, chlorzoxazone, cyclobenzaprine, metaxalone
	Benzodiazepines	Diazepam
Adjuvants for cancer pain	For bone pain	Biphosphonates, calcitonin
	For bowel obstruction	Scopolamine, octreotide, corticosteroids

Note. SSRI, selective serotonin reuptake inhibitor; NSRI, norepinephrine–serotonin reuptake inhibitor.

adjuvant analgesics." These include antidepressants (tricyclics, selective serotonin or serotonin and norepinephrine reuptake inhibitors, bupropion), corticosteroids (mainly dexamethasone), and alpha-2-receptor agonists (clonidine, tizanidine). Other adjuvant analgesics are indicated only for specific pain syndromes. Anticonvulsants (e.g., gabapentin, topiramate, levetiracetam, lamotrigine), local anesthetics (e.g., intravenous or topical lidocaine, oral mexiletine, and NMDA receptor antagonists (ketamine, dextromethorphan, amantadine) are used in neuropathic pain.

Other Analgesic Approaches

Although the range and effectiveness of the pharmacological therapies for pain offer extraordinary opportunities for the patient with chronic pain, pharmacotherapy should not be considered a uniform first-line approach for pain. The assessment of the patient should allow a thoughtful positioning of drug treatment overall, and opioid treatment specifically, in relation to the large number of nonpharmacological treatments now available. Some patients are reasonable candidates for drug therapy alone; others should receive drugs only as part of a multimodality strategy, and still others should not be offered pharmacotherapy because the risk:benefit ratio for other treatments is better. These decisions often evolve over time and require ongoing evaluation of outcomes. By gaining insight into the available approaches for pain, clinicians can make reasoned decisions about the selection of patients for treatment and referral when appropriate.

CONCLUSION

Issues at the interface between pain and chemical dependence are complex and clinically relevant. In a striking paradox, concern about abuse and addiction contributes to undertreatment at the same time that a tendency to prescribe abusable drugs, without addressing the risk of abuse and addiction, may be contributing to bad therapeutic outcomes. Clinicians would be best served by gaining the skills to assess pain comprehensively, learning about the range of approaches available to treat pain in diverse populations, and approaching the problem of opioid therapy from the perspective of balance. At the level of patient care, a balanced perspective implies that clinicians acquire both the skills to optimize the principles of prescribing and the skills necessary to perform risk assessment and management. The goals are to relieve pain and improve quality of life, while minimizing the risk of all adverse outcomes.

REFERENCES

Adams, L. L., Gatchelm, R. J., Robinson, R. C., Polatin, P., Gajraj, N., Deschner, M., & Noe, C. (2004). Development of a self-report screening instrument for assessing potential opioid medication misuse in chronic pain patients. *J Pain Symptom Manage, 27*(5), 440–459.

American Pain Society. (2003). *Principles of analgesic use in the treatment of acute pain and cancer pain.* Glenview, IL: Author.

American Psychiatric Association. (2000). *Diagnostic and statistical manual for mental disorders* (4th ed., text rev.). Washington, DC: Author.

Arner, S., & Myerson, B. A. (1988). Lack of analgesic effects of opioids on neuropathic and idiopathic forms of pain. *Pain, 33,* 11–23.

Bruera, E., Fainsinger, R., MacEachern, T., & Hanson, J. (1992). The use of methylphenidate in patients with incident cancer pain receiving regular opiates. *Pain, 50,* 75–77.

Bruera, E. B., & Neumann, C. M. (1999). Role of methadone in the management of pain in cancer patients. *Oncology, 13,* 1275–1291.

Chabal, C., Erjavec, M. K., Jacobson, L., Mariano, A., & Chaney, E. (1997). Prescription opiate abuse in chronic pain patients: Clinical criteria, incidence, and predictors. *Clin J Pain, 12,* 150–155.

Coambs, R. B., & Jarry, J. L. (1996). The SISAP: A new screening instrument for identifying potential opioid abusers in the management of chronic nonmalignant pain in general medical practice. *Pain Res Manag, 1,* 155–162.

Colliver, J. D., & Kopstein, A. N. (1991). Trends in cocaine abuse reflected in emergency room episodes reported to DAWN. *Public Health Rep, 106,* 59–68.

Compton, P., Darakjian, J., & Mitto, K. (1998). Screening for addiction in patients with chronic pain and "problematic" substance use: Evaluation of a pilot assessment tool. *J Pain Symptom Manage, 16,* 355–363.

Davis, A. M., & Inturrisi, C. E. (1999). d-Methadone blocks morphine tolerance and N-methyl-D-aspartate-induced hyperalgesia. *J Pharmacol Exp Ther, 289,* 1048–1053.

de Stoutz, N. D., Bruera, E., & Suarez-Almazor, M. (1995). Opioid rotation for toxicity reduction in terminal cancer patients. *J Pain Symptom Manage, 10,* 378–384.

Dole, V. P. (1972). Narcotic addiction, physical dependence and relapse. *N Engl J Med, 286,* 988–991.

Edwards, W. T. (1990). Optimizing opioid treatment of postoperative pain. *J Pain Symptom Manage, 5,* S24–S36.

Fine, P. G., Marcus, M., Just De Boer, A., & Van der Oord, B. (1991). An open label study of oral transmucosal fentanyl citrate (OTFC) for the treatment of breakthrough cancer pain. *Pain, 45,* 149–153.

Friedman, D. P. (1990). Perspectives on the medical use of drugs of abuse. *J Pain Symptom Manage, 5*(Suppl), 2–5.

Friedman, R., Li, V., & Mehrotra, D. (2003). Treating pain patients at risk: evaluation of a screening tool in opioid-treated pain patients with and without addiction. *Pain Med, 4,* 182–185.

Fultz, J. M. (1975). Guidelines for the management of hospitalized narcotic addicts. *Ann Intern Med, 82,* 815–818.

Gfoerer, J., & Brodsky, M. (1992). The incidence of illicit drug use in the United States, 1962–1989. *Br J Addict, 87,* 1345–1351.

Gonzales, G. R., & Coyle, N. (1992). Treatment of cancer pain in a former opioid abuser: Fears of the patient and staff and their influence on care. *J Pain Symptom Manage, 7,* 246–249.

Halpern, L. M., & Robinson, J. (1985). Prescribing practices for pain in drug dependence: A lesson in ignorance. *Adv Alcohol Subst Abuse, 5,* 135–162.

Hernandez-Diaz, S., & Rodriguez, L. A. (2000). Association between nonsteroidal antiinflammatory drugs and upper gastrointestinal tract bleeding/perforation: An overview of epidemiologic studies published in the 1990s. *Arch Intern Med, 160*, 2093–2099.

Hill, H. E., Haertzen, C. A., & Davis, H. (1962). An MMPI factor analytic study of alcoholics, narcotic addicts and criminals. *Qualitative J Stud Alcohol, 23*, 411–431.

Hill, H. E., Haertzen, C. A., & Glaser, R. (1960). Personality characteristics of narcotic addicts as indicated by the MMPI. *J Gen Psychol, 62*, 127–139.

Hoskin, P. J., & Hanks, G. W. (1991). Opioid agonist–antagonist drugs in acute and chronic pain patients. *Drugs, 41*, 329–344.

Houde, R. W. (1979). Analgesic effectiveness of the narcotic agonist–antagonists. *Br J Clin Pharmacol, 7*, 297S–308S.

Indelicato, R. A., & Portenoy, R. K. (2002). Opioid rotation in the management of refractory cancer pain. *J Clin Oncol, 20*, 348–352.

Kaiko, R. F., Foley, K. M., Grabinski, P. Y., Heidrich, G., Rogers, A. G., Inturrisi, C. E., & Reidenberg, M. M. (1983). Central nervous system excitatory effects of meperidine in cancer patients. *Ann Neurol, 13*, 180–185.

Kirsh, K. L., Whitcomb, L. A., Donaghy, K., & Passik, S. D. (2002). Abuse and addiction issues in medically ill patients with pain: Attempts at clarification of terms and empirical study. *Clin J Pain, 4*(Suppl), S52–S60.

Kornick, C. A., Kilborn, M. J., Santiago-Palma, J., Schulman, G., Thaler, H. T., Keefe, D. L., et al. (2003). QTc interval prolongation associated with intravenous methadone. *Pain, 105*, 499–506.

La Corte, R., Caselli, M., Castellino, G., Bajocchi, G., & Trotta, F. (1999). Prophylaxis and treatment of NSAID-induced gastroduodenal disorders. *Drug Safety, 20*, 527–543.

Loeb, D. S., Ahlquist, D. A., & Talley, N. J. (1992). Management of gastroduodenopathy associated with use of nonsteroidal anti-inflammatory drugs. *Mayo Clin Proc, 67*, 354–364.

Lussier, D., & Portenoy, R. K. (2003). Adjuvant analgesics in pain management. In D. Doyle, G. W. Hanks, R. N. MacDonald, & N. I. Cherny (Eds.), *Oxford textbook of palliative medicine* (pp. 349–377). Oxford, UK: Oxford University Press.

Macaluso, C., Weinberg, D., & Foley, K. M. (1988). Opioid abuse and misuse in a cancer pain population. *J Pain Symptom Manage, 3*, S24.

Mamdani, M., Rochon, P. A., Juurlink, D. N., Kopp, A., Anderson, G. M., Naglie, G., et al. (2000). Observational study of upper gastrointestinal haemorrhage in elderly patients given selective cyclo-oxygenase-2 inhibitors or conventional nonsteroidal anti-inflammatory drugs. *Br Med J, 325*, 624–629.

Martin, W. R., & Jasinski, D. R. (1969). Physiological parameters of morphine dependence in man—tolerance, early abstinence, protracted abstinence. *J Psychiatr Res, 7*, 9–13.

Merskey, H., & Bogduk, N. (1994). *Classification of chronic pain* (2nd ed.). Seattle, WA: IASP Press.

Musto, D. F. (1999). *The American disease: Origins of narcotics control.* New York: Oxford University Press.

Nghiemphu, L. P., & Portenoy, R. K. (2000). Opioid tolerance: A clinical perspective. In E. B. Bruera & R. K. Portenoy (Eds.), *Topics in palliative care* (Vol. 5, pp. 197–212). New York: Oxford University Press.

Passik, S. D., Kirsh, K. L., & Portenoy, R. K. (2002). Substance abuse issues in palliative care. In A. Berger, R. K. Portenoy, & D. E. Weissman (Eds.), *Principles and practice of palliative care and supportive oncology* (pp. 593–603). Philadelphia: Lippincott/ Williams & Wilkins.

Passik, S. D., & Portenoy, R. K. (1998). Substance abuse disorders. In J. C. Holland (Ed.), *Psycho-oncology* (pp. 576–586). New York: Oxford University Press.

Perry, S., & Heidrich, G. (1982). Management of pain during débridement: A survey of U.S. burn units. *Pain, 13,* 267–280.

Peterson, G. M., Randall, C. T. C., & Paterson, J. (1990). Plasma levels of morphine and morphine glucuronides in the treatment of cancer pain: Relationship to renal function and route of administration. *Eur J Clin Pharmacol, 38,* 121–124.

Plummer, J. L., Cherry, D. A., Cousins, M. J., Gourlay, G. K., Onley, M. M., & Evans, K. H. (1991). Long-term spinal administration of morphine in cancer and non-cancer pain: A retrospective study. *Pain, 44,* 215–220.

Plummer, J. L., Gourlay, G. K., Cherry, D. A., & Cousins, M. J. (1988). Estimation of methadone clearance: Application in the management of cancer pain. *Pain, 33,* 313–322.

Portenoy, R. K. (1994). Opioid tolerance and efficacy: Basic research and clinical observations. In G. Gebhardt, D. Hammond, T. Jensen (Eds.), *Proceedings of the VII World Congress on Pain: Progress in pain research management* (Vol. 2, pp. 595–619). Seattle: IASP Press.

Portenoy, R. K., & Lesage, P. (1999). Management of cancer pain. *Lancet, 353,* 1695–1700.

Portenoy, R. K., Payne, D., & Jacobsen, P. (1999). Breakthrough pain: Characteristics and impact in patients with cancer pain. *Pain, 81,* 129–134.

Redmond, D. E., & Krystal, J. H. (1984). Multiple mechanisms of withdrawal from opioid drugs. *Ann Rev Neurosci, 7,* 443–478.

Regier, D. A., Myers, J. K., Kramer, M., Robins, L. N., Blazer, D. G., Hough, R. L., et al. (1984). The NIMH Epidemiologic Catchment Area program: Historical context, major objectives, and study population characteristics. *Arch Gen Psychiatry, 41,* 934–941.

Rinaldi, R. C., Steindler, E. M., Wilford, B. B., & Goodwin, D. (1988). Clarification and standardization of substance abuse terminology. *JAMA, 259,* 555–557.

Rock, P. E. (Ed.). (1977). *Drugs and politics.* New Brunswick, NJ: Transaction.

Rosenblum, A., Joseph, H., Fong, C., Kipnis, S., Cleeland, C., & Portenoy, R. K. (2003). Prevalence and characteristics of chronic pain among chemically dependent patients in methadone maintenance and residential treatment facilities. *JAMA, 289,* 2370–2378.

Savage, S. R., Joranson, D. E., Covington, E. C., Schnoll, S. H., Heit, H. A., & Gilson, A. M. (2003). Definitions related to the medical use of opioids: Evolution towards universal agreement. *J Pain Symptom Manage, 26,* 655–667.

Sjogren, P. (1997). Clinical implications of morphine metabolites. In R. K. Portenoy & E. B. Bruera (Eds.), *Topics in palliative care* (Vol. 1, pp. 163–175). New York: Oxford University Press.

Smith, T. J., Staats, P. S., Deer, T., Stearns, L. J., Rauck, R. L., Boortz-Marx, R. L., et al. (2002). Randomized clinical trial of an implantable drug delivery system compared with comprehensive medical management for refractory cancer pain: impact on pain, drug-related toxicity, and survival. *J Clin Oncol, 20,* 4040–4049.

Verhaak, P. F., Kerssens, J. J., Dekker, J., Sorbi, M. J., & Bensing, J. M. (1998). Prevalence of chronic benign pain disorder among adults: A review of the literature. *Pain, 77,* 231–239.

Weissman, D. E., & Haddox, J. D. (1989). Opioid pseudoaddiction—an iatrogenic syndrome. *Pain, 36,* 363–366.

Wikler, A. (1980). *Opioid dependence: Mechanisms and treatment.* New York: Plenum Press.

World Health Organization. (1996). *Cancer pain relief, with a guide to opioid availability* (2nd ed.). Geneva: Author.

World Health Organization. (1969). *Expert Committee on Drug Dependence, 16th report* (Technical Report No. 407). Geneva: Author.

Zimmerman, H., & Maddrey, W. (1995). Acetaminophen (paracetamol) hepatotoxicity with regular intake of alcohol: Analysis of instances of therapeutic misadventure. *Hepatology, 22,* 767–773.

CHAPTER 18

Alcoholism and Substance Abuse in Older Adults

SHELDON ZIMBERG

People over 65 years of age are the fastest growing population in the United States. The U.S. Public Health Service's Healthy People 2000 initiative noted that 13% of the population is 65 years of age or older. It was noted that alcoholism and substance abuse are substantial problems in the general population, including elderly people (Menninger, 2002).

Although there have been substantial increases in services for younger alcoholics and substance abusers, including detoxification facilities, outpatient clinics, and inpatient rehabilitation over the years, few specialized programs for elderly people have been developed. Clinical experience has shown that because of increased resistance to acknowledge an alcohol or substance use problem and lack of emphasis in existing treatment programs on the life issues they experience, few elderly are willing to go to existing treatment facilities (Barrick & Conners, 2002). A substantial number of senior citizens have alcohol problems, in the range of 10–15%. Illicit drug use among the elderly is rare, but prescription drug misuse and abuse is substantial (Reid & Anderson, 1997; Zimberg, 1995).

In addition to patient resistance, among health care workers, there is a low index of suspicion about these conditions in elderly patients and negative attitudes, such as "Why bother to treat an older person? The alcohol is all that he or she has left." This attitude can be considered a form of ageism. It is particularly unfortunate, since elderly patients can be diagnosed and effectively treated, if the stresses of aging are recognized and dealt with in an "aging-specific" treatment approach utilized by myself and others to treat this population

(Zimberg, 1996). The availability of treatment services is further complicated by the lack of knowledge of addictive disorders among primary care physicians and geriatric specialists, and the reciprocal lack of knowledge of aging-related problems among addiction specialists.

In this chapter, I discuss the prevalence of alcoholism and prescription drug abuse among elderly persons, diagnostic approaches, and therapy directed at the maladaptations to aging that often lead to alcohol and prescription drug misuse. In addition, I present a section on the recognition and treatment of elderly alcoholics admitted to general hospitals, since so many such patients are often not diagnosed and not treated or are inappropriately treated.

PREVALENCE OF ALCOHOLISM AND PRESCRIPTION DRUG MISUSE IN ELDERLY PEOPLE

Prevalence studies of alcoholism in elderly people in the community have been reported in the range from 4 to 20% (Atkinson, Ganzini, & Bernstein, 1992; Bridgewater, Leigh, James, & Potter, 1987; Cahalan, Cisin, & Crossley, 1969). A study in the Washington Heights area in Manhattan indicated an alcoholism rate of 105/1000 residents among elderly widowers (Bailey, Haberman, & Alksne, 1965). The researchers asked questions about problems associated with drinking rather than quantity–frequency questions, which often give unreliable information. The elderly widowers had the highest rates of alcohol problems found. Another community-based study of United Automobile Workers in Baltimore found that 10% of men and 20% of women over age 60 were heavy escape drinkers and considered to be alcoholics (Siassi, Crocetti, & Spiro, 1973).

In studies in primary care settings, outpatient treatment, medical and psychiatric inpatient treatment, and emergency rooms, elderly patients show rates of alcoholism in the 15 to 20% range (Adams, Barry, & Fleming, 1996; Adams, Magruder-Habid, Trued, & Broome, 1992; Adams, Zhung, Barhoriak, & Rimm, 1993; McCusker, Cherubin, & Zimberg, 1971; Moore, 1972; Zimberg, 1969). A particularly significant study of hospital admissions under Medicare showed that elderly patients with alcoholism or alcohol-related medical conditions were admitted at a rate of 48 per 10,000 population, similar to the rates of admission for myocardial infarction for this age group (Adams et al., 1993).

As indicated previously, illicit drug use of heroin, cocaine, marijuana, and other substances is relatively rare. The major concern, however, is with prescription and over-the-counter drug misuse and abuse. Many elderly individuals are on multiple prescription drugs, at times supplemented by over-the-counter analgesics, antihistamines, laxatives, cold preparations, and sedatives. These multiple drugs can produce side effects through interactions and can cause problems for elderly people who are using and abusing alcohol. Confusion with drug effects, complicated by drug–drug interactions, is a major part of the problem in diagnosing alcohol dependence or abuse in elderly people (Schuckit, 1979).

The class of drugs most subject to misuse and abuse is the benzodiazapines. These drugs are prescribed for anxiety and depression; however, their liability to tolerance and dependence creates problems for patients, and demands are often made on the prescribing physicians to give more. These drugs also cause cognitive impairments and confusion that suggest dementia. It is particularly problematic when benzodiazepines are also used with alcohol, and by those with alcohol problems. Such a combination of benzodiazepines and alcohol use is common and often complicates treatment of the alcohol problem. Benzodiazepines represent the most widely used psychiatric prescription drugs among elderly patients in primary care and psychiatric settings, and can cause problems by leading to organicity, drug interactions, and addiction. Their use, with the liabilities indicated, creates more problems than they solve and is particularly inappropriate when other drugs, such as selective serotonin reuptake inhibitors, have been found to be safe and effective in geriatric patients with anxiety and depression (Kennedy, 2000; Rigler, 2000; Zimberg, 1995), and their use is preferable to benzodiazepines in most cases.

TYPOLOGY AND DIAGNOSIS OF ELDERLY ALCOHOLICS

Typology

Work done more than two decades ago by Simon, Epstein, and Reynolds (1968) and Gaitz and Baer (1971) found distinctions between elderly alcoholics, with and without organic mental syndromes, and also typed an early- versus late-onset typology. These authors suggested that the patients with significant organic deficits did poorly in treatment and died at an earlier age. Simon and colleagues also noted that in the psychiatric inpatient population of elderly persons they studied, 23% had alcohol problems; 16% became alcoholic before age 60, and 7% after age 60. Rosin and Glatt (1971) had similar findings and showed that the early-onset group had personality characteristics similar to younger alcoholics, whereas the late-onset group developed drinking problems in reaction to bereavement, depression, retirement, loneliness, and physical illness. They suggested that late-onset alcoholism was related to the stresses of aging.

In my work with elderly alcoholics (Zimberg, 1974), I found this typology to exist in the elderly patients I encountered in mental health clinics, home care programs, nursing homes, senior citizen centers, and inpatient medical services in general hospitals. It was also noted that the early-onset group experienced serious stresses of aging, and that reaction to these stresses perpetuated drinking problems as the group aged (Schonfeld & Dupree, 1991).

There have been suggestions that people tend to drink less as they get older, that alcoholism is a self-limiting disease, and that as people age, the alcohol problems "burns out" (Drew, 1968). Those experiencing serious stresses of aging may continue problematic drinking as a maladaptation to the stresses of aging. With further study of the elderly alcoholic population, I noted a subgroup of early-onset alcoholics who had had alcoholism treatment when they were younger and had experienced remissions, but relapsed as they got older. This group, also described by Carruth, Williams, Mysak, and Boudreau (1975), can be considered an early-onset group with late-onset relapse.

Diagnosis

Part of the resistance to developing programs for elderly alcoholics has been the difficulties in making a diagnosis. There is often confusion regarding patients with dementia, drug–drug interactions, greater denial by patients and family, and less acute medical problems associated with alcoholism. Graham (1986) noted that there are fewer social, legal, occupational, and interpersonal consequences of alcoholism, because the elderly persons are often not working, live alone, and consume lesser quantities of alcohol, so that there is less alcohol dependence and withdrawal.

In recent years, there have been advances in the diagnosis of alcohol problems in the elderly population. A geriatric version of the Michigan Alcoholism Screening Test was developed (Blow et al., 1992). This 24-question screening instrument is reported to have good sensitivity and specificity. It can be useful as a screening instrument in large populations, but it is cumbersome to use in a clinical interview.

A useful and more practical tool, the CAGE Questionnaire (Ewing, 1984), has been found useful in diagnosing alcohol problems in general alcoholic populations and also in the aged (Reid & Anderson, 1997; Rigler, 2000). A "yes" answer to any one of the four questions indicates a suspected alcohol problem; two "yes" responses are a strong indicator of an alcohol problem. I have used the CAGE (Zimberg, 1996) and have found it useful, with questions 1 and 3 most commonly being answered positively among elderly alcoholics.

Laboratory testing can assist in the diagnosis of alcohol problems in elderly persons and includes liver function tests and elevated values of the mean corpuscular volume (MCV) and mean corpuscular hemoglobin (MCH), which are part of the complete blood count (CBC). A newer test of the level of carbohydrate-deficient transferrin may prove useful as well (DuPont, 1999). Although, these laboratory tests are by no means diagnostic in younger alcoholics, a study of elderly alcoholics indicated that 70% of the 200 patients studied had abnormalities in the MCV, MCH, and liver function tests (Hunt, Finlayson, Morse, & Davis, 1988). This represented a much higher percentage of these abnormal blood studies in elderly alcoholics than in younger alcoholics.

I (Zimberg, 1996) conducted a pilot study of identified elderly alcoholics on a medical service in a New York City hospital. Of the 15 patients interviewed, all answered "yes" to questions 1 and 3 of the CAGE. In addition, all had abnormal MCV or MCH and/or abnormal liver function tests. Thus, these patients could be readily identified in a medical setting.

The other area of concern regarding diagnosis of elderly alcoholics is the lack of diagnostic signs so common in younger alcoholics, as I indicated earlier. I developed a list of key questions that can be asked of patients and their families (Zimberg, 1995). These questions are listed in Table 18.1. As can be seen, the questions relate to behavioral, cognitive, social, and activities of daily living that can be seriously affected by excessive alcohol consumption in a elderly individual. The use of benzodiazepines is also commonly seen in such patients. An accident or a fall can be the precipitating event that brings the alcohol problem to the attention of family members and, if serious enough, result in hospitalization (Surock & Shimkin, 1988).

Therefore, the ability to diagnose an alcohol problem in an older person is possible and relatively easy to accomplish. The use of the CAGE, laboratory testing, and the use of the key questions with the patient and with family can facilitate this diagnostic process. Since the evidence of a relatively high prevalence of alcohol problems in the elderly has been established, it is necessary to increase the index of suspicion among health care professionals, utilizing the diagnostic tools indicated to make the diagnosis and engage the patient in treatment or referral for treatment.

The other diagnostic concern with the elderly alcoholics in looking for

---

TABLE 18.1. Approach to Interview and Assessment

1. Has there been any recent marked change in behavior or personality?
2. Are there recurring episodes of memory loss and confusion?
3. Has the person tended to become more socially isolated and stay at home most of the time?
4. Has the person become more argumentative and resistant to offers of help?
5. Has the person tended to neglect personal hygiene, not been eating regularly, and not keep appointments, especially doctor's appointments?
6. Has the individual been neglecting his or her medical treatment regimen?
7. Has the individual been neglecting to manage his or her income effectively?
8. Has the individual been in trouble with the law?
9. Has the individual caused problems with neighbors?
10. Has the individual been subject to excessive falls or accidents?
11. Does the individual frequently use benzodiazepines (Valium, Librium, Xanax, etc.)?
12. Has drinking been associated with any of the above situations?

coexisting psychiatric disorders, particularly depression, cognitive impairment, and prescription drug misuse. I have found that at least 50% of the elderly alcoholics I have treated are clinically depressed and in need of antidepressant treatment (Zimberg, 1996).

TREATMENT

Engaging in Treatment

Once the diagnosis of an alcohol problem has been made and problems associated with the stresses of aging and any coexisting psychiatric problems determined, the patient should be told about these problems, including an alcohol problem. The other problems should be indicated along with the alcohol problem as requiring treatment. This contrasts the confrontation necessary with a younger alcoholic, where often the alcohol problem is the major concern that must be dealt with first.

Elderly individuals have greater denial of an alcohol problem, and dealing with the alcohol problem in the context of stresses of aging is more readily accepted and often engenders a willingness to accept treatment. Labeling an elderly patient an "alcoholic" will often result in the patient refusing to engage in treatment.

Detoxification

Most elderly people with alcohol problems do not consume large amounts of alcohol that will result in withdrawal if the drinking stops. However, some patients may require detoxification. The patient should have a medical evaluation, or his or her primary care physician should be contacted. If the patient is not suffering from serious medical problems, outpatient detoxification is often possible (Evans, Street, & Lynch, 1996). Benzodiazepines are the drugs of choice (Kraemer, Conigliaro, & Saitz, 1999; Saitz & O'Malley, 1997).

I prescribe diazepam, 10–15 mg daily, with a reduction of half a tablet every other day, while monitoring blood pressure and pulse. The patient should be seen at least three or four times during this period of ambulatory detoxification. A long-acting benzodiazepine is preferred because of its built-in tapering effect after the last dose.

If the patient has serious medical problems, the detoxification should be done in a hospital. Patients dependent on benzodiazepines, or a combination of alcohol and benzodiazepines, should be detoxified in a hospital setting. Most elderly people find it more acceptable to be detoxified on a general medical service rather than a specialized inpatient detoxification unit, and will often refuse to be admitted to such a unit.

Alcohol-Specific Approach to Treatment

The treatment approach commonly used to treat alcohol-dependent individuals involves confronting them with the diagnosis and suggesting treatment leading to abstinence. Detoxification is used, if indicated, and the treatment contract is established with the patient. This treatment is directed at the alcohol problem, with cognitive therapy that involves relapse prevention and supportive therapy to establish a positive relationship with the patient. Referral to Alcoholics Anonymous (AA) is often made to encourage peer support and role models of recovery (Zimberg, 1999b).

Pharmacological treatment, such as disulfiram, can be used with very resistant patients, particularly if taking the disulfiram is observed (Kranzler, 2000). The use of naltrexone to reduce craving for alcohol has been found useful (Weinrieb & O'Brien, 1997). Clearly, the emphasis of this alcohol-specific approach is centered on the use of alcohol and developing more effective ways to function without alcohol.

With elderly people, such an approach has not been successful in my experience, except for the subgroup of elderly alcoholics treated for their alcohol problem in an alcohol-specific way during their younger years. The reason for this lack of success, and therefore for the very few elderly patients in treatment at traditional alcohol programs, is that the stresses of aging are the major factors leading to alcohol problems in older people. The inability to adapt the alcohol-specific approach to the needs of the elderly has perpetuated the gap between the awareness of the problem and the availability of effective treatment (Graham, 1986; Schonfeld & Dupree, 1991).

Aging-Specific Approach to Treatment

The aging-specific approach involves identifying an alcohol problem among other problems associated with aging: loneliness, retirement, deteriorating health, loss of loved ones, cognitive impairments, and depression. Depression is also a condition in the elderly that is often underdiagnosed (Zimberg, 1996).

Some early clinical literature on treating elderly alcoholics emphasized the stresses of aging, pointing the way toward a more effective treatment approach. An article by Droller (1964) reported on seven elderly alcoholic patients. This family physician visited elderly alcoholics at home. He found that in addition to medical and supportive treatment, primarily social treatment was most beneficial and reduced or eliminated the alcohol problem.

Rosin and Glatt (1971), who treated 103 elderly alcoholics, found that environmental manipulation, medical services, day hospital treatment, and home visiting by staff or good neighbors were the most beneficial services. Here again, the therapeutic efforts that were directed at the stresses of aging proved the most effective.

In more recent years, Kofoed, Tolson, Atkinson, Toth, and Turner (1987) found that aging-specific treatment was more effective than mainstreaming patients in standard alcoholism treatment in an outpatient setting. Another study that compared an elder-specific approach to traditional alcoholism treatment in an inpatient unit found that the elder-specific approach produced 2.1 times more abstinence and was slightly less costly (Kashner, Rudell, Ogden, Guggenheim, & Karson, 1992). Other studies have found that aging-specific approaches are more effective than treating elderly alcoholic in mixed-age groups (Liberto, Oslin, & Ruskin, 1992; Rigler, 2000; Schonfeld & Dupree, 1999). Taken together with my experience treating elderly alcoholics in different settings, this suggests that an aging-specific approach that deals with both the stresses of aging and the alcohol can be more effective than the traditional alcohol-specific approach in engaging patients in treatment and producing better outcomes.

Patients should have a complete physical examination, including laboratory tests and a psychiatric evaluation. If detoxification is needed, the approach described earlier for outpatient or inpatient should be utilized.

The ideal approach is to use group therapy when possible. However, this group approach should not be insight-oriented or deal with alcohol use as the major problem. It can be a mixed group of elderly persons with a variety of social and psychological problems, and organic mental disorders and physical disorders, not just alcoholism. Patients with alcoholism should be told they have an alcohol problem, along with the other problems that they may be experiencing, and that their problems relate to difficulties in adjusting to their current situation.

The group should meet at least once a week for 90 minutes. Some socialization time and having cookies, coffee, and tea should be available prior to the formal group session. The approach utilized by the group leader should be supportive and directed at problem solving, utilizing various group member's experiences with similar problems in their lives. Drinking should be one of the problem areas discussed. Members of the group should be encouraged to discuss their own problems and give advise to other group members. This self-help and help others approach leads to members' elevated self-esteem and helps them overcome feeling of helplessness and despair. The reality is that most elderly persons have achieved experiences and wisdom during their lives that should be recognized, and they should be encouraged to utilize these assets. Our society, with rapid technological advances and quick obsolescence, often relegates elderly people to the sidelines of life. Encouraging utilization of their life experiences can be a very therapeutic and counter the many of stresses of aging exhibited by the patients.

In addition to the socialization period, formal group sessions, outings, and trips can be planned. Patients should be actively involved in deciding where to go and participate in the planning of trips. The more independence the patients can show, the greater the therapeutic value.

Staffing of the group program should include a group leader who is knowledgeable about alcoholism and geriatrics, ideally a psychiatrist, a nurse, or social worker, or an alcoholism counselor helping patients with practical problems, such as economic and housing needs, and relationships to friends, relatives, and neighbors. Helping a patient make doctor appointments and attend to other needs should be continued until the patient is able to accomplish theses activities on his or her own (Zimberg, 1995).

The most important goal of the aging-specific approach to treatment of alcoholism is not necessarily producing abstinence. This fact creates resistance among the clinicians used to the alcohol-specific approach, where abstinence is the goal of treatment. The aging-specific approach is not designed as a harm reduction technique either. The paradox of the aging-specific approach directed mainly at the psychosocial stresses of aging is that it often results in abstinence achieved early in treatment and is more easily maintained, with few, if any, relapses to drinking. Abstinence is encouraged and occurs in the context of reduction of the maladaptations to aging, the treatment of coexisting depression, and improved self-esteem, with more opportunities to feel worthwhile.

Current experiences support the findings of the early clinicians working with elderly alcoholics in the 1960s and 1970s that psychosocial treatments are better for alcohol problems that are caused or exacerbated by the psychosocial stresses of aging. This observation can be applied equally well to both early-onset and late-onset elderly alcoholics. Both groups respond to the aging-specific approach (Zimberg, 1974).

Pharmacological Treatment

Pharmacological treatment of alcohol withdrawal in elderly persons involves use of tapering doses of long-acting benzodiazepines, as indicated earlier. I have found that the use of benzodiazepines can be safe and effective. Ambulatory detoxification can be carried out in those elderly alcoholics who do not have serious cardiovascular disease, or other serious medical or neurological problems. A physical examination is necessary prior to starting an outpatient detoxification. Patients should not be maintained on benzodiazepines because of the drug's dependence liability, adverse cognitive effects, and the availability of other, safer drugs to treat anxiety.

Depression is a common problem among elderly alcoholics. The use of selective serotonin reuptake inhibitor drugs, such as sertraline, or tricyclics, such as nortriptyline, has been found effective in treating depression in the elderly (Kennedy, 2000). The elderly alcoholic patient should not be actively drinking and should be alcohol-free for 2–3 weeks to determine whether the observed depression is alcohol induced. If alcohol is not a cause, starting on antidepressant medication can be very effective in helping patients maintain abstinence, motivating them to increase their activities and get involved in stimulating and worthwhile efforts that will enhance their self-esteem. Both the depression and the alcohol use are thus effectively treated.

In some cases of elderly alcoholics who appear severely depressed, it may be possible to establish a differential diagnosis in a shorter period of time than the 2–3 weeks indicated. A dual-diagnosis typology has been developed, with a questionnaire that can determine whether the depression is alcohol-induced or independent of alcohol use (Zimberg, 1999a).

The questions involve determining the presence of depression during periods of sobriety, whether depression occurs after the onset of drinking, but not at other times, and whether there is a previous history of depression. This information can lead to a determination of coexisting depression and the start of antidepressant medication sooner. The patient should be alcohol-free at the time the antidepressant medication is started.

Disulfiram has been available for the treatment of alcoholics for 50 years. Its value in controlled studies has been found to be equivocal. However, studies using disulfiram with observed administration or under the supervision of employee assistance programs, or with patients on probation or on parole, has been found useful (Brewer, Meyers, & Johnsen, 2000). The conventional wisdom regarding the use of disulfiram in elderly alcoholics has been that the drug is too dangerous to use. However, in my experience, in elderly alcoholics who have proved resistant to other treatment efforts and are not suffering from significant cardiovascular or liver disease, and who do not have serious cognitive impairment, the smaller dose of disulfinam (125 mg/day) given under supervision has been safe and effective.

The long-acting opiate antagonist naltrexone has been found to be effective in reducing craving and alcohol use in the alcohol-dependent patient (Weinrieb & O'Brien, 1997). A study of naltrexone in elderly alcoholics has shown a similar beneficial effect (Oslin, Liberto, O'Brien, Krois, & Norbeck, 1997). I have used this drug at a dose of 50 mg/day and have given patients a card to warn about the use of opiates for pain. In patients who have intense craving and have not responded to the psychosocial treatment of the stresses of aging, naltrexone can be safely used.

Another drug that decreases craving, acamprosate, functions as a modulator of glutamate in the central nervous system (Zornoza, Cano, Polache, & Granero, 2003). It has been used extensively in Europe and received Food and Drug Administration (FDA) approval for this indication in mid-2004. No studies on the elderly have been done. If effective, this may be an additional pharmacological treatment (Whitworth et al., 1996).

It should be noted that most elderly alcoholics respond to the aging-specific approach, often with the use of antidepressants. For the minority of patients who are treatment-resistant, usually the early-onset type, the pharmacological options discussed should be considered.

Location of Treatment

The group approach I have described has been generally very effective. This can be provided wherever elderly alcoholics are found in psychiatric clinics, inpatient alcoholism programs, geriatric clinics, and senior citizen centers or nursing homes. The approach can also be provided individually in primary care physicians' or psychiatrists' offices. I provide the aging-specific approach individually in my office, with generally high recovery rates.

The essence of the aging-specific approach includes determining whether there is an alcohol problem, what stresses of aging are affecting the patient, the presence of coexisting depression or other psychiatric conditions, and relationship to families and friends. Many elderly patients look forward to the visit to the doctor's office, and this interest can be utilized to engage patients in treating not only the alcohol problem but also other problems that they may be experiencing.

ELDERLY ALCOHOLICS IN GENERAL HOSPITALS

Elderly alcoholics can be found in significant numbers in general hospitals (Adams et al., 1993 Gerke, Hapke, Rumpf, & John, 1997; Moore et al., 1989). They are usually more frequently found on medical–surgical services rather than in inpatient detoxification or psychiatric units.

The presence of elderly alcoholics in relatively large numbers presents a particular challenge to consultation–liaison psychiatrists and addiction psychiatrists working in general hospitals. Diagnostic approaches indicated for elderly alcoholics can be readily applied in a general hospital setting. A study that compared readiness to deal with alcohol problems in alcohol-dependent patients in the general hospital and such patients in the general population found that the general hospital patients seemed more willing to engage in treatment (Rumpf, Hapke, Meyer, & John, 1999). However, my experience with identifying and referring elderly alcoholics for treatment after discharge, by using alcohol nurse coordinators, resulted in very few successful referrals. This failure resulted in part because of the lack of an aging-specific program at this hospital's alcoholism clinic and the fact that the patients were referred to a clinician at the alcoholism clinic who was anonymous as far as the patients were concerned. They also resisted going to an alcoholism clinic. In contrast, in my experience, patients seen at the general hospital by me and referred to myself for outpatient care accepted the referral and followed up treatment.

To be able to engage elderly alcoholics in the general hospital, treatment programs must be available to meet their needs. First, there should be a high index of suspicion of alcohol problems among elderly persons admitted to general hospitals. Administering the CAGE and reviewing blood studies should be part of an alcohol screening effort. Information from relatives, friends neighbors, and home attendants, if possible, should be obtained. A staff member involved in an aging-specific treatment program should see the patient in the hospital and have the patient referred to him- or herself at the treatment site.

A particularly egregious situation exists for alcoholic patients in some general hospitals, particularly patients admitted to the surgical services. Undiagnosed alcoholic elderly patients admitted with an acute surgical emergency, such as a hip fracture, are operated on promptly, and on the first postoperative day may develop acute alcohol withdrawal that produces serious morbidity and, in some cases, death. I have observed such instances frequently. There are no data to determine how frequent such a complication occurs, but it is a preventable one!

Part of every evaluation for emergency surgical and medical admissions of the elderly should be screening for alcoholism, as indicated, not simply asking whether the patient drinks alcohol. If there is a suspicion of an alcohol problem use of a benzodiazepine taper on admission or postoperatively should be instituted.

The problem of using benzodiazepines in surgical patients is complicated by a lingering belief among some physicians that ethanol, including intravenous ethanol, should be used to treat or prevent alcohol withdrawal. A recent study documents this inappropriate use of ethanol, which can be particularly dangerous in elderly alcoholics (Rosenbaum & McCanty, 2002).

The low index of suspicion of alcohol problems in the elderly and the use of ethanol for detoxification represent a problem in diagnosis and treatment, with potentially serious consequences. The need to educate the medical community about the diagnosis and treatment of elderly alcoholics is important, since diagnostic clues exist and effective treatment is possible.

CONCLUSION

Alcoholism and prescription drug abuse in the elderly are common problems. They often are not diagnosed or treated. This chapter presents tools that can be helpful in the diagnosis of alcoholism in the elderly and suggests psychosocial treatment based on an aging-specific approach as being most effective. Pharmacological treatments, including benzodiazepines for detoxification, antidepressants for coexisting depression, disulfiram as a deterrent, and the anticraving drugs naltrexone and acamprosate, were presented.

The general hospital can be a place to identify, to provide detoxification, and to engage elderly patients in a friendly way. The morbidity and mortality of alcohol withdrawal syndrome in patients admitted for medical and surgical emergencies can be prevented if the alcohol screening is done early and benzodiazepine detoxification is carried out soon after admission in patients likey to go into withdrawal.

REFERENCES

Adams, W. L., Barry, K. L., & Fleming, M. F. (1996). Screening for problem drinking in older primary care patients. *JAMA, 276,* 1964–1967.

Adams, W. L., Magruder-Habid, K., Trued, S., & Broome, H. L. (1992). Alcohol abuse in elderly emergency department patients. *J Am Geriatr Soc, 40,* 1236–1240.

Adams, W. L., Zhung, Y., Barhoriak, J. J., & Rimm, A. A. (1993). Alcohol related hospitalizations of elderly people. *JAMA, 270,* 1222–1225.

Atkinson, R. M., Ganzini, L., & Bernstein, M. J. (1992). Alcohol and substance use disorders in the elderly. In J. Birren, R. Sloane, & G. Cohen (Eds.), *Handbook of mental health and aging* (pp. 515–555). San Diego, CA: Academic Press.

Bailey, M. B., Haberman, P. W., & Alksne, H. (1965). The epidemiology of alcoholism in urban residential area. *Q J Stud Alcohol, 26,* 19–40.

Barrick, C., & Conners, G. J. (2002). Relapse prevention and maintaining abstinence in older adults with alcohol use disorders. *Drugs Aging, 19,* 584–593.

Blow, F. C., Brower, K. J., Schulenberg, J. E., Demo-Daranger, L. M., Young, M. S., & Beresford, T. P. (1992). The Michigan Alcoholism Screening Test: A new elderly specific screening instrument. *Alcohol Clin Exp Res, 16,* 372–377.

Brewer, C., Meyers, R., & Johnsen, J. (2000). Does disulfiram help to prevent relapse in alcohol abuse? *CNS Drugs, 14,* 329–341.

Bridgewater, R., Leigh, S., James, O. F. W., & Potter, J. F. (1987). Alcohol consumption and dependence in elderly patients in an urban community. *Br Med J, 295,* 884–885.

Cahalan D., Cisin, J. H., & Crossley, H. M. (1969). *American drinking practices.* New Brunswick, NJ: Rutgers Center of Alcoholic Studies.

Carruth, B., Williams, E. P., Mysak, S., & Boudreaux, L. (1975, July). Community care providers and the older problem drinker. *Grassroots,* pp. 1–5.

Drew, L. R. H. (1968). Alcohol as a self limiting disease. *Q J Stud Alcohol, 29,* 956–967.

Droller, H. (1964). Some aspects of alcoholism in the elderly. *Lancet, 2,* 137–139.

DuPont, R. L. (1999). Diagnostic testing: Laboratory and psychologial. In M. Galanter & H. D. Kleber (Eds.), *Textbook of substance abuse treatment* (2nd ed., pp. 521–528). Washington, DC: American Psychiatric Press.

Evans, D. J., Street, S. D., & Lynch, D. J. (1996). Alcohol withdrawal at home: Pilot project for frail elderly people. *Can Fam Physician, 42,* 937–945.

Ewing, J. H. A. (1984). Detecting alcoholism: The CAGE Questionnaire. *JAMA, 252,* 1905–1907.

Gaitz, C. M., & Baer, P. E. (1971). Characteristics of elderly patients with alcoholism. *Arch Gen Psychiatry, 24,* 327–378.

Gerke, P., Hapke, U., Rumpf, H.-J., & John, U. (1997). Alcohol related diseases in general hospital patients. *Alcohol Alcohol, 32,* 179–184.

Graham, K. (1986). Identifying and measuring alcohol abuse among the elderly: Serious problems with exisiting instrumentation. *J Stud Alcohol, 47,* 322–326.

Hunt, R. D., Finlayson, R. E., Morse, R. M., & Davis, L. J. (1988). Alcoholism in elderly persons: Medical aspects and prognosis in 216 patients. *Mayo Clin Proc, 63,* 753–760.

Kashner, T. M., Rudell, D. E., Ogden, S. R., Guggenheim, F. G., & Karson, C. N.

(1992). Outcomes and costs of two VA inpatient treatment programs for older alcoholic patients. *Hosp Community Psychiatry, 43*, 985–989.

Kennedy, G. J. (2000). *Geriatric mental health care.* New York: Guilford Press.

Kofoed, L. L., Tolson, R. L., Atkinson, R. M., Toth, R. F., & Turner, J. A. (1987). Treatment compliance of older alcoholics: An elder specific approach is superior to "mainstreaming." *J Stud Alcohol, 48*, 47–51.

Kraemer, K. L., Congliaro, J., & Saitz, R. (1999). Managing alcohol withdrawal in the elderly. *Drugs Aging, 14*, 409–425.

Kranzler, H. (2000). Pharmacotherapy of alcoholism: Gaps in knowledge and opportunities for reasearch. *Alcohol Alcohol, 35*, 537–547.

Liberto, J. G., Oslin, D. W., & Ruskin, P. E. (1992). Alcoholism in older persons: a review of the literature. *Hosp Community Psychiatry, 43*, 975–984.

McCusker, J., Cherubin, C. F., & Zimberg, S. (1971). Prevalence of alcoholism in general municipal hospital population. *NY State J Med, 71*, 751–754.

Menninger, J. A. (2002). Assesment and treatment of alcoholism and substance related disorders in the elderly. *Bull Menninger Clin, 66*, 166–183.

Moore, R. A. (1972). The diagnosis of alcoholism in a psychiatric hospital: A trial of the Michigan Alcoholism Sceening Test (MAST). *Am J Psychiatry, 128*, 1565–1569.

Moore, R. D., Bune, L. R., Geller, G., Mamon, J. A., Stokes, J., & Levine, D. M. (1989). Prevalence, detection and treatment of alcoholism in hospitalized patients. *JAMA, 261*, 403–407.

Oslin, D., Liberto, J., O'Brien, J., Krois, S., & Norbeck, J. (1997). Natrexone as an adjunctive treatment for older patients with alcohol dependence. *Am J Geriatr Psychiatry, 5*, 324–232.

Reid, M. C., & Anderson, P. A. (1997). Geriatric substance use disorders. *Med Clin North Am, 81*, 999–1016.

Rigler, S. K. (2000). Alcoholism in the elderly. *Am Fam Physician, 61*, 1710–1716.

Rosenbaum, M., & McCanty, T. (2002). Alcohol prescription by surgeons in the prevention and treatment of delirium tremors: Historic and current practice. *Gen Hosp Psychiatry, 24*, 257–259.

Rosin, A. J., & Glatt, M. M. (1971). Alcohol excess in the elderly. *Q J Stud Alcohol, 32*, 53–59.

Rumpf, H.-J., Hapke, U., Meyer, C., & John, U. (1999). Motivation to change drinking behavior: Comparison of alcohol-dependent individuals in a general hospital and a general population sample. *Gen Hosp Psychiatry, 21*, 348–353.

Saitz, R., & O'Malley, S. S. (1997). Pharmacotherapies for alcohol abuse: Withdrawal and treatment. *Med Clin North Am, 81*, 881–907.

Schonfeld, L., & Dupree, L. W. (1991). Antecedants of drinking for early and late onset elderly alcohol abusers. *J Stud Alcohol, 52*, 587–592.

Schonfeld, L., & Dupree, L. W. (1999). Alcohol use and misuse in older adults. *Rev Clin Gerontol, 9*, 151–162.

Schuckit, M. (1979). Geriatric alcoholism and drug abuse. *Gerontologist, 17*, 168–174.

Siassi, I., Crocetti, G., & Spiro, H. R. (1973). Drinking paterns and alcoholism in a blue collar population. *Q J Stud Alcohol, 34*, 197–226.

Simon, A., Epstein, L. J., & Reynolds, L. (1968). Alcoholism in the geriatric mentally ill. *Geriatrics, 23*, 125–131.

Surock, G. S., & Shimkin, E. E. (1988). Benzodiazepine sedatives and the risk of falling in a community cohort. *Arch Intern Med, 148,* 2441–2445.

Weinrieb, R. M., & O'Brien, C. P. (1997). Naltrexone in the treatment of alcoholism. *Annu Rev Med, 48,* 447–487.

Whitworth, A. B., Fischer, F., Lesch, O. M., Nimmerrichter, A., Oberbauer, H., Platz, T., et. al. (1996). Comparison of acamprosate and placebo in long-term treatment of alcohol dependence. *Lancet, 347,* 1438–1442.

Zimberg, S. (1969). Outpatient geriatric psychiatry in an urban ghetto with nonprofessional workers. *Am J Psychiatry, 125,* 1697–1702.

Zimberg, S. (1974). The two types of problem drinkers: Both can be managed. *Geriatrics, 29,* 135–138.

Zimberg, S. (1995). The elderly. In A. M. Washton (Ed.), *Psychotherapy and substance abuse: A practitioner's handbook* (pp. 413–427). New York: Guilford Press.

Zimberg, S. (1996). Treating alcoholism: An age-specific intervention that works for older patients. *Geriatrics, 51,* 45–49.

Zimberg, S. (1999a). A dual diagnosis typology to improve diagnosis and treatment of dual disorder patients. *J Psychoactive Drugs, 31,* 47–51.

Zimberg, S. (1999b). Individual psychotherapy: Alcohol. In M. Galanter & H. D. Kleber (Eds.), *Textbook of substance abuse treatment* (2nd ed., pp. 335–342). Washington, DC: American Psychiatric Press.

Zornoza, T., Cano, M. J., Polache, A., & Granero, L. (2003). Pharmacology of acamprosate: An overview. *CNS Drug Rev, 9,* 359–374.

CHAPTER 19

HIV/AIDS and Substance Use Disorders

CHERYL ANN KENNEDY
JAMES M. HILL
STEVEN J. SCHLEIFER

Since its appearance in 1981, the human immunodeficiency virus/acquired immune deficiency syndrome (HIV/AIDS) pandemic has been the focus of global attention and remains a serious public health threat throughout the world. By the end of 2004, over 40 million people worldwide, including 2.5 million children under age 15, were living with HIV/AIDS, mostly in Africa and Asia (UNAIDS, 2004). Showing a decrease from prior years, 22% of the 43,171 new cases of HIV/AIDS reported in the United States in 2003 had injection drug use (IDU) as the major risk factor for transmission. The majority of those with HIV/AIDS in the United States are minorities: African Americans and Latinos (Centers for Disease Control and Prevention, 2003). Among non-injecting drug users (NIDUs) there are clear links between substance abuse and high-risk behaviors in both men and women, especially those who use crack cocaine (Astemborski, Vhalov, Warren, Solomon, & Nelson, 1994; De Souza, Diaz, Sutmoller, & Bastos, 2002; Edlin et al., 1994). Use of mind-altering substances, such as alcohol, other sedatives, stimulants, and club drugs, plays an increasing, albeit less direct, role in HIV risk and disease progression. Impaired states induced by alcohol and other drugs can influence sexual behavior and lead to risky, unsafe sexual practices that increase risk of HIV exposure (Kennedy et al., 1993; National Institute of Drug Abuse, 2002). HIV infection among IDUs has been reported in nearly 180 countries worldwide and presents the risk of spreading to 40 more. Once the virus has been introduced into a local community of IDUs, spread is ordinarily rapid. Drug-using populations are fueling the epidemic around the world. There is increasing evidence that these individuals are at higher risk for accelerated and more severe neurocognitive dysfunction compared to non-drug-using HIV-infected populations (Nath et al., 2002).

NEUROPSYCHIATRIC COMPLICATIONS OF AIDS

Early in the HIV epidemic, the extent to which neuropsychiatric complications occurred in patients was not appreciated. It is now widely understood that cognitive, affective, and behavioral symptoms may often be manifestations of HIV infection in the central nervous system (CNS). These symptoms are the initial manifestation of AIDS in 7–20% of patients, with the frequency increasing as the disease progresses (Reger, Welsh, Razani, Martin, & Boone, 2002). Neurological involvement may range from subtle changes to severe global impairment. HIV-associated dementia (also referred to as HIV-associated motor complex, HIV encephalopathy, or AIDS–dementia complex) has been described as progressive and is the most common of the neurological manifestations of HIV infection (Bouwman et al., 1998). It is currently estimated that up to one-third of the adults and more than one-half of the children with HIV will eventually develop a dementing disease, and that HIV is the leading cause of dementia in people less than 60 years of age (Janssen, Nwanyanwu, Selik, & Stehr-Green, 1992; Koutsilieri, Scheller, Sopper, ter Meulen, & Riederer, 2002). When working with substance users with HIV, clinical expertise is essential for accurate diagnosis and optimal management of the neurological and neuropsychiatric complications. The symptom overlap between the neurological effects of drug use and HIV-associated illnesses presents an important clinical challenge.

Early detection of HIV-associated dementia is based on careful tracking of mental status and cognitive changes. A recent meta-analysis of 41 neuropsychological studies of HIV disease revealed that motor functioning, executive skills, and information-processing speed were the functions showing the greatest decline as disease progressed (Reger et al., 2002). Differentiating these CNS effects of HIV from those related to drug and alcohol is difficult, in that there is neurological deficit overlap. Abnormal findings on measures of dexterity, sensory processing, attention, concentration, language, verbal and nonverbal memory, abstraction, and problem solving have been demonstrated with chronic alcohol, cocaine, opiate, and polysubstance abuse (Ling, Compton, Rawson, & Wesson, 1996). In addition to the actual drug used and chronicity of use, age at use (Klisz & Parsons, 1977), history of impairment preceding use, gender (Fabian, Parsons, & Sheldon, 1985; Glenn & Parsons, 1992), and educational level (Grant & Reed, 1985) may further mediate neuropsychological findings. These factors have led to some controversy as to the increased risk of developing dementia in HIV patients with comorbid substance abuse disorders (SUDs). Some investigators (Bouwman et al., 1998) have reported that substance users with HIV are at a higher risk for dementia than are individuals with other risk behaviors, but this finding has been not found by others (Qureshi, Hanson, Jones, & Janssen, 1998; DeRonchi et al., 2002). Although the results of these studies vary, it is generally accepted that neuropsychological impairments associated with substance use can vary from mild to severe, and may be stabilized or reversed by abstinence (Selby & Azrin, 1998). In the AIDS patient, the impairment is progressive and, by the terminal phase of the disease, severe. It is critical that physicians treating substance users who develop AIDS be alert, because these patients may suffer from both drug- and infection-related cognitive impairment. It is also important for physicians to consider the diagnosis of HIV in all substance users with cognitive impairment. They must be aware that timing of the effects of HIV on cognition is variable and not fully understood.

The clinical significance of the seroconversion and asymptomatic phases are debatable, but the physician caring for people in high-risk groups should know of possible CNS effects to increase the likelihood of early detection. Headaches and photophobia may be frequent in the seroconversion-related mononucleosis-like syndrome associated with HIV (Tindall & Cooper, 1991). Although this early syndrome is apparently common, it is frequently indistinguishable from other viral infections and may not be recognized. The virus can be detected in cerebrospinal fluid shortly after infection and it has been asserted that cognitive changes could begin during the asymptomatic phase of infection that usually lasts a decade or more (Bornstein et al., 1991; Lunn et al., 1991). There has been controversy over the possibility that cognitive decline can occur before the onset of other medical symptoms. After controlling for substance abuse, psychiatric history, use of psychoactive medications, and neurological problems, HIV-positive asymptomatic patients show little difference in cognitive functioning when compared with controls (Damos, John, Parker, & Levine, 1997). It is now generally accepted that caution should be exercised in assigning cognitive deficits to asymptomatic HIV-positive patients, but given the erratic health care utilization of substance users, which is a potential barrier to early HIV detection and intervention, professionals working with this group should have a low threshold for considering neurological and cognitive symptoms as possible complications of undiagnosed HIV.

Early detection and monitoring of cognitive changes are critical, because these symptoms may be reversed and possibly prevented with antiretroviral therapy (ART; Moore, Keruly, Gallant, & Chaisson, 1998; Price et al., 1999; Sacktor & McArthur, 1997). The impact of ART has added support to the hypothesis that, in most cases, HIV-associated dementia is the result of the effect of the virus on the CNS rather than that of a secondary opportunistic infection or process. Many believe that this effect is achieved by indirect mechanisms, since productive infection within the CNS is confined predominantly to macrophages and microglia (Kolson, Lavi, Gonzalez, & Scarano, 1998;

Lipton & Gendelman, 1995; Price, 1995). After infection with HIV, CNS macrophages and microglia may be activated and induced to produce various proinflammatory cytokines that may contribute to neuronal dysfunction or death (Glass, Fedor, Wesselingh, & McArthur, 1995; Portegies, 1995). Regardless of the intermediary steps involved in the link of the HIV to CNS functioning, if brain infection is involved in the pathogenesis of HIV-associated dementia, ART may be critical to prevention and treatment.

Recently there has been increased focus on mechanisms underlying neurodegeneration in patients with combined HIV and substance use. Although studies assessing neuropsychological functioning in HIV-infected asymptomatic substance users have failed to offer consistent evidence of cognitive deficits, neuropathological studies comparing HIV-infected substance users to nonusers have shown a marked severity of HIV encephalitis in substance users (Bell, Brettle, & Chiswick, 1998), with significant loss of dopaminergic neurons in the substantia nigra (Reyes, Faraldi, Senseng, Flowers, & Fariello, 1991). Since most drugs of abuse have dopaminergic activation properties, recent work in this area has focused on the possibility that drugs of abuse may destabilize the dopaminergic system and result in a synergistic neurotoxicity when combined with HIV (Nath et al., 2002). This work adds further support for the importance of achieving abstinence or limiting drug intake in HIV-infected patients.

Although most HIV-associated dementia is from the effect of the virus on the CNS, it has long been recognized that such cognitive changes can also result from other mechanisms, including opportunistic infections (Price, Sidits, & Brew, 1991), HIV-related CNS neoplasms (DeAngelis, 1991; Remick et al., 1990; Shapshak et al., 1991), CNS effects of systemic illness (Holtzman, Kaku, & So, 1989), and CNS effects of antivirals and other medications used to treat related infections. Mass lesions and infectious processes in the CNS, including *Cryptococcus neoformans*, toxoplasmosis, cytomegalovirus, and lymphoma, are thought to account for approximately 30% of the CNS complications of AIDS (Navia, Jordon, & Price, 1986). Neuroimaging procedures, cerebrospinal fluid exams, serological titers, toxic screens, and stereotaxic biopsy techniques are helpful in evaluating AIDS patients with CNS dysfunction and are useful in establishing whether such potentially reversible conditions are involved with any cognitive decline. Accurate diagnosis of such underlying conditions is the first step in managing AIDS patients with CNS dysfunction.

If HIV-associated dementia is established, antiretroviral drugs should be considered, because they have reportedly lessened some cognitive losses. Psychotropics should be considered for specific symptom management. Given the sensitivity to psychotropic side effects in patients with CNS compromise, such treatments should be started with low doses and carefully monitored. Finally, supportive and insight-oriented psychotherapy with neuropsychoeducation may assist the patient and significant others with coping and adaptation.

SUBSTANCE USE AND RISK OF HIV INFECTION

A variety of exposure and host factors influence seroconversion and disease progression. These may include altered baseline host immune capacity and viral load in the seropositive person. The presence of host-concurrent infections, most notably viral (*Herpes simplex*, cytomegalovirus, the hepatitides) and bacterial infections in the bloodstream (endocarditis, others), may contribute to altered immunity. In the case of skin or mucosal ulcerations or inflammation from repeated injection sites or sexually transmitted diseases, breaches can afford easy entry of microorganisms. Clearly, some practices in drug use and sexual behavior carry more risk than others for disease transmission. In general, infections have increased prevalence in substance-using populations, and since substance users often do not restrict their use to a single drug, some risk effects may be synergistic.

Heroin use by injection is a key element in the progression of the HIV epidemic. IDUs, as well as other substance abusers, have further increased risk due to social and sexual contact with other high-risk individuals. Use of other agents contributes substantially to behavioral risk through disinhibiting effects on the primary modes of transmission: sexual contact and injecting drug use (Booth, Kwiatkowski, & Chitwood, 2000; Woods et al., 1996). Stall, McKusick, Wiley, Coates, and Ostrow (1986) found that homosexual men with high-risk sexual behaviors were at least twice as likely to use drugs during sexual encounters as men considered at low risk for HIV exposure. Stimulant users, particularly, crack cocaine smokers and injecting stimulant users (cocaine, amphetamine), incur considerable risk for HIV. Cocaine injectors inject more frequently to maintain a quickly decaying "high." As with other disinhibiting drugs, users are apt to engage in risky sexual behavior fueled by these drugs' stimulant properties. Consistent with an earlier report, Seidman, Sterk-Elifson, and Aral (1994), in a national study of 27,000 current drug users, found that sexual risk behaviors for HIV transmission were significantly higher in crack cocaine smokers and crack-smoking IDUs than in nonsmoking IDUs, and that the alarmingly low rate of condom use (< 20%) was additionally associated with concurrent alcohol use (Booth et al., 2000). Female substance abusers are at particular risk for transmission through sexual risk behaviors (Booth, Koester, & Pinto, 1995), which include turning to commercial sex work as a primary means of support. The use of crack cocaine is a strong predictor of risky sexual behaviors among women (Hoffman, Klein, Eber, & Crosby, 2000). Alcohol abuse has been increasingly recognized as a major cofactor in HIV transmission risk. Higher alcohol consumption in homosexual and bisexual men has been associated with increased HIV seroconversion (Penkower et al., 1991) and NIDU ambulatory alcoholics had higher than expected HIV seroprevalence rates associated with more risky sexual behaviors (Avins et al., 1994).

Co-abuse of cocaine and alcohol has been associated with the highest risk (Wang, Collins, Kohler, DiClemente, & Wingood, 2000). The widespread use of alcohol and other drugs among adolescents presents a significant threat to adolescent health, associated with motor vehicle accidents, homicides, and suicides, as well as medical, psychological, and social morbidity (Singh, Kochaneck, & MacDorman, 1996). The use of alcohol and other drugs significantly increases adolescent risk behaviors for HIV transmission (Boyer & Ellen, 1994; Rotheram-Borus, Rosario, Reid, & Koopman, 1995). Cases of AIDS and rates of HIV infection are rapidly rising among adolescents, particularly in those from risk groups not easily accessed (Kennedy & Eckholdt, 1997; Mofenson, & Flynn, 2000).

Opioids

In addition to the exceptionally high risk of HIV transmission in opiate abusers who inject and share needles, compromised immune function as a result of exposure to opiates may add to risk of infection and disease progression. Brown, Stimmel, Taub, Kochwa, and Rosenfield (1974) and others (Govitaprong, Suttitum, Kotchabhakdi, & Uneklabh, 1998) found reduced lymphocyte stimulation in response to various mitogens in heroin addicts, suggesting a possible impairment in cell-mediated immunity. Addicts also have a significant reduction in numbers of T-cells when compared with nonaddicts (McDonough et al., 1980). A review of the literature defining the connection between AIDS and opiate use concluded that numerous aspects of the drug culture may have differential, even offsetting effects in terms of the potential to regulate either HIV-1 expression or host-regulation responses (Donahue & Vlahov, 1998).

Opioids may incur considerable risk to some users; opiate addicts who enter methadone treatment are significantly less likely to become HIV infected in the first place (Metzger et al., 1993). In experimental studies of immunity, opiates have been found to have a variety of effects that are primarily immunosuppressive (McCarthy, Wetzela, Slikera, Eisenstein, & Rogers, 2001). There is evidence that chronic exposure to morphine may reduce HIV replication, while withdrawal, mediated by the stress effects, may lead to acute immunosuppression and disease exacerbation (Donahoe & Vlahov, 1998). For those already HIV-infected, consistent participation in methadone maintenance treatment was associated with high probability and consistency of use of ART (Sambamoorthi, Warner, Crystal, & Walkup, 2000). More recent availability of oral outpatient opiate detoxification agents, buprenorphine and the buprenorphine–naloxone combination, opens up new modalities to assist physicians and patients in achieving drug-free or less harmful drug-using states (Ling et al., 1998; O'Connor et al., 1998).

Alcohol

Alcoholics, many of whom use multiple drugs, are at increased risk of exposure to HIV through high-risk behavior. Alcohol use is increasing worldwide, particularly in countries in transition and throughout the developing world, where it is contributing to an increasing number of health and social problems (Monteiro, 2001). Homosexual and bisexual men who drank high volumes of alcohol had increased HIV seroconversion rates (Penkower et al., 1991). Nearly 20 years of studies have linked alcohol with high-risk behavior of all types, including sexual behavior (Stall et al., 1986; Baldwin, Maxwell, Fenaughty, Trotter, & Stevens, 2000). In a study of alcohol treatment centers, non-IDUs had higher than expected seroprevalence for HIV that was associated with a high prevalence of risky sexual behaviors (Avins et al., 1994). In a large study of sexually transmitted disease clinic attendees, alcohol was frequently used and was associated with other risk factors for HIV infection (Zenilman et al., 1994). Studies of alcohol abusers have described a range of immune alterations (Arria, Tarter, & Van Theil, 1991; Cook, 1998). Since alcoholism and medical morbidity often coexist, it is difficult to distinguish immune alterations associated with alcoholism per se from those associated with alcohol-related morbidity, such as liver disease or other comorbid medical conditions. Acute exposure to alcohol has demonstrable immune effects, and chronic alcohol abusers, who may have adapted to ethanol effects, show immune alterations of modest scope, unless they have developed secondary liver disease or other comorbid medical conditions (Cook, 1998; Schleifer, Keller, Shiflett, Benton, & Eckholdt, 1999). The immune effects that have been observed in alcoholics, many of which may relate to the secondary complications, include suppressed natural killer cell activity (NKCA) (Irwin et al., 1990; Ochshorn-Andelson et al., 1994; Ristow, Starkey, & Hass, 1982), shifts in CD4+ and CD8+ lymphocyte subsets, suggesting abnormal activation (Cook, 1998), and altered monocytic and phagocytic activity (Cook, 1998; Schleifer et al., 1999). Studies from our laboratory found that, compared with chronic alcoholics with no evidence of medical compromise, those with only minor such changes showed decreased CD45RA+ (inducer–suppressor/naive) cells, decreased HLA-DR+ (activated) T-cells, and an increased proportion of circulating CD56+ natural killer (NK) cells (Schleifer, Benton, Keller, & Dhaibar, 2002). Improvement of CD4+ cell count has been demonstrated after cessation of alcohol use in some HIV-positive alcoholics (Pol, Artru, Thepot, Berthelot, & Nalpas, 1996).

Important in assessing the role of substances of abuse, and especially alcohol, in immune change, is the role of comorbid depressive disorders. Irwin and colleagues (1990) found decreased NKCA in patients with alcoholism that was exacerbated significantly in patients with both alcoholism and major depression. We have found that comorbid major depression may account for many of the immune changes found in alcoholics (Schleifer, Keller, & Czaja, 2003). It should also be noted that exposure to alcohol and other drugs may influence the symptomatic and pathological course of HIV-associated CNS disturbance either through additive effects on CNS function (Fein, Biggins, & MacKay, 1995) or neurotoxic interactions with the viral effects (Tabakoff, 1994). Alcohol consumption remains a risk factor for medication adherence and can modify liver metabolism, both of which could lead to drug-resistant virus (Kresina et al., 2002). Other researchers have found alcohol consumption prevalent in their HIV-positive, drug-using population, and have found that it significantly negatively impacts immunological and viral response to ART (Miguez, Shor-Posner, Morales, Rodriguez, & Burbano, 2003).

Marijuana

The contribution of cannabinoid use to human disease remains unclear and is a subject of considerable debate. A large study in California suggested that mortality rates in the general population are not increased by marijuana use; however, marijuana use was associated with increased mortality in persons with HIV disease (Sidney, Beck, Tekawa, Quesenberry, & Friedman, 1997). Whether these reflect direct effects on the disease process or lifestyle differences associated with marijuana use remains to be determined (Klein, Newton, Snella, & Friedman, 2001; Sidney et al., 1997). Both the clinical and the experimental data remain unclear as to whether marijuana use contributes negatively to the course of HIV disease. Correspondingly, it is unclear whether cannabinoids are useful adjuncts to the management of AIDS-related symptoms and syndromes, such as the AIDS-wasting syndrome, nausea, vomiting, anorexia, and glaucoma.

Stimulants

Stimulant users, particularly crack cocaine smokers or injecting stimulant users (cocaine, amphetamine) incur considerable risk for HIV. There is little definitive evidence of cocaine effects on T-cell function (MacGregor, 1988). In contrast, a few studies have associated both cocaine and amphetamines with increased NK activity (Swerdlow et al., 1991; Van Dyke, Stesin, Jones, Chuntharapai, & Seaman, 1986). Considering the prevalence of cocaine and other stimulant use, and its role as a behavioral risk factor for HIV transmission, the effects of cocaine use and withdrawal require further investigation. One study reported only limited effects of cocaine withdrawal on immune-related markers in pregnant women (Johnson, Knisely, Christmas, Schnoll, & Ruddy, 1996). Finally, the role of the most ubiquitous substance of abuse, tobacco, cannot be underestimated. Tobacco exposure has pervasive effects on health, including reported effects on the course of HIV, and has been associated with leukocytosis, shifts in T-cell subsets, decreased NKCA, and mitogen response; some studies also suggest immune activation under certain conditions (McAllister-Sistilli et al., 1998).

Behavior–Immune Interactions

Other factors that are present in alcoholics and drug users may further compromise the immune system and increase the risk for poor outcomes in HIV disease. Malnutrition is an important immunosuppressive factor influencing various components of the immune system (Chedid, 1995; MacGregor, 1988). Immune effects associated with life stress, poor coping mechanisms, and depression, which are highly prevalent in alcoholics and other substance abusers (Schuckit & Bogard, 1986), may further exacerbate AIDS risk and disease progression in these populations. Depressive symptoms have been linked with increased risk for mortality in HIV (Mayne, Vittinghoff, Chesney, Barrett, & Coates, 1996). Evans and colleagues (1995) have shown that the stress of HIV, even if asymptomatic, may adversely affect the immune system. In one study, psychological distress was independently associated with shorter time to AIDS among HIV-infected IDUs, especially among those with the lowest CD4+ counts (Golub et al., 2003).

So-called "club drugs," including 3,4-methylenedioxymethamphetamine (MDMA, Ecstasy), an amphetamine analogue with stimulant properties, and gamma-hydroxybutyrate (GHB), an analogue of gamma-aminobutyric acid with sedative properties, have become increasingly popular, and their use is widespread. These drugs are often used at all-night dance parties or "raves," clubs, and bars. Other drugs in this group include flunitrazepam (Rohypnol—or "Roofies," a long-acting, potent benzodiazepine not marketed in the United States), ketamine, methamphetamine, and hallucinogenics. The sedatives in the group, GHB and Rohypnol, have become known as "date-rape" drugs. All of these drugs enhance the risk of unsafe, novel, or repeated sexual behaviors that increase the risk of acquiring HIV and other sexually transmitted infections.

In one ART adherence study of current and former drug users, the strongest predictor of poor adherence and lack of viral suppression was active cocaine use. Depressive symptoms and the tendency to use alcohol and drugs to cope with stress were also predictive of nonadherence (Arsten et al., 2002). A longitudinal study of HIV-positive drug and alcohol users found strong temporal association of ART adherence and viral suppression when users switched to nonuse (Lucas, Gebo, Chaisson, & Moore, 2002). Interventions to treat affective disorders in substance users may have both medical and psychosocial benefits. Recent studies have begun to systematically investigate the links among immunologically relevant psychosocial predictors, psychosocial interventions, and the course of disease. Attention to a wider range of immune measures other than CD4+ cells alone and more extensive psychosocial assessments have found associations between specific stressors and depression and the course of HIV (Burack et al., 1993; Cole, Kemeny, Taylor, Visscher, & Fahey, 1996; Evans et al., 1995; Goodkin et al., 1994).

AIDS IN DRUG ADDICTION TREATMENT

Vigorous behavioral change strategies are required in the treatment of alcohol and drug abuse in those infected with or at risk for HIV infection. AIDS education, prevention, and behavioral training should be a regular and ongoing component of drug treatment. Evaluators must use recognized general treatment principles, such as those in the "Practice Guideline for Treatment of Patients with Substance Use Disorders" (American Psychiatric Association, 1995) and widely accepted placement criteria (American Society of Addiction Medicine, 2003). Drug addiction is a chronic, relapsing disease and may require ongoing or repeated treatments. In one 12-year study, 29% of drug injectors remained persistent injectors and had the highest mortality rates (Galai, Safaeian, Vlahov, Bolotin, & Celentano, 2003). Overall care of those with HIV is likely to be improved by integration of case management, medical, and substance abuse treatment (Knowlton et al., 2001).

BASIC COMPONENTS OF HIV/AIDS PREVENTION/ TREATMENT IN DRUG ABUSE TREATMENT SETTINGS

Effective management of these cases requires a multidisciplinary team that can implement an individualized treatment plan structured to succeed within the constraints of available resources and motivational forces:

- Assessment of HIV risk behavior with frequent reassessments
- Complete physical examination
- Psychiatric assessment and indicated treatment
- HIV testing
- Safe sex training for all. This includes explicit discussion of proper use of barrier methods and techniques (latex condoms, gloves, and dental dams), and stressing the importance of using barrier methods for all penetrative sexual practices or when body fluids are transmitted or exchanged (Centers for Disease Control and Prevention, 1993).

Active alcohol and drug abusers encountered in any health care settings should be offered appropriate referrals and encouraged to enter treatment. Cultural competency presents the primary hurdle in altering risk behaviors, particularly since community-based outreach programs have proved to be the most effective (Kwiatowski, Booth, & Lloyd, 2000). For the users who cannot or will not enter treatment, specific counseling methods can be employed to communicate effective harm reduction techniques. IDUs must learn the hazards of needle sharing and, for those who do not stop injecting, emphasis must be placed on use of a new, sterile needle for each injection to prevent blood-borne infections. Methods of needle decontamination, such as flushing with bleach, can reduce some exposure risk, but are not as safe as using a sterile, unused needle for each injection (Gostin, Lazzarini, Jones, & Flaherty, 1997).

Counseling for noninjecting substance abusers is no less important—especially when sex partners may be IDUs (see "Prevention and Public Health"). Alcoholics, especially females and stimulant users, should be specifically targeted for counseling on sexual practices during intoxicated states. Commercial sex work, often found linked with drug use to support habits (Edlin et al., 1994) or bartering sex to obtain drugs, further adds to risk by introducing multiple partners (Catania et al., 1992, 1995) and circumstances where safe sex practices are unlikely to be easily maintained.

HIV TESTING: CLINICAL CONSIDERATIONS

The Centers for Disease Control and Prevention (CDC) has suggested since 1988 that all patients admitted to substance abuse treatment programs be screened for the presence of the HIV antibody. Screening and treatment for HIV infection are often linked to substance abuse programs. Literature on the behavioral impact of HIV testing is mixed. For some who are HIV positive, testing and notification are catalysts for needle use risk reduction among IDUs in treatment (Casadonte, Des Jarlais, Friedman, & Rotrose, 1990) or other forms of behavioral change (Cleary et al., 1991). Comprehensive counseling must accompany testing. For some individuals, either a positive or negative HIV test can be a powerful motivating factor for continued treatment for the addictive disorder (Perry, Fishman, Jacobsberg, Young, & Frances, 1991). Health professionals can help facilitate positive motivation by stressing the beneficial effects that drug abstinence and other healthy lifestyle changes can have on the course of HIV infection, particularly in the context of effective ART regimens. Watkins, Metzger, Woody, and McLellan (1993) found that knowledge of HIV status was an important determinate of condom use among IDUs.

Information on HIV status can aid physicians in evaluating patients with nonspecific medical, neurological, and psychiatric symptoms and assist in the prompt recognition and treatment of infection (Stimmel, 1988). CD4+ lymphocyte counts and lymphocyte subsets, and viral load and viral resistance testing can be used to stage treatment protocols for antiretroviral medications. In the immune compromised, some opportunistic infections can be prevented with pharmacotherapy; others can be prevented through environmental manipulations (e.g., avoidance of undercooked or contaminated food or water).

The CDC (1997, 2001) has extensive recommendations on the use of ART in HIV-positive pregnant or nursing women to reduce mother-to-infant transmission (MIT). In the United States, the number of reported MIT-acquired AIDS cases fell 43% from 1992 to 1996, likely because of providing zidovudine (AZT) to HIV-infected mothers, better guidelines for prenatal HIV counseling and testing, and changes in obstetrical management (Centers for Disease Control and Prevention, 1997; Wilfert, 1999). Management of the HIV-positive pregnant woman who is undergoing treatment for an SUD is best done with a specialty team or in a specially designed program (Lindberg, 1996).

HIV Testing: Guidelines for Counseling

Pretest Counseling

- Get written informed consent.
- Assess knowledge, attitude, and past experience with HIV/AIDS and HIV testing.
- Assess individual risk factors.
  - Determine substance use (what, how, where, with whom, how much and how often?).
  - Determine sexual behaviors, barrier use (condoms, gloves, dental dams).
- Explain antibody test in clear, easy-to-understand language.
- Assess degree of risk.
- Inform of the risk status.
- Counsel on specific, effective means of reducing future risk behavior.

Posttest Counseling: Positive Result

- Anticipate emotional and behavioral responses to a positive test result.
- Evaluate social support systems and coping strategies.
- Advise of treatment options and available services.
- Make referrals.
  - Medical evaluation.
  - Psychiatric evaluation: acute reaction, risk for suicide, past or current depression, other mental disorder, positive family history for mental disorder.
- Provide opportunity to ask questions, respond to the results.
- Provide information about symptoms associated with altered immunity and the effects of alcohol and drugs on the immune system (Stimmel, 1988).

Reactions run the gamut and many immediately react as if they had an imminently terminal condition. Delayed emotional reactions are common as well. There are reports of knowledge of positive HIV status having severe adverse psychological effects, including suicidal behavior (Glass, 1988). Hospitalized patients may be especially vulnerable to suicidal ideation and intent (Alfonso et al., 1994).

Posttest Counseling: Negative Result

- Emphasize test limitations.
- Emphasize the need for continued HIV precautions.
- Emphasize the need for retesting.
- Preemptively address erroneous conclusions about negative tests in high-risk individuals.
- Have a low threshold for specialized referral to mental health services, especially for individuals from groups that have endured multiple and ongoing losses to the AIDS epidemic or from particularly marginalized groups.

Residential treatment programs should make information about HIV available and provide a variety of support mechanisms for those affected, including access to medical and mental health services. Ethical issues raised by HIV testing are not readily resolved. For example, if an individual is found to be HIV antibody positive, is there a duty to warn the sexual partner(s)? How will these sorts of issues affect the therapeutic relationship? Because public health regulations regarding these matters vary from state to state, practitioners must consult local public health requirements and guidelines.

Clinical Assessment and Management

The many physical and emotional effects of AIDS complicate the contemporaneous treatment of chemical dependence. The presence of those with AIDS in drug treatment units elicits complex feelings in staff and others if their status is known. Issues of death and dying may dominate, and patients may express feelings of hopelessness and question the value or practicality of abstinence from drug and alcohol use. Issues of medical regimen compliance and drug adherence versus control become critical features in treatment. Arrangements for aftercare and placement of patients with AIDS following inpatient detoxification or residential drug treatment may be difficult.

Combined diagnoses complicate treatment. Retention may be a problem: In one study, those with HIV who were receiving ambulatory psychiatric treatment were more likely to drop out of treatment if they drank or used drugs (Kennedy, Skurnick, & Lintott, 1994). The patient's family and significant others who could be instrumental in motivating drug-addicted individuals for treatment may, in the face of HIV, overlook or be reluctant to confront the substance abuse problem. Physicians and other health workers may minimize an individual's addiction in light of overwhelming physical illness. Those with long-term addictions and multiple disabilities may be marginalized and may have long been estranged from families or other support mechanisms. Many have alienated health care providers by inconsistent compliance and subsequent crisis use of the system, when life-threatening infections or overdoses occur.

It is important not to focus on substance abuse issues alone to the point of excluding AIDS-related psychological needs. Anxiety and depression, complicated at times by cognitive impairment, frequently accompany HIV/AIDS. As noted, suicidal ideation is common. These symptoms need frequent reevaluation through treatment. Patients overwhelmed by illness, grief, and a sense of loss require a supportive, insight-oriented, and psychodynamically sound approach. Depressive symptoms have been associated with increased mortality from HIV infection (Mayne et al., 1996) and underscore the need for psychiatric services for this population. Consultation–liaison psychiatrists may be particularly valuable in the care of patients with HIV and addiction, regardless of setting. A working knowledge of current therapies and scientific advances for HIV infection is important. Psychiatrists are in a unique position to assist those living with or dying of HIV/AIDS to receive the type and level of care desired (Kennedy & Hill, 1997). Disclosure to others about lifestyle, risk behaviors, seropositivity, or complicated needs for care may be very difficult. Significant others may benefit from referral to AIDS support resources. Women may have special issues and suffer more psychological distress than men (Kennedy, Skurnick, Foley, & Louria, 1995). Nonjudgmental attitudes that convey a true sense of willingness to help have a better chance of building successful rapport with patients and may achieve a higher level of adherence to medical recommendations and lifestyle changes.

Patients do best with coordinated care at centers where there are specialized services, integrated care management, and a track record with HIV. A psychiatrist or therapist may be in a pivotal position to help coordinate and promote cooperation among the various caregivers. Pitfalls for mental health professionals, addictions counselors, and other staff include countertransference issues linked to fear of contagion, addictophobia, racism, fear of homosexuality, denial of helplessness, and need for professional omnipotence. Mechanisms such as displacement and reaction formation can result in failure to maintain appropriate empathic distance from the patients. Therapists need to be alert to the how the overwhelming emotional issues may impact, strain, and push traditional boundries observed in psychotherapy. The therapist must avoid becoming overwhelmed by what he or she feels the patient is experiencing. Taking a moralistic attitude toward the patient's drug use and sexual behaviors will undermine treatment. Therapists must confront their own feelings and attitudes toward drug addiction, homosexuality, and AIDS.

Legal Issues

Issues of confidentiality arise when treating individuals with drug addiction and HIV infection. Federal law protects the confidentiality of patient records for those persons under treatment for drug abuse. This includes drug-abusing patients who have AIDS. (There is, however, no general federal confidentiality protection for medical records of AIDS patients not being treated for drug abuse.) These federal regulations protect both oral and written communications (Pascal, 1987). The more recent Health Insurance Portability Assurance Act (2003) provides for the electronic transmission of health information and is concerned with medical record privacy and the U.S. standards for the protection and privacy of personal health information. In the acute delivery of health care, use of universal precautions obviates the need to identify specifically any individual as HIV positive. Disclosure to those outside the clinical setting is permitted only with the patient's written consent. Reporting of HIV status to public health authorities may be required in some states and may be disclosed without patient consent to the extent required by law. In all other situations, disclosure without the patient's consent must be obtained through a court order, based on a finding of good cause (Pascal, 1987). All employers should be aware of the provisions of the Americans with Disabilities Act.

Once a health care provider has knowledge of a positive HIV test, he or she is obligated to inform the individual. Failure to do so may make the provider liable for any harm that results to the individual or to his or her sexual partners (Pascal, 1987). Because HIV is communicable and AIDS can be fatal, situations may arise in which the physician or therapist is aware of a danger posed to a third party, such as a sexual partner. HIV-positive patients must be counseled on their responsibilities and encouraged to voluntarily self-report to third parties who may be at risk for infection (Pascal, 1987). Some states have partner notification programs or requirements. If a substance abuse program considers it indicated to warn a third party concerning a patient's HIV status, the patient's consent or a court order must be obtained to comply with federal confidentiality regulations. A policy of universal education for all patients, their spouses, significant others, and caregivers is often used and is consistent with the consensus public health viewpoint that education, prevention, and voluntary measures are the best approaches to stemming the AIDS epidemic, and that punitive approaches are counterproductive (Pascal, 1987).

Single parents of minor children and, especially, pregnant women have special issues regarding custody and care should the mother or other primary caregiver become disabled, incapacitated, or die. At the end stages of illness, patients may experience cognitive deficits; thus, issues of competency and future planning should be addressed in a timely and appropriate manner. Again, consultation psychiatrists are in a unique position to assist patients who are grappling with such difficult and serious matters. Many avenues and alternatives can be explored. Patients themselves prefer that physicians broach these subjects, and earlier rather than later (Kennedy & Hill, 1997).

PREVENTION AND PUBLIC HEALTH

Prevention is the strongest defense against spread of this blood-borne and sexually transmitted infection. Behavioral change studies indicate that some IDUs are attempting risk reduction, especially in needle sharing (Des Jarlais & Friedman, 1987; Des Jarlais, Friedman, Choopanya, Varichseni, & Ward, 1992; Selwyn & Cox, 1985). There is evidence that IDUs can reduce their risk by altering needle-sharing behaviors. Attending a methadone-maintenance program promotes risk reduction (Des Jarlais & Friedman, 1987). More recently, IDUs with AIDS knowledge reported that their consistent use of sterile new needles depended on availability (Des Jarlais et al., 1992; Gostin et al., 1997). When sterile needles are unavailable, however, they use whatever is available. Needle sharing is common but not universal among IDUs. Sharing practices are influenced by many factors, including economics, regional drug norms, needle availability, length of habit, drug of choice (i.e., heroin, cocaine, or drug combinations), and others. A large national survey of the regulation of syringes and needles concluded that deregulation of syringe sale and possession would reduce the morbidity and mortality associated with blood-borne infections, including HIV, among IDUs, their sexual partners, and their children (Gostin et al., 1997). Regulations vary throughout the United States, but despite a U.S. General Accounting Office (1993) report and numerous other government task force recommendations pointing out that new infections in IDUs plateau where needle exchanges have been tried, widespread support or federal backing for such strategies has been lacking. International studies show that needle exchange coupled with other risk-reduction education and available treatment slots has been successful (Des Jarlais et al., 1992). One evaluation of an experimental U.S. needle exchange program showed that it was quickly adopted by IDUs, and an increase in injection and use did not occur (Watters, Estilo, Clark, & Lorvick, 1994). Lurie and Drucker (1997) estimated that from 4,000 to 10,000 HIV infections in the United States, which cost between $250,000 and $500,000 each, and untold amounts of human misery might have been prevented by needle exchange programs.

Prevention strategies to reduce the risk of exposure to contaminated needles include cessation of injection drug use, cessation of needle sharing, and implementation of harm reduction methods, methadone maintenance, outpatient detoxification, and drug-free treatment programs and needle exchange programs. Male IDUs are especially important for the spread of HIV into the general population. Murphy (1988) found that male IDUs reported a greater percentage of non-IDU heterosexual contacts than did female IDUs. Similar findings were reported by Des Jarlais and colleagues (1987). In contrast, female IDUs may be at particular risk for being exposed to HIV as a result of heterosexual behaviors and needle sharing. Des Jarlais and colleagues reported that female IDUs were more likely than male IDUs to have sexual contacts that were also IDUs and tended to be needle sharers. Women who shared needles had twice as many IDU sexual partners as those who did not, whereas the majority of sexual partners of male needle sharers were not themselves needle sharers. Kennedy and colleagues (1993) found that high-risk women (those with HIV-positive male partners) were more likely to insist on condom use for sex if they were employed. Skurnick, Abrams, Kennedy, Valentin, and Cordell (1998) also found that heterosexual couples who practiced safe sex at a study entry were less likely to relapse into unsafe behaviors in 6 months if the female was employed. Unsafe sexual practices, most notably anal sex, are implicated in sexual transmission of HIV within heterosexual couples (Skurnick et al., 1998).

CONCLUSION

IDUs and other drug users are primary sources of HIV transmission to other adults and to children in the general population. Health care providers have a major responsibility to provide education, promote prevention, and provide treatment to this group. HIV counseling, testing, referral to drug treatment, and mental health and health services must be readily available. Those drug users who are unable to abstain from injecting may benefit from therapeutic educational strategies about risk reduction. Public health measures may have to be addressed through policy change. Counselors involved in the treatment of drug-addicted individuals must explicitly discuss issues of safe sex and condom usage, as well as openly discuss the effects of drug use and intoxication on sexual behavior and HIV risk. Furthermore, knowledge of medical, mental health, and social services resources is required for those caring for addicted individuals. Professionals should be aware of the wide range of presenting signs and symptoms of HIV infection, as well as treatment choice options and difficult, end-of-life decisions regarding care, treatments and legal issues, including estate planning and care of minor children.

The extraordinary rates of HIV infection among substance users suggest that these individuals will occupy an increasing proportion of health care resources, particularly as the disease is stretched into a chronic, ongoing state as those who are infected live longer. Numerous behavioral epidemiological studies have shown that both injection-related risk factors (years of injecting drugs, type of drug injected, direct and indirect sharing of injection paraphernalia) and sex-related risk factors (lack of condom use, multiple sex partners, survival sex) lead to the spread of HIV, hepatitis B virus (HBV), and hepatitis C virus (HCV). In order to interrupt the spread, the capacity of outreach workers to be able to refer to drug treatment programs (especially for IDUs), and increased access to health and social services for those who are using drugs or are HIV infected, need to be expanded (Estrada, 2002). Treatment slots for those with HIV infection or AIDS will be increasingly required in alcohol and drug treatment programs. As the incidence of HIV infection increases among the drug-using, -abusing, and -dependent, the potential for spread into other segments of the population increases. For a successful battle against one part of the AIDS epidemic, additional resources for drug education, prevention, treatment, rehabilitation, and research are urgently needed.

REFERENCES

Alfonso, C. A., Cohen, M. A. A., Aladjem, A. D., Morrison, F., Powell, D. R., Winter, R. A., & Orlowski, B. K. (1994). HIV seropositivity as a major risk factor for suicide in the general hospital. *Psychosomatics, 35*, 368–373.

American Psychiatric Association. (1995). Practice guideline for the treatment of patients with substance use disorders: Alcohol, cocaine, opioids. *Am J Psychiatry, 152*, 5–59.

American Society of Addiction Medicine. (2003). *Patient placement criteria for the treatment of substance related disorders* (3rd ed., ASAM PPC-2). Chevy Chase, MD: Author.

Arria, A. M., Tarter, R. E., & Van Thiel, D. H. (1991). Vulnerability to alcoholic liver disease. *Recent Dev Alcohol, 9*, 185–204.

Arsten, J. H., Demas, P. A., Grant, R. W., Gourevitch, M. N., Farzadegan, H., Howard, A. A., & Schoenbaum, E. E. (2002). Impact of active drug use on antiretroviral therapy adherence and viral suppression in HIV-infected drug users. *J Gen Intern Med, 17*, 377–381.

Astemborski, J., Vlahov, D., Warren, D., Solomon, L., & Nelson, K. E. (1994). The trading of sex for drugs or money and HIV seropositivity among female intravenous drug users. *Am J Public Health, 84*, 382–387.

Avins, A. L., Woods, W. J., Lindan, C. P., Hudes, E. S., Clark, W., & Hulley, S. B. (1994). Infection and risk behaviors among heterosexuals in alcohol treatment programs. *JAMA, 271*, 515–519.

Baldwin, J. A., Maxwell, C. J., Fenaughty, A. M., Trotter, R. T., & Stevens, S. (2000). Alcohol as a risk factor for HIV transmission among American Indian/Alaskan Native drug users. *Am Indian Alsk Native Ment Health Res, 1*, 1–16.

Bell, J. E., Brettle, R. P., & Chiswick, A. (1998). HIV encephalitis, proviral load and dementia in drug users and homosexuals with AIDS: Effect of neocortical involvement. *Brain, 121*, 2043–2052.

Booth, R. E., Koester, S. K., & Pinto, F. (1995). Gender differences in sex-risk behaviors, economic livelihood, and self-concept among drug injectors and crack smokers. *Am J Addict, 4,* 313–322.

Booth, R. E., Kwiatkowski, C. F., & Chitwood, D. D. (2000). Sex related HIV risk behaviors: Differential risks among injection drug smokers, crack smothers, and injection drug users who smoke crack. *Drug Alcohol Depend, 58,* 219–226.

Bornstein, R., Nasrallah, H., Para, M., Fass, R., Whitacre, C., & Rice, R. (1991). Rate of CD4 decline and neuropsychological performance in HIV infection. *Arch Neurol, 48,* 704–707.

Bouwman, F. H., Skolasky, R. L., Hes, D., Selnes, O. A., Glass, J. D., Nance-Sprosso, T. E., et al. (1998). Variable progression of HIV-associated dementia. *Neurology, 50,* 1814–1820.

Boyer, C. B., & Ellen, J. M. (1994). HIV risk in adolescents: The role of sexual activity and substance use behaviors. In R. J. Battjes, Z. Sloboda, & W. C. Grace (Eds.), *The context of HIV risk among drug users and their sexual partners* (NIDA Research Monograph No. 143, pp. 135–154). Washington, DC: U.S. Government Printing Office.

Brown, S., Stimmel, B., Taub, R. N., Kochwa, S., & Rosenfield, R. E. (1974). Immunologic dysfunction in heroin addicts. *Arch Intern Med, 134,* 1001–1006.

Burack, J. H., Barret, D. C., Stall, R. D., Chesney, M. A., Ekstrand, M. L., & Coates, T. J. (1993). Depressive symptoms and CD4 lymphocyte decline among HIV-infected men. *JAMA, 270,* 2568–2575.

Casadonte, P., Des Jarlais, D., Friedman, S. R., & Rotrose, J. P. (1990). Psychological and behavioral impact of learning HIV test results. *Int J Addict, 25,* 409–426.

Catania, J. A., Binson, D., Dolcini, M. M., Stall, R., Choi, K., Pollack, L. M., et al. (1995). Risk factors for HIV and other sexually transmitted diseases and prevention practices among U.S. heterosexual adults: Changes from 1990 to 1992. *Am J Public Health, 85,* 1492–1499.

Catania, J. A., Coates, T. J., Stall, R., Turner, H., Peterson, J., Hearst, N., et al. (1992). AIDS-related risk factors and condom use in the United States. *Science, 258,* 1101–1106.

Centers for Disease Control and Prevention. (1993). Update: Barrier protection against HIV infection and other sexually transmitted diseases. *Morb Mortal Wkly Rep, 42,* 589–599.

Centers for Disease Control and Prevention. (1997). Update: Perinatally acquired HIV/AIDS-United States. *Morb Mortal Wkly Rep, 45,* 1086–1092.

Centers for Disease Control and Prevention. (2001). Revised guidelines for HIV counseling, testing, and referral and revised recommendations for HIV screening of pregnant women. *Morb Mortal Wkly Rep, 50*(RR-19), 1–85.

Centers for Disease Control and Prevention. (2004). *HIV/AIDS Surveillance Report, 2003* (Vol. 15, pp. 5–8). Atlanta, GA: Author.

Chedid, A. (1995). Alcoholic liver disease, malnutrition, and the immune response. In R. R. Watson (Ed.), *Alcohol, drugs of abuse and immune function* (pp. 87–103). Boca Raton, FL: CRC Press.

Cleary, P. D., VanDevanter, N., Rogers, T.F., Singer, E., Shipton-Levy, R., Steilen, M., et al. (1991). Behavior changes after notification of HIV infection. *Am J Public Health, 81,* 1586–1590.

Cole, S. W., Kemeny, M. E., Taylor, S. E., Visscher, B. R., & Fahey, J. L. (1996). Accelerated course of human immunodeficiency virus infection in gay men who conceal their homosexual identity. *Psychol Med, 58,* 219–231.

Cook, R. T. (1998). Alcohol abuse, alcoholism, and damage to the immune system—A review. *Alcohol: Clin Expe Res, 22,* 1927–1942.

Damos, D. L., John, R. S., Parker, E. S., & Levine, A. M. (1997). Cognitive function in asymptomatic HIV infection. *Arch Neurol, 54*(2), 179–185.

DeAngelis, L. M. (1991). Primary CNS lymphoma: A new clinical challenge. *Neurology, 41,* 619.

DeRonchi, D., Faranca, I., Berardi, D., Scudellari, P., Borderi, M., Manfredi, R., & Fratiglioni, L. (2002). Risk factors for cognitive impairment in HIV-1 infected persons with different risk behaviors. *Arch Neurol, 59*(2), 812–818.

Des Jarlais, D. C., & Friedman, S. (1987). HIV infection among intravenous drug users: Epidemiology and risk reduction. *AIDS, 1,* 67–76.

Des Jarlais, D. C., Friedman, S. R., Choopanya, K., Varichseni, S., & Ward, T. (1992). International epidemiology of HIV and AIDS among injecting Drug Users. *AIDS, 6,* 1053–1068.

Des Jarlais, D. C., Wish, E., Friedman, S. R., Stoneburner, R., Yancovitz, S. R., Mildvan, D., et al. (1987). Intravenous drug use and the heterosexual transmission of the human immunodeficiency virus: Current trends in New York City. *NY State J Med, 3,* 283–286.

De Souza, C. T., Diaz, T., Sutmoller, F., & Bastos, F. I. (2002). The association of socioeconomic status and use of crack/cocaine with unprotected anal sex in a cohort of men who have sex with men in Rio de Janeiro, Brazil. *J Acquir Immune Defic Syndr, 29,* 95–101.

Donahue, R. M., & Vlahov, D. (1998). Opiates as potential cofactors in progression of HIV-1 infections to AIDS. *J Neuroimmunol, 15,* 77–87.

Edlin, B. R., Irwin, K. L., Faruque, S., McCoy, C. B., Word, C., Serrano, Y., et al. (1994). Intersecting epidemics—crack cocaine use and HIV infection among inner city young adults: Multicenter crack cocaine and HIV infection study team. *N Engl J Med, 331,* 1422–1427.

Estrada, A. L. (2002). Epidemiology of HIV/AIDS, hepatitis B, hepatitis C, and tuberculosis among minority injection drug users. *Public Health Reporter, 117*(Suppl), S126–S134.

Evans, D. L., Leserman, J., Perkins, D. O., Stern, R. A., Murphy, C., Tamul, K., et al. (1995). Stress-associated reductions of cytotoxic T-lymphocytes and natural killer cells in asymptomatic HIV infection. *Am J Psychiatry, 152,* 543–550.

Fabian, M. S., Parsons, O. A., & Sheldon, M. D. (1985). Effects of gender and alcoholism on verbal and visual–spatial learning. *J Nerv Ment Dis, 172,* 16–20.

Fein, G., Biggins, C. A., & MacKay, S. (1995). Alcohol abuse and HIV infection have additive effects on frontal cortex function as measured by auditory evoked potential P3A latency. *Biol Psychiatry, 37,* 183–195.

Galai, N., Safaeian, M., Vlahov, D., Bolotin, A., & Celentano, D. D. (2003). Longitudinal patterns of drug injection behavior in the ALIVE Study cohort, 1988–2000: Description and determinants. *Am J Epidemiol, 158,* 695–704.

Glass, J. D., Fedor, H., Wesslingh, S. L., & McArthur, J. C. (1995). Immunocytochemical quantitation of HIV in the brain: Correlations with HIV-associated dementia. *Ann Neurol, 38,* 755–762.

Glass, R. M. (1988). AIDS and suicide [Editorial]. *JAMA, 259,* 1369–1370.

Glenn, S. W., & Parsons, O. A. (1992). Neuropsychological efficiency measures in male and female alcoholics. *J Stud Alcohol, 53,* 546–552.

Golub, E. T., Astemborski, J. A., Hoover, D. R., Anthony, J. C., Vlahov, D., & Strathdee, S. A. (2003). Psychological distress and progression to AIDS in a cohort of injection drug users. *J Acquir Immune Defic Syndr, 32,* 429–434.

Goodkin, K., Mulder, C. L., Blaney, N. T., Ironson, G., Kumar, M., & Fletcher, M. A. (1994). Psychoneuroimmunology and human immunodeficiency virus type 1 infection revisited. *Arch Gen Psychiatry, 51,* 246–247.

Gostin, L. O., Lazzarini, S., Jones, S., & Flaherty, K. (1997). Prevention of HIV/AIDS and other blood-borne diseases among injection drug users. *JAMA, 277,* 53–62.

Govitrapong, P., Suttitum, T., Kotchabhakdi, N. & Uneklabh, T. (1998). Alterations of immune functions in heroin addicts and heroin withdrawal subjects. *J Pharmacol Exp Ther, 286,* 883–889.

Grant, I., & Reed, R. (1985). Neuropsychology of alcohol and drug abuse. In A. I. Alterman (Ed.), *Substance abuse and psychopathology* (pp. 289–341). New York: Plenum Press.

Health Insurance Portability and Accountability Act. (2003). Office for Civil Rights. Washington, DC: Department of Health and Human Services. Retrieved December, 27, 2003, from *www.hhs.gov/ocr/hipaa*

Hoffman, J. A., Klein, H., Eber, M., & Crosby, H. (2000). Frequency and intensity of crack use. *Drug Alcohol Depend, 58,* 227–236.

Holtzman, D. M., Kaku, D. A., & So, Y. T. (1989). New onset seizures associated with human immunodeficiency virus infection: Causation and clinical features in 100 cases. *Am J Med, 87,* 173–180.

Irwin, M., Caldwell, C., Smith, T. L., Brown, S., Schuckit, M. A., & Gillin, J. C. (1990). Major depressive disorder, alcoholism, and reduced natural killer cell cytotoxicity. *Arch Gen Psychiatry, 47,* 713–719.

Janssen, R. S., Nwanyanwu, O. C., Selik, R. M., & Stehr-Green, J. K. (1992). Epidemiology of human immunodeficiency virus encephalopathy in the United States. *Neurology, 42,* 1472–1476.

Johnson, T. R., Knisely, J. S., Christmas, J. T., Schnoll, S. H., & Ruddy, S. (1996). Changes in immunologic cell surface markers during cocaine withdrawal in pregnant women. *Brain Behav Immun, 10,* 324–336.

Kennedy, C. A., & Eckholdt, H. M. (1997). Diagnosis of AIDS in U.S. adolescents: 1983–1993. In L. Sherr (Ed.), *AIDS and adolescents* (pp. 51–61). London: Harwood Academic.

Kennedy, C. A., & Hill, J. M. (1997, March). *Barriers to advance directives in hospitalized AIDS patients.* Paper presented at the annual meeting of the American Psychosomatic Association, Santa Fe, NM.

Kennedy, C. A., Skurnick, J. H., Foley, M., & Louria, D. (1995). Gender differences in HIV-related psychological distress in heterosexual couples. *AIDS Care, 7,* S33–S38.

Kennedy, C. A., Skurnick, J. H., & Lintott, M. (1994, May). *Evaluation of factors related to retention of HIV positive patients in ambulatory psychiatric treatment.* Poster presented at the annual meeting of the American Psychiatric Association, Philadelphia.

Kennedy, C. A., Skurnick, J., Wan, J. Y., Quattrone, G., Sheffet, A., Quinones, M., et al. (1993). Psychological distress, drug and alcohol use as correlates of condom use in HIV-serodiscordant heterosexual couples. *AIDS, 7,* 1493–1499.

Klein, T. W., Newton, C., Snella, E., & Friedman, H. (2001). Marijuana, the cannabinoid system, and immunolmodulation. In R. Ader, D. L. Felten, & N. Cohen (Eds.), *Psychoneuroimmunology* (3rd ed., pp. 415–432). San Diego, CA: Academic Press.

Klisz, D. K., & Parsons, O. A. (1977). Hypothesis testing in younger and older alcoholic. *J Stud Alcohol, 38,* 1718–1729.

Knowlton, A. R., Hoover, D. R., Chung, S. E., Celentano, D. D., Vlahov, D., & Latkin, C. A. (2001). Access to medical care and service utilization among injection drug users with HIV/AIDS. *Drug Alcohol Depend, 64,* 55–62.

Kolson, D. L., Lavi, E., Gonzalez, M., & Scarano, F. (1998). The effects of human immuno deficiency virus in the central nervous system. *Adv Virus Res, 50,* 1–47.

Koutsilieri, E., Scheller, C., Sopper, S., ter Meulen, V., & Riederer, P. (2002). The pathogenesis of HIV-induced dementia. *Mech Ageing Dev, 123,* 1047–1053.

Kresina, T. F., Flexner, C. W., Sinclair, J., Correia, M. A., Stapleton, J., Adeniyi-Jones, S., et al. (2002). Alcohol use and HIV pharmacotherapy. *AIDS Res Hum Retroviruses, 18,* 757–770.

Kwiatkowski, C., Booth, R. E., & Lloyd, L. A. (2000). The effects of offering free treatment to street-recruited opioid injectors. *Addiction, 95,* 697–704.

Lindberg, C. (1996). *HIV and pregnancy: Information for service providers.* New Brunswick, NJ: New Jersey Women and AIDS Network.

Ling, W., Charvuvastra, C., Collins, J. F., Batki, S., Brown, L. S., Kintaudi, P., et al. (1998). Buprenorphine maintenance treatment of opiate dependence: A multicenter, randomized clinical trial. *Addiction, 93,* 475–486.

Ling, W., Compton, P., Rawson, R., & Wesson, D. (1996). Neuropsychiatry of alcohol and drug abuse. In B. Fogel, R. Schiffer, & S. Rao (Eds.), *Neuropsychiatry* (pp. 679–722). Baltimore: Williams & Wilkins.

Lipton, S. A., & Gendelman, H. E. (1995). Seminars in medicine of the Beth Israel Hospital, Boston: Dementia associated with the acquired immunodeficiency syndrome. *N Engl J Med, 332,* 934–940.

Lucas, G. M., Gebo, K. A., Chaisson, R. E., & Moore, R. D. (2002). Longitudinal assessment of the effects of drug and alcohol abuse on HIV-1 treatment outcomes in an urban clinic. *AIDS, 16,* 767–774.

Lunn, S., Skydsbjerg, M., Schulsinger, H., Parnas, J., Pedersen, J., & Mathiesen, L. (1991). A preliminary report on the neuropsychologic sequelae of human immunodeficiency virus. *Arch Gen Psychiatry, 48,* 139–142.

Lurie, P., & Drucker, E. (1997). An opportunity lost: HIV infections associated with lack of a national needle-exchange programme in the USA. *Lancet, 349,* 604–608.

MacGregor, R. (1988). Alcohol and drugs as co-factors for AIDS. *Adv Alcohol Subst Abuse, 7,* 47–51.

Mayne, T. J., Vittinghoff, E., Chesney, M. A., Barrett, D. C., & Coates, T. J. (1996).

Depressive affect and survival among gay and bisexual men infected with HIV. *Arch Intern Med*, 156, 2233–2238.

McAllister-Sistilli, C. G., Caggiula, A. R., Knopf, S., Rose, C. A., Miller, A. L., & Donny, E. C. (1998). The effects of nicotine on the immune system. *Psychoneuroendocrinology*, 23, 175–187.

McCarthy, L., Wetzela, M., Slikera, J. K., Eisenstein, T. K., & Rogers, T. J. (2001). Opioids, opioid receptors, and the immune response. *Drug Alcohol Depend*, 62, 111–123.

McDonough, R. J., Madden, J. J., Falek, A., Shafer, D. A., Pline, M., Gordon, D., et al. (1980). Alteration of T- and null lymphocyte frequencies in the peripheral blood of human opiate addicts: *In vivo* evidence for opiate receptor sites on T-lymphocytes. *J Immunol*, 125, 2539–2543.

Metzger, D. S., Woody, G., McLellan, T., O'Brien, C. P., Druley, P., Navaline, H., et al. (1993). Human immunodeficiency virus seroconversion among intravenous drug users in- and out-of-treatment: An 18-month prospective follow-up. *J Acquir Immune Defic Syndr*, 6, 1049–1056.

Miguez, M. J., Shor-Posner, G., Morales, G., Rodriguez, A., & Burbano, X. (2003). HIV treatment in drug abusers: Impact of alcohol use. *Addict Biol*, 8, 33–37.

Mofenson, L. M., & Flynn, P. M. (2000, March). *The challenge of adolescent HIV infection: From prevention to treatment* [Seminar S221]. Paper presented at the annual meeting of the American Academy of Pediatrics, Chicago.

Monteiro, M. G. (2001). A World Health Organization perspective on alcohol and illicit drug use and health. *Eur Addict Res*, 3, 98–100.

Moore, R., Keruly, J., Gallant, J., & Chaisson, R. (1998). *Decline in mortality rates and opportunistic disease with combination antiretroviral therapy* [Abstract 32192]. Paper presented at the 12th World AIDS Conference, Geneva, Switzerland.

Murphy, D. L. (1988). Heterosexual contacts of intravenous drug abusers: Implications for the next spread of the AIDS epidemic. *Adv Alcohol Subst Abuse*, 7, 89–97.

Nath, A., Hauser, K. F., Wojna, V., Booze, R. M., Maragos, W., Prendergast, M., et al. (2002). Molecular basis for interactions of HIV and drugs of abuse. *J Acquir Immune Defic Syndr*, 31, S62–S69.

National Institute of Drug Abuse. (2002). Club drugs: Community Drug Alert Bulletin: Some fact about club drugs. Retrieved December 27, 2003, from *www.165.112.78.61/clubalert/clubdrugalert.html/*

Navia, B. A., Jordon, B. D., & Price, R. W. (1986). The AIDS dementia complex: I. Clinical features. *Ann Neurol*, 19, 517–524.

O'Connor, P. G., Oliveto, A. H., Shi, J. M.., Triffleman, E. G., Carroll, K. M., Kosten, T. R., et al. (1998). A randomized trial of buprenorphine maintenance for heroin dependence in a primary care clinic for substance users verus a methadone clinic. *Am J Med*, 105, 100–105.

Ochshorn-Andelson, M., Bodner, G., Toraker, P., Albeck, H., Ho, A., & Kreek, M. J. (1994). Effects of ethanol on human natural killer cell activity: In vitro and acute, low-dose in vivo studies. *Alcohol: Clin Exp Res*, 18, 1361–1367.

Pascal, C. B. (1987). Selected legal issues about AIDS for drug abuse treatment programs. *J Psychoactive Drugs*, 19, 1–12.

Penkower, L., Dew, M. A., Kingsley, L., Becker, J. T., Satz, P., Schaerf, F. W., &

Sheridan, K. (1991). Behavioral, health and psychosocial factors and risk for HIV infection among sexually active homosexual men: The multicenter AIDS cohort study. *Am J Public Health, 81,* 194–196.

Perry, S., Fishman, B., Jacobsberg, L., Young, J., & Frances, A. (1991). Effectiveness of psychoeducational interventions in decreasing emotional distress after HIV antibody testing. *Arch Gen Psychiatry, 48,* 143–147.

Pol, S., Artru, P., Thepot, V., Berthelot, P., & Nalpas, B. (1996). Improvement of the CD4 cell count after alcohol withdrawal in HIV-positive alcoholic patients [Letter]. *AIDS, 10,* 1293–1294.

Portegies, P. (1995). *The neurology of HIV-1 infection.* London: MediTech Media.

Portegies, P., de Gans, J., Lange, J. M., Derix, M. M., Speelman, H., Bakker, M., et al. (1989). Declining incidence of AIDS dementia complex after introduction of zidovudine treatment. *Br Med J, 299,* 819–821.

Price, R. W. (1995). Management of AIDS dementia complex and HIV-1 infection of the nervous system. *AIDS, 9,* S221–S236.

Price, R. W., Sidtis, J. J., & Brew, B. J. (1991). AIDS dementia complex and HIV-1 infection: A view from the clinic. *Brain Pathol, 1,* 155–160.

Price, R. W., Yiannoutsos, C. T., Clifford, D. B., Zaborski, L., Tselis, A., Siditis, J. J., et al. (1999). Neurological outcomes in late HIV infection: Adverse impact of neurological impairment on survival and protective effect of antiviral therapy. *AIDS, 13,* 1677–1685.

Qureshi, A. I., Hanson, D. L., Jones, J. L., & Janssen, R. S. (1998). Estimation of the temporal probability of human immunodeficiency virus (HIV) dementia after risk stratification for HIV-infected persons. *Neurology, 50,* 392–397.

Reger, M., Welsh, R., Razani, J., Martin, D. J., & Boone, K. B. (2002). A meta-analysis of the neuropsychological sequelae of HIV infection. *J Int Neuropsychol Soc, 8,* 410–424.

Remick, S. C., Diamond, C., Migliozzi, J. A., Solis, O., Wagner, J. R., Haase, R. F., & Ruckderschel, J. C. (1990). Primary central nervous system lymphoma in patients with and without the acquired immune deficiency syndrome: A retrospective analysis and review of the literature. *Medicine, 69,* 345–360.

Reyes, M. G., Faraldi, F., Senseng, C. S., Flowers, C., & Fariello, R. (1991). Nigral degeneration in acquired immune deficiency syndrome (AIDS). *Acta Neuropathol, 82,* 39–44.

Ristow, S. S., Starkey, J. R., & Hass, G. M. (1982). Inhibition of natural killer cell activity in vitro by alcohols. *Biochem Biophys Res Community, 105,* 1315–1521.

Rotheram-Borus, M. J., Rosario, M., Reid, H., & Koopman, C. (1995). Predicting patterns of sexual acts among homosexual and bisexual youths. *Am J Psychiatry, 152,* 588–595.

Sacktor, N. C., & McArthur, J. C. (1997). Prospects for therapy of HIV-associated neurologic disease. *J Neurovirol, 3,* 89–101.

Sambamoorthi, U., Warner, L. A., Crystal, S., & Walkup, J. (2000). Drug abuse, methadone treatment and health services use among injection drug users with AIDS. *Drug Alcohol Depend, 60,* 77–89.

Schleifer. S. J., Benton, T. S., Keller, S. E., & Dhaibar, Y. (2002). Immune measures in alcohol-dependent persons with minor health abnormalities. *Alcohol, 26,* 35–41.

Schleifer, S. J., Keller, S., & Czaja, S. (2003, June). *Major depression, alcoholism and immunity in alcohol dependent persons.* Paper presented at the annual meeting of the Psychoneuroimmunology Research Society, Amelia Island, FL.

Schleifer, S. J., Keller, S. E., Shiflett, S., Benton, T., & Eckholdt, H. (1999). Immune changes in alcohol-dependent patients without medical disorders. *Alcohol Clin Exp Res, 23,* 1199–1206.

Schuckit, M., & Bogard, B. (1986). Intravenous drug use in alcoholics. *J Clin Psychiatry, 47,* 11–16.

Seidman, S. N., Sterk-Elifson, C., & Aral, S. O. (1994). High-risk sexual behavior among drug-using men. *Sex Transm Dis, 21,* 173–180.

Selby, M. J., & Azrin, R. L. (1998). Neuropsychological functioning in drug abusers. *Drug Alcohol Depend, 50,* 39–45.

Selwyn, P. A., & Cox, C. P. (1985, November). *Knowledge about AIDS and high risk behavior among intravenous drug abusers in New York City.* Paper presented at the annual meeting of the American Public Health Association, Washington, DC.

Shapshak, P., Sun, N. C., Resnick, L., Thornwaite, J. T., Schiller, P., Yoshioka, M., et al. (1991). HIV-1 propagates in human neuroblastoma cells. *J Acquir Immune Defic Syndr, 4,* 228–232.

Sidney, S., Beck, J. E., Tekawa, I. S., Quesenberry, C. P., & Friedman, G. C. D. (1997). Marijuana use and mortality. *Am J Public Health, 87,* 585–590.

Singh, G. K., Kochaneck, K. D., & MacDorman, M. F. (1996). Advance report of final mortality statistics, 1994 (Monthly Vital Statistics Report No. 45, 3, S, pp. 1–13). Hyattsville, MD: National Center for Health Statistics.

Skurnick, J. H., Abrams, J., Kennedy, C. A., Valentin, S., & Cordell, J. (1998). Maintenance of safe-sex behavior by HIV-serodiscordant heterosexual couples. *AIDS Educ Prev, 10,* 493–505.

Skurnick, J. H., Kennedy, C. A., Perez, G., Abrams, J., Vermund, S. H., Denny, T., et al. (1998). Behavioral and demographic risk factors for transmission of human immunodeficiency virus type 1 in heterosexual couples: Report from the heterosexual HIV transmission study. *Clin Infect Dis, 26,* 855–864.

Stall, R., McKusick, R., Wiley, J., Coates, T. J., & Ostrow, D. G. (1986). Alcohol and drug use during sexual activity and compliance with safe sex guidelines for AIDS: The AIDS Behavior Research Project. *Health Educ Q, 13,* 359–371.

Stimmel, B. (1988). To test or not to test: The value of routine testing for antibodies to the human immunodeficiency virus (HIV). *Adv Alcohol Subst Abuse, 7,* 2.

Swerdlow, N. R., Hauger, R., Irwin, M., Koob, G. F., Britton, K. T., & Pulvirenti, L. (1991). Endocrine, immune, and neurochemical changes in rats during withdrawal from chronic amphetamine intoxication. *Neuropsychopharmacology, 5,* 23–33.

Tabakoff, B. (1994). Alcohol and AIDS: Is the relationship all in our heads? *Alcohol Clin Exp Res, 18,* 415–416.

Tindall, B., & Cooper, D. A. (1991). Primary HIV infection: Host responses and intervention strategies. *AIDS, 5,* 1–7.

UNAIDS. (2004). AIDS epidemic update: Geneva: World Health Organization.

U.S. General Accounting Office. (1993). *Report to the Chairman, House Select Committee on Narcotics Abuse and Control.* Washington, DC: Author.

Van Dyke, C., Stesin, A., Jones, R., Chuntharapai, A., & Seaman, W. (1986). Cocaine increases natural killer cell activity. *J Clin Invest, 77,* 1387–1390.

Wang, M. Q., Collins, C. B., Kohler, C., DiClemente R. J., & Wingood G. (2000).

Drug use and HIV-risk-related sex behaviors: A street outreach study of black adults. *South Med J, 93,* 186–190.

Watkins, K. E., Metzger, D., Woody, G., & McLellan, A. T. (1993). Determinants of condom use among intravenous drug users. *AIDS, 7,* 719–723.

Watters, J. K., Estilo, M. J., Clark, G. L., & Lorvick, J. (1994). Syringe and needle exchange as HIV/AIDS prevention for injection drug users. *JAMA, 271,* 115–120.

Wilfret, D., & Workshop Participants. (1999). Consensus statement: Science, ethics, and the future of research into maternal infant transmission of HIV-1. *Lancet, 353,* 832–835.

Woods, W. J., Avins, A. L., Lindan, C. P., Hudes, E. S., Boscarino, J. A., & Clark, W. W. (1996). Predictors of HIV-related risk behaviors among heterosexuals in alcoholism treatment. *J Stud Alcohol, 57,* 486–493.

Zenilman, J. M., Hook, E. W., Shepherd, M., Smith, P., Rompalo, A. M., & Celentano, D. D. (1994). Alcohol and other substance use in STD clinic patients: Relationships with STDs and prevalent HIV infection. *Sex Transm Dis, 21,* 220–225.

CHAPTER 20

Addictive Disorders in Women

SHEILA B. BLUME
MONICA L. ZILBERMAN

Why write a chapter on women? Alcoholism and other addictions have traditionally been considered problems of men. The classical studies that have shaped our understanding of the nature and course of these diseases, from Jellinek's (1952) research on phases of alcoholism to Vaillant's (1995) 45-year longitudinal study of alcohol abuse in an inner-city and college cohort, limit themselves to male subjects. The earliest screening tools were developed for men. (The first version of the Michigan Alcohol Screening Test contained a question about the subject's wife, which only later was changed to "spouse.") Treatment methods and programs were also initially designed for male patients, and it was not unusual for women suffering from addictive disorders to be housed on general psychiatric wards, while men were in special units. Male-oriented treatment models, like the so-called boot camps for addicts in the criminal justice system, were "adapted" for women simply by subjecting them to the same program, including masculine clothing and haircuts. Early studies that included information about women often failed to analyze or report these data (Blume, 1980). Although there has been improvement, gender bias in addiction research remained evident in the 1990s (Brett, Graham, & Smythe, 1995).

In spite of these limitations, a growing body of research has identified male–female differences in the way addictions develop and in treatment needs. This chapter summarizes some of the more clinically relevant features of addictive disorders in women. A number of recent reviews are available (Blume & Zilberman, 2004; Center on Addiction and Substance Abuse, 1996; Graham & Schultz, 1998; Zilberman & Blume, 2004), as are several federal publications on the treatment of women (Substance Abuse and Mental Health Services Administration, 2001a; U.S. Department of Health and Human Services, 1993, 1994).

EPIDEMIOLOGY

In general, men are more likely to report any use of psychoactive substances, including alcohol and nicotine. However, changes in use differ by gender. For example, over the last 30 years, the proportion of U.S. men who smoke has fallen at a much greater rate than the corresponding decrease among women, so that the difference is progressively smaller (27 vs. 23%). Among adolescents ages 12–17, girls already outnumber boys in rates of tobacco use (14 vs. 13%). Furthermore, while reduction in the rate of smoking has been detected among boys, the same is not true for girls (Substance Abuse and Mental Health Services Administration, 2001b).

Table 20.1 summarizes data on rates of substance use disorders. These rates were estimated for noninstitutionalized U.S. adults, ages 15–54, from a diagnostic interview based on criteria according to the revised third edition of *Diagnostic and Statistical Manual of Mental Disorders* (DSM-III-R; American Psychiatric Association, 1987), administered to more than 8,000 subjects in the early 1990s as part of the National Comorbidity Survey (Warner, Kessler, Hughes, Anthony, & Nelson, 1995). The overall higher prevalence in men masks subgroup gender differences. Women ages 45–54 reported a higher lifetime prevalence of drug dependence (other than alcohol or nicotine) than did men (3.8% compared to 2.1% for men), whereas the 12-month prevalence is similar between the sexes at this age (0.8% for women, 0.6% for men). This finding

TABLE 20.1. Relative Prevalence of Addictive Disorders in the United States, Ages 15–54

Disorder	Males (%)	Females (5)	Male:female ratio
Lifetime abuse/dependence			
Any substance	35.4	17.9	2.0:1
Alcohol	32.6	14.62	2.2:1
Other drug[a]	14.6	9.4	1.6:1
12-month abuse/dependence			
Any substance	16.1	6.6	2.4:1
Alcohol	14.1	5.3	2.7:1
Other drug[a]	5.1	2.2	2.3:1

Note. Date from the National Comorbidity Study (Warner et al., 1995).
[a] Excludes nicotine; includes nonmedical use of prescription psychotropics.

reflects the higher prevalence of prescription drug dependence in women, whereas men have higher rates of dependence on illicit drugs.

Among young people, ages 15–24, the male rate of 12-month drug dependence (4.5%) is about twice the female rate (2.1%). However, among young people who have used a drug within the past 12 months, the rates are almost equal (males 13.6%, females 10.6%).

Demographic risk factors for alcohol problems in women have been found to be age-dependent in a large general population sample. Women ages 21–34 years reported the highest problem rates. Among them, those who were never married, childless, and not employed ("roleless") were at highest risk. For women ages 35–49, those who were divorced or separated, had children not living with them, and were unemployed ("lost role"), and for women ages 50–64, those who were married, had children not living with them, and were not working outside the home ("role entrapment") had the highest problem rates. The last group is reminiscent of the so-called "empty nest" syndrome described among older women (Blume & Zilberman, 2004).

A prominent risk factor for both alcohol and other drug abuse/dependence in women is a history of physical and/or sexual abuse (Center on Addiction and Substance Abuse, 1996; Simpson & Miller, 2002). In data derived from the Epidemiologic Catchment Area (ECA) study in the early 1980s, it was found that the lifetime prevalence of alcohol abuse/dependence increased threefold and that of other drug abuse/dependence increased fourfold in women who reported a history of sexual assault (Blume & Zilberman, 2004).

Several researchers documented the influence of male "significant others" on the substance use patterns of women (e.g., Amaro & Hardy-Fanta, 1995). Men are likely to introduce women to the use of drugs and to supply drugs to their female partners.

Rates of both alcohol and other drug abuse/dependence are thought to be particularly high among lesbian women (McKirnan & Peterson, 1989) and women in the criminal justice system (Center on Addiction and Substance Abuse, 1996). Among women convicted of homicide, rates of alcohol abuse/ dependence were increased nearly fiftyfold above rates in the general population (Eronen, 1995). Among Jewish Americans who voluntarily participated in two studies, an overrepresentation of women compared to men was found (Vex & Blume, 2001).

PHYSIOLOGICAL FACTORS

Pharmacology

Early research on the pharmacology of alcohol and other drugs was performed on male subjects and thought to apply to both sexes. More recently, however, it has been found that given equal doses of alcohol (even if corrected for body weight), women reach higher blood alcohol levels than men. This fact is partly related to alcohol's distribution in total body water, because women have a greater proportion of fat and less body water than do men. In addition, men have higher levels of the enzyme alcohol dehydrogenase (ADH) in the gastric mucosa, leading to increased metabolism in the stomach (first-pass metabolism) and less absorption into the male bloodstream. Other differences include greater variability in blood alcohol concentrations, faster alcohol metabolism, and reduced acute tolerance to alcohol in women compared to men, leading to more intense and less predictable reactions to alcohol consumption in women than in men (Blume & Zilberman, 2004).

Gender differences in the pharmacology of other drugs are less well studied. The differences in body composition noted previously produce longer half-lives in lipid-soluble drugs such as diazepam and oxazepam in women. Intranasal cocaine administration produces higher subjective effects accompanied by higher plasma levels in men compared to women. Variations in women's plasma levels according to menstrual cycle phases have also been reported (Zilberman & Blume, 2004).

Health Effects

Chronic heavy alcohol use has been linked to many serious medical complications in both sexes (National Institute on Alcohol Abuse and Alcoholism, 2000). However, many of these complications develop more rapidly in women, with a lower level of alcohol intake. Included are hepatic steatosis and cirrhosis, hypertension, anemia, malnutrition, gastrointestinal hemorrhage, peptic ulcer, and both peripheral myopathy and cardiomyopathy. Both human immunodeficiency virus (HIV) infection and other sexually transmitted diseases are linked to substance use disorders in women (Center on Addiction and Substance Abuse, 1996). Seventy percent of currently HIV-infected women acquired the virus either through injection drug use or during sexual relations with a drug-injecting partner, compared to less than half of HIV-infected men. Addicted women, particularly those dependent on crack cocaine or heroin, often become infected by exchanging sex for drugs or by engaging in prostitution to obtain money for drugs.

Alcohol and other drug use is closely linked to smoking in women. Mortality for lung cancer in U.S. women surpassed breast cancer mortality in 1986 to become the leading cause of cancer death. The risks for coronary artery disease, obstructive lung disease, peptic ulcer, and early menopause, as well as cancers of the mouth, larynx, esophagus, stomach, bladder, and cervix are increased in female smokers (Zilberman & Blume, 2004), as is the risk for breast cancer in female drinkers (National Institute on Alcohol Abuse and Alcoholism, 2000).

Effects on Reproductive Functioning

Whereas single doses of alcohol have little effect on sex hormone levels in women, chronic heavy drinking leads to inhibition of ovulation, infertility, and a variety of reproductive and sexual dysfunctions (Blume & Zilberman, 2004).

Consumption of alcohol by women suppresses both sexual arousal and orgasmic function in a dose–response fashion. The physiological reality is contrary to the widely held cultural belief that alcohol is an aphrodisiac for women (Blume, 1991). This belief often leads alcoholic women to expect that they need alcohol to perform and enjoy the sexual act, in spite of their alcohol-related sexual problems. The clinician can help such women by explaining that their drinking has depressed rather than enhanced their sexual responsiveness, and that in the presence of a loving relationship, they will find sex more enjoyable in recovery than they did while drinking (Gavaler, Rizzo, & Rossaro, 1993).

Cocaine and amphetamines are widely believed by their users to be sexual stimulants, whereas chronic use is often associated with loss of sexual desire and inhibited orgasm. In addition, cocaine use has been associated with menstrual alterations, galactorrhea, infertility, hyperprolactinemia, and increased levels of luteinizing hormones in women (Mendelson, Sholar, Siegel, & Mello, 2001). Heroin use has been reported to suppress both ovulation and sexual desire, as has abuse of sedative drugs (Zilberman & Blume, 2004).

Fetal Alcohol and Drug Effects

Fetal alcohol syndrome (FAS), a combination of birth defects producing life-long disability, is currently estimated to affect about 1–3 infants for every 1,000 live births in the United States. FAS is thus among the three most frequent birth defects resulting in mental retardation, with a prevalence similar to Down syndrome and spina bifida. A diagnosis of FAS is based on the co-occurrence of pre- and postnatal growth deficiency, structural facial abnormalities, and central nervous system dysfunctions, including poor coordination, mental retardation, and/or behavioral dyscontrol. In addition, a wide variety of other birth defects affecting vision, hearing, and other body systems are often seen in these children. Although the full FAS syndrome is seen almost exclusively in the offspring of alcoholic women who drink heavily (an average of six or more drinks per day) during pregnancy, women who drink at lower levels are at risk for fetal alcohol effects such as miscarriage, low birthweight, birth defects, and behavioral abnormalities (Warren et al., 2001). The prevalence of fetal alcohol effects is thought to be many times greater than that of FAS.

Fetal damage is also associated with other drug use and abuse (Singer et al., 2002). Cigarette smoking during pregnancy is implicated as an important factor in miscarriage, low birthweight, and sudden infant death syndrome. Unfortunately, many young women believe that cocaine facilitates a quick and less painful delivery, whereas it actually produces obstetric complications that cause damage to the newborn, as well as birth defects secondary to its deleterious effects on fetal circulation. Pregnant heroin addicts are customarily treated with methadone as a maintenance drug rather than detoxification to abstinence, as a safer regimen for the fetus. With good prenatal care, such patients can be brought to term and experience normal deliveries. However, their infants require treatment for neonatal opiate withdrawal (U.S. Department of Health and Human Services, 1993).

Whether or not birth defects occur, untreated substance abuse/dependence in a new mother will interfere with maternal–infant bonding, parenting, and family life. Thus, pregnancy is a critical time for case finding and intervention. Among the approximately 4 million pregnancies in the United States annually, approximately 12% of women smoke (Ibrahim, Floyd, Merritt, & De Couble, 2000), 23% use alcoholic beverages, and 4.4% use other substances (Substance Abuse and Mental Health Services Administration, 2002).

GENETIC INFLUENCES

A great deal of research has been devoted to the effort to differentiate genetic from environmental factors in the etiology of alcoholism, as well as other drug dependencies. Almost all implicate a combination of nature and nurture (Kendler, Walters, & Neale, 1995). Of interest here is that some studies show different patterns of alcoholism heredity for men and women (Prescott, Aggen, & Kendler, 1999).

Studies of possible genetic markers in children of alcoholics have largely been confined to males, or to a small number of women. Daughters of alcoholic parents have also been found to have more positive and pleasant mood reactions to a single dose of alprazolam, suggesting that they may be at greater risk for abuse of this drug. Regarding the heritability of drug use disorders, there is indication that genetic influences are stronger for males than for females, while environmental factors are more evident in females than in males (Blume & Zilberman, 2004; Zilberman & Blume, 2004).

In addition, some research suggests that there is a genetic link between alcoholism in male relatives and major depressive disease in women, in a combination of genetic and environmental causation (Cadoret et al., 1996). A study in female twin pairs suggests separate heredity but common environmental risk factors for comorbid alcoholism and major depression in women (Kendler, Heath, Neale, Kessler, & Eaves, 1993).

PSYCHOLOGICAL FACTORS

The role of psychological factors in the etiology of substance use disorders has been a subject of uncertainty for many years. Long-term longitudinal studies of male alcoholics have found that psychiatric disorders and symptoms are more likely to be the result of alcoholism than to have been predisposing factors (Vaillant, 1995). However, the lack of similar studies in women leaves the question open. The strong association between childhood physical and sexual abuse and later addictive disease in women, alluded to in the section "Epidemiology," suggests mediation through psychological symptoms such as low self-esteem, depression, shame, guilt, and feelings of sexual inadequacy. One of the few longitudinal studies that did include women, a 27-year follow-up of a college drinking study, looked at risk factors for later drinking problems. These factors were different for males and females. Although women who had alcohol-related problems in college had a higher prevalence of later problems than did their female classmates, the women at highest risk for problems later in life were those who reported in college that they drank to relieve shyness, to feel gay, to get along better on dates, and to get high. This pattern suggests psychological dependence as a risk factor for women (Blume & Zilberman, 2004).

Another approach to the study of psychological factors is to examine gender differences in the patterns of comorbid psychiatric disorders in identified alcoholics and other drug addicts. Both in general population studies and in clinical populations, female alcoholics and addicts have higher rates of comorbid psychiatric disorders in general, and higher rates of depressive and anxiety disorders in particular, compared to males (Zilberman, Tavares, Blume, & el-Guebaly, 2003). In fact, the only comorbid diagnoses found more frequently in addicted males are residual attention deficit disorder, antisocial personality disorder, and pathological gambling (Lesieur, Blume, & Zoppa, 1986). Eating disorders (Walfish, Stenmark, Sarco, Shealy, & Krone, 1992) and posttraumatic stress disorder (commonly related in women to sexual abuse) (Kessler, Sonnega, Bromet, Hughes, & Nelson, 1995) are seen frequently in women with addictions.

Of particular interest from the point of view of etiology is the question concerning which disorders occur first (primary) and which develop subsequently (secondary). As mentioned earlier, Vaillant (1995) found that alcoholism was usually primary in men. However, in the general population ECA study, it was found that among adults with lifetime diagnoses of both alcohol abuse/dependence and major depression, depression was primary in 66% of the women compared to only 22% of men. Likewise, in an inpatient alcoholism treatment population, it was found that depression was primary in 66% of the women with comorbid major depression compared to 41% of men. Similar findings were reported for alcoholic research volunteers (Roy et al., 1991) and dual-diagnosed adolescents. Longitudinal survey evidence in women also tends to support a relationship between earlier reports of depression and later increases in alcohol use or chronicity of alcohol problems. Interestingly, alcohol use at time 1 in these longitudinal studies in women also predicted later depression (Blume & Zilberman, 2004). Similar findings have been reported in a longitudinal study of adolescents (Brook, Brook, Zhang, Cohen, & Whiteman, 2002).

Taken together, the previous discussion suggests some link between primary depression and secondary alcoholism in women. Because alcohol is not an effective antidepressant (Vaillant, 1995), the link is probably not simple self-medication. Further research is needed to elucidate this relationship. However, the relationship highlights the need to take careful psychiatric histories in all women suffering from addictive disorders, with special emphasis on the temporal development of comorbid disorders. Patients whose depression preceded their addiction or occurred during a prolonged period of abstinence are likely to have a primary depressive disorder requiring specific treatment, whereas depression secondary to addiction is more likely to improve spontaneously with recovery from the addiction. In addition, patients with primary depression should be warned about the possibility of recurrence and carefully educated to recognize early symptoms of a recurrent major depressive episode. Vigorous treatment of such an episode during remission of the patient's addiction can avoid alcohol/drug relapse and promote further progress in the patient's recovery.

SOCIOCULTURAL FACTORS

As pointed out in the section "Genetic Influences," environmental factors are particularly important in the etiology of addictive disorders in women. Sociocultural influences include general cultural and subcultural norms for alcohol, tobacco, and other drug use; culturally based attitudes and beliefs about such use (including popular media stereotypes of users and abusers); peer pressure; prescription practices; laws regulating availability and use; and the economics of supply, demand, price, and disposable income. In all societies that allow alcohol and/or drug use, these norms, attitudes, stereotypes, peer pressures, and even laws (dating as far back as the Code of Hammurabi in 2000 B.C.E.) differ for males and females.

Social attitudes act as a double-edged sword for women. On the one hand, the expectation that women will drink lower quantities of alcoholic beverages and drink less frequently is protective (Blume & Zilberman, 2004). On the other hand, the intense stigma linked to stereotypes of alcoholic and addicted women creates serious problems for women who drink and/or use other drugs (Blume, 1991). Behavior tolerated in men is considered scandalous for women. Compare the expression "drunk as a lord" with its feminine equivalent, "drunk as a lady." In addition, the drinking/drugging woman is considered promiscuous. Society believes, contrary to fact, that alcohol is a sexual stimulant for women, so that a woman under the influence who says "no" really means "yes." Although a general population survey of nearly 1,000 women failed to find evidence that women who drink become less particular in their choice of sexual partner, even if drinking heavily, women's drinking is a frequent rationalization for sexual assault, including date rape (Blume, 1991). In a study of beliefs about rape, young adults considered a rapist who is intoxicated less responsible for the crime, whereas they considered a victim who has been drinking more to blame. It is not surprising, then, that alcoholic women are much more likely to be victims of violent crime, including rape, than are matched controls. These women are also more likely to report spousal violence than are control women. Society's view of alcohol/drug-abusing women is one of moral and sexual degradation, making them acceptable targets for sexual aggression (Blume, 1991).

Another result of this stigma is denial on the personal, family, and societal levels. A woman in the early stage of alcohol/drug dependence, accepting the cultural stereotype, denies that she may have a problem ("I'm not like that!"). Families also deny that the difficulty with their mother, daughter, sister, or wife could be alcoholism or addiction ("She's not like that!"). Physicians and other health professionals often fail to diagnose alcoholism in patients who do not resemble social stereotypes. Alcoholic patients least likely to be correctly identified in a large general hospital study were those with higher incomes and educational levels, those with private insurance, and those who were female (Blume & Zilberman, 2004).

As the disease progresses in the addicted woman, intense guilt and shame often drive the sufferer into hiding, so that the alcoholic woman is far more likely to drink alone than is the alcoholic man. If she lives alone or is a single parent with small children, there may be no significant others in her social network able to recognize her problem and intervene. Although alcoholic women frequently seek medical help for a variety of complaints ranging from infertility, depression, anxiety, or insomnia to hypertension and peptic ulcer, their guilt, shame, and denial require that the interviewing professional screen actively for alcohol/drug problems. Undetected alcohol/drug use disorders can lead to inappropriate symptomatic treatment, with the danger of adding dependence on prescription sedatives, analgesics, or tranquilizers to the patient's problems. Failure in diagnosis in women of childbearing age may lead to the appearance of preventable birth defects in their offspring. Finally, delay in diagnosis allows the development of late-stage physical, psychological, and social complications, making eventual treatment more costly, more difficult, and less successful. Early diagnosis and adequate treatment of substance use disorders in women is also an important component in the prevention of teen pregnancy, acquired immune deficiency syndrome, hepatitis, suicide, and other negative outcomes.

CLINICAL FEATURES OF ADDICTIVE DISORDERS IN WOMEN

Table 20.2 summarizes the more important features that have been described in the literature as differentiating addictive disorders in women from their occurrence in men. In general, alcoholic women are less likely to report "acting out" behaviors such as breaking the law, problems with the criminal justice system, or feeling "out of control." Women more commonly report problems with health and family, and psychological symptoms such as depression and low self-esteem. Because of the differences in self-identified problems and clinical manifestations, investigators developed several screening tools designed specially to identify alcoholism in women. These include the T-ACE (Sokol, Martier, & Ager, 1989), TWEAK (Russell, Martier, & Sokol, 1994), SWAG (Spak & Hallstrom, 1996) and Health Questionnaire (Blume & Russell, 1993). Laboratory testing has also been found helpful in screening for alcoholism in women. In a cohort of 100 early-stage alcoholic women, it was found that a screening criterion of either an elevated gamma-glutamyl transferase (GGT) or an increased mean corpuscular volume (MCV) correctly identified two-thirds of the women. The same two laboratory tests were found useful in screening an obstetric population and predicting birth defects (Blume & Zilberman, 2004).

Although the clinical presentation of any individual patient depends on a combination of physical, psychological, and social factors, sex differences in symptoms and problems are themselves subject to social and cultural influences. Thus, sex differences may be expected to change over time as society itself changes.

Mortality rates for alcoholic women are high compared to both the general population of women and alcoholic men (Klatsky, Armstrong, & Friedman,

---

TABLE 20.2. Features of Addictive Disorders in Women, Compared to Men

- Start substance use later (A).
- Disease progresses more rapidly (A, C).
- Drink significantly less than males (A, C, O).
- "Significant other" more likely to be substance abuser (A, C, O).
- Higher rates of comorbid psychiatric disorders (A, C).
- Higher rates of comorbid prescription drug dependence (A).
- More likely to make suicide attempts (A).
- More likely to have a history of physical and sexual abuse (A, C, O).
- More often date the onset of pathological alcohol/drug use to a specific stressful event (A, C).
- More likely to report previous psychiatric treatment (A).
- Higher mortality rate (A).

Note. See Blume and Zilberman (2004); White, Brady, and Sonne (1996); Lewis, Bucholz, Spitznagel, and Shayka (1996); and Griffin, Weiss, and Mirin (1989). A, reported for alcoholism; C, reported for cocaine; O, reported for other drugs.

1992). In a longitudinal study of 5,000 treated alcoholics, the mortality rate for men was three times the expected rate, whereas for women it was 5.2 times the comparable rate in the general public (Lindberg & Agren, 1988).

TREATMENT OF ADDICTIVE DISORDERS IN WOMEN

Although utilization of treatment resources for alcoholism has increased during recent years, women remain underrepresented in treatment. When women do look for help, they are more likely to use mental health services and other facilities not specific to addiction (Weisner & Schmidt, 1992). The reasons for this, including social stigma, denial, and the frequent failure to diagnose women, have been mentioned. In addition, however, the most common current, organized case-finding methods (e.g., drinking driver programs, drug courts, and employee assistance programs) are primarily useful for identifying male alcoholics/addicts. Appropriate settings for identifying women in need of treatment would be medical settings of all kinds (including mental health facilities) and family counseling services. Unfortunately, organized screening in health facilities is the exception rather than the rule, and women identified in these settings are usually in late stages of addiction.

Research on the effectiveness of treatment for women has employed a wide variety of methods (Ashley, Marsden, & Brady, 2003). In general, adult women and men treated together in the same specialized addiction programs do about equally well (Vannicelli, 1986). A recent study reported that although problem-drinking women started off more symptomatic than men, they actually did better than men at the 8-year follow-up in different interventions. Particularly, women seem to benefit from maintained Alcoholics Anonymous (AA) attendance (Timko, Moos, Finney, & Connell, 2002). Studies of special women´s programming have shown positive effects, although few have employed random assignment techniques. Research supports the value of adding child care, mother–child residential programming, all-female counseling groups, and supplemental women-focused educational sessions (e.g., sexual and reproductive counseling, assertiveness, parenting, and communication skills training) (Ashley et al., 2003). Comprehensive programming, combining several of these specific components, is also effective. Whether women-only programs are superior to mixed programs is still not well established. The only published random-assignment study found a superior outcome in a 2-year follow-up of 100 alcoholic women randomly assigned to a specialized women's clinic compared to 100 assigned to a mixed-sex treatment (Dahlgren & Willander, 1989). A women-only self-help program, Women for Sobriety, is thriving in some parts of the country (Kaskutas, 1996), while the number of women utilizing AA is also growing, and women-only AA groups are available in some areas. Based on what is known about the characteristics of addicted women, Table 20.3 sum-

TABLE 20.3. Special Considerations in Women's Treatment

- Psychiatric assessment for comorbid disorders; date of onset for each (primary/secondary).
- Attention to past history and present risk of physical and sexual assault.
- Assessment of prescription drug abuse/dependence.
- Comprehensive physical examination for physical complications and comorbid disorders.
- Need for access to health care (including obstetric care).
- Psychoeducation to include information on substance use in pregnancy.
- Child-care services for women in treatment.
- Parenting education and assistance.
- Evaluation and treatment of significant others and children.
- Positive female role models (among treatment staff; self-help).
- Attention to guilt, shame, and self-esteem issues.
- Assessment and treatment of sexual dysfunction.
- Attention to the effects of sexism in the previous experience of the patient (e.g., underemployment, lack of opportunity, and rigid sex roles).
- Avoidance of iatrogenic drug dependence.
- Special attention to the needs of minority women, lesbian women, and those in the criminal justice system.

marizes the special emphases that have been found helpful in treating these women. For pregnant women, the provision of prenatal care, along with women-centered programming, has been shown to improve both treatment retention and birth outcomes (Ashley et al., 2003).

The good news is that specific program components for women can be added to existing programs, and staff sensitivity can be improved by training. The bad news is that, in a large survey, only 19% of addiction programs reported providing special programming for pregnant or postpartum women, and only 28% offered women's programming at all (Office of Applied Studies, 2000). We can and must do better.

PREVENTION

Effective primary prevention of alcohol, tobacco, and other drug dependence in women has received little research attention, with the exception of specific public education campaigns to prevent FAS. Such efforts have proven more effective in persuading light and moderate drinkers to abstain during pregnancy than in persuading the heaviest alcohol consumers. Thus, screening in medical and obstetric practice remains essential.

In designing educational approaches in the schools and for the general public, it is important to remember the double-edged sword quality of societal attitudes. The goal of reducing the social stigma attached to the female addict must be balanced against that of preserving the cultural expectation that women will practice abstinence or moderation. Straightforward information should be provided about women's sensitivity to alcohol; principles for the safe use of prescribed psychoactive drugs; the health effects of tobacco, alcohol, and other drugs particular to women (e.g., breast cancer, birth defects, and obstetric complications); the dangers of using substances to "medicate" feelings of inadequacy or sexual problems; and the special risks of women from alcoholic families. These general education efforts are particularly important, because the alcoholic beverage industry has targeted women as a "growth market," linking drinking in their advertisements with youth, beauty, sexual attractiveness, and success. Such advertising sends messages that can alter the cultural norms that protect women. Likewise, cigarette advertising aimed at women stressing slimness and "liberation" (e.g., the slogan "You've come a long way baby") tends to make smoking more socially acceptable for women and adolescent girls. Because smoking is more strongly associated with the use of illegal drugs in girls than boys (Center on Addiction and Substance Abuse, 1996), smoking among adolescent girls should be a priority prevention target.

In addition to general population efforts, specific alcohol/drug prevention techniques should be aimed at high-risk groups such as adolescent and adult daughters of alcoholics/addicts, victims of physical and sexual abuse, women entering new social groups with different drinking customs (e.g., college freshmen and women entering the military), women undergoing stressful life transitions (e.g., divorce, widowhood, childbirth, and reentry into the labor force), and women acting as caretaker for a chronically ill relative. Such risk groups can be helped to develop self-esteem and coping skills that do not involve substance use.

Laws and their applications also exert an important influence on substance use disorders in women. Recently, the resources of the criminal justice system have been used to initiate prosecution of women who use alcohol and other drugs during pregnancy. Such women have been charged with "prenatal child abuse" or "delivery of controlled substances to a minor" (via the umbilical cord). Although many cases have been thrown out of court, and many convictions have been reversed on appeal, the result of these policies has been less often prevention of substance use than deterring pregnant substance users from seeking either prenatal or addiction treatment (Harris & Paltrow, 2003).

In summarizing this overview of use and abuse of psychoactive substances by girls and women in the United States, it is clear that our society has strong feelings about such use but has not translated those feelings into an adequate investment in prevention, treatment, and research. Let us hope that a renewed focus on the problems of women will stimulate medical and social policymakers to rethink the priority devoted to this issue.

REFERENCES

Amaro, H., & Hardy-Fanta, C. (1995). Gender relations in addiction and recovery. *J Psychoactive Drugs, 27*, 325–333.

American Psychiatric Association. (1987). *Diagnostic and statistical manual of mental disorders* (3rd ed., rev.). Washington, DC: Author.

Ashley, O. S., Marsden, M. E., & Brady, T. M. (2003). Effectiveness of substance abuse treatment programming for women: A review. *Am J Drug Alcohol Abuse, 29*(1), 19–54.

Blume, S. B. (1980). Researches on women and alcohol. In *Alcohol and women* (Research Monograph No. 1, DHEW Publication No. ADM 80-835, pp. 121–151). Washington, DC: U.S. Department of Health, Education and Welfare.

Blume, S. B. (1991). Sexuality and stigma: The alcoholic woman. *Alcohol Health Res World, 15*(2), 139–146.

Blume, S. B., & Russell, M. (1993). Alcohol and substance abuse in the practice of obstetrics and gynecology. In D. E. Stewart & N. L. Stotland (Eds.), *Psychological aspects of women's health care: The interface between psychiatry and obstetrics and gynecology* (pp. 391–409). Washington, DC: American Psychiatric Press.

Blume, S. B., & Zilberman, M. L. (2004). *Alcohol and women.* In J. Lowinson, P. Ruiz, R. B. Millman, & J. G. Langrodet (Eds.), *Substance abuse: A comprehensive textbook* (4th ed., pp. 1049–1063). Philadelphia: Lippincott/Williams & Wilkins.

Brett, P. J., Graham, K., & Smythe, C. (1995). An analysis of specialty journals on alcohol, drugs and addictive behaviors for sex bias in research methods and reporting. *J Stud Alcohol, 56*, 24–34.

Brook, D. W., Brook, J. S., Zhang, C., Cohen, P. & Whiteman, M. (2002). Drug use and the risk of major depressive disorder, alcohol dependence and substance use disorders. *Arch Gen Psychiatry, 59*, 1039–1044.

Cadoret, R. J., Winokur, G., Langbehn, D., Troughton, E., Yates, W. R., & Stewart, M. A. (1996). Depression spectrum disease: I. The role of gene–environment interaction. *Am J Psychiatry, 153*, 892–899.

Center on Addiction and Substance Abuse. (1996). *Substance abuse and American women.* New York: Author.

Dahlgren, L., & Willander, A. (1989). Are special treatment facilities for female alcoholics needed?: A controlled 2-year follow-up study from a specialized female unit (EWA) versus a mixed male/female treatment facility. *Alcohol Clin Exp Res, 13*(4), 499–504.

Eronen, M. (1995). Mental disorders and homicidal behavior in female subjects. *Am J Psychiatry, 152*(8), 1216–1218.

Gavaler, J. S., Rizzo, A., & Rossaro, L. (1993). Sexuality of alcoholic women with menstrual cycle function: Effects of duration of alcohol abstinence. *Alcohol Clin Exp Res, 17*, 778–781.

Graham, A. W., & Schultz, T. K. (Eds.). (1998). *Principles of addiction medicine: Women, infants and addiction* (2nd ed., pp. 1171–1238). Chevy Chase, MD: American Society of Addiction Medicine.

Griffin, M. L., Weiss, R. L., & Mirin, S. M. (1989). A comparison of male and female cocaine abusers. *Arch Gen Psychiatry, 46*, 122–126.

Harris, L. H., & Paltrow, L. (2003). MSJAMA: The status of pregnant women and fetuses in US criminal law. *JAMA, 289*(13), 1697–1699.

Ibrahim, S. H., Floyd, R. L., Merritt, R. K., & De Couble, P. (2000). Trends in pregnancy-related smoking rates in the United States 1987–1996. *JAMA, 283*(3), 361–366.

Jellinek, E. M. (1952). Phases of alcohol addiction. *Q J Stud Alcohol, 13*, 673–684.

Kaskutas, L. A. (1996). Pathways to self-help among women for sobriety. *Am J Drug Alcohol Abuse, 22*(2), 259–280.

Kendler, K. S., Heath, A. C., Neale, M. C., Kessler, R. C., & Eaves, L. J. (1993). Alcoholism and major depression in women: A twin study of the causes of comorbidity. *Arch Gen Psychiatry, 50*(9), 690–698.

Kendler, K. S., Walters, M. S., & Neale, M. C. (1995). The structure of the genetic and environmental risk factors for six major psychiatric disorders in women. *Arch Gen Psychiatry, 52*, 374–383.

Kessler, R. C., Sonnega, A., Bromet, E., Hughes, M., & Nelson, C. B. (1995). Posttraumatic stress disorder in the national comorbidity survey. *Arch Gen Psychiatry, 52*(12), 1048–1060.

Klatsky, A. L., Armstrong, M. A., & Friedman, G. D. (1992). Alcohol and mortality. *Ann Intern Med, 117*, 646–654.

Lesieur, H. R., Blume, S. B., & Zoppa, R. M. (1986). Alcoholism, drug abuse, and gambling. *Alcohol Clin Exp Res, 10*(1), 33–38.

Lewis, C. E., Bucholz, K. K., Spitznagel, E., & Shayka, J. J. (1996). Effects of gender and comorbidity on problem drinking in a community sample. *Alcohol Clin Exp Res, 20*(3), 466–476.

Lindberg, S., & Agren G. (1988). Mortality among male and female hospitalized alcoholics in Stockholm 1962–1983. *Br J Addict, 83*, 1193–1200.

McKirnan, D. J., & Peterson, P. L. (1989). Alcohol and drug use among homosexual men and women: Epidemiology and population characteristics. *Addict Behav, 14*, 545–553.

Mendelson, J. H., Sholar, M. B., Siegel, A. J., & Mello, N. K. (2001). Effects of cocaine on luteinizing hormone in women during the follicular and luteal phases of the menstrual cycle and in men. *J Pharmacol Exp Ther, 296*, 972–979.

National Institute on Alcohol Abuse and Alcoholism. (2000). *Tenth special report to the U.S. Congress on alcohol and health* (NIH Publication No. 00-1583, pp. 197–338). Washington, DC: U.S. Department of Health and Human Services.

Office of Applied Studies. (2000). Uniform Facility Data Set (DHHS Publication No. [SMA] 00-3463). Rockville, MD: Substance Abuse and Mental Health Services Administration.

Prescott, C. A., Aggen, S. H., & Kendler, K. S. (1999). Sex differences in the sources of genetic liability to alcohol abuse and dependence in a population-based sample of U.S. twins. *Alcohol Clin Exp Res, 23*, 1136–1144.

Roy, A., DeJong, J., Lamparski, D., Adinoff, B., George, T., Moore, V., et al. (1991). Mental disorders among alcoholics. *Arch Gen Psychiatry, 48*, 423–427.

Russell, M., Martier, S. S., & Sokol, R. J. (1994). Screening for pregnancy risk-drinking: Tweaking the tests. *Alcohol Clin Exp Res, 18*, 1156–1161.

Simpson, T. L., & Miller, W. R. (2002). Concomitance between childhood sexual and physical abuse and substance use problems: A review. *Clin Psychol Rev, 22*, 27–77.

Singer, L. T., Arendt, R., Minnes, S., Farkas, K., Salvator, A., Kirchner, H. L., & Kliegman, R. (2002). Cognitive and motor outcomes of cocaine-exposed infants. *JAMA, 287*, 1952–1960.

Sokol, R. J., Martier, S. S., & Ager, J. W. (1989). The T-ACE questions: Practical prenatal detection of risk-drinking. *Am J Obstet Gynecol, 160*, 863–870.

Spak, F., & Hallstrom, T. (1996). Screening for alcohol dependence and abuse in women: Description, validation, and psychometric properties of a new screening instrument, SWAG, in a population study. *Alcohol Clin Exp Res, 20*(4), 723–731.

Substance Abuse and Mental Health Services Administration. (2001a). *Benefits of residential substance abuse treatment for pregnant and parenting women: Highlights from a study of 50 demonstration programs of the Center for Substance Abuse Treatment.* Rockville, MD: U.S. Department of Health and Human Services.

Substance Abuse and Mental Health Services Administration. (2001b). *Summary of findings from the 2000 National Household Survey on Drug Abuse* (Office of Applied Studies, NHSDA Series H-13, DHHS Publication No. [SMA] 01-3549). Rockville, MD: U.S. Department of Health and Human Services.

Substance Abuse and Mental Health Services Administration. (2002). *National Household Survey on Drug Abuse Survey Report 5/17/02.* Retrieved April 10, 2003, from *www.samhsa.gov/oas/2k2/preg/preg.htm*

Timko, C., Moos, R. H., Finney, J. W., & Connell, E. G. (2002). Gender differences in help-utilization and the 8-year course of alcohol abuse. *Addiction, 97*(7), 877–889.

U.S. Department of Health and Human Services. (1993). *Pregnant, substance-using women* (DHSS Publication No. [SMA] 93-1998). Rockville, MD: Author.

U.S. Department of Health and Human Services. (1994). *Practical approaches in the treatment of women who abuse alcohol and other drugs* (DHSS Publication No. [SMA] 94-3006). Rockville, MD: Author.

Vaillant, G. E. (1995). *The natural history of alcoholism revisited.* Cambridge, MA: Harvard University Press.

Vannicelli, M. (1986). Treatment considerations. In *Women and alcohol: Health-related issues* (Research Monograph No. 16, Publication No. ADM 86-1139, pp. 130–153). Washington, DC: U.S. Department of Health and Human Services.

Vex, S. L., & Blume, S. B. (2001). The JACS Study I: Characteristics of a population of chemically dependent Jewish men and women. *J Addict Dis, 20*(4), 71–89.

Walfish, S., Stenmark, D. E., Sarco, D., Shealy, J. S., & Krone, A. M. (1992). Incidence of bulimia in substance misusing women in residential treatment. *Int J Addict, 27*(4), 425–433.

Warner, L. A., Kessler, R. C., Hughes, M., Anthony, J. C., & Nelson, C. B. (1995). Prevalence and correlates of drug use and dependence in the United States. *Arch Gen Psychiatry, 52*(3), 219–228.

Warren, K. R., Calhoun, F. J., May, P. A., Viljoen, D. L., Li, T. K., Tanaka, H., et al. (2001). Fetal alcohol syndrome: An international perspective. *Alcohol Clin Exp Res, 25*, 202S–206S.

Weisner, C., & Schmidt, L. (1992). Gender disparities in treatment for alcohol problems. JAMA, 268(14), 1872–1876.

White, K. A., Brady, K. T., & Sonne, S. (1996). Gender differences in patterns of cocaine use. Am J Addict, 5(3), 259–261.

Zilberman, M. L., & Blume, S. B. (2004). Drugs and women. In J. Lowinson, P. Ruiz, R. B. Millman, & J. G. Langrodet (Eds.), Substance abuse: A comprehensive textbook (4th ed., pp. 1064–1079). Philadelphia: Lippincott/Williams & Wilkins.

Zilberman, M. L., Tavares, H., Blume, S. B., & el-Guebaly, N. (2003). Substance use disorders: Sex differences in psychiatric comorbidities. Can J Psychiatry, 48(1), 5–15.

PART V

TREATMENTS FOR ADDICTIONS

TREATMENTS FOR ADDICTION

CHAPTER 21

Individual Psychodynamic Psychotherapy

LANCE M. DODES
EDWARD J. KHANTZIAN

Individual psychotherapy is widely used in treatment of addicts, though it is perhaps still underappreciated in comparison with group modalities, including self-help groups. Many addicts benefit from a combination of simultaneous individual and group treatments, and some require the individual psychotherapy to be able to remain with other treatments (Khantzian, 1986). Furthermore, a significant number cannot, or choose not to, make use of other treatment and can only be treated successfully with individual psychotherapy. This chapter rearticulates and extends ideas that we and others have developed previously, based on our understanding and treatment experience with addicted individuals over many years (Dodes, 1984, 1988, 1990, 1996, 2002, 2003; Dodes & Khantzian, 1991; Flores, 2004; Kaufman, 1994; Khantzian, 1980, 1986, 1995, 1999a, 1999b, 2001, 2003; Khantzian, Dodes, & Brehm, 2005; Walant, 1995).

The rationale for individual psychotherapy with addicts arises from an understanding of the psychological factors that contribute to addiction. Contemporary psychodynamic formulations stress the role of conflict, the object meaning of alcohol or drugs, deficits and dysfunctions in ego functioning, and narcissistic deficits as important factors in reliance on substances (Dodes & Khantzian, 1991). These deficits and dysfunctions result in self-regulation disturbances involving affects, self-esteem maintenance, and the capacity for self-care and self–other relations. These areas of psychological vulnerability or dysfunction contribute significantly to addictions and are targeted in psychotherapy (Khantzian, 1986, 1995, 1999b, 2001).

Although we believe that there are indications for referring addicts to psychotherapy, often patients themselves begin the treatment of their addiction with psychotherapy (perhaps particularly those who are more psychologically oriented). Others start individual psychotherapy after first seeking treatment through self-help groups or a more educationally based treatment program, such as that offered in many inpatient settings and outpatient clinics. In either case, via exploring their emotional issues, patients begin to understand not only their own psychology but also the place of substance abuse in their emotional lives. This understanding not only addresses the reasons for their continued problems even when chemical free but also, by placing the substance problem in the context of their emotional lives, provides a strong internal basis for avoiding relapse.

Another route into individual psychotherapy for addicted patients is via repeated treatment failures in other, less introspective settings. Some of these patients repeatedly relapse, despite clear and conscious motivation to abstain, because they are unaware of the internal, largely unconscious factors that lead them to resume substance use. Failing to recognize the role of unconscious processes causes patients to attribute their behavior to lack of willpower, which contributes further to their self-devaluation. Learning about themselves in individual psychotherapy thus contributes not only to a more stable chemical-free state and to overall general improvement in emotional function but also to diminished shame concerning their addiction.

Many addicts may also successfully pursue individual psychotherapy in conjunction with other treatment (e.g., Alcoholics Anonymous [AA], Narcotics Anonymous [NA], or a professionally led group therapy). In such cases, the individual work aims for the usual goals of insight and emotional growth, while the other modalities focus on supporting the patient's chemical-free state.

A number of studies substantiate the value of individual psychotherapy with addicts. Woody and colleagues (1983) noted that in seven investigations with methadone-treated patients, where patients were randomly assigned to psychotherapy or a different treatment (most often drug counseling), five of the studies showed better outcome in the psychotherapy group. Woody's own group also found that patients who received psychotherapy and drug counseling had better results than did patients who received drug counseling alone, when measured in terms of number of areas of improvement, less use of illicit opiates, and lower doses of methadone required. This group (Woody, McLellan, Luborsky, & O'Brien, 1986) noted further that the patients with the most disturbed global psychiatric ratings benefited particularly from psychotherapy, as compared with drug counseling. A number of investigators documented early a high correlation between psychiatric disorders, especially depression, and addiction (Khantzian & Treece, 1985; Rounsaville, Weissman, Kleber, & Wilber, 1982). These findings have been substantiated in a more recent series of clinical and epidemiological studies (Carroll & Rounsaville, 1992; Halikas, Crosby,

Pearson, Nugent, & Carlson, 1994; Kessler et al., 1997; Kleinman, Miller, & Millman, 1990; Penick et al., 1994; Regier et al., 1990; Rounsaville et al., 1991; Schuckit & Hesselbrock, 1994; Schuckit, Irwin, & Brown, 1990; Wilens, Biederman, Spencer, & Frances, 1994).

Brown (1985) found that 45% of a group of abstinent alcoholics in AA sought psychotherapy, and more than 90% of them found it helpful. Rounsaville, Gawin, and Kleber (1985) also reported positive results in a preliminary study treating outpatient cocaine abusers with a modified interpersonal psychotherapy along with medication trials. Woody and colleagues (1986) reported that when psychotherapists were integrated in the treatment team, the entire staff reduced their stress as a result of the successful management of the most psychiatrically troubled patients. More recently, Woody, McLellan, Luborsky, and O'Brien (1995) validated the benefit of psychotherapy in community programs. In contrast, Carroll and colleagues (1994), as well as Kang and colleagues (1991), reported less benefit from psychotherapy in ambulatory cocaine abusers. In the latter studies, the authors underscored the importance of the severity of illness, stages of recovery, and level of care. Finally, when psychotherapy was added to paraprofessional drug counseling in an inpatient setting (Rogalski, 1984), patients improved in compliance with treatment as measured in decreased number of discharges against medical advice, disciplinary discharges, or unauthorized absences.

In addition to these studies that statistically examined effects of psychotherapy, a significant psychodynamic literature reports on the treatability of addicted patients with psychodynamic or psychoanalytically oriented psychotherapy (Brown, 1985; Dodes, 1984, 1988, 1990, 1996, 2002, 2003; Flores, 2004; Johnson, 1992; Kaufman, 1994; Khantzian, 1986, 1999a, 1999b, 2001; Krystal, 1982; Krystal & Raskin, 1970; Silber, 1974; Treece & Khantzian, 1986; Walant, 1995; Woody, Luborsky, McLellan, & O'Brien, 1989; Wurmser, 1974). The experience of treating addicted individuals in psychodynamic therapy has also provided our best information about the psychology of addiction, which in turn serves as the theoretical basis for technical approaches to the therapy of these patients.

Indications for psychodynamic psychotherapy depend on the patient's capacity to benefit, as well as on his or her motivation. Addicted individuals who are able to achieve and maintain sobriety with substance abuse counseling and/or self-help groups, and who are unaware of conflict, anxiety, depression, or other symptoms, are unlikely to seek psychotherapy. Addicted patients who are able to develop a therapeutic alliance, who have the capacity to be at least moderately introspective, and who have emotional suffering are candidates for psychotherapy as much as are nonaddicts with similar characteristics. Some of these patients use psychotherapy to help them to achieve abstinence; others use it to help them maintain abstinence, and both groups can also use their therapy to help their overall emotional health once they achieve abstinence.

PSYCHODYNAMIC BASIS FOR PSYCHOTHERAPY OF ADDICTED PATIENTS

There have been a number of major contributions to understanding the psychology of the addictions, particularly over the past 25 years (Khantzian et al., 2005). The most frequently described function of substance use is the management of intolerable or overwhelming affects. The idea that certain substances are preferentially chosen on the basis of their specific ability to address (ameliorate, express) certain affective states is termed the "self-medication hypothesis" (Khantzian, 1985b, 1997). Various authors described connections between certain affects and the use of alcohol or particular drugs, for example, use of narcotics to manage rage or loneliness, and use of cocaine and other stimulants to manage depression, boredom, and emptiness, or to provide a sense of grandeur (Khantzian, 1985b; Milkman & Frosch, 1973; Wurmser, 1974). In a more general way, Krystal and Raskin (1970) spoke of a "defective stimulus barrier" in addicts, causing them to be susceptible to flooding with intolerable affective states that are traumatic. They described a normal process of affective development in which affects are differentiated, desomatized, and verbalized, and pointed to defects in this development in (some) addicted individuals. These defects leave some addicts with the inability to use affects as signals, a critical capacity for managing them. Without this signal capacity, drugs may be used to ward off affective flooding. Others have noted the quality of addicts' relatedness to their alcohol or drugs as akin to human object relationships. The chemical becomes a substitute for a longed-for or needed figure—one that has omnipotent properties or is completely controllable and available (Krystal & Raskin, 1970; Wieder & Kaplan, 1969; Wurmser, 1974).

Related to these views are observations about the narcissistic pathology of addicts. Wurmser (1974) described a "narcissistic crisis" in addicts. He noted that for some addicts, collapse of a grandiose self or of an idealized object provides the impetus for substance use in an effort to resolve feelings of narcissistic frustration, shame, and rage. Kohut (1971) also referred to the narcissistic function of alcohol or drugs in addiction as a replacement for defective psychological structure, particularly that arising from an inadequate idealized self-object.

From another perspective, Khantzian (1978, 1995, 1999b) and Khantzian and Mack (1983) described defective self-care functions in addicts—the group of ego functions involved with anticipation of danger, appropriate modulated response to protect oneself, and sufficient positive self-esteem to care about oneself. These defective self-care functions may be seen in many substance abusers who characteristically place themselves in danger or fail to protect their health and well-being. In turn, this problem may be related to inadequate attention to the protection of the child by his or her parent, resulting in the failure to internalize self-care functions.

In addition to this ego deficit psychology, several investigators described a generally defective capacity to be aware of affective states in certain addicts. Some addicts appear to be "alexithymic," that is, unable to name or describe emotions in words. Krystal (1982) described substance use in some of these patients as a search for an external agent to soothe them, associated with their lack of sense of ability to soothe themselves. McDougall (1984) described patients whose use of words and ideas is without affective meaning, and who use alcohol or drugs to disperse emotional arousal and thus avoid affective flooding. Although the final appearance of this affective intolerance has the quality of an ego deficit, its underlying basis is understood to be a defensive avoidance of intolerable feelings. Krystal (1982) described this defense as arising secondary to psychological trauma in either childhood or adult life.

Khantzian (1999a) wrote about the preverbal origins of distress found among some substance abusers. He described a case in which early experience that remained out of conscious awareness created a nameless pain that recurred in response to a current stimulus (a film), leading to an alcoholic relapse. Of equal importance, when the early experience of abandonment again recurred in the setting of a group therapy, it could be clearly interpreted, understood, and borne rather than managed through substance abuse. Along similar lines, Walant (1995) stressed infantile origins of problems with interpersonal contact and interdependence that could predispose to addictive adaptations. Along similar lines, more recently, Flores (2004) has elaborated on addictions as an attachment disorder for some patients.

Finally, addiction may play a central role in seeking restoration of inner control of one's affective state (Dodes, 1990, 1996, 2002). This need for control in addicts involves a narcissistic vulnerability to being traumatized by the experience of helplessness or powerlessness. The use of substances is seen as a way to correct the experience of helplessness; that is, by taking an action (using alcohol or drugs) that can alter their internal affective state, addicts may reassert the power to control their inner experience, undoing and reversing the feeling of powerlessness. Because a sense of control of inner experience is a central aspect of narcissism, the intense aggressive drive to achieve this control when it is felt to be threatened may appropriately be considered narcissistic rage. According to this view, narcissistic rage arising from feelings of powerlessness gives addiction its most defining characteristics, namely, its insistent, compulsive, unrelenting quality and its relative unresponsiveness to realistic factors. This also offers an explanation for why, like narcissistic rage in general, the addictive drive may well overwhelm other aspects of the personality (Dodes, 1990).

More recently, Dodes (1996) expanded this view to place addictions within the category of those psychological problems currently and historically known as compulsions. He pointed out that although addictions and compulsions are clearly similar to each other in their "compulsive" quality, they have always, incorrectly, been seen as fundamentally different, namely, because compulsions are experienced as ego-dystonic—as things one feels compelled to do although one does not consciously wish to do them, whereas addictions have been experienced as ego-syntonic—as things one does because one consciously wants to do them. However, addictions commonly move from being ego-syntonic to ego-dystonic as people wish to stop their behavior, and compulsions often shift from being ego-dystonic to ego-syntonic as people make a virtue of their compelled behavior. Another false distinction has been that compulsions are viewed as compromise formations between a forbidden wish and an opposing (superego) force. But addictions have been viewed as the result of either an ego function (e.g., self-medication) or a deficit in ego function (e.g., self-care deficiencies), rather than being centrally viewed as compromises. However, in his formulation of addiction (an action driven to correct helplessness and to express the narcissistic rage engendered by this helplessness), Dodes described an inherent compromise formation. This compromise is expressed in the defensive *displacement* of the reassertion of power and the expression of rage to the addictive behavior. For instance, Dodes described a man who had an alcoholic binge after he was unable to fire his son from his company, despite the fact the son had embezzled a large amount of money. This man felt it was morally wrong to fire his son, even though he felt a strong impetus to do so, and as a consequence, he rendered himself helpless. This was intolerable, but since he could not allow himself to act directly (fire his son), he displaced the need to be empowered to his drinking, which therefore acquired a compulsive character. The addictive behavior, then, reflected a psychological compromise between doing what he was driven to do, and forbidding himself to do it. Dodes concluded that, with no distinction based on ego-syntonicity or on the psychology of the two diagnoses, addictions are fundamentally the same as compulsions. The important implication of this finding is that addictions should be seen as treatable in traditional psychodynamic psychotherapy as much as are compulsions, which have traditionally been understood to be amenable to a psychodynamic or psychoanalytic approach (Dodes, 1996, 2002, 2003).

TECHNICAL ASPECTS OF PSYCHOTHERAPY WITH ADDICTS

There are a number of special considerations in the psychodynamic psychotherapy of addicted individuals (Dodes & Khantzian, 1991). From the formulations discussed previously, it is clear that various meanings and roles of drugs or alcohol need to be considered in understanding the patient. In addition, addicts are frequently still abusing substances at the time they are first seen, which poses an immediate threat to their emotional and physical health, their relationships, and their overall capacity to function. This threat makes it necessary to address the question of abstinence from substance use first, when beginning treatment.

The first step is diagnosing substance abuse or dependence and informing the patient of the diagnosis, since the patient may fail to perceive the extent of the problem or may present with overt denial or minimization. The manner in which this is accomplished is also an important first step in establishing a positive therapeutic relationship, a basic element for all subsequent phases of treatment. To make the diagnosis and have a basis for showing it clearly to the patient, it is necessary to take a detailed history of the problems that have been caused by the patient's use of drugs or alcohol. In taking this history, it is useful to inquire systematically about trouble in the areas of work, medical health, relationships with friends, relationships with family (adults and children), legal problems, and intrapsychic problems (depression, shame, anxiety). It is often helpful to ask specifically what the patient is like when he or she drinks or uses drugs and the details of what happens at these times, as well as the effects the patient seeks from substance use. This involves exploring both the "positive" and negative effects he or she experiences from the use of drugs or alcohol. In the first instance, it is often reassuring and alliance building to ask, "What does the drug do for you?" Inquiring in this way, the patient is more apt to feel understood and not judged. Both the patient and therapist are provided an opportunity to appreciate how drugs or alcohol become compelling, such as enabling social contact, or relieving anxiety, agitation, depression or rage. On the maladaptive side, does he or she become more belligerent, moody, withdrawn, or sad? Might the patient have had more or better relationships with friends if she had never had a drink or a drug? Patients often deny trouble in their marriages but when the matter is explored in detail will acknowledge that their spouses would prefer that they drink less or have asked them on more than one occasion to cut down or stop. Upon reflection, they may recognize that their use of alcohol or drugs has silently become a source of chronic tension in their relationships. Once the patient clarifies or even lists the areas of difficulties that are due to alcohol or drugs, it is often possible for him to acknowledge the global impact of substance abuse on his life.

Focusing on the diagnosis of alcoholism or other drug abuse is more than a merely cognitive process. The realization that she is out of control in this area of life is a significant psychological step in itself. Brown (1985), in her work with alcoholic patients, stresses loss of control as a core issue and focus of psychotherapy. It is a blow to the narcissistic potency of the patient; as such, it may be usefully investigated, because it bears on the patient's important feelings and issues concerning powerlessness and mastery (Dodes, 1988). Mack (1981) felt that an alcoholic's recognition of failure to be in control of his or her drinking is a first step in the assumption of responsibility.

Through all this early diagnostic and at times confrontational work, as in therapy in general, the therapist's attitude must be exploratory without being judgmental. The patient's denial or minimization is often closely connected with his shame, and throughout this initial evaluation the patient is simultaneously evaluating the therapist—in particular, the therapist's attitude toward the patient and his addictive problem. To put it another way, the patient is faced with her own projections onto the therapist, and it is important that the therapist not accede to the role of a harsh or punitive superego that might be invisibly imposed.

Transference manifestations may also arise from narcissistic deficits, leading to idealizing and mirroring relationships or fearful, guarded positions against being overcontrolled or overwhelmed. Common countertransference difficulties with substance abusers revolve around frustration, anger, and guilt, as patients' failures to abstain challenge the therapeutic potency of the treatment professional. These countertransference feelings may result in withdrawal, inappropriately critical attitudes, or overinvolvement (when therapists attempt to reverse their desire to withdraw). The severe nature of the risks facing addicts makes the work with them both particularly challenging and rewarding. It is important for the therapist to be able to view both the overt behavior and the inner psychopathology of the addict with the same combination of objectivity and compassion that is brought to any patient.

Developing a therapeutic alliance early in therapy is also made difficult by the patient's frequently ambivalent relationship toward abstention from drinking or drug use at the same time that the therapist is appropriately concerned with the patient's achieving abstinence. It may be ineffective and even counterproductive to be seen as requiring (vs. suggesting) something the patient does not consciously feel is in his best interest. Once the patient concurs with the diagnosis, he or she has a necessary, though not always sufficient, basis for an alliance with the therapist to achieve abstinence. In fact, the psychological issues in abstention are complex.

We (Dodes, 1984; Khantzian, 1980) have addressed issues in abstention with alcoholics. Patients' achievement of abstinence hinges not only on the place of substance use in their psychological equilibrium but also critically on the alliance with, and transference to, the therapist. Many patients quickly achieve abstinence upon beginning psychotherapy, in spite of the evident importance to them of their drugs or alcohol. But others may continue to use substances, although not in a way that is malignantly out of control or that creates an emergency. In a number of these cases, we have helped patients establish abstinence over time, psychotherapeutically. When the therapist focuses on the patient's failure to perceive the danger to herself that is contained in the continued abuse, the therapist's caring concern may be internalized by the patient, providing a nucleus for the introjection of a healthy "self-care" function (Dodes, 1984). However, the patient's ability to perceive the therapist in a benign way that may be internalized depends on absence or resolution of negative transference feelings at the beginning of treatment.

For some patients, early achievement of abstinence is possible because of a genuine therapeutic alliance with the therapist. In other cases, abstinence may be achieved early on because of unconscious wishes to merge with, or be held by, a therapist who is idealized, or because of a compliant identification with the aggressor (Dodes, 1984). When the patient does not initially abstain, subsequent confrontation may produce abstention, because the patient finally perceives the confrontation as a longed-for message of caring that was absent or insufficient in his childhood (Khantzian & Mack, 1983, also described this kind of parental insufficiency in their discussion of the origin of self-care deficits). From a practical standpoint, the clinical choices involved must depend on the immediate risks to the patient. If patients drink only intermittently and are able to participate genuinely in the process of psychotherapy, we have found that the psychotherapy can continue. Indeed, the psychotherapy provides an opportunity to explore the issues in the continued drinking, including problems with self-care and the transference implications of the failure to abstain. However, when drinking becomes continually destructive, patients are generally unable to participate in the process, requiring early confrontation around the need to be hospitalized or to interupt therapy. Over the course of an ongoing psychotherapy, the capacity for abstinence may vary, depending in part on shifts in the therapeutic relationship (Dodes, 1984). We discuss the question of relapses in an abstinent patient later.

Once the patient achieves abstinence, the therapy may broaden to explore all areas of her psychological life, as in any psychotherapy. Some authors writing about alcoholism, however, recommend a kind of staging of the therapy. Prochaska and Di Clemente (1985), based on a cognitive-behavioral paradigm, introduced the "stages of change" model to help individuals shift from a "precontemplative" stage (denial) to a "contemplative" (acknowledgment) stage, to initiate a process of engaging in treatment and preventing relapse. Not inconsistent with the psychodynamic approach, the first phase is directed toward helping the patient develop an identity as an alcoholic (Brown, 1985) focusing on the drinking, on ways to stay sober, and on mourning the losses incurred as a result of drinking (Bean-Bayog, 1985). Kaufman (1994) similarly stresses the importance of abstinence, stabilization, and relapse prevention and then, in advanced recovery, the importance of addressing issues of intimacy and autonomy. In our experience, however, it is generally unnecessary and potentially counterproductive to attempt to direct the therapeutic process according to a preconceived agenda. As with any patient, imposing one's own focus risks interfering with the free evolution of the patient's thoughts toward deeper and more meaningful understanding of the issues. In our opinion, although some addicts (like some patients in general) require a more supportive rather than an exploratory approach, or special approaches based on some of the dynamic factors described earlier, this decision should be based on an individual assessment of the patient's psychology rather than on a generalization for all substance abusers. The approach in treatment may, and should, vary according to the stage of treatment and the status of the patient's abstinence.

The idea of imposing structure in psychotherapy with addicts arises in part from concerns about the ability of such patients to tolerate the process of therapy. At the heart of this thought is the worry that exploring the important issues in their lives will lead addicts to resume their substance abuse. Actually, the reverse is often the case: Patients who do not deal with the issues that trouble them may be at much greater risk of continued substance use or relapse. Nonetheless, there may be difficulties with pursuing psychotherapy. At times, therapists fail to attend appropriately to the life-threatening nature of continued substance abuse (Bean-Bayog, 1985) or fail to make the diagnosis (Brown, 1985), overlooking the ongoing deterioration of their patients' lives. Alcoholics may also try to use therapy to aid their denial of their alcoholism.

However, these concerns largely hinge on failures of the therapist and may be avoided by a therapist who is attentive to these issues (Dodes, 1988, 1991). For instance, as described earlier, attention must be paid initially to the question of abstinence (whether or not it can be achieved). Likewise, if a patient misuses the treatment to rationalize continued drug or alcohol use, an appropriately responsive therapist would recognize this misuse and bring it into the treatment process to identify and deal with it. Addicts have a wide variety of characterological structures, strengths, and weaknesses, and are in general as capable of dealing with the issues and strong transference feelings that may arise in a psychotherapy as patients with other presenting problems. Brown's (1985) concern that a psychodynamic psychotherapy may distract the alcoholic patient from his or her task of establishing an identity as an alcoholic may also be taken principally as a reminder to the therapist to attend to the patient's alcoholism rather than a contraindication to psychotherapy (Dodes, 1988).

In fact, in the ongoing therapy of addicts, once the patient achieves abstinence, the therapist should always be alert to the meanings and purposes of the patient's substance use as these become clearer. Part of the advantage of psychotherapy with addicts is that it offers an ongoing opportunity for patients to take firmer control over their addiction, based on understanding and tolerating the feelings and issues that contribute to it. The therapist's continual attentiveness to improved understanding of the patient's drug use also avoids the problem of distracting the patient from his or her addiction.

Of course, any therapist can be fooled: Patients who deny, minimize, or distort the facts about their substance use may render its diagnosis and treatment impossible for any therapist. This is a limitation to psychotherapy, as it is to other attempted interventions.

Having considered early issues of abstinence and allowing the focus of the therapy to broaden, we may now consider how the dynamics of addicts may necessitate a modification of approach. In the case of alexithymic patients, Krystal (1982) and Krystal and Raskin (1970) proposed a preparatory stage in which patients' affects are identified and explained—with the goal of increasing ego function, which includes improving the use of affects as signals and improving affect tolerance. McDougall (1984) focused on the countertransference problems produced with such patients. She described feelings of boredom and helplessness, with consequent emotional withdrawal by the therapist, and pointed to the need for the therapist to provide a consistent holding environment that may last for years before patients are able to acknowledge their emotions. She also offered an understanding of this process in terms of the patient's creating a "primitive communication that is intended, in a deeply unconscious fashion, to make the analyst experience what the distressed and misunderstood infant had once felt" (p. 399).

A contemporary psychodynamic understanding of addicted patients, however, does not usually suggest this sort of modification of approach but, rather, a need to attend to one or another aspect of the meaning and role of the addiction for a patient. For instance, for some patients it is particularly important to attend to the object-substitute meanings of alcohol or drugs. In some patients, narcissistic vulnerabilities are of paramount importance, for instance, the collapse of idealized objects, as described by Wurmser (1974), or the role of particular affective states in precipitating substance use, mentioned by a number of authors. With some patients, self-care deficits, as described by Khantzian and Mack (1983), are of great significance. From a different perspective, the active nature of addictive behavior in seizing control against an intolerable feeling of helplessness, as described by Dodes (1990), is often an important focus. In such cases, it is important to address patients' experiences of helplessness and powerlessness as major factors in precipitating substance use.

With patients whose affect management and self-care are seriously impaired (Khantzian, 1986, 1995), it is important for the therapist to be especially active. Excessive passivity with such patients can be dangerous. It is necessary in these cases to empathically draw the patients' attention to ways in which they render themselves vulnerable as a result of their self-care deficits, and to point out how these self-care deficits render them susceptible to addictive behavior. With some patients, it is necessary to explore the details of current life situations to help them recognize their feelings and see that these feelings may serve as "guides to appropriate reactions and self-protective behavior rather than signals for impulsive action and the obliteration of feelings with drugs" (Khantzian, 1986, p. 217).

Consistent with the need to maintain an active stance, the therapist may at times need to serve as a "primary care" physician—especially at the start of treatment, when he or she must often play multiple roles to ensure that the patient receives appropriate care from a number of sources (Khantzian, 1985a, 1988). This task may include decisions about (and active involvement in arranging) hospitalization and detoxification, involvement with AA or NA, professionally led group treatments, or pharmacological treatment. However, such an active approach, although possibly life saving, may interfere with the later development of a traditional psychotherapeutic relationship because of the transference and countertransference issues it induces, particularly in regard to the patient's realistic gratitude. If this gratitude becomes a prominent interfering factor, referral to another therapist for continued psychotherapy may be required (Khantzian, 1985a).

Just as with the initial attention to abstinence, therapy must focus on relapses when they occur. Relapses (or the patient's awareness that he feels a greater urge to use alcohol or drugs) provide an opportunity to learn about the factors leading to substance use. Frequently patients are unaware of these factors; their lack of awareness contributes to their feelings of frustration and helplessness, and leaves them unprepared for further relapses. A careful, even microscopic, investigation of the feelings, relationships, and events that preceded the relapse are often revealing. Once these issues and affects are clarified, they often contribute to an understanding of the patient's psychology in general, because they center on areas felt to be intolerable by the patient. Commonly, patients bring up their increased thinking about drugs or alcohol when there is an impending relapse. At other times, the therapist may infer an increased risk based on what he or she knows of the patient's history and emotional life. Conveying this perception to patients is one way to help them learn to attend to their affects, thoughts, and behaviors, and utilize them as signals. Often, abstinent addicts have dreams about alcohol or drugs that can indicate that something current in their lives is reviving the association with substance use, warning of the risk of relapse.

Finally, we should mention organicity. Some treatment providers view addicted patients as too impaired in brain functioning, as a result of drug or alcohol abuse ("wet brain"), to be able to utilize a dynamic psychotherapy until after a lengthy time of abstinence. Certainly some patients exhibit impaired memory and capacity for skilled cognitive functions immediately after stopping drug or alcohol use. However, in our experience this limitation is frequently mild or not significant for all but the most severely affected addicts (e.g., alcoholics with hepatic failure and elevated blood ammonia levels). In fact, as regularly observed in inpatient treatment centers, patients can do significant work to understand themselves and the dynamic issues in their families and can also return to complex tasks within the span of a few weeks immediately following detoxification. The implication for psychotherapy is that it is rarely necessary to wait an extended time to begin because of organic factors. Patients who are truly impaired because their drug or alcohol use is so continuous that they are always either high/drunk or withdrawing should not be in psychotherapy to begin with, because they require hospitalization to break the pattern before they will be able to attend to the work of the treatment.

PSYCHOTHERAPY AND SELF-HELP GROUPS

Rosen (1981) looked at role of therapy in helping patients to separate from their attachment to AA, which he viewed as having elements of a symbiosis. He noted the striking fact that AA, unlike psychoanalytically oriented psychotherapy, provides no mechanism for termination. He saw a critical aspect of the role of psychotherapy as helping to work out separation and termination from AA.

Patients in a combined treatment of psychotherapy and a 12-step group often engage differently with each element; that is, patients may split their transference projections, expectations, and attachments, engaging the therapy and the self-help group at separate psychological levels (Dodes, 1988). Patients' attachment to AA may provide opportunity for needed internalization of self-care and self-valuing, with AA serving as a valuing, idealized object (or transitional object); important elements of the narcissistic (idealizing and mirroring) transference may be assigned to AA. The degree to which the transference is split in this way varies in different patients. It is critical for the therapist to be aware of this split, because a patient's sobriety may hinge on an idealization of AA or its "Higher Power" concept, and this sobriety may be lost if the idealization is prematurely challenged (Dodes, 1988). Consequently, the therapist may first have to help the patient to increase his tolerance of affects and "await internalization of sufficient narcissistic potency" (Dodes, 1988, p. 289) before too closely examining the defenses and functions of AA.

In our opinion, the need for a nondynamic, supportive approach through AA may lessen eventually either as a consequence of the patient's growth, including internalization of a sense of adequate narcissistic potency, or as a consequence of greater insight into the psychology of the addictive behavior. However, this does not always occur, leading to the need to attend AA meetings indefinitely (Dodes, 1984). Other long-term AA members remain involved because of social and interpersonal factors, or because of their interest in helping others, even though they may not require AA for sobriety.

Dodes (1988) suggested that the fear of disrupting the idealizing transference to AA (and consequently losing the sobriety that is dependent on this transference) underlies the fear of psychotherapy among some patients and treatment providers. A careful therapist, however, will avoid this pitfall. Overall, the combination of psychodynamic psychotherapy and AA or NA is useful for many patients (Dodes, 1988; Khantzian, 1985a, 1988).

The disease concept is closely linked with self-help groups and has traditionally been difficult to reconcile with psychoanalytically oriented psychotherapy. Mack (1981) noted that this concept led to "oversimplified physiological models and a territorial smugness . . . which . . . precludes a sophisticated psychodynamic understanding of the problems of the individual alcoholic" (p. 129). The term "disease" itself has not been well or clearly defined, a fact addressed by Shaffer (1985). However, it is possible to integrate the disease concept with a traditional psychoanalytic psychotherapy (Dodes, 1988). In the first place, focusing on the addictive behavior specifically as an illness may be useful, because it helps to avoid the kind of failure to address the problem that some have worried about with psychotherapy. Moreover, acknowledgment of a disease or diagnosis often arouses feelings about being unable to control oneself that may be quite important to explore (Dodes, 1988, 1990).

In order to integrate a disease concept with a psychodynamic psychotherapy, Dodes (1988) suggested that the "disease" (e.g., alcoholism) be defined to the patient as having two parts: the patient's history of alcoholism, and the patient's being at permanent risk of repeating this behavior in the future. This definition does not impede psychological exploration of the meanings of the patient's drinking. The risk of repetition of drinking that is so central to the disease idea may be troublesome for dynamic exploration only if it has the quality of something that is inexplicable in dynamic terms. However, this risk is actually the same as the regressive potential of any patient in psychotherapy. Addicts, like all other individuals in psychotherapy, never totally eliminate the potential of resuming old pathological defenses and behaviors, and of regressing. Their risk of resuming substance abuse is therefore just an example of this general rule.

CONCLUSION

This chapter has presented a description of individual psychodynamic psychotherapy with addicts, based on a contemporary psychoanalytical understanding of their vulnerabilities and disturbances. We emphasized disturbances in ego function and narcissistic difficulties that affect addicts' capacities to regulate their feeling life, self-esteem, and relationships. A major psychotherapeutic task for addicted patients is to bring into their awareness their emotional difficulties and the way their problems predispose them to relapse into drug/alcohol use and dependence. We have reviewed implications for technique with regard to characteristic central issues for addicts and the need in certain cases for active intervention. We explored strategies for establishing abstinence, including the value of working with self-help groups such as AA and NA. Finally, we have emphasized a flexible approach with regard to the timing, sequencing, and integration of psychotherapy in relation to other interventions and needs based on patient characteristics and clinical considerations.

REFERENCES

Bean-Bayog, M. (1985). Alcoholism treatment as an alternative to psychiatric hospitalization. *Psychiatr Clin North Am*, 8, 501–512.

Brown, S. (1985). *Treating the alcoholic: A developmental model of recovery*. New York: Wiley.

Carroll, K. M., & Rounsaville, B. J. (1992). Contrast of treatment seeking and untreated cocaine abusers. *Arch Gen Psychiatry, 49,* 464–471.

Carroll, K. M., Rounsaville, B. J., Gordon, L. T., Nich, C., Jatlow, P., Bisighini, R. M., & Gawin, F. H. (1994). Psychotherapy and pharmacotherapy for ambulatory cocaine abusers. *Arch Gen Psychiatry, 51,* 177–187.

Dodes, L. M. (1984). Abstinence from alcohol in long-term individual psychotherapy with alcoholics. *Am J Psychother, 38,* 248–256.

Dodes, L. M. (1988). The psychology of combining dynamic psychotherapy and Alcoholics Anonymous. *Bull Menninger Clin, 52,* 283–293.

Dodes, L. M. (1990). Addiction, helplessness, and narcissistic rage. *Psychoanal Q, 59,* 398–419.

Dodes, L. M. (1991). Psychotherapy is useful, often essential, for alcoholics. *Psychodynamic Lett, 1*(2), 4–7.

Dodes, L. M. (1996). Compulsion and addiction. *J Am Psychoanal Assoc, 44,* 815–835.

Dodes, L. M. (2002). *The heart of addiction.* New York: HarperCollins.

Dodes, L. M. (2003). Addiction and Psychoanalysis. *Can J Psychoanal, 11,* 123–134.

Dodes, L. M., & Khantzian, E. J. (1991). Psychotherapy and chemical dependence. In D. Ciraulo & R. Shader (Eds.), *Clinical manual of chemical dependence* (pp. 345–358). Washington, DC: American Psychiatric Press.

Flores, P. (2004). *Addiction as an attachment disorder.* Northvale, NJ: Aronson.

Halikas, J. A., Crosby, R. D., Pearson, V. L., Nugent, S. M., & Carlson, G. A. (1994). Psychiatric comorbidity in treatment seeking cocaine abusers. *Am J Addict, 3,* 25–35.

Johnson, B. (1992). The psychoanalysis of a man with active alcoholism. *J Subst Abuse Treat, 9,* 111–123.

Kang, S. Y., Kleinman, P. H., Woody, G. E., Millman, R. B., Todd, T. C., Kemp, J., & Lipton, D. S. (1991). Outcome for cocaine abusers after once-a-week psychosocial therapy. *Am J Psychiatry, 148,* 630–635.

Kaufman, E. (1994). *Psychotherapy of addicted persons.* New York: Guilford Press.

Kessler, R. C., Crum, R. M., Warner, L. A., Nelson, C. B., Schulenberg, J., & Anthony, J. C. (1997). Lifetime co-occurrence of DSM-III-R alcohol abuse and dependence with other psychiatric disorders in the National Comorbidity Survey. *Arch Gen Psychiatry, 54,* 313–321.

Khantzian, E. J. (1978). The ego, the self and opiate addiction: Theoretical and treatment considerations. *Int Rev Psychoanal, 5,* 189–198.

Khantzian, E. J. (1980). The alcoholic patient: An overview and perspective. *Am J Psychother, 34,* 4–19.

Khantzian, E. J. (1985a). Psychotherapeutic interventions with substance abusers: The clinical context. *J Subst Abuse Treat, 2,* 83–88.

Khantzian, E. J. (1985b). The self-medication hypothesis of addictive disorders: Focus on heroin and cocaine dependence. *Am J Psychiatry, 142,* 1259–1264.

Khantzian, E. J. (1986). A contemporary psychodynamic approach to drug abuse treatment. *Am J Drug Alcohol Abuse, 12,* 213–222.

Khantzian, E. J. (1988). The primary care therapist and patient needs in substance abuse treatment. *Am J Drug Alcohol Abuse, 14*(2), 159–167.

Khantzian, E. J. (1995). Self-regulation vulnerabilities in substance abusers: Treatment implications. In S. Dowling (Ed.), *The psychology and treatment of addictive behavior* (pp. 17–41). New York: International Universities Press.

Khantzian, E. J. (1997). The self-medication hypothesis of substance use disorders: A reconsideration and recent applications. *Harv Rev Psychiatry, 4,* 231–244.

Khantzian, E. J. (1999a). Preverbal origins of distress, substance use disorders and psychotherapy. In E. J. Khantzian (Ed.), *Treating addictions as a human process* (pp. 629–637). Northvale, NJ: Aronson.

Khantzian, E. J. (1999b). *Treating addictions as a human process.* Northvale, NJ: Aronson.

Khantzian, E. J. (2001). Reflections on group treatment as corrective experiences for addictive vulnerability. *Int J Group Psychother, 51,* 11–20.

Khantzian, E. J. (2003). Addictive vulnerability: An evolving psychodynamic perspective. *Neuro-Psychoanalysis, 5,* 5–21.

Khantzian, E. J., Dodes, L. M., & Brehm, N. M. (2005). Determinants and perpetuators of substance abuse and dependence: Psychodynamics. In J. H. Lowinson, P. Ruiz, R. B. Millman, & J. G. Langrod (Eds.), *Substance abuse: A comprehensive textbook* (4th ed., pp. 97–107). Baltimore: Williams & Wilkins.

Khantzian, E. J., & Mack, J. (1983). Self-preservation and the care of the self. *Psychoanal Stud Child, 38,* 209–232.

Khantzian, E. J., & Treece, C. (1985). DSM-III psychiatric diagnosis of narcotic addicts. *Arch Gen Psychiatry, 42,* 1067–1071.

Kleimman, P. K., Miller, A. B., & Millman, R. B. (1990). Psychopathology among cocaine abusers entering treatment. *J Nerv Ment Dis, 178,* 442–447.

Kohut, H. (1971). *The analysis of the self.* Madison, CT: International Universities Press.

Krystal, H. (1982). Alexithymia and the effectiveness of psychoanalytic treatment. *Int J Psychoanal Psychother, 9,* 353–378.

Krystal, H., & Raskin, H. (1970). *Drug dependence: Aspects of ego function.* Detroit, MI: Wayne State University Press.

Mack, J. (1981). Alcoholism, A.A., and the governance of the self. In M. H. Bean & N. E. Zinberg (Eds.), *Dynamic approaches to the understanding and treatment of alcoholism* (pp. 128–162). New York: Free Press.

McDougall, J. (1984). The "disaffected" patient: Reflections on affect pathology. *Psychoanal Q, 53,* 386–409.

Milkman, H., & Frosch, W. A. (1973). On the preferential abuse of heroin and amphetamines. *J Nerv Ment Dis, 156,* 242–248.

Penick, E. C., Powell, B. J., Nickel, E. J., Bingham, S. F., Rieseenmy, K. R., Read, M. R., & Campbell, J. (1994). Co-morbidity of lifetime psychiatric disorder among male alcoholic patients. *Alcohol Clin Exp Res, 18,* 1289–1293.

Prochaska, J. O., & DiClemente, C. C. (1985). Common processes of change in smoking, weight control, and psychological distress. In S. Shiffman & T. A. Willis (Eds.), *Coping and substance abuse* (pp. 345–363). New York: Academic Press.

Regier, D. A., Farmer, M. E., Rae, D. S., Locke, B. Z., Keith, S. J., Judd, L. L., & Goodwin, K. K. (1990). Comorbidity of mental disorders with alcohol and other drug abuse: Results from the Epidemiologic Catchment Area (ECA) study. *JAMA, 264,* 2511–2518.

Rogalski, C. J. (1984). Professional psychotherapy and its relationship to compliance intreatment. *Int J Addict, 19,* 521–539.

Rosen, A. (1981). Psychotherapy and Alcoholics Anonymous: Can they be coordinated? *Bull Menninger Clin, 45,* 229–246.

Rounsaville, B. J., Anton, S. F., Carroll, K., Budde, D., Prusoff, B., & Gawin, F. (1991). Psychiatric diagnosis of treatment-seeking cocaine-abusers. *Arch Gen Psychiatry, 48,* 43–51.

Rounsaville, B. J., Gawin, F. H., Kleber, H. D. (1985). Interpersonal psychotherapy (IPT) adapted for ambulatory cocaine abusers. *Am J Drug Alcohol Abuse, 11,* 171–191.

Rounsaville, B. J., Weissman, M., Kleber, H., & Wilber, C. (1982). Heterogeneity of psychiatric diagnosis in treated opiate addicts. *Arch Gen Psychiatry, 39,* 161–166.

Schuckit, M. A., & Hesselbrock, V. (1994). Alcohol dependence and anxiety disorders: What is the relationship? *Am J Psychiatry, 151,* 1723–1734.

Schuckit, M. A., Irwin, M., & Brown, S. A. (1990). The history of anxiety symptoms among 171 primary alcoholics. *J Stud Alcohol, 51,* 34–41.

Shaffer, H. J. (1985). The disease controversy: Of metaphors, maps and menus. *J Psychoactive Drugs, 17,* 65–76.

Silber, A. (1974). Rationale for the technique of psychotherapy with alcoholics. *Int J Psychoanal Psychother, 3,* 28–47.

Treece, C., & Khantzian, E. J. (1986). Psychodynamic factors in the development of drug dependence. *Psychiatr Clin North Am, 9,* 399–412.

Walant, K. B. (1995). *Creating the capacity for attachment: Treating addictions and the alienated self.* Northvale, NJ: Aronson.

Wieder, H., & Kaplan, E. (1969). Drug use in adolescents. *Psychoanal Study Child, 24,* 399–431.

Wilens, T. E., Biederman, J., Spencer, T. J., & Frances, R. J. (1994). Comorbidity of attention deficit hyperactivity and psychoactive substance use disorders. *Hosp Community Psychiatry, 45,* 421–435.

Woody, G. E., Luborsky, L., McLellan, A. T., & O'Brien, C. P. (1989). Individual psychotherapy for substance abuse. In T. B. Karasu (Ed.), *Treatment of psychiatric disorders: A task force report of the American Psychiatric Association* (pp. 1417–1430). Washington, DC: American Psychiatric Press.

Woody G. E., Luborsky, L., McLellan, A. T., O'Brien, C. P., Beck, A. T., Blaine, J., et al. (1983). Psychotherapy for opiate addicts: Does it help? *Arch Gen Psychiatry, 40,* 639–645.

Woody, G. E., McLellan, A. T., Luborsky, L., & O'Brien, C. P. (1986). Psychotherapy for substance abuse. *Psychiatr Clin North Am, 9,* 547–562.

Woody, G. E., McLellan, A. T., Luborsky, L., & O'Brien, C. P. (1995). Psychotherapy in community methadone programs. *Am J Psychiatry, 152,* 1302–1308.

Wurmser, L. (1974). Psychoanalytic considerations of the etiology of compulsive drug use. *J Am Psychoanal Assoc, 22,* 820–843.

CHAPTER 22

Cognitive Therapy

JUDITH S. BECK
BRUCE S. LIESE
LISA M. NAJAVITS

Kim is a 32-year-old woman with a complex history of substance abuse that began when she was 13 years old. At various times, Kim has experimented with most illicit substances (including marijuana, heroin, LSD, Ecstasy, and cocaine) and she has been dependent on nicotine, alcohol, amphetamines, and barbiturates. She also suffers from chronic depression. She has been treated intermittently for depression since age 15 and has cycled in and out of substance treatment programs since age 19. Kim has never been married. She works as a night janitor at a fast-food restaurant.

Currently, Kim smokes marijuana several times daily. She says, "I smoke so much, I don't even get high anymore." She smokes to deal with feelings of depression, emptiness, and loneliness. She views herself as hopeless but says she has no plans to kill herself, because she is afraid of dying. She has gained over 50 pounds in the last few years, and she says she wants to "do nothing but sit around the house all day."

Kim meets criteria for avoidant personality disorder with dependent and borderline features. She describes constant boredom and isolation. Nonetheless, she refuses to take social or occupational risks, saying "If I put myself out there, I'll only get burned." She has a history of numerous failed relationships and jobs.

Eventually Kim joins a self-help group for women with depression, where she admits to daily marijuana use. Another group member, Jenna, explains that she, too, was a heavy marijuana smoker at one time. Jenna warns Kim that she will only feel better when she quits smoking marijuana.

After listening, Kim feels motivated to stop but finds it impossible to quit. After only a few days of abstinence, she feels more depressed and anxious, so she picks up smoking again.

For over a decade cognitive therapy has been refined to help people like Kim who are addicted to a variety of substances, including alcohol, cocaine, opioids, marijuana, prescription medications, nicotine, and other psychoactive substances (A. T. Beck, Wright, Newman, & Liese, 1993; Carroll, 1998, 1999; Liese & Beck, 1997; Liese & Franz, 1996; Najavits, Liese, & Harned, 2004; Newman & Ratto, 1999). Cognitive therapy is also used for compulsive gambling, shopping, and sexual behaviors. Applications of cognitive therapy to substance-abusing adolescents (Fromme & Brown, 2000; Waldron, Slesnick, Brody, Turner, & Peterson, 2001), dual diagnosis patients (e.g., Barrowclough et al., 2001; Najavits, 2002a; Weiss, Najavits, & Greenfield, 1999), older patients (Schonfeld et al., 2000), and other important subgroups are additional recent developments. Patients like Kim have taught us a great deal about the development, maintenance, and treatment of addictive behavior (Liese & Franz, 1996). Currently, cognitive-behavioral therapy (CBT) approaches to substance abuse are considered among the most empirically studied, well-defined, and widely used approaches (Carroll, 1999; Thase, 1997).

The cognitive therapy of substance abuse is quite similar to cognitive therapy for other psychological problems, including depression (A. T. Beck, Rush, Shaw, & Emery, 1979), anxiety (A. T. Beck & Emery, with Greenberg, 1985), and personality disorders (A. T. Beck, Freeman, & Associates, 1990; Young, 1999). Each places emphasis on collaboration, case conceptualization, structure, patient education, and the application of standard cognitive-behavioral techniques. In addition, when working with substance abuse patients, cognitive therapists focus on the cognitive and behavioral sequences leading to substance use, management of cravings, avoidance of high-risk situations, case management, mood regulation (i.e., coping), and lifestyle change. The cognitive therapy of substance abuse is an integrative, collaborative endeavor. Patients are encouraged to seek adjunctive services (e.g., 12-step and other programs) to reinforce their progress in cognitive therapy.

In cognitive therapy of substance abuse, thoughts are viewed as playing a major role in addictive behavior (e.g., substance use), negative emotions (e.g., anxiety and depression), and physiological responses (including some withdrawal symptoms). Although strategies and interventions vary based on the individual and particular substance, the basic conceptualization of the patient in cognitive terms remains constant (A. T. Beck et al., 1993; see Figure 22.1 for the basic cognitive model of substance abuse).

Cognitive therapists assess the development of their patients' beliefs about themselves, their early life experiences, exposure to substances, the development of substance-related beliefs, and their eventual reliance on substances

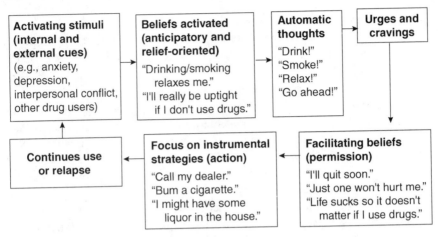

FIGURE 22.1. The cognitive model of substance abuse. From A. T. Beck, Wright, Newman, and Liese (1993, p. 47). Copyright 1993 by The Guilford Press. Adapted by permission.

(Liese & Franz, 1996; see Figure 22.2). An important assumption is that substance abuse is in large part learned and can be modified by changing cognitive-behavioral processes.

Our model for cognitive therapy of substance abuse has been substantially influenced by other cognitive behaviorists. For example, Marlatt and colleagues (Dimeff & Marlatt, 1998; Marlatt & Gordon, 1985) presented an important model of relapse prevention that has contributed greatly to our own work. Identifying high-risk situations, understanding the decision chain leading to substance use, modifying substance users' dysfunctional lifestyles, and learning from lapses to prevent full-fledged relapses are all integral to the relapse prevention model and the cognitive models of addiction.

There are numerous CBT approaches for substance abuse (Najavits et al., 2004), and the past several years have seen a variety of major empirical studies on CBT for substance abuse (e.g., Crits-Christoph et al., 1999; Maude-Griffin et al., 1998; Project MATCH Research Group, 1997; Rawson et al., 2002; Waldron et al., 2001). In this chapter, we focus primarily on the cognitive therapy model defined by Aaron T. Beck and colleagues. The cognitive therapy model, or some of its various components, is often part of other CBTs.

We address four key topics: cognitive case conceptualization; principles of treatment; treatment planning (including specific cognitive and behavioral interventions); and comparison to some other major psychosocial treatments for substance abuse. Our patient, Kim, is used as an example throughout.

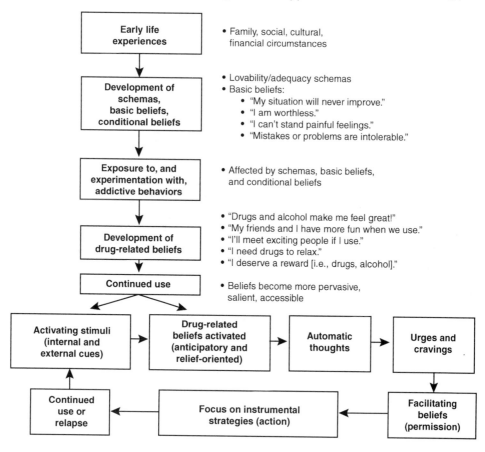

FIGURE 22.2. The cognitive developmental model of substance abuse. From Liese and Franz (1996, p. 482). Copyright 1996 by The Guilford Press. Reprinted by permission.

THE COGNITIVE CONCEPTUALIZATION DIAGRAM

Cognitive therapy begins with a formulation of the case, using a standardized form for structuring the case conceptualization (J. S. Beck, 1995). An example using Kim's current difficulties is provided in Figure 22.3. She holds fundamental beliefs that she is helpless and incompetent, bad, unlovable, and vulnerable. These beliefs originated in childhood and became stronger and stronger as time went on. The next to last of eight children in a poor family, Kim was emotionally neglected by a depressed, alcoholic mother. Her father was cold, distant, and uninterested in Kim. He abandoned the family when Kim was 7 and never contacted them again. Kim had few friends, felt rejected by her family, did poorly in school, and dropped out when she was halfway through 11th grade.

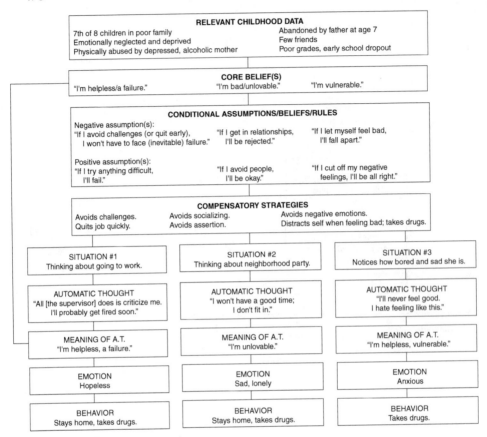

FIGURE 22.3. Cognitive conceptualization diagram. From J. S. Beck (1995, p. 139). Copyright 1995 by Judith S. Beck. Adapted by permission.

Kim's core beliefs of helplessness, badness, and vulnerability have caused her great pain, and over the years, she has developed rules (i.e., conditional assumptions) for survival. One such conditional assumption is, "If I avoid challenges, I won't have to face failure." Thus, Kim uses a typical compensatory strategy: She avoids applying for any but the most menial jobs. She then quits these jobs when small problems arise, believing she is helpless to solve problems. Likewise, she tries only halfheartedly in substance abuse treatment programs and drops out prematurely, believing she cannot abstain from substances. She also avoids conflicts with others, believing that she does not deserve to get what she wants.

Kim's core beliefs of badness and unlovability permeate virtually all of her relationships. In addition to her conditional belief, "If I try to get what I want from a relationship, I'll fail" (which stems from a core belief of helplessness), she also believes, "If I assert myself or let others get too close, they'll reject me, because nobody could possibly love me." Therefore, she uses compensatory strategies such as isolating herself, avoiding assertion, avoiding intimacy, and, perhaps most obvious, taking substances. Most of her social contacts are with other substance abusers who manipulate and take advantage of her.

Kim also has a core belief that she is vulnerable, especially to negative emotion. Her conditional assumption is, "If I start to feel bad, my emotions will get out of control and overwhelm me." She avoids even mildly challenging situations in which she predicts she will feel sad, rejected, or helpless. Avoidance itself, however, often leads to boredom and frustration, which increases her sense of failure and helplessness.

Kim discovered at an early age that she could feel better by drinking alcohol and taking substances. As a result, she failed to develop healthier coping strategies (e.g., learning to tolerate bad moods, solving problems, asserting herself, or looking at situations more realistically). For much of her life, she has tried to cope with a combination of avoidance and substance use.

The cognitive conceptualization diagram in Figure 22.3 demonstrates how Kim's thinking in specific situations leads to substance use. In situation 1, for example, Kim thinks about going to work. She has a mental image of her supervisor looking at her "with a mean face" and she thinks, "All he ever does is criticize me. I'll probably get fired soon." This is an *automatic thought*, because it seems to pop into Kim's mind spontaneously. Prior to receiving therapy, Kim had little awareness of her automatic thoughts; she was much more aware of her subsequent negative emotions. As a result, she felt helpless, and her behavioral response was to stay home and take substances.

Why does Kim consistently have these thoughts of failure and helplessness? Kim's negative core beliefs about herself influence every perception. She *assumes* she will fail, never thinking to question such beliefs about herself. Given this tendency, it is no surprise that Kim avoids challenges. She thinks it is just a matter of time until her failure becomes apparent.

In situation 2 (see Figure 22.3), Kim considers whether to attend a party given by neighbors. Because of her core belief that she is unlovable, she automatically thinks, "I won't have a good time. I don't fit in." Accepting these thoughts as true, she feels sad and chooses to stay home and get high. Whereas many automatic thoughts have a grain of truth, they are usually distorted in some way. Had Kim evaluated her thoughts critically, she might have concluded that she could not predict the future with certainty, that several neighbors had seemed pleasant in the past, and that the reason for the neighbors on the street to have the party was to get to know one another better. Kim's core belief of unlovability once again leads her to accept negative thoughts as true and to use her dysfunctional strategies of avoidance and substance use.

In situation 3, Kim becomes aware of how bored and sad she feels. She thinks, "I'll never feel good. I hate feeling like this." Her negative prediction and intolerance of dysphoria are again linked to her core beliefs of helplessness and vulnerability. Again, she copes with her anxiety by turning to substances.

The cognitive conceptualization diagram can serve as an aid to identify quickly the most central beliefs and dysfunctional strategies of substance abusers, to recognize how their beliefs influence their perceptions of current situations, and to explain why they respond emotionally and behaviorally in such ineffective ways. An important part of the cognitive approach is to help patients begin to question the validity of their perceptions and the accuracy of automatic thoughts that lead to substance abuse.

A first step in therapy is to help patients recognize that their negative automatic thoughts are not completely valid. When they test their thinking and modify it to more closely resemble reality, they feel better. A later step is to help them use the same kind of evaluative process with their core beliefs, to guide them in understanding that such beliefs are ideas, not necessarily truths. Once they see themselves in a more realistic light, they begin to perceive situations differently, feel better emotionally, and use more functional strategies learned in therapy. When this occurs, they become less likely to "need" substances for mood regulation, because they have developed internal strategies for coping.

Cognitive therapy for substance abuse, therefore, aims to modify thoughts associated with substance use (both surface-level "automatic thoughts" and deep-level "core beliefs"). The goal is to develop new behaviors to take the place of dysfunctional ones. An additional focus, described later in this chapter, is practical problem solving and modifying the patient's lifestyle to decrease the likelihood of relapse. The modification of patients' long-term negative beliefs about the self is crucial to their ability to see alternative explanations for distressing events, to use more functional coping strategies learned in therapy, and to create better lives.

At some point, cognitive therapists may explore childhood issues that relate to patients' core beliefs and addictive behavior. Such exploration helps both clinicians and patients understand how patients came to such rigid, global, and inaccurate negative ideas about themselves.

Figure 22.4 reflects the basic cognitive model of substance abuse as applied to Kim's substance abuse behavior. It illustrates the cyclical nature of substance abuse. Kim, like most substance abusers, believes that taking substances is an automatic process, beyond her control. This diagram helps her identify the sequence of events leading to an incident of substance use and identifies potential points of intervention in the future. In this example, Kim feels hopeless, because she predicts she will lose her job. As she searches for a way to cope with her dysphoria, a basic substance-related belief emerges ("If I feel bad, I should smoke") and she thinks, "I might as well use." She then experiences cravings and gives herself permission to use ("My life is crummy. I deserve to feel

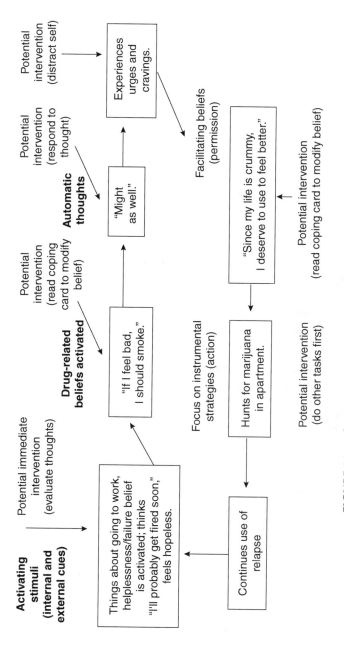

FIGURE 22.4. Cognitive model of substance abuse applied to case example.

better"); she hunts for her marijuana and smokes a joint. This typical sequence of events takes place in seconds, and Kim initially believes it is automatic. By breaking it down into a series of steps, Kim can learn a variety of ways to intervene at each stage along the way.

PRINCIPLES OF TREATMENT

A cognitive therapist could use hundreds of interventions with any given patient at any given time. In this section, we discuss cognitive therapy principles that apply to all patients, using substance abuse examples.

1. Cognitive therapy is based on a unique cognitive conceptualization of each patient.
2. A strong therapeutic alliance is essential.
3. Cognitive therapy is goal-oriented.
4. The initial focus of therapy is on the present.
5. Cognitive therapy is time-sensitive.
6. Therapy sessions are structured, with active participation.
7. Patients are taught to identify and respond to dysfunctional thoughts.
8. Cognitive therapy emphasizes psychoeducation and relapse prevention.

Principle 1: Cognitive Therapy Is Based on a Unique Cognitive Conceptualization of Each Patient

Conceptualization of the case includes analysis of the current problematic situations of substance abusers and their associated thoughts and reactions (emotional, behavioral, and physiological). Therapists and patients look for meanings expressed in patients' automatic thoughts to identify their most basic, dysfunctional core beliefs about themselves, their world, and other people (e.g., "I am weak," "The world is a hostile place").

They also identify patterns of behavior that patients develop to cope with these negative ideas. Such patterns might include taking substances, preying on people, and distancing from others. The connection between their core beliefs and compensatory strategies becomes clearer when therapists and patients identify the conditional assumptions that drive patients' behavior (e.g., "If I try to do anything difficult, I'll probably fail because I'm so weak").

Therapists and patients look at patients' developmental histories to understand how they came to hold such strong, rigid, negative core beliefs. They also explore how these beliefs might not be true today and, in some cases, were not completely true even in childhood. They look at patients' enduring patterns of interpretation that have caused them to process information so negatively.

Therapists also draw diagrams of scenarios in which patients take substances (Figure 22.4) to illustrate the cyclical process of substance use and the many opportunities to intervene and avert a relapse.

Principle 2: A Strong Therapeutic Alliance Is Essential

Successful treatment relies on a caring, collaborative, respectful therapeutic relationship. Effective therapists explain their therapeutic approach, encourage patients to express skepticism, help them test the validity of their doubts, provide explanations for their interventions, share their cognitive formulation to make sure they have an accurate understanding of the patient, and consistently ask for feedback.

Therapists who are very collaborative typically find that they can establish sound therapeutic relationships with most substance abuse patients. However, even the most skilled therapists, who embody the essential characteristics of warmth, empathy, caring, and genuine regard, find it challenging to develop good relationships with occasional patients who are suspicious, manipulative, or avoidant. Therapists are encouraged to examine relationship problems with the same careful cognitive exploration of session-related behavior as is done for all other behaviors. See Figure 22.5 for a cognitive conceptualization diagram of missed sessions and dropout.

An effective therapist seeks to avoid activating patients' core beliefs through his or her own behavior in therapy and helps patients test the validity of their ideas about the therapist. For example, Kim's therapist asked for evidence when Kim said she believed the therapist was judging her as "bad" for having a substance abuse problem. Of course, effective therapists need to examine their own thoughts, feelings, and behaviors periodically to ensure that they are not viewing their patients in a negative light. When therapists maintain true nonjudgmental attitudes, they can sincerely tell patients that they are not negatively evaluating them. They can further explain that they view patients as using substances to try to cope with the difficulties inherent in their lives.

At times, a persistent problem in the therapeutic relationship arises from a clash of patient and therapist beliefs. Therapists are advised to do conceptualization diagrams of patients and of themselves to identify dysfunctional ideas they may have about interacting with difficult people.

For example, one substance abuse patient held the core belief, "If I show any weakness, others will hurt me," and a related assumption, "If I listen to my therapist, he'll see me as weak." As a result, the patient was very controlling in the session, kept criticizing the therapist, and would not do any self-help assignments suggested by the therapist. The problem persisted, at least in part, because the therapist too had a broad assumption, "If people don't listen to me, it means they don't value me, and therefore don't deserve my best effort." The

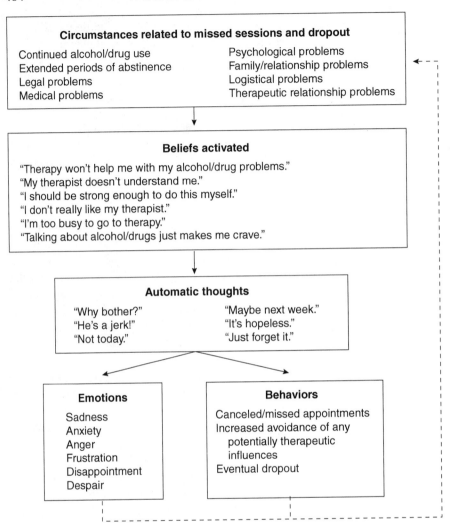

FIGURE 22.5. Cognitive conceptualization of missed sessions and dropouts.

therapist became irritated with the patient, expressing dissatisfaction through body language and tone of voice. The patient, already hypervigilant for possible harm from others, perceived the therapist's negative attitude and dropped out of therapy prematurely.

Liese and Franz (1996) have identified common dysfunctional beliefs of therapists that interfere with delivering therapy to substance abuse patients. Although many patients may minimize their substance use, confronting them in a harsh manner is likely to result in diminished therapeutic efficacy and dropping out.

When patients report no substance use during the previous week, it is often useful to inquire about times when they felt cravings. Thus, therapists can obtain relevant cognitive material to help patients continue effective responses in the coming week.

Because patients with substance problems have high dropout rates (Simpson, Joe, Rowan Szal, & Greener, 1997), it is essential to build a strong therapeutic relationship. Liese and Beck (1997) describe how cognitive therapy skills can maximize retention in treatment. Figure 22.5 presents their model for missed sessions and dropout.

Therapists increase the alliance by emphasizing that they and the patient are on the same team, working toward long-term goals. The patient can learn that therapy is not an adversarial relationship. The therapist and patient collaboratively make most of the decisions about therapy. However, therapists should know that a common compensatory strategy of substance abuse patients is avoidance (e.g., minimizing difficulties in abstaining from substances). It is important, therefore, to help patients recognize in a nonconfrontational manner that the advantages of avoidance are clearly outweighed by the disadvantages.

Principle 3: Cognitive Therapy Is Goal-Oriented

At the first session and periodically thereafter, therapists ask patients to set goals. They identify objectives in specific behavioral terms by asking, "How would you like to be different by the end of therapy?" It is important to give patients feedback about their goals, because they sometimes harbor unrealistic expectations. Therapists also help to identify short-term goals and propose ways the patient can meet those goals.

For example, Kim's therapist helped her specify her goal of "being happy" in behavioral terms: getting a job she enjoyed, entering into a romantic relationship, getting along with her family, and staying abstinent. He helped her set smaller goals along the way. A first step in getting a new job was to improve her attendance at her current job, so she could get a good letter of reference.

Therapists also question patients about the degree to which they *really* want to meet their goals. A helpful technique is the advantage–disadvantage analysis (Figure 22.6), adapted from Marlatt and Gordon (1985). In this exercise, the therapist explores the benefits of achieving a goal, while also reframing the disadvantages.

For some patients, a goal of harm reduction is more acceptable and achievable than complete abstinence (Fletcher, 2001; Marlatt, Tucker, Donovan, & Vuchinich, 1997). While abstinence is generally the safest goal, a decrease in substance use is more desirable than early dropout from therapy, which can occur if the therapist tries too early or too strongly to impose a total ban on all substances.

Advantages of Abstinence	Advantages of Taking Drugs (with reframe)
1. Feel better about myself. 2. Feel more in control. 3. Get to work on time. 4. More likely to keep my job. 5. Save money. 6. Better for my health. 7. Not get so criticized by my sister. 8. Not hang around other "druggies" so much. 9. Spend my time better.	1. Escape from feeling bad (**BUT** it's only a temporary escape and I don't really solve my problems). 2. Have people to hang out with (**BUT** they're druggies and I don't really like them). 3. It's hard work to quit (**BUT** I'll do it step-by-step with my therapist).
Disadvantages of Abstinence (with reframe)	**Disadvantages of Taking Drugs**
1. I may feel bored and anxious (**BUT** it's only temporary and it's good to learn to stand bad feelings). 2. I don't know what to do with my time (**BUT** I can learn in therapy how to spend time better). 3. I won't be able to hang out with my "friends" (**BUT** I do want to meet new "nondruggie" friends).	1. Seems to make me depressed. 2. Costs money. 3. Bad for my health. 4. Makes me feel like I'm not in control of my life. 5. Makes me feel unmotivated. 6. Hard to solve my real problems. 7. May make me lose my job. 8. Makes relationship with my sister worse. 9. Stops me from going out and making new friends. 10. Makes me feel like I'm wasting time. 11. Makes me feel stuck, like I'm not getting anywhere.

FIGURE 22.6. Advantages–disadvantages analysis.

Principle 4: The Initial Focus of Therapy Is on the Present

Therapists initially emphasize current and specific problems that are distressing to the patient. When the patient has a comorbid diagnosis, it is important to address problems related to both. For example, Kim needed help in problem solving about a critical supervisor at work and in learning alternate coping strategies (instead of using substances) when she was distressed about a work problem. She and her therapist discussed how to respond to the hurt she felt when the supervisor rebuked her for lateness, how to decrease her anger by rehearsing a coping statement addressing her activated core belief, how to use anger management techniques such as controlled breathing and time-out, and how to talk to the supervisor in a reasonable manner.

The therapist also helped Kim respond to automatic thoughts. Through a combination of Socratic questioning and modeling, Kim learned to change the thought, "I should tell my supervisor off," with "He's just trying to do his job; I want to keep this job; I can just say OK for now and stay calm." Toward the middle of therapy, the therapist and Kim began discussing her past as well—to see how she developed her ideas about relationships, and how they related to her current difficulties.

Principle 5: Cognitive Therapy Is Time-Sensitive

The course of therapy for substance abuse patients varies depending on the severity of the substance use. Weekly or even twice-weekly sessions are recommended until symptoms are significantly reduced. With effective treatment, patients stabilize their moods, learn more tools, and gain confidence in using alternate coping strategies. At this point, therapist and patient may experiment with decreasing sessions. For example, in a major study of cognitive therapy for cocaine dependence (Crits-Christoph et al., 1997), the frequency of sessions went from once a week to once every 2 weeks, then to once every 3 or 4 weeks. After termination, an "open door" approach is helpful, in which patients are invited to return to therapy if they are tempted to use substances again.

Principle 6: Therapy Sessions Are Structured, with Active Participation

Typically, therapists use a structured format, unless it interferes with the therapeutic alliance. Usually therapists first check the patient's mood and recent amount and type of substance use (including, if possible, objective assessment of these). They explore the patient's progress or worsening, and elicit the patient's feelings about coming to therapy that day. Next the therapist sets an agenda and decides with the patient what problems to focus on in the session. Standard items include the successes and difficulties the patient experienced during the past week and upcoming situations that could lead to substance use or dropout.

The therapist then makes a bridge from the previous session, asking the patient to recall the important things they discussed. If the patient has difficulty remembering the content, they problem-solve to help the patient make better use of future sessions. Encouraging patients to take notes and review these during the week helps them integrate the lessons of therapy. Also, during this part of the session, the therapist reviews the therapy homework completed during the week. If therapists suspect that patients have reacted badly to a previous session, they may ask for feedback about the session.

Next, they address specific topics of concern to the patient. As they discuss the first problem, they collect information about it, conceptualize how it arose, evaluate thoughts about it, modify relevant beliefs, and problem-solve as needed. In the context of discussing the problem, the therapist teaches the patient skills in various domains: interpersonal (e.g., assertiveness), mood management (e.g., relaxation, anger management), behavioral (e.g., alternate behaviors when cravings start), and cognitive (e.g., worksheets on dysfunctional cognitions).

Homework is customized to the patient. Typically, it includes monitoring substance use and mood, responding to automatic thoughts and beliefs, practicing new skills, and problem solving.

Throughout the session, the therapist summarizes the material the patient has presented and checks comprehension by asking about the "main message." At the end of the session, they summarize what occurred, checking that the patient understands and is likely to do the homework. Finally, the therapist asks for feedback. Skillful questioning of the patient's honest reactions and non-defensive problem solving by the therapist promote progress and lessen dropout.

Adhering to this structure has many benefits: The most important issues are discussed; there is continuity between sessions; substance use is monitored; and problems are directly addressed. In addition, patients learn new skills and are more likely to use these in the coming week. The structure also ensures that patient and therapist understand the lessons of the session, and that the patient is given the opportunity to provide feedback, so therapy can be modified if needed.

Principle 7: Patients Are Taught to Identify and Respond to Dysfunctional Thoughts

The therapist emphasizes the cognitive model at each session—that patients' thoughts influence how they react emotionally, physiologically, and behaviorally, and that by correcting their dysfunctional thinking, they can feel and behave better. The therapist does not assume that automatic thoughts are distorted; instead, therapist and patient investigate whether a given thought is valid. When thoughts *are* accurate (e.g., "I want a fix"), they either problem-solve (discuss ways to respond to the thought) or explore the validity of the conclusion the patient has drawn (e.g., "Wanting a fix shows I am weak"). When evaluating thoughts, the therapist primarily uses questioning rather than persuading the patient, and standard tools such as the Dysfunctional Thought Record (J. S. Beck, 1995) are used when possible.

Principle 8: Cognitive Therapy Emphasizes Psychoeducation and Relapse Prevention

From the first session, the goal is to maximize patients' learning. The therapist encourages patients to write down important points during the session or does the writing for them, if necessary. When patients are illiterate, the therapist uses ingenuity to create a system for helping them remember (e.g., audiotaping the session, a brief summary of the session, or brainstorming whom the patient might ask to read therapy notes).

The therapist teaches patients how to best use the new strategies. The goal is to make the patient her own best "cognitive therapist." For example, the therapist teaches Kim how to identify her negative thoughts when she feels upset, how to respond to these thoughts, how to examine her behaviors, how to use coping strategies when she has cravings, how to communicate effectively, how to avoid high-risk situations, and many more cognitive, behavioral, mood-stabilizing, and general life skills.

Prior to termination, relapse prevention is emphasized. The therapist and patient review skills; predict difficulties; note early warning signs of relapse; and discuss how to limit a lapse from becoming a relapse. They agree on when the patient needs to return to therapy, that is, if a lapse is imminent (instead of just after it occurs). Finally, they develop a plan for patients to continue to work on their goals, preferably with the support of friends and family.

TREATMENT PLANNING

The first step in treatment planning is to complete a thorough diagnostic assessment based on the criteria of the *Diagnostic and Statistical Manual of Mental Disorders* (DSM-IV-TR; American Psychiatric Association, 2000). It is essential to evaluate comorbid Axis I and Axis II disorders, as well as medical complications.

According to research (Kessler et al., 1996), many patients with substance use disorders have a co-occurring psychiatric disorder. The treatment plan should address both. For example, Kim's therapist conceptualized that she was medicating her depression with marijuana. In addition to treating her substance use, the therapist focused on the depression itself, using standard cognitive therapy strategies to reduce her depressive symptoms: activity scheduling, responding to negative cognitions (e.g., "I can't do anything right"), and problem solving (e.g., about work problems and loneliness), among others (see A. T. Beck et al., 1979; J. S. Beck, 1995). She was also referred to a psychiatrist for a medication consultation.

Kim also had an Axis II diagnosis: avoidant personality disorder with dependent and borderline features. One important implication of any personality disorder is the strong likelihood that associated dysfunctional beliefs (e.g., "I am helpless; I am bad") might arise in the therapy session itself. Her therapist planned treatment to avoid intense schema activation early in therapy that might have led to premature dropout. Adding elements from cognitive therapy for personality disorders may be helpful for Axis II issues (Beck et al., 1990; Young, 1999).

A second key step in treatment planning is to identify the patient's motivation for change. Prochaska, DiClemente, and Norcross (1992) describe five stages of change: the precontemplation stage (in which patients are only minimally, if at all, distressed about their problems and have little motivation to change), the contemplation stage (in which they have sufficient motivation to consider their problems and think about change, although not necessarily enough to take action), the preparation stage (in which they want help to make changes but may not feel they know what to do), the action stage (in which they start to change their behavior), or the maintenance stage (in which they are motivated to continue to change).

Kim, for example, was at the contemplation stage when she entered therapy. Her therapist helped her identify the problems associated with her substance use, some of which she had avoided focusing on before therapy. Her therapist also helped her do an advantages–disadvantages analysis of marijuana use (Figure 22.6). He helped her "reframe" or find a functional response to her dysfunctional ideas of not changing. These techniques helped move Kim from the contemplation to the preparation stage. Had her therapist started with a treatment plan that emphasized immediate change of substance use behaviors, it is likely that Kim would have resisted, tried only halfheartedly, or dropped out of therapy altogether.

Part of every treatment plan involves socializing patients to the cognitive model, so that they begin to view their reactions as stemming from their (often distorted) perceptions of situations. Once her therapist taught her to ask herself what was going through her mind just before she reached for a joint, Kim could understand how her automatic thoughts influenced her emotional and behavioral reactions. Later, he taught her how to identify the more complex sequence (Figure 22.4) leading to substance use and helped her identify how she could intervene at each stage.

An essential element in treatment planning is evaluating the strength of the therapeutic alliance. Substance abuse patients often enter treatment with dysfunctional beliefs about therapy, such as the following:

"My therapist may try to force me to do things I don't like."
"This therapy may do more harm than good."
"He probably thinks he knows everything."
"She'll think I'm a failure if I use again."
"I'm better off without therapy."

The treatment plan should include the identification and testing of these dysfunctional beliefs. Otherwise, patients may drop out prematurely. A good treatment plan also specifies patients' problems (or, positively framed, their goals) and the concrete steps needed to ameliorate them. Kim and her therapist discussed her work problems. They did a combination of problem solving and correcting distortions related to work themes, such as getting to work on time, boredom on the job, fear of criticism, and relating to coworkers. Eventually she sought a new job, when it became clear that the disadvantages of the job (low pay and lack of stimulation) still outweighed the positive aspects. Her therapist encouraged her in the job search.

The work problem was one of the first problems they tackled, because Kim was motivated to work on it, it was closely connected to her marijuana use, and it seemed they might make improvements on it in a short period. Later in therapy, they addressed situations that were even more difficult: getting along with her family, meeting new friends, and developing broader interests.

Her therapist continuously assessed Kim's readiness to change her substance abuse by measuring the strength of her beliefs. At the beginning of therapy, she believed that her marijuana use might contribute to her work problems, her social isolation, and her lack of motivation. However, she also believed that nothing, including therapy, could help. After several weeks, she began to see things differently, especially when she recognized that some initial behavioral activation and responding to automatic thoughts improved her mood. Now she was ready to explore how she came to use marijuana, to start monitoring her substance use, to learn strategies to manage cravings, to avoid high-risk situations, to respond to substance-related beliefs, to join a self-help group, and to make some lifestyle changes. These strategies are described next.

Teaching Patients to Observe Substance Use Sequences

Kim's therapist used a blank version of Figure 22.4, asking Kim to fill in the boxes after thinking about a recent episode of marijuana use. For the first time, it became clear to Kim that her behavior was at least somewhat voluntary. Previously she had believed that her use was completely out of her control.

The therapist reviewed how a typical activating stimulus gave rise to negative thoughts, which led to feelings of hopelessness. They discussed how she could learn to intervene. First, she could respond to her negative thoughts to reduce her dysphoria. Even if that did not work, she could still respond to her substance-related beliefs. She could, for example, read a coping card they developed in session. Such a card might contain "what to do if I want to smoke." These coping cards are not merely affirmations but jointly composed statements that the patient endorses in session. They might include the following:

1. Go for a walk.
2. Call a friend.
3. Go out for coffee.
4. Watch a movie.
5. Read my Narcotics Anonymous book.

If Kim's automatic thoughts about substance use continued, she would have another opportunity to respond. Upon experiencing cravings, she could tell herself to ignore these sensations and distract herself. For example, she might create a coping card that said:

"If I feel cravings, *they are just cravings*. I don't have to attend to them. They'll go away. I can stand them. I've stood cravings in the past. I'll be *very* glad in a few minutes that I ignored them. When I ignore them, I get stronger!"

If she recognized her permission-giving beliefs, she could read another coping card that might say:

"Don't reach for a joint. Wait 5 minutes. I am strong enough to wait. In the meantime, do what's on my 'to do' list."

If she found herself focusing on strategies to get substances, she could try another waiting period or do other tasks outlined in therapy. A careful analysis of the substance-taking sequence, along with potential interventions, gave Kim hope that she could conquer this problem.

Kim and her therapist developed the coping cards over several sessions. First they discussed what Kim wished she could tell herself at each stage. Before writing the cards, the therapist asked Kim how much she believed each statement. When the strength of her belief was less than 90–100%, they reworded the statement or discussed it further to increase its validity. They observed that if Kim did not believe an idea strongly in the session, it was unlikely to work in "real life"; thus, they needed more compelling beliefs.

Monitoring Progress

Progress is monitored in several ways. Most obvious is the patient's report of substance use, obtained at each session. Urine and Breathalyzer tests can also motivate a decrease in use and an increase in the validity of self-reports. When patients do use, they are encouraged to see it not as an indication of failure, but rather as an opportunity to learn from the experience and to make future abstinence more likely. A variety of self-report instruments exist for substance abuse, such as the Timeline Followback (Sobell & Sobell, 1993). For substance abuse instruments that can be downloaded directly from the Web, see the appendices at the end of this chapter. Reports from others, such as family members or probation officers, may also be particularly important for patients with low motivation or a history of lying about their use.

When a patient has a comorbid Axis I or II disorder, progress is also measured by instruments such as the Beck Depression Inventory (A. T. Beck & Steer, 1993b), the Beck Anxiety Inventory (A. T. Beck & Steer, 1993a), the Brief Symptom Inventory (Derogatis, 1992), and other instruments relevant to particular symptoms. Improvements in scores provide an opportunity to reinforce positive changes that patients have made in their thinking and behavior in the past week. Worsening scores raise a red flag, and careful questioning about recent events and perceptions often reveals agenda items to prevent the resumption of substance use in the coming week.

It is also important to monitor how patients spend their time. Kim, for example, made some changes early in therapy: less time watching television alone and fewer visits to substance-using friends. Had her therapist not been vigilant about checking weekly on these improvements, he might have missed significant backsliding many weeks later, which could have led to a relapse.

Another aspect of monitoring is assessment of old, dysfunctional beliefs versus newer, more functional ideas. At each session, the therapist assessed how much Kim believed substance-related ideas such as "I can't stand to feel bored" and "Smoking marijuana is the only way to feel better," and how much she believed the new ideas they had developed, such as "My life will improve if I don't use" and "I can feel better by answering my negative thoughts and completing my 'to do' list." This monitoring helped the therapist intervene early when Kim's dysfunctional beliefs occasionally resurfaced strongly.

Dealing with High-Risk Situations

Marlatt and Gordon (1985) observed that exposure to activating stimuli, or triggers, makes substance use more likely. In high-risk situations, activating stimuli trigger substance-related beliefs, leading to cravings. These stimuli are idiosyncratic; what triggers one patient may not trigger another.

Triggers can be internal or external. Internal cues include negative mood states such as depression, anxiety, loneliness, and boredom, or physical factors such as pain, hunger, or fatigue. Although many patients use substances to regulate negative moods, many also use substances when they already feel good, to "celebrate" or to feel great.

External cues occur outside the individual: people, places, or things related to substance use, such as relationship conflicts or seeing substance paraphernalia. In one study, Cummings, Gordon, and Marlatt (1980) found that 35% of relapses were precipitated by negative emotional states, 20% by social pressure, and 16% by interpersonal conflict.

The therapist helps patients identify the high-risk situations in which their substance-related beliefs and cravings occur. They are encouraged to avoid these situations and are taught relationship skills to handle conflict and pressure to use. For example, they might rehearse how Kim could respond when a friend offers her a drink.

Managing Cravings and Urges

Patients should learn both cognitive and behavioral techniques for managing cravings. Distraction is often helpful, and patients can devise a list of things they can easily do (e.g., exercise, read, and talk on the telephone). Thought stopping can reduce urges. Snapping a rubber band and yelling "Stop!" while envisioning a stop sign helped Kim manage her craving. Grounding is another strategy that aids distraction from cravings and intense negative emotions; one can teach mental, physical, and soothing grounding methods (see Najavits, 2002a, for a description and handouts).

The therapist can help patients identify beliefs that encourage the use of substances to deal with cravings, for example, "I can't stand the craving"; "If I have cravings, I have to give in." Socratic questioning, examining past experiences of resisting craving, reflecting on the relative difficulty versus impossibility of tolerating cravings, and other cognitive techniques can modify these dysfunctional ideas.

Case Management and Lifestyle Change

Helping patients solve their real-life problems is an essential part of cognitive therapy. Patients who abuse substances often have complex medical, legal, employment, housing, and family difficulties. Therapists should refer patients for assistance when needed. Therefore, they need to be aware of community resources and social services. Sometimes they can help identify people in patients' social network who can help them work through such practical problems.

In some cases, however, it is necessary to help patients directly in session to take steps to improve their lives. Examining employment ads in the newspaper, for example, or completing forms (e.g., for public housing) with the patient is often an important part of treatment. For examples of case management for substance abuse, including dual diagnosis, see Drake and Noordsy (1994), Najavits (2002b), and Ridgely and Willenbring (1992).

Some lifestyle change is usually necessary for substance abuse patients to eliminate substance use and to maintain progress. Often the therapist needs to help the patient repair important supportive relationships and develop new relationships with people who do not use. Many substance abusers are deficient in relationship skills and need to learn these through discussion and role plays. Patients often have dysfunctional beliefs about relationships, and modification of these beliefs is a necessary step in learning to relate well to others.

Patients sometimes need help identifying how they can build a new, nonusing network of friends. The therapist can discuss contact with nonusers in the patient's environment, as well as encourage new activities to meet new people.

Self-help groups can be a valuable adjunct to therapy—for meeting new, nonusing people, reinforcing functional beliefs, and building a healthier lifestyle. Therapists should be aware of self-help groups in their area and encourage patients to attend. AA, NA, SMART Recovery, and Moderation Management are a few examples of groups that can be of significant benefit to patients. See the appendices at the end of this chapter for websites and phone numbers. Therapists can help patients who are reluctant to attend self-help groups by eliciting their automatic thoughts and aiding them in responding to these thoughts. Problem solving may be needed to help the patient choose groups or activities, find transportation, and manage anxiety about new experiences.

Reducing Dropout

Studies have shown that approximately 30–60% of substance abuse patients drop out of therapy (Wierzbicki & Pekarik, 1993). Many factors account for this high rate, including continued substance use; legal, medical, relationship, or psychological problems; practical problems (e.g., transportation, finances); dissatisfaction with therapy; and problems with the therapeutic alliance (Liese & Beck, 1997). Early in therapy, therapist and patient should predict potential difficulties that might interfere with regular attendance in therapy and either problem-solve in advance or collaboratively develop a plan for contact (usually by phone) if the patient misses a session.

Kim's therapist, for example, helped her with problems such as changing her work schedule and transportation, which otherwise would have impeded her attendance. Both straightforward problem solving and responding to negative thinking ("I'll be too tired to come after work"; "It's not worth taking two buses") were necessary to avoid missed sessions.

To maximize regular attendance, the therapist needs to monitor the strength of the therapeutic relationship at each session. Negative changes in patients' body language, voice, and degree of openness usually signal that dysfunctional beliefs (about themselves or therapy) have been activated. A list of 50 common beliefs leading to missed sessions and dropout (Liese & Beck, 1997) is a valuable guide for therapists. Testing negative thoughts immediately can prevent a negative reaction that otherwise might have resulted in the patient missing the next session. Kim had many such cognitions, especially early in therapy: "I'm not smart enough for this therapy"; "I can't do this." A therapist who still suspects a patient may miss the next session may be able to turn the tide by phoning the patient the day before the session and demonstrating care and concern.

Formulating an accurate cognitive conceptualization of the patient from the start enables the therapist to plan interventions to avoid inadvertent activation of dysfunctional beliefs within and between sessions. Kim's therapist, for example, recognized how overwhelmed Kim became when faced with even minor challenges. She therefore took care to explain concepts simply, to limit the amount of material each session, to check her understanding frequently, and to suggest homework that she could do. Thus, she avoided undue activation of Kim's beliefs of inadequacy and helped maintain her therapy attendance.

COMPARISON WITH OTHER MODELS

It may be helpful to compare cognitive therapy for substance abuse with some other widely known approaches, specifically, motivational enhancement therapy and dialectical behavior therapy.

Motivational enhancement therapy (MET; Miller, Zweben, DiClemente, & Rychtarik, 1995) derives from several different theories, including client-centered, cognitive-behavioral, and systems theories, and the social psychology of persuasion. The treatment is guided by five principles: The therapist should express empathy, develop discrepancy between the patient's goals and current problem behavior, avoid argumentation, roll with resistance rather than opposing it directly, and support self-efficacy by emphasizing personal responsibility and the hope of change. Specific strategies include reflective listening, affirmation, open-ended questions, summarizing, and eliciting self-motivational statements (e.g., asking evocative questions, inquiring about pros and cons of behavior, and exploring goals). The therapist also addresses ambivalence that may interfere with motivation and uses assessment instruments that are presented to the patient to increase motivation for change (e.g., alcohol/drug use, functional analysis of behavior, readiness to change, life problems, and biomedical impact).

MET differs from cognitive therapy for substance abuse in several ways. First, MET is primarily designed as a process-oriented method to increase motivation. It was not designed to teach specific new skills or coping strategies (such as cognitive therapy skills of identifying dysfunctional cognitions, rehearsal of new responses to cognitions, identification of alternative coping strategies, mood monitoring, social skills training, and lifestyle changes). Second, and likely because of the difference in goals, MET is typically much shorter. For example, in Project MATCH, MET was four sessions. Indeed, MET is primarily thought of as a precursor to or combination with other therapies for substance abuse, including cognitive therapy (e.g., Barrowclough et al., 2001).

Dialectical behavior therapy (DBT) by Linehan (1993) is a CBT designed for borderline personality disorder (BPD). It comprises twice weekly group sessions and weekly individual sessions, and as-needed phone coaching. DBT teaches a variety of skills, in part inspired by Eastern philosophy, including mindfulness, distress tolerance, emotion regulation, interpersonal effectiveness, and self-management (Linehan, 1993). After positive outcomes with patients with BPD, it was adapted for substance abuse patients with BPD in the late 1990s (Dimeff, Rizvi, Brown, & Linehan, 2000; Linehan et al., 1999, 2002). The adaptation for substance abuse includes several new skills, including alternate rebellion, adaptive denial, burning bridges to drug use, and building a life worth living. DBT differs from cognitive therapy in several ways. First, cognitive therapy for substance abuse was designed for a very broad spectrum of substance abuse patients, whereas DBT focuses on patients with the dual diagnosis of BPD and substance abuse. Thus, some precepts that may be especially helpful for BPD may not apply to the typical substance abuse patient without BPD. For example, under the "four-session rule" in DBT, if a client misses four or more sessions, she loses access to the therapy. Also, a patient in DBT must agree to a lengthy course of treatment (e.g., two full rounds of the DBT skills modules, and sessions three times per week). In cognitive therapy, such imperatives are not required. Second, and again, likely due to the nature of BPD, therapists use a team or community-of-therapists approach, and therapists are asked to be available after hours for phone coaching of clients. Cognitive therapy follows more traditional therapist roles. Finally, whereas both DBT and cognitive therapy focus on teaching new coping skills, the skills themselves differ to some degree. For example, cognitive therapy focuses much more formally on changing cognitions through the use of structured tools for cognitive change such as the Dysfunctional Thoughts Record.

CONCLUSION

Cognitive therapy can be an effective treatment for substance abuse patients. It requires accurate conceptualization of the patient, a sound treatment plan based on this case formulation, a strong therapeutic relationship, and specialized interventions. Structuring the therapy session, problem solving of current difficulties, education about the sequence of substance use, planning for high-risk situations, monitoring of substance use, lifestyle change, and intensive case management are important facets of treatment.

Kim could easily have become an unemployed "revolving door" user and a burden to family, friends, and society. Cognitive therapy helped her to engage in therapy, work through dysfunctional beliefs about herself and the therapist, develop functional goals, learn new skills to solve problems, tolerate negative emotion, persist when she felt hopeless, engage in alternative behaviors when she craved substances, and develop a healthier lifestyle. Hard work by both the therapist and substance abuse patient can pay off handsomely.

APPENDIX 22.1. SUBSTANCE ABUSE RECOVERY RESOURCES*

Resource	Website	Phone
National Drug Information, Treatment and Referral Line	www.drughelp.org	800-662-HELP
National Clearinghouse for Alcohol and Drug Information	www.health.org	800-729-6686
Alcohol and Drug Healthline	www.samsha.gov	800-821-4357
Alcoholics Anonymous	www.alcoholics-anonymous.org	800-637-6237
Cocaine Anonymous	www.ca.org	310-559-5833
Narcotics Anonymous	www.na.org	818-773-9999

Resource	Website	Phone
Marijuana Anonymous	www.marijuana-anonymous.org	800-766-6779
Nicotine Anonymous	www.nicotine-anonymous.org	415-750-0328
Smart Recovery	www.smartrecovery.org	440-951-5357
Secular Organization for Sobriety/Save Our Selves	www.secularsobriety.org	323-666-4295
Harm Reduction Coalition	www.harmreduction.org	510-444-6969
Moderation Management Network	www.moderation.org	212-871-0974
Women for Sobriety	www.womenforsobriety.org	215-536-8026

*From Najavits (2002a). Copyright 2002 by the Guilford Press. Adapted by permission.

APPENDIX 22.2. SUBSTANCE ABUSE ASSESSMENT RESOURCES*

Resource	Website	Phone
National Institute on Alcohol Abuse and Alcoholism	www.niaaa.nih.gov/publications	—
Substance Abuse and Mental Health Services Administration	store.health.org and www.samsha.gov (click "publications," then "substance abuse treatment resources")	800-729-6686
National Institute on Drug Abuse	www.nida.nih.gov (click "publications")	—
Free screening online for alcoholism	www.alcoholscreening.org	—
University of New Mexico Center on Alcoholism, Substance Abuse, and Addictions	casaa.unm.edu/inst/inst.html	
To locate substance abuse home-test kits	www.thomasregister.com (enter "alcohol drug test" for list of companies that provide home test kits for substance abuse)	—

*From Najavits (2004). Copyright 2004 by The Guilford Press. Adapted by permission.

REFERENCES

American Psychiatric Association. (2000). *Diagnostic and statistical manual of mental disorders* (4th ed., text rev.). Washington, DC: Author.

Barrowclough, C., Haddock, G., Tarrier, N., Lewis, S. W., Moring, J., O'Brien, R., et al.. (2001). Randomized controlled trial of motivational interviewing, cognitive behavioral therapy, and family intervention for patients with comorbid schizophrenia and substance use disorders. *Am J Psychiatry, 158,* 1706–1713.

Beck, A. T., Emery, G., with Greenberg, R. L. (1985). *Anxiety disorders and phobias: A cognitive perspective.* New York: Basic Books.

Beck, A. T., Freeman, A., & Associates, (1990). *Cognitive therapy of personality disorders.* New York: Guilford Press.

Beck, A. T., Rush, A. J., Shaw, B. F., & Emery, G. (1979). *Cognitive therapy of depression.* New York: Guilford Press.

Beck, A. T., & Steer, R. A. (1993a). *Beck Anxiety Inventory manual.* San Antonio, TX: Psychological Corporation.

Beck, A. T., & Steer, R. A. (1993b). *Beck Depression Inventory manual.* San Antonio, TX: Psychological Corporation.

Beck, A. T., Wright, F. D., Newman, C. F., & Liese, B. S. (1993). *Cognitive therapy of substance abuse.* New York: Guilford Press.

Beck, J. S. (1995). *Cognitive therapy: Basics and beyond.* New York: Guilford Press.

Carroll, K. (1998). *A cognitive-behavioral approach: Treating cocaine addiction* (NIH Publication No. 98-4308). Rockville, MD: National Institute on Drug Abuse.

Carroll, K. M. (1999). Behavioral and cognitive behavioral treatments. In B. S. McCrady & E. E. Epstein (Eds.), *Addictions: A comprehensive guidebook* (pp. 250–267). New York: Oxford University Press.

Crits-Christoph, P., Siqueland, L., Blaine, J., Frank, A., Luborsky, L., Onken, L. S., et al. (1997). The NIDA Cocaine Collaborative Treatment Study: Rationale and methods. *Arch Gen Psychiatry, 54,* 721–726.

Crits-Christoph, P., Siqueland, L., Blaine, J., Frank, A., Luborsky, L., Onken, L. S., et al. (1999). Psychosocial treatment for cocaine dependence: The National Institute on Drug Abuse Collaborative Cocaine Treatment Study. *Arch Gen Psychiatry, 56,* 493–502.

Cummings, C., Gordon, J. R., & Marlatt, G. A. (1980). Relapse: Prevention and prediction. In W. R. Miller (Ed.), *The addictive behaviors: Treatment of alcoholism, substance abuse, smoking and obesity* (pp. 291–321). Oxford, UK: Pergamon Press.

Derogatis, L. R. (1992). *Brief Symptom Inventory.* Baltimore: Clinical Psychometric Research, Inc.

Dimeff, L., Rizvi, S. L., Brown, M., & Linehan, M. M. (2000). Dialectical behavioral therapy for substance abuse: A pilot application to methamphetamine-dependent women with borderline personality disorder. *Cognit Behav Pract, 7,* 457–468.

Dimeff, L. A., & Marlatt, G. A. (1998). Preventing relapse and maintaining change in addictive behaviors. *Clin Psychol: Sci Pract, 5,* 513–525.

Drake, R. E., & Noordsy, D. L. (1994). Case management for people with coexisting severe mental disorder and substance use disorder. *Psychiatr Ann, 24,* 427–431.

Fletcher, A. (2001). *Sober for good: New solutions for drinking problems—advice from those who have succeeded.* Boston: Houghton Mifflin.

Fromme, K., & Brown, S. A. (2000). Empirically based prevention and treatment approaches for adolescent and young adult substance use. *Cog Behav Pract, 7,* 61–64.

Kessler, R. C., Nelson, C. B., McGonagle, K. A., Edlund, M. J., Frank, R. G., & Leaf, P. J. (1996). The epidemiology of co-occurring addictive and mental disorders: Implications for prevention and service utilization. *Am J Orthopsychiatry, 66*(1), 17–31.

Liese, B. S., & Beck, A. T. (1997). Back to basics: Fundamental cognitive therapy skills for keeping substance-dependent individuals in treatment. In L. S. Onken, J. D. Blaine, & J. J. Boren (Eds.), *Beyond the therapeutic alliance: Keeping substance-dependent individuals in treatment* (NIDA Research Monograph No. 165, DHHS Publication No. 97-4142, pp. 207–230). Washington, DC: U.S. Government Printing Office.

Liese, B. S., & Franz, R. A. (1996). Treating substance use disorders with cognitive therapy: Lessons learned and implications for the future. In P. Salkovskis (Ed.), *Frontiers of cognitive therapy* (pp. 470–508). New York: Guilford Press.

Linehan, M. M. (1993). *Skills training manual for treating borderline personality disorder.* New York: Guilford Press.

Linehan, M. M., Dimeff, L. A., Reynolds, S. K., Comtois, K. A., Welch, S. S., Heagerty, P., & Kivlahan, D. R. (2002). Dialectal behavioral therapy versus comprehensive validation therapy plus 12-step for the treatment of opioid dependent women meeting criteria for borderline personality disorder. *Drug Alcohol Depend, 67,* 13–26.

Linehan, M. M., Schmidt, H., Dimeff, L. A., Craft, J. C., Kanter, J., & Comtois, K. A. (1999). Dialectical behavioral therapy for patients with borderline personality disorder and drug-dependence. *Am J Addict, 8,* 279–292.

Marlatt, G. A., Tucker, J., Donovan, D., & Vuchinich, R. (1997). Help-seeking by substance abusers: The role of harm reduction and behavioral-economic approaches to facilitate treatment entry and retention. In L. Onken & J. Blaine & J. Boren (Eds.), *Beyond the therapeutic alliance: Keeping the drug-dependent individual in treatment* (pp. 44–84). Rockville, MD: U.S. Department of Health and Human Services.

Marlatt, G. A., & Gordon, J. R. (Eds.). (1985). *Relapse prevention: Maintenance strategies in the treatment of addictive behavior.* New York: Guilford Press.

Maude-Griffin, P. M., Hohenstein, J. M., Humfleet, G. L., Reilly, P. M., Tusel, D. J., & Hall, S. M. (1998). Superior efficacy of cognitive-behavioral therapy for urban crack cocaine abusers: Main and matching effects. *J Consult Clin Psychol, 66,* 832–837.

Miller, W. R., Zweben, A., DiClemente, C. C., & Rychtarik, R. G. (Eds.). (1995). *Motivational enhancement therapy manual* (Vol. 2). Rockville, MD: U.S. Department of Health and Human Services.

Najavits, L. M. (2002a). *Seeking safety: A treatment manual for PTSD and substance abuse.* New York: Guilford Press.

Najavits, L. M. (2002b). *A woman's addiction workbook.* Oakland, CA: New Harbinger.

Najavits, L. M. (2004). Assessment of trauma, PTSD, and substance use disorder: A practical guide. In J. P. Wilson & T. M. Keane (Eds.), *Assessing psychological trauma and PTSD* (2nd ed., pp. 466–491). New York: Guilford Press.

Najavits, L. M., Liese, B. S., & Harned, M. (2004). Cognitive-behavioral therapy. In J. H. Lowinson, P. Ruiz, R. B. Millman, & J. G. Langrod (Eds.), *Substance abuse: A comprehensive textbook* (4th ed., pp. 723–732). Baltimore: Williams & Wilkins.

Newman, C. F., & Ratto, C. L. (1999). Cognitive therapy of substance abuse. In E. T. Dowd & L. Rugle (Eds.), *Comparative treatments of substance abuse* (Vol. 1, pp. 96–126). New York: Springer.

Prochaska, J. O., DiClemente, C. C., & Norcross, J. C. (1992). In search of how people change: Applications to addictive behaviors. *Am Psychol, 47*, 1102–1114.

Project MATCH Research Group. (1997). Matching alcoholism treatments to client heterogeneity: Project MATCH posttreatment drinking outcomes. *J Stud Alcohol, 58*, 7–29.

Rawson, R. A., Huber, A., McCann, M., Shoptaw, S., Farabee, D., Reiber, C., & Ling, W. (2002). A comparison of contingency management and cognitive-behavioral approaches during methadone maintenance treatment for cocaine dependence. *Arch Gen Psychiatry, 59*, 817–824.

Ridgely, M. S., & Willenbring, M. L. (1992). Application of case management to drug abuse treatment: Overview of models and research issues. (NIDA Research Monograph, Vol. 127, pp. 12–33). Rockville, MD: U.S. Department of Health and Human Services.

Schonfeld, L., Dupree, L. W., Dickson-Fuhrmann, E., Royer, C. M., McDermott, C. H., Rosansky, J. S., et al. (2000). Cognitive-behavioral treatment of older veterans with substance abuse problems. *J Geriatr Psychiatry Neurol, 13*, 124–129.

Simpson, D. D., Joe, G. W., Rowan Szal, G. A., & Greener, J. M. (1997). Drug abuse treatment process components that improve retention. *J Subst Abuse Treat, 14*(6), 565–572.

Sobell, M. B., & Sobell, L. C. (1993). *Problem drinkers: Guided self-change treatment.* New York: Guilford Press.

Thase, M. E. (1997). Cognitive-behavioral therapy for substance abuse disorders. In L. J. Dickstein, M. B. Riba, & J. Oldham (Eds.), *American Psychiatric Press review of psychiatry* (Vol. 16, pp. 145–171). Washington, DC: American Psychiatric Press.

Waldron, H. B., Slesnick, N., Brody, J. L., Turner, C. W., & Peterson, T. R. (2001). Treatment outcomes for adolescent substance abuse at 4- and 7-month assessments. *J Consult Clin Psychol, 69*, 802–813.

Weiss, R. D., Najavits, L. M., & Greenfield, S. F. (1999). A relapse prevention group for patients with bipolar and substance use disorders. *J Subst Abuse Treat, 16*, 47–54.

Wierzbicki, M., & Pekarik, G. (1993). A meta-analysis of psychotherapy dropout. *Professional Psychol: Res Pract, 24*, 190–195.

Young, J. E. (1999). *Cognitive therapy for personality disorders: A schema-focused approach* (3rd ed.). Sarasota, FL: Professional Resource Press.

CHAPTER 23

Group Therapy, Self-Help Groups, and Network Therapy

MARC GALANTER
FRANCIS HAYDEN
RICARDO CASTAÑEDA
HUGO FRANCO

Treatment modalities that employ social networks, such as group therapy, self-help programs, and adaptations of individual office-based psychotherapy (such as network therapy, described below), are of particular importance in treating alcoholism and drug abuse. Family therapy is described elsewhere in this volume (Chapter 24). One reason is that the addictions are characterized by massive denial of illness, and rehabilitation must begin with a frank acknowledgment of the nature of the patient's addictive process. The consensual validation and influence necessary to achieve such pronounced attitude change are most effectively gained through group influence. Indeed, for this purpose, a fellow addict carries the greatest amount of credibility. Another reason for employing social networks is that they provide an avenue for maintaining ties to the patient beyond the traditional therapeutic relationship. Furthermore, therapists are not in the position to confront, cajole, support, and express feeling in a manner that can influence the abuser to return to abstinence; a group of fellow addicts or members of the patient's family can do so quite directly.

This chapter explores the impact of group treatment in a number of disparate settings. We look at therapy groups directed specifically at the treatment of addiction, at 12-step programs such as Alcoholics Anonymous (AA), and Narcotics Anonymous (NA), and at institution-based self-help for substance abusers. The role of the clinician varies considerably in relation to each of these modalities; in each case, the mental health professional is provided with an unusual opportunity to step out of the traditional role of the psychodynamic therapist or the psychopharmacologist and examine the ways in which social influence is wrought through the group setting.

GROUP THERAPY FOR ALCOHOLISM AND DRUG ABUSE

How to Refer a Patient to Group Therapy

Adequate matching of the treatment needs of an addicted individual with the most appropriate group therapy format is important. Psychotherapeutic groups for alcoholics, for example, generally fare better when all members are alcoholics, and the focus of the group is on the characteristic behaviors and consequences of this problem. Usually each group includes from 5 to 12 members who meet one to three times a week. Criteria for exclusion include severe sociopathy or lack of motivation for treatment, acute or poorly controlled psychotic disorders, and the presence of transient or permanent severe cognitive deficits. Those patients who, because of their dual problems—addiction and mental illness—cannot be integrated into single-problem group formats must be treated within specialized dual-diagnosis groups and treatment settings (Galanter, Castañeda, & Ferman, 1988; Minkoff & Drake, 1991). Vannicelli (1982) observed that often patients are eventually excluded from the addiction group if they are unable to commit themselves to working toward abstinence. Polyaddicted individuals frequently are better integrated within multifocused groups. While dependent and nonsociopathic individuals are more easily engaged in interactional group models, individuals with sociopathic and other character problems are better retained in coping skills groups (Cooney, Kadden, Litt, & Getter, 1991; Poldrugo & Forti, 1988).

Group Treatment Modalities

Group treatment for alcoholism and other addictions was developed out of general disappointment with the results of individual therapy (Cooper, 1987). Table 23.1 presents brief descriptions of different group modalities for treatment of addicted individuals.

Leadership Style and Group Aims

The optimum style for a leader conducting a group for substance abusers appears to be one in which the focus is group- rather than leader-determined, in which the leader not only is knowledgeable about substance abuse but also acts as a facilitator of interpersonal process, and in which the group members seek to understand each other from their own perspective.

TABLE 23.1. Different Group Modalities for Treatment of Alcoholics

Category	Technique	Goals	Curative factors
Interactional	Interpretation of interactional process; promotion of self-disclosure and emotion expression	Promotion of understanding and resolution of interpersonal problems	Increased awareness of own relatedness
Modified interactional	Processing of interactional problems, but strong emphasis on ancillary supports for abstinence such as AA and Antabuse	Promotion of abstinence and improvement of interpersonal difficulties	Incorporation of specific resources to support abstinence and improvement of interpersonal relatedness
Behavioral	Reinforcement of abstinence-promoting behaviors; punishment of undesirable behaviors	Specific behavior modification	Prevention of specific responses
Insight-oriented psychotherapy	Exploration and interpretation of group and individual processes	Promotion of ability to tolerate distressing feelings without resorting to alcohol	Increased insight and improved ability to tolerate stress
Supportive	Specific support offered to individuals, to enable them to draw on their own resources	Promotion of adaptation to alcohol-free living	Improvement in self-confidence, and incorporation of specific recommendations

Groups differ in their aims and the style of their leaders. Some groups allow for discussion of issues other than addiction in the hope that group members will identify the association between the addictive behavior and all other problems. Other groups focus primarily on relapse prevention through the identification and discussion of all problems, even if unrelated to the addictive behavior. Groups also vary according to the degree of support offered to members—from confrontational groups that give support only when a patient espouses the views of the group leader to supportive groups that accept and explore individual attitudes and beliefs.

Despite the obvious importance of group style and the need for clearly described group techniques, little has been written that provides group leaders with specific group strategies (Vannicelli, Canning, & Griefen, 1984). The question of the group's style (defined as the way in which the group's goals and processes are linked) is not merely one of academic importance. For example, Harticollis (1980) found that psychoanalytical groups are widely regarded as inadequate and are not recommended for active substance abusers because of the counterproductive degree of anxiety that they generate. An early study by Ends and Page (1957) demonstrated that the style of a group of alcoholics predicted treatment outcome. In this study, alcoholics were assigned to one of several groups of different design. Group styles varied from one group described as relatively unfocused and "client centered," whose leader avoided a dominant role and instead promoted interpersonal processes among the group members, to another group based on learning theory, whose leader assumed a dominant role, offered only conditional support, and focused strongly on punishment and reward. At follow-up, those alcoholics treated in the client-centered group fared far better than those included in the confrontational group.

Descriptions of Some Representative Group Models

Exploratory and Supportive Groups

An interesting model, the modified dynamic group psychotherapy, developed by Khantzian allows for the identification of individuals' vulnerabilities and problems within a context of "safety." Abstinence is strongly endorsed, and the group, which requires an active style of leadership, promotes mutual support and outreach, and constantly strives to identify and manage contingencies for relapse (Khantzian, Halliday, & McAuliffe, 1990). According to Cooper (1987), psychotherapeutic groups based on exploration and interpretation aim at forging an increased ability in their members to tolerate higher levels of distressing feelings, without resorting to mood-altering substances. In contrast, purely supportive treatment groups aim at helping addicted group members to tolerate abstinence and assist them in remaining chemical-free, without necessarily understanding the determinants of their addiction.

Interactional Group Model

Yalom, Bloch, and Bond (1978) described an important group style in which therapy is conducted in weekly, 90-minute meetings of 8–10 members who, under the leadership of two trained group therapists, are encouraged to explore their interpersonal relationships with the group leaders and the other members. An effort is made to create an environment of safety, cohesion, and trust, where members engage in in-depth self-disclosure and affective expression. The goal of the group is not abstinence but the understanding and working through of interpersonal conflicts. (However, "improvement" without abstinence is often illusory.) In fact, groups of alcoholics are oriented away from an explicit discussion of drinking. The leaders emphasize that they do not see the group as the main instrument for achieving abstinence, and patients are encouraged to attend AA or to seek other forms of treatment for this purpose. Within this format, a group member can be described as "improved" along a series of 19 possible areas of growth, irrespective of the severity of his or her drinking.

This interactional model was further developed by Vannicelli (1982; Vannicelli et al., 1984), who, unlike Yalom and colleagues (1978), recommends that the group leaders strongly support abstinence as being essential to the patient's eventual emotional stability. The group leaders firmly endorse simultaneous use of other supports, such as AA and Antabuse (disulfiram) therapy. In contrast to working with neurotics, whose anxieties provide motivation and direction for treatment, the leaders of such a group of alcoholics are forced to intervene to provide limits and focus, without generation of more anxiety than necessary. The group therapists resist members' inquiries into the leaders' drinking habits by instead exploring the patients' underlying concerns about whether they will be helped and understood. Patients who miss early group sessions are actively sought out and brought back into the group. Confrontation (particularly of actively drinking members) is used sparingly and only with the aim of providing better understanding of the behavior, thus promoting growth and the necessary goal of activity changes.

Interpersonal Problem-Solving Skill Groups

According to Jehoda (1958), interpersonal problem-solving skill groups are based on the premise that the capacity to solve problems in life determines quality of mental health. Several empirical studies lend some support to this assumption, suggesting that there is a relation between cognitive interpersonal problem-solving skills and psychological adjustment. These groups have been implemented for alcoholics (Intagliata, 1978) and heroin addicts (Platt, Scura, & Harmon, 1960) with some degree of success. Usually problem-solving skills groups are run for a limited number of sessions (frequently 10) and are organized to teach a multistep approach to interpersonal problem solving. Most often, such steps include the following: (1) Recognize that a problem exists; (2) define the problem; (3) generate several possible solutions; and (4) select the best alternative after determining the likely consequences of each of the available possible solutions to the problem. Follow-up studies determined that groups with this format were effective in generating specific skills such as anticipating and planning ahead for problems, even following participants' discharge from the treatment programs. The value of problem-solving skills groups with respect to other primary modalities of addiction treatment, however, remains to be determined. It is unclear, for instance, whether these groups contribute to the overall rates of abstinence achieved in inpatient and outpatient treatment programs.

Educational Groups

Educational groups represent important ancillary treatment modalities in substance abuse treatment, not only for addicts but also for their relatives and
other social contacts. The obvious purpose of these groups is to provide information on issues relevant to specific addictions, such as the natural course and
medical consequences of alcoholism, the implications of intravenous addiction
for sexual contacts and the family, the availability of community resources, and
so forth. Often, educational groups provide opportunities for cognitive reframing and behavioral changes along specific guidelines. These groups are
often welcomed by some treatment-resistant addicts and alcoholics who cannot
cooperate with other forms of therapy. More often than not, educational groups
offer structured, group-specific, didactic material delivered by different means,
including videotapes, audiocassettes, or lectures; these presentations are followed by discussions led by an experienced and knowledgeable leader.

Activity Groups

Like educational groups, activity groups constitute another important ancillary
modality in the treatment of alcoholics and other addicts. Unlike educational
groups, however, patient participation is the main goal of activity groups, which
can evolve around a variety of occupational and recreational avenues. In a safe
and sober context, the addict can expedite socialization, recreation, and self-
and group expression. Activity groups are often the source of valuable insight
into patients' deficits and assets, both of which may go undetected by treatment
staff members concerned with more narrowly focused treatment interventions,
such as psychotherapists and nurses. When appropriately designed, activity
groups may constitute invaluable sources of self-discovery, self-esteem, and
newly acquired skills that facilitate sober social interactions.

Other groups also promote the acquisition of specific skills, such as those
devoted to reviewing relapse prevention techniques and those aimed at building social skills. These groups are particularly helpful in the early stages of the
rehabilitation process of the alcoholic patient.

Groups with Methadone-Maintenance Patients

Groups with methadone-maintenance patients experience problems that relate
more to the structure of the therapy than to the group content. Encouragement
is always needed for patients to participate in these groups. Often, groups for
these patients are an efficient way of coping with problems under professional
guidance and peers' support (Ben-Yehuda, 1980). These groups generally go
through several stages: the development of *esprit de corps*, the division of labor,

the establishment of group cohesion, and the development of outside-the-group relations.

Relationship of Group Therapy to Individual Treatment

It is not a surprise that group therapists maintain that group treatment is the treatment of choice for alcoholics and other addicts (Matano & Yalom, 1991). In support of this, group therapists such as Kanas (1982) stress not only the difficulty that these patients have in developing an "analyzable transference neurosis" in individual therapy but also their tendency to display impulsive acting out—both of which are characteristics better addressed in the anxiety-diffusing context of a group setting. Alcoholics, for example, are often seen as being orally fixated, with resulting narcissistic, passive–dependent, and depressive personality traits (Feibel, 1960). Platt and colleagues (1960) and Feibel (1960) pointed out that individual insight-oriented psychotherapy is often said to be contraindicated in addicts, because the following problems often present in these patients: intolerance of anxiety, episodes of rage and self-destructive behavior as a result of frustrated infantile needs, poor impulse control, and (probably most important) the tendency to develop a primitive transference toward the therapist.

Pfeffer, Friedland, and Wortis (1949) described an undeniable advantage of group therapy over individual treatment, namely, the easily generated peer pressure, which can often promote behavioral changes and a reduction of denial of addiction and interpersonal difficulties. In addition, peer-generated support often satisfies narcissistic and dependence needs. Primitive, intense transferences are often avoided in the group setting because of diffusion among the other members of the group and the "relative transparency of the group leaders" (Kanas, 1982, p. 1016). The tendency to leave treatment prematurely in individual therapy is often countered by the group's ability to promote a reduction of anxiety and to generate a therapeutic alliance not only with the leader but also with the other group members. As stated previously, it is important when deciding between group and individual therapy to assess both the patient's ability to tolerate and benefit from social interactions and his or her level of cognitive and psychological functioning. Patients with moderate cognitive deficits, or paranoid or other psychotic disorders, are likely to become isolated or hostile and to leave the group setting prematurely.

The following is a clinical example of the success of group therapy in a case in which individual therapy had no impact:

> At the time of referral, Mr. A, a 45-year-old white male, was employed as an administrator. He was married and had children. His chief complaints were frequent mood changes of many years' duration and unprovoked

bouts of anger, often directed at his wife, children, and coworkers. Although he had no history of psychiatric or medical problems, he reluctantly acknowledged that his wife thought he drank too much and that his boss had strongly demanded that he do something about his angry outbursts and poor job attendance. The patient was referred for individual therapy, but initial attempts at establishing a therapeutic relationship failed. He displayed markedly narcissistic personality traits, which resulted in an often disruptive relationship with the therapist, and he had difficulty in recognizing any interpersonal and mood problems associated with his alcohol consumption. The patient, however, acknowledged drinking more and more often than was "healthy" for him. His motivation for treatment derived from his determination to maintain his current employment and his interest in learning how to avoid depressive thinking.

Both the patient and the therapist felt that no progress was being made in individual therapy, and the therapist then referred the patient to alcoholism group treatment. In the group, the patient was exposed to other group members' descriptions of their problems of mood and social relations. On two occasions during the beginning phases of his involvement with the group, he came to the group while intoxicated. The threat of expulsion from the group in the face of these intoxications brought into focus the similar situation he faced at work, where his drinking was also jeopardizing his ability to remain employed. Confronted by group members and therapists alike, he eventually identified a relationship between his drinking and his angry outbursts at home and at work. From the outset, his drinking was interpreted by other group members as a reflection of his alcoholism rather than the expression of psychological conflicts. After a few months in treatment, this patient finally felt that he indeed was an alcoholic. The absence of drinking was associated with a total remission of depressive moods. He eventually made a commitment to abstinence, and he remained in group treatment for several years.

Management of Group Members Who Do Not Remain Abstinent

Drinking by some group members is to be expected in alcoholic groups. Full-blown slips or covert drinking by any group member interrupts the group process, elicits drinking-related thoughts and behaviors in other members, and requires specific and prompt intervention by the group leader. Often, however, a well-managed drinking episode represents an invaluable learning opportunity for all group members. A slip is not in itself cause for dismissal from the group. A resumption of drinking illustrates to all members the importance of prompt identification and interruption of denial, and the need constantly to ensure the effectiveness of selected measures for maintaining abstinence. Responsibility for the slip should be defined to the group as resting entirely on the patient who is drinking and not on any past event or interaction between other group members.

Drinking can assume different forms, depending on whether it is acknowledged or denied by the person and whether or not, despite the drinking, the group member professes adherence to the group norms regarding abstinence and self-disclosure. Those patients who keep drinking and express no intention to stop should be asked to leave the group. Dismissal from the group is best explained to the patient and to the other group members as justified by the person's present drinking behavior. Readmission into the group once the patient is willing to accept the group norms, including a commitment to achieving abstinence, should always be offered to a patient who is leaving the group. A different approach is to be adopted with patients who express a desire to end the relapse and agree to participate in a discussion within the group of their active drinking. Initially, any information from any source (within or outside the group) that a group member is drinking should be immediately shared with all members. If the patient is intoxicated, he or she needs to be asked to leave the group and to return sober to the following session. The next meeting should serve as an occasion to explore feelings about drinking behavior and denial. At this point, the group norms are reiterated; if necessary, specific contingency contracts with the drinking member are drawn up.

Another presentation of the problem is the patient who drinks yet refuses to acknowledge it. It should be part of the group contract that any important information concerning drinking behavior by a group member should be shared with the group. In the face of contrasting versions of a patient's behavior, clarification should be sought from the patient in a way that facilitates "voluntary" disclosure. Eventually, it may be necessary to confront the patient directly; if denial persists, the patient should leave the group.

Other Group Treatment Considerations

Group psychotherapy based on interpersonal and interpretive approaches rests in part on the self-medication hypothesis, which contends that substance abuse should be understood as the outcome of efforts at self-medication of distressing symptoms (Cooper, 1987; Khantzian, 1989). Recent challenges to this theory, however, suggest that drug abuse (particularly abuse of cocaine) may not necessarily be related to attempts at self-medication (Castañeda, Galanter, & Franco, 1989). Accordingly, it is advisable that group leaders be knowledgeable about addiction and able to anticipate that addicted group members may display drug-seeking behaviors that can best be regarded as conditioned responses (triggered by specific internal or environmental cues, such as the sight of a bottle or feelings of euphoria and celebration) rather than attempts on the part of the addict at dealing with emotional conflict (Galanter & Castañeda, 1985).

SELF-HELP, 12-STEP GROUPS, AND 12-STEP FACILITATION

Role of Self-Help Groups in Addiction Treatment

Self-help groups represent a widely available resource for the treatment of alcoholism, as well as other forms of chemical dependence. AA and other 12-step organizations such as NA and Cocaine Anonymous (CA) have not only provided a large population of addicts with support and guidance but also have contributed conceptually to the field of understanding and treating substance abuse. However, important questions for the clinician and the researcher need to be answered before the proper role of 12-step programs in the treatment of addicts can be established. In what ways are such self-help programs compatible with professional care? In what ways do these groups achieve their effects? For which patients are they most useful? Familiarity with self-help groups is essential both for the clinician providing care for substance abusers and for the researcher attempting to understand psychosocial factors involved in the outcome of addictions.

History of Self-Help Programs

Self-help groups can be understood as a grassroots response to a perceived need for services and support (Levy, 1976; Tracy & Gussow, 1976). In this sense, AA is the prototypical organization; it provided a model for the other successful groups such as NA and CA, as well as for its more closely related offspring such as Al-Anon, Alateen, and Children of Alcoholics. Levy (1976) proposed a rough division of self-help groups in two types of organizations: type I groups, which are truly mutual help organizations and include all 12-step programs, and type II groups, which more frequently operate as foundations and place more emphasis on promoting biomedical research, fundraising, public education, and legislative and lobbying activities. Type I and type II groups are by no means totally exclusive, because type I associations promote public education, and type II groups sometimes provide direct services.

The development of AA has exerted a major influence on the self-help movement in general. The next section is concerned only with the development of AA and related 12-step programs for addictions, which are clearly defined as type I associations.

Origins and Growth of Alcoholics Anonymous

AA's principal founder, "Bill W," in accordance with the AA tradition of anonymity, was himself an alcoholic. Bill was spiritually influenced by a drinking friend, Edwin Thatcher, who belonged to the Oxford Group, an evangelical religious sect (Kurtz, 1982). Thatcher, usually referred to as Ebby, attributed his abstinence to his involvement with the Oxford Group, which displayed many of the characteristics later adopted by AA, such as open confessions and guidance from members of the group. Bill W continued to drink despite his encounter with Ebby in 1934, but he felt that there was a kinship of common suffering among alcoholics. During his final hospital detoxification, he experienced an altered state of consciousness characterized by a strong feeling of proximity with God, which gave him a sense of mission to help other alcoholics to achieve sobriety.

Bill's initial efforts to influence other alcoholics were unsuccessful until, in May 1935, he met another member of the Oxford Group, "Dr. Bob," who a month later achieved sobriety and became the cofounder of AA. The number of alcoholics who experienced spiritual recovery and achieved sobriety in AA progressively increased; in 1939, when group membership reached 100, they published *Alcoholics Anonymous*, the book that became the bible for the movement (Galanter, 1989). AA institutionalized practices such as a 90-day induction period, sponsorship relationships, the "12 Steps," and recruitment for the fellowship. The expansion and stability of the organization resulted from its "12 Traditions," which avoid concentration of power within the organization, prevent involvement of AA with other causes, maintain the anonymity of its membership, and preserve the neutrality of the association in relation to controversial issues. Its membership continued to grow; AA, now a global organization, is reported to have more than 75,000 informal groups in the United States and 114 other countries, with a membership estimated at 1.5 million. The birth and development of NA illustrate how AA provided a model to other self-help programs for addictions.

History and Approach of Narcotics Anonymous

Although the NA program was first applied to drug addiction at the U.S. Public Health Service Hospital at Lexington, Kentucky, in 1947, it was an NA group independent of any institution and formed by AA members who were addicts in Sun Valley, California, in 1953, that expanded and gave NA its current form (Peyrot, 1985). The Sun Valley NA group did not identify itself with a program organized in New York City in 1948 by Dan Carlson, an addict formerly exposed to the Lexington program, because the Sun Valley founders felt that NA should strictly adhere to AA's 12 Steps and 12 Traditions by not identifying itself with any specific agency and not accepting government funds.

There are a few differences between AA and NA. NA members usually use illegal drugs, in contrast to most AA members until recently, who could be described as traditional alcoholics. Also, instead of using the term "alcoholism," NA refers to its problem as "addiction" and addresses the entire range of abusable psychoactive substances. There is, however, a clear overlap of approach and membership between the organizations, despite their complete independence of each other. Following in the footsteps of AA, NA has experienced fast-paced growth. It became an international organization, present in at least

36 countries, with a probable membership of 250,000. According to the NA World Service Office, which publishes NA literature and centralizes information within NA, the growth rate of the organization's membership has been 30–40% a year (Wells, 1987). The growth of NA and other 12-2tep programs demonstrates the organizational strength and appeal of the AA model.

How 12-Step Programs Work

Participation in a 12-step program can start at the moment the addict meets a member of an organization, reads its literature, or simply attends meetings (e.g., an open meeting or an institutional meeting run by AA or NA speakers) (Galanter, 1989). A desire to stop drinking and/or abusing other drugs is the only requirement for membership. Total abstinence becomes a goal from the outset of the participation in the fellowship. Initial participation turns into an induction period, which, in the case of AA, for instance, lasts 90 days and encourages daily attendance at meetings. The member is exposed to the 12-step approach to recovery; the first step consists of admitting powerlessness over the addiction, and consequently breaking with denial. Seeking sponsorship from another member who has been sober for months (preferably more than a year) is also encouraged. Sponsors are usually of the same sex if the group is large enough, so that emotional entanglements can be avoided to keep from distracting members from the purpose of attaining and maintaining sobriety. Open meetings usually consist of talks by a leader and two or three speakers who share their experiences of how the 12-step program related to their recovery.

The 12-step program is an attempt to effect changes in addicts' lives that go beyond just stopping the use of substances—changes in personal values and interpersonal behavior, as well as continued participation in the fellowship. The 12 steps are studied and followed with the guidance of a sponsor and participation in meetings focused on each step. Each step involves changes in behavior and attitudes that may profoundly affect the addict's life. To achieve the ninth step, for instance, the addict makes amends to people formerly harmed by his or her behavior. These amends may result in changes in the way the person relates to others and interprets the problems that have affected past and present relationships. For instance, an alcoholic man may "talk" to a deceased father whom he formerly hated and attempt a "conciliation" with his image of his dead father. The 12th step encourages propagation of the group's philosophy and consequently fosters the individual's recovery by providing opportunities to others to recover and expand the fellowship.

Traditionally, 12-step meetings are open to all members, but they may be directed to special-interest groups (e.g., gays, women, minority groups, and physicians). Meetings can be of different types, such as discussions, 12-step study, and testimonials; some may be open to nonmembers, and others may be for members only. If the recovery progresses, the member will learn strategies to avoid relapse (e.g., "One day at a time"), obtain help from other members, and eventually help fellow addicts in their recovery. By helping other addicts and by sponsoring newcomers to the program, the individual is helping him- or herself by becoming more involved with the recovery process and the organization's philosophy.

Why 12-Step Programs Work

It is still unclear why 12-step programs can help people exposed to them. From an existential perspective, AA, for instance, encourages acceptance of one's finitude and essential limitation by conveying the idea of powerlessness over alcohol. On the other hand, one can go beyond this limitation by relating to others and sharing some of the painful aspects of human existence. Kurtz (1982) emphasized that consistency in thought and action is crucial to maintaining a conscious effort to be honest with oneself and others. This effort produces an increased awareness of one's own needs for growth. AA stresses the need for consistency in thought and action in all stages of its recovery program.

From a learning theory perspective, the group selectively reinforces social and cognitive behaviors that usually are incompatible with the addictive behavior. Attendance at meetings is basically incompatible with using the same time to drink or abuse other drugs. Achievements resulting from sobriety are generously praised, and strategies of self-monitoring and self-control are constantly reinforced through constant interactions with others attempting to remain sober. AA enhances self-monitoring of emotions and behaviors by helping the addict to detect reactions to certain internal and external stimuli (craving, distress with interpersonal problems, denial in the presence of depressive feelings, unrealistic goals when under pressure, etc.). In addition to self-monitoring, self-control is enhanced as alcoholics learn a new repertoire of cognitive and social behaviors, such as attending more meetings when craving increases, using the 12 steps to cope with stressful life events, and obtain group support to face painful feelings about themselves and others. Other theoretical perspectives used to understand 12-step programs include operant and social learning views; however, because experimentation with the processes involved in participation in 12-step programs is an almost impossible proposition, the use of learning models remains largely descriptive and speculative.

OUTCOME STUDIES

Group Treatment Outcomes

The immense popularity of group treatment and self-help for alcoholics and other substance abusers preceded the availability of significant numbers of controlled outcome studies (Bowers & al-Rheda, 1990; Cooney et al., 1991; Kang,

Kleinman, & Woody, 1991; Poldrugo & Forti, 1988; Yalom et al., 1978). Yalom and colleagues (1978) reported significant improvement at 8-month and 1-year follow-ups of both alcoholics and neurotics treated in weekly interactional group therapy. Improvement was measured along specific variables, however, and not according to the quality of abstinence eventually attained by the group members. In an early report, Ends and Page (1957) compared the outcome effects on alcoholics of several group therapy designs, including groups based on learning theory, client-centered (supportive) groups, psychoanalytical groups, and nonpsychotherapy discussion groups. They found that both client-centered and psychoanalytical groups yielded better outcomes than did discussion groups and groups based on learning theory, as measured by improvement in self-concept at a 1-year follow-up. Client-centered groups also were associated with lower rates of readmission than all other groups in this and a subsequent study. Mindlin and Belden (1965) studied the attitudes of hospitalized alcoholics before and after participation in group psychotherapy, occupational groups, or no-group treatment, and found that group psychotherapy significantly improved motivation for treatment and attitude toward alcoholism.

The 1998 report by the Institute of Medicine, *Bridging the Gap between Research and Practice*, has spurred on the development and evaluation of evidence-based therapies (Marinelli-Casey, Domier, & Rawson, 2002). The past 10 years have seen a large increase in the number and quality of clinical trials (e.g., Charney, Paraherakis, & Gill, 2001; Magura et al., 2003; Marques & Formigoni, 2001; Meyers, Miller, Smith, & Tonigan, 2002; Ouimett et al., 2001; Petry, Martin, & Finocche, 2001). Many of these studies examine heretofore understudied populations, such as those with co-occurring substance dependence and other major mental illness, serious medical conditions, and or polysubstance dependence. Studies have been designed to test the effectiveness of a variety of group treatment approaches. The feasibility of their transfer from both research to clinical settings and individual to group formats has been investigated (Carise, Cornely, & Gurel, 2002; Carroll et al., 2002; Foote et al., 1999; Hanson, Leshner, & Tai, 2002; Petry & Simcic, 2002; Van Horn & Bux, 2001). While some of the more ambitious protocols, such as those developed via the Clinical Trials Network (CTN), are still undergoing various phases of implementation, there is widespread optimism that group therapy will soon be established on much firmer empirical foundation than was true in the past.

Some of the approaches that have been receiving significant attention in terms of adaptation to group format, standardization, and dissemination, include motivational enhancement therapy (MET; Miller, Zweben, DiClemente, & Rychtarik, 1994), cognitive-behavioral coping skills therapy (CBST, often referred to as "relapse prevention"; Kadden et al., 1995; for an update, see Longabaugh & Morgenstern, 1999), and 12-step facilitation (TSF, discussed below).

Self-Help and Treatment Outcome

Alcoholics Anonymous

AA has received more attention from investigators studying outcome variables than other 12-step programs. Consequently, most of our knowledge about the impact of 12-step programs on the lives of addicts is limited to the effects of AA on some samples of alcoholics. The structure of 12-step organizations and their emphasis on anonymity make scientific research on these groups a very difficult task (Glaser & Osborne, 1982). Investigators have studied outcome variables related to participation in AA, such as severity of drinking, personality traits, attendance at meetings, total abstinence versus controlled drinking as a therapeutic goal, and concomitance of AA attendance with professional care (Elal-Lawrence, Slade, & Dewey, 1987; Seixas, Washburn, & Eisen, 1988; Thurstin, Alfano, & Nerviano, 1987; Thurstin, Alfano, & Sherer, 1986).

The first variable to deserve attention is that those alcoholics who join AA are not representative of the total population of alcoholics receiving treatment (Emrick, 1987). AA members tend to be, as common sense would indicate, more sociable and affiliative. Studies also suggest that AA members have more severe problems resulting from their drinking and experience more guilt regarding their behavior. Attendance at meetings has been associated in some studies (Emrick, 1987) with better outcome, although the nature of this association remains unclear. Thurstin and colleagues (1986) found no clear personality traits that might seem to be associated with AA membership, but they reported that success among members appears to be related to less depression, less anxiety, and better sociability. AA seems not to benefit those who can become nonproblem users, and it may actually be detrimental to patients who can learn to control their drinking (Emrick, 1987). AA members who receive other forms of treatment concomitantly with their participation in AA meetings probably do better.

As noted earlier, several problems make it difficult to study outcome factors related to participation in 12-step programs. One is the changing composition of AA membership: more women, younger people, and multiply addicted alcoholics that have been joining the organization. The heterogeneity of addictive disorders, the anonymity of membership, the impossibility of experimentation with components of the programs, the self-selection factor in affiliation, and the lack of appropriate group controls all impose serious methodological difficulties in evaluating outcome variables. For clinical purposes, the benefit of membership in self-help groups has to be empirically evaluated for each individual patient.

12-Step Facilitation

TSF is a manualized individual counseling method developed for use in Project MATCH (Anonymous, 1997), a large multicenter study of the effect of customizing alcoholism treatment to individual needs. It describes a type of therapy in which the goal is to engender patients' active participation in AA. It regards such active involvement as the main treatment element promoting sobriety. The study found it to be effective and equal to other treatments employed, namely, MET and CBST (Nowinski, Baker, & Carroll, 1995).

Institutional Self-Help Treatment Groups

Most ambulatory programs for substance abuse treatment are modeled after ones used in general psychiatric clinics. They rely primarily on professionally conducted individual and small-group therapy. Whether there are more cost-effective options or more potent ones has yet to be fully explored. One alternative approach to conventional institutional treatment is based on psychological influence in a self-help group context and is designed to allow for decreased staffing. Such an approach to group treatment is designed to draw on the principles of zealous group psychology observed in freestanding self-help approaches to addictive illness, such as those of AA and the drug-free therapeutic communities, but at the same time serves as the primary group-based modality employed in an institutional treatment setting. In other words, it can be employed in institutional settings, such as hospitals and clinics, and still capture the psychological effect of freestanding self-help groups.

In a study conducted on this treatment model (Galanter, 1982, 1983), primary therapists were social workers and paraprofessionals experienced in alcoholism treatment, supervised by attending psychiatrists. One social worker and one paraprofessional treated patients in the experimental self-help treatment program, and two members of each of the latter disciplines treated the controls; the self-help program therefore operated at half the usual staffing level. The program included an alcohol clinic attached to an inpatient detoxification unit.

The control and the experimental self-help programs illustrate the contrast between institution-based self-help groups and conventional care. In the study (Galanter, 1982, 1983), the programs operated simultaneously and independently in the outpatient department. Therapists in each program were encouraged to perfect their respective clinical approaches, and each group of therapists received clinical supervision appropriate to its needs and experience. Differences between the two programs are outlined here to illustrate the operation of institutionally grounded self-help group care.

ORIENTATION PROGRAM

In the control (traditional) group setting, two primary therapists served as coleaders of a group for their own patients, and attendance in each session ranged between 8 and 15 patients. In the self-help program, the same format was used, but groups were led by patients of the primary therapists who had established sobriety and had demonstrated a measure of social stability over several months. These "senior patients" monitored the progress of patients in the orientation group and were supervised by the primary therapists, who attended the orientation for part of each session, participating in a limited fashion only. A patient in crisis might be invited to return to the orientation group, if this invitation was seen as helpful.

GROUP THERAPY

Weekly group meetings were oriented toward practical life issues among controls, but insight was encouraged; progress toward abstinence was a major theme. The two primary therapists served as facilitators for the group, using their own empathic manner to encourage mutual acceptance and support. When confrontation was necessary, the therapists undertook it in a forthright but supportive manner. In the self-help program, groups met with the same frequency, but senior patients assumed the leadership role. Primary therapists attended part of each session and participated intermittently; they served, however, primarily in a coordinating capacity for these groups and supervised the senior patients. Patients were encouraged to deal with unusual problems by recourse to their peers in the program, either in their therapy group or through senior patients.

PEER THERAPY

Self-help program patients were made aware that the primary source of support in the clinic was the peer group. New patients were encouraged to seek out peers and senior patients who would be available to assist them through the program. Senior patients were supervised in assisting with crises when this assistance was judged clinically appropriate by the primary therapists. The senior patient program was operated in the self-help modality. Potential senior patients were screened for sobriety and social stability, and assisted in patient management of the program for a time-limited period. Those who served as group leaders met weekly as a group with the primary therapists, focusing on their therapeutic functions in the unit. Under supervision of the therapists, they directed orientation, therapy, and activity groups. Their interventions in more difficult patients' problems were reviewed with the primary therapists, and they referred self-help patients to their respective primary therapists for more troublesome problems. Other senior patients had administrative functions in the program.

Meetings of the full patient complement also took place in the self-help program. A monthly evening meeting open to all patients served as a focus for group spirit and as a context for organizing recreational activities. The meetings were run collaboratively by staff and senior patients, with programwide activities and patients' progress as the focus. Socialization at the time of these meetings focused on the status of patients' recovery.

OUTCOME AND COMMENTS

Two outcome studies (Galanter, 1982, 1983) of this project found that the experimental program, with half the staffing of the traditional modality, was quite viable in a municipal hospital alcoholism treatment program. Furthermore, retention of inpatients upon transfer to the alcohol clinic was 38% greater than in the control (non-self-help) program; rates of abstinence in outpatients were no less, and social adjustment over the course of a 12-month follow-up was enhanced. The self-help format appears therefore to offer a format for institutional treatment that is less expensive and potentially more effective.

The following case example illustrates the ethos of the self-help program:

A 36-year-old outpatient came to the clinic intoxicated, without a scheduled visit, and asked to speak with a senior patient whom he knew well. He had been in outpatient treatment for 8 months, and had been abstinent for the last 4 months. Five days earlier, he had begun drinking subsequent to a crisis in his family and had missed his group meeting. He gave a history of falling down a staircase earlier in the day, bruising his head. The senior patient he had asked to see and another senior patient were present, and they encouraged him to seek a medical evaluation. The case was then reviewed with the primary therapist, who saw him briefly, wrote a referral for medical assessment, and returned him to the two senior patients' care. After an hour, the senior patients prevailed on him to go with one of them to the emergency service. One of them took him on the following afternoon to a meeting of an AA group he had previously attended. The patient was able to maintain abstinence until his next weekly group therapy meeting, at which time a group member offered to get together with him during the ensuing week to provide him with some encouragement.

Given a need for increased substance abuse treatment services, it is important to note that counseling staff members (social workers and counselors) comprise 66% of the staffs in all federally assisted alcoholism treatment facilities, which constitute the bulk of publicly supported programs (Vischi, Jones, Shank, & Lima, 1980). The question then arises as to whether these counseling staffers are used in the most cost-effective way. One problematic aspect of this issue is illustrated by the finding of Paredes and Gregory (1979) that in alcoholism treatment programs, the economic resources invested in alcoholism treatment are not positively correlated with outcome. They concluded that the type and quantity of therapeutic resources invested are related to the characteristics of the agencies themselves rather than to a treatment strategy conceived for optimal cost-effectiveness.

Two issues common to most small-group therapies for substance abuse in the clinic setting are relevant here. In the first place, whether behavioral, insight-oriented, or directive, they all focus on the concerns of a relatively small number of patients involved in the therapy group (typically 6 to 10), to the exclusion of other program participants. Second, it is generally agreed that such small-group therapy for alcoholics offers a better outcome when conducted in the context of a multimodal program. Such a program may integrate treatment components to implement a carefully structured plan, as described by Hunt and Azrin (1973).

These two aspects of small-group therapy may be considered in relation to a self-help–oriented treatment program such as the one described previously. With regard to group size, such a program introduces the option of the patients' strong identification with and sense of cohesion in a treatment network of many more than 6 to 10 patients. In fact, it encourages affiliative feelings among the full complement of self-help patients, providing an experience of a large, zealous group (Galanter, 1989). This cohesion is promoted by therapeutic contact with a number of senior patients who are involved in the therapy groups; by programwide patient-run activities, such as the orientation groups open to patients in crisis; and in monthly large-group meetings, also open to all patients. This broader identification forms the bulwark of a self-help orientation.

Self-Help Groups and the Clinician

The relationship between professional treatment and membership in a 12-step group has been less than systematically addressed. Clark (1987) proposed guidelines to orient the clinician. Clearly, acquaintance with 12-step programs is essential for the clinician to orient patients regarding their needs and to respond to possible conflicts between the nature and goals of professional care and the demands of participation in self-help organizations. Clinicians treating addicts can learn about 12-step programs by attending local meetings, by becoming familiar with the fellowship's literature, and by exploring their patients' experiences in the context of their membership in these organizations.

One point deserving emphasis is that physicians should be aware of the danger of prescribing habit-forming substances to addicts because of not only the inherent dangers involved in the use of these substances but also the goals of programs that demand complete avoidance of chemical solutions for life's problems (Zweben, 1987). When psychotropic medication is strongly recommended, the benefits and risks involved in their use should be carefully discussed with the patient in the context of the goals of 12-step programs. An occasional sponsor may be opposed to any medication, even when a patient clearly needs pharmacological treatment to alleviate disabling behavioral or physical conditions. In this situation, the clinician has to address the nature of the conflict involved in the treatment by making the needed medical treatment compatible with the program philosophy. This desirable goal can only be achieved when the clinician is well informed about the nature of 12-step programs and can help the patient to integrate the rationale for medical treatment with the general goals of his or her membership in the self-help program. Avoidance of prescribing drugs with habit-forming potential, willingness to educate patients about the nature of their problems, and a positive attitude toward 12-step organizations make it easier for clinicians to integrate their interventions with the orientation of the fellowship. Candidates for controlled drinking should not be encouraged to participate in abstinence-oriented programs, because the incompatibility of the goals of professional treatment with a 12-step orientation may prove to be very detrimental to therapy (Emrick, 1987).

Clinicians should, in general, encourage their patients to get exposed to 12-step programs, but they should remember that a large number of addicts who never participate in these organizations can make good use of professional treatment and successfully recover. Because the composition of the membership of self-help groups continually changes, it is possible for patients treated with psychotropic medication, including methadone, to benefit from participation in these groups (Obuchowsky & Zweben, 1987).

THE NETWORK THERAPY TECHNIQUE

Overview

This approach can be useful in addressing a broad range of addicted patients characterized by the following clinical hallmarks of addictive illness: First, when they initiate consumption of their addictive agent, be it alcohol, cocaine, opiates, or depressant drugs, they frequently cannot limit that consumption to a reasonable and predictable level; this phenomenon has been termed "loss of control" by clinicians who treat alcohol- or drug-dependent persons (Jellinek, 1963). Second, they consistently demonstrate relapse to the agent of abuse, that is, they attempted to stop using the drug for varying periods of time but returned to it, despite a specific intent to avoid it.

This treatment approach is not necessary for those abusers who can, in fact, learn to set limits on their use of alcohol or drugs; their abuse may be treated as a behavioral symptom in a more traditional psychotherapeutic fashion. Nor is it directed at those patients for whom the addictive pattern is most unmanageable (e.g., addicted people with unusual destabilizing circumstances such as homelessness, severe character pathology, or psychosis). These patients may need special supportive care (e.g., inpatient detoxification or long-term residential treatment).

Key Elements of Network Therapy

Three elements are essential to the network therapy technique. The first is a cognitive-behavioral approach to relapse prevention, independently reported to be valuable in addiction treatment (Marlatt & Gordon, 1985). Emphasis in this approach is placed on triggers to relapse and behavioral techniques for avoiding them, rather than on exploring underlying psychodynamic issues.

Second, support of the patient's natural social network is engaged in treatment. Peer support in AA has long been shown to be an effective vehicle for promoting abstinence, and the idea of the therapist's intervening with family and friends in starting treatment was employed in one of the early ambulatory techniques specific to addiction (Johnson, 1986). The involvement of spouses (McCrady, Stout, Noel, Abrams, & Fisher-Nelson, 1991) has since been shown to be effective in enhancing the outcome of professional therapy.

Third, the orchestration of resources to provide community reinforcement suggests a more robust treatment intervention by providing a support for drug-free rehabilitation (Azrin, Sisson, & Meyers, 1982). In this relation, Khantzian (1988) points to the "primary care therapist" as one who functions in direct coordinating and monitoring roles in order to combine psychotherapeutic and self-help elements. It is this overall management role over circumstances outside, as well as inside, the office session that is presented to trainees to maximize the effectiveness of the intervention.

Starting a Network

Patients should be asked to bring their spouse or a close friend to the first session. Alcoholic patients often dislike certain things they hear when they first come for treatment and may deny or rationalize, even if they voluntarily sought help. Because of their denial, a significant other is essential to both history taking and implementing a viable treatment plan. A close relative or spouse can often cut through the denial in a way that an unfamiliar therapist cannot, and can therefore be invaluable in setting a standard of realism in dealing with the addiction.

Once the patient comes for an appointment, establishing a network is a task undertaken with active collaboration of patient and therapist. The two, aided by those parties who join the network initially, must search for the right balance of members. The therapist must carefully promote the choice of appropriate network members, however, just as the platoon leader selects those who will go into combat.

Defining the Network's Task

As conceived here, the therapist's relationship to the network is like that of a task-oriented team leader rather than that of a family therapist oriented toward insight. The network is established to implement a straightforward task: aiding the therapist in sustaining the patient's abstinence. It must be directed with the same clarity of purpose that a task force is directed in any effective organization. Competing and alternative goals must be suppressed or at least prevented from interfering with the primary task.

Unlike family members involved in traditional family therapy, network members are not led to expect symptom relief for themselves or self-realization. This lack of expectation prevents the development of competing goals for the network's meetings. It also provides the members protection from having their own motives scrutinized, and thereby supports their continuing involvement, without the threat of an assault on their psychological defenses.

Adapting Individual Therapy to the Network Treatment

Of primary importance is the need to address exposure to substances of abuse or to cues that might precipitate alcohol or drug use (Galanter, 1993). First, both patient and therapist should be sensitive to this matter and explore these situations as they arise. Second, a stable social context in an appropriate social environment—one conducive to abstinence with minimal disruption of life circumstances—should be supported. Considerations of minor disruptions in place of residence, friends, or job need not be a primary issue for the patient with character disorder or neurosis, but they cannot go untended here. For a considerable period, the substance abuser is highly vulnerable to exacerbations of the addictive illness and in some respects must be viewed with the considerable caution with which one treats the recently compensated psychotic.

Study on Training Naive Therapists

A course of training for psychiatric residents naive to addiction and ambulatory treatments was undertaken over a period of 2 academic years. Before beginning treatment, the residents were given a structured treatment manual for network therapy and participated in a 13-session seminar on application of the network therapy technique. Cocaine-abusing patients were eligible for treatment in this study, if they could come for evaluation with a friend or family member who could participate in their treatment. In all, 22 patients were enrolled. The treating psychiatric residents were able to establish requisite networks for 20 of these patients (i.e., a network with at least one member). The networks had an average of 2.3 members, and the most typical configuration included family members and friends. Supervisors' evaluation of videotapes of the network sessions employing standardized instruments indicated good adherence to the manualized treatment, with effective use of network therapy techniques. The outcome of treatment (Galanter, Dermatis, Keller, & Trujillo, 2002; Galanter, Keller, & Dermatis, 1997; Keller, Galanter, & Weinberg, 1997) reflected retention and abstinence rates as good as, or better than, comparable ambulatory care carried out by therapists experienced in addiction treatment. The study demonstrated the feasibility of teaching the network technique to therapists naive to addiction treatment.

REFERENCES

Anonymous. (1997). Matching alcoholism treatments to client heterogeneity: Project MATCH posttreatment drinking outcomes. *J Stud Alcohol, 58*, 7–29.

Azrin, N. H., Sisson, R. W., & Meyers, R. (1982). Alcoholism treatment by disulfiram and community reinforcement therapy. *J Behav Ther Exp Psychiatry, 13*, 105–112.

Ben-Yehuda, N. (1980). Group therapy with methadone-maintained patients: Structural problems and solutions. *Int J Group Psychother, 30*, 331–345.

Bowers T. G., & al-Rheda, M. R. (1990) A comparison of outcome with group/marital and standard/individual therapies with alcoholics. *J Stud Alcohol, 51*, 301–309.

Carise, D., Cornely, W., & Gurel, O. (2002). A successful researcher–practitioner collaboration in substance abuse treatment. *J Subst Abuse Treat, 23*, 157–162.

Carroll, K. M., Nich, C., Sifry, R. L., Nuro, K. F., Frankforter, T. L., Ball, S. A., et al. (2002). A general system for evaluating therapist adherence and competence in psychotherapy research in the addictions. *Drug Alcohol Depend, 57*, 225–238.

Castañeda, R., Galanter, M., & Franco, H. (1989). Self-medication among addicts with primary psychiatric disorders. *Compr Psychiatry, 30*, 80–83.

Charney, D. A., Paraherakis, A. M., & Gill, K. J. (2001). Integrated treatment of comorbid depression and substance use disorders. *J Clin Psychiatry, 62*, 672–677.

Clark, H. W. (1987). On professional therapists and Alcoholics Anonymous. *J Psychoactive Drugs, 19*, 233–242.

Cooney, N. L., Kadden, R. M., Litt, M. D., & Getter, H. (1991). Matching alcoholics to coping skills or interactional therapies: Two year-follow-up results. *J Consult Clin Psychol, 59*, 598–601.

Cooper, D. E. (1987). The role of group psychotherapy in the treatment of substance abusers. *Am J Psychother, 41*, 55–67.

Elal-Lawrence, G., Slade, P. D., & Dewey, M. E. (1987). Treatment and follow-up variables discriminating abstainers, controlled drinkers and relapsers. *J Stud Alcohol, 48*, 39–46.

Emrick, C. D. (1987). Alcoholics Anonymous: Affiliation processes and effectiveness as treatment. *Alcohol Clin Exp Res, 11*, 416–442.

Ends, E. J., & Page, C. W. (1957). A study of three types of group psychotherapy with hospitalized male inebriates. *Q J Stud Alcohol, 18*, 263–277.

Feibel, C. (1960). The archaic personality structure of alcoholics and its indications for therapy. *Int J Group Psychother, 10*, 39–45.

Foote, J., DeLuca, A. Magura, S., Warner, A., Grand, A., Rosenblum, A., & Stahl, S. (1999). A group motivational treatment for chemical dependency. *J Subst Abuse Treat, 17*, 181–192.

Galanter, M. (1982). Overview: Charismatic religious sects and psychiatry. *Am J Psychiatry, 139*, 1539–1548.

Galanter, M. (1983). Engaged members of the Unification Church: The impact of a charismatic group on adaptation and behavior. *Arch Gen Psychiatry, 40*, 1197–1202.

Galanter, M. (1989). *Cults: Faith, healing and coercion.* New York: Oxford University Press.

Galanter, M. (1993). Network therapy for addiction: A model for office practice. *Am J Psychiatry, 150,* 28–36.

Galanter, M., & Castañeda, R. (1985). Self-destructive behavior in the substance abuser. *Psychiatr Clin North Am, 8,* 251–261.

Galanter, M., Castañeda, R., & Ferman, J. (1988). Substance abuse among general psychiatric patients: Place of presentation, diagnosis and treatment. *Am J Drug Alcohol Abuse, 14,* 211–235.

Galanter, M., Dermatis, H., Keller, D., & Trujillo, M. (2002). Network therapy for cocaine abuse: Use of family and peer supports. *Am J Addict, 11,* 161–166.

Galanter, M., Keller, D., & Dermatis, H. (1997). Network therapy for addiction: Assessment of the clinical outcome of training. *Am J Drug Alcohol Abuse, 23,* 355–367.

Glaser, F. B., & Osborne, A. (1982). Does AA really work? *Br J Addict, 77,* 123–129.

Hanson, G. R., Leshner, A. I., & Tai, B. (2002). Putting drug abuse research to use in real-life settings. *J Subst Abuse Treat, 23,* 69–70.

Harticollis, P. (1980). Alcoholism, borderline and narcissistic disorders: A psychoanalytic overview. In W. Fann (Ed.), *Phenomenology and treatment of alcoholism* (pp. 93–110). New York: Spectrum.

Hunt, G. M., & Azrin, N. H. (1973). A community-reinforcement approach to alcoholism. *Behav Res Ther, 11,* 91–104.

Intagliata, J. C. (1978). Increasing the interpersonal problem-solving skills of an alcoholic population. *J Consult Clin Psychol, 46,* 489–498.

Jehoda, M. (1958). *Current concepts in positive mental health.* New York: Basic Books.

Jellinek, E. M. (1963). *The disease concept of alcoholism.* New Haven, CT: Hillhouse.

Johnson, V. E. (1986). *Intervention: How to help someone who doesn't want help.* Minneapolis, MN: Johnson Institute.

Kadden, R., Carroll, K. M., Donovan, D., Cooney, N., Monti, P., Abrams, D., et al. (1995). *Cognitive-behavioral coping skills therapy manual: A clinical research guide for therapists treating individuals with alcohol abuse and dependence.* Rockville, MD: National Institute on Alcohol Abuse and Alcoholism.

Kanas, N. (1982). Alcoholism and group psychotherapy. In E. Kauffman & M. Pattison (Eds.), *Comprehensive textbook of alcoholism* (pp. 1011–1021). New York: Gardner Press.

Kang, S. Y., Kleinman, P. H., & Woody, G. E. (1991). Outcomes for cocaine abusers after once-a-week psychosocial therapy. *Am J Psychiatry, 131,* 160–164.

Keller, D. S., Galanter, M., & Weinberg, S. (1997). Validation of a scale for network therapy: a technique for systematic use of peer and family support in addition treatment. *Am J Drug Alcohol Abuse, 23,* 115–127.

Khantzian, E. J. (1988). The primary care therapist and patient needs in substance abuse treatment. *Am J Drug Alcohol Abuse, 14*(2), 159–167.

Khantzian, E. J. (1989). The self-medication hypothesis for substance abusers. *Am J Psychiatry, 30,* 81–83.

Khantzian, E. J., Halliday, K. S., & McAuliffe, W. E. (1990). *Addiction and vulnerable self.* New York: Guilford Press.

Kurtz, E. (1982). Why AA works. *J Stud Alcohol, 43,* 38–80.

Levy, L. H. (1976). Self-help health groups: Types and psychological processes. *J Appl Behav Sci, 12,* 310–322.

Longabaugh, R., & Morgenstern, J. (1999). Cognitive-behavioral coping-skills therapy for alcohol dependence: Current status and future directions. *Alcohol Res Health, 23*, 78–85.

Magura, S., Laudet, A. B., Mahmood, D., Rosenblum, A., Vogel, H. S., & Knight, E. L. (2003). Role of self-help processes in achieving abstinence among dually diagnosed persons. *Addict Behav, 28*, 399–413.

Marinelli-Casey, P., Domier, C. P., & Rawson, R. A. (2002). The gap between research and practice in substance abuse treatment. *Psychiatr Serv, 53*, 984–987.

Marlatt, G. A., & Gordon, J. R. (Eds.).(1985). *Relapse prevention: Maintenance strategies in the treatment of addictive behaviors*. New York: Guilford Press.

Marques, A. C., & Formigoni, M. L. (2001). Comparison of individual and group cognitive-behavioral therapy for alcohol and/or drug-dependent patients. *Addiction, 96*, 835–846.

Matano R. N., & Yalom, I. D. (1991). Approaches to chemical dependency: Chemical dependency and interactive group therapy—a synthesis. *Int J Group Psychother, 41*, 269–293.

McCrady, B. S., Stout, R., Noel, N., Abrams, D., & Fisher-Nelson, H. (1991). Effectiveness of three types of spouse-involved behavioral alcoholism treatment. *Br J Addict, 86*, 1415–1424.

Meyers, R. J., Miller, W. R., Smith J. E., & Tonigan, J. S. (2002). A randomized trial of two methods for engaging treatment-refusing drug users through concerned significant others. *J Consult Clin Psychol, 70*, 1182–1185.

Miller, W. R., Zweben, A., DiClemente, C. C., & Rychtarik, R. G. (1994). *Motivational enhancement therapy manual: A clinical research guide for therapists treating individuals with alcohol abuse and dependence*. Rockville MD: National Institute on Alcohol Abuse and Alcoholism.

Mindlin, D. F., & Belden, E. (1965). Attitude changes with alcoholics in group therapy. *CA Ment Health Rev Digest, 3*, 102–103.

Minkoff, K., & Drake, R. E. (Eds.). (1991). *Dual diagnosis of major mental illness and substance abuse disorder*. San Francisco: Jossey-Bass.

Nowinski, J., Baker, S., & Carroll, K. M. (1995). *Twelve step facilitation therapy manual: A clinical research guide for therapists treating individuals with alcohol abuse and dependence*. Rockville, MD: National Institute on Alcohol Abuse and Alcoholism.

Obuchowsky, M. A., & Zweben, J. E. (1987). Bridging the gap: The methadone client in 12-step programs. *J Psychoactive Drugs, 19*, 301–302.

Ouimette, P., Humphreys, K., Moos, R. H., Finney, J. W., Cronkite, R., & Federman. B. (2001). Self-help group participation among substance use disorder patients with posttraumatic stress disorder. *J Subst Abuse Treat, 20*, 25–32.

Paredes, A., & Gregory, D. (1979). Therapeutic impact and fiscal investment in alcoholism services. In M. Galanter (Ed.), *Currents in alcoholism* (Vol. 4, pp. 441–456). New York: Grune & Stratton.

Petry, N. M., Martin, B., & Finocche, C. (2001). Contingency management in group treatment: A demonstration project in an HIV drop-in center. *J Subst Abuse Treat, 21*, 89–96.

Petry, N. M., & Simcic, F., Jr. (2002). Recent advances in the dissemination of contingency management techniques: Clinical and research perspectives. *J Subst Abuse Treat, 23*, 81–86.

Peyrot, M. (1985). Narcotics Anonymous: Its history, structure, and approach. *Int J Addict, 20,* 1509–1522.

Pfeffer, A. Z., Friedland, P., & Wortis, S. B. (1949). Group psychotherapy with alcoholics. *Q J Stud Alcohol, 10,* 198–216.

Platt, J. J., Scura, W., & Harmon, J. R. (1960). Problem-solving thinking of youthful incarcerated heroin addicts: The archaic personality structure of alcoholics and its indications for group therapy. *Int J Group Psychother, 10,* 39–45.

Poldrugo, F., & Forti, B. (1988). Personality disorders and alcoholism treatment outcome. *Drug Alcohol Depend, 21,* 171–176.

Seixas, F., Washburn, S., & Eisen, S. V. (1988). Alcoholism, Alcoholics Anonymous attendance, and outcome in a prison system. *Am J Drug Alcohol Abuse, 14,* 515–524.

Thurstin, A. H., Alfano, A. M., & Nerviano, V. J. (1987). The efficacy of AA attendance for aftercare of inpatient alcoholics: Some follow-up data. *Int J Addict, 22,* 1083–1090.

Thurstin, A. H., Alfano, A. M., & Sherer, M. (1986). Pretreatment MMPI profiles of AA members and non-members. *J Stud Alcohol, 47,* 468–471.

Tracy, G. S., & Gussow, Z. (1976). Self-help health groups: A grass roots response to a need for services. *J Appl Behav Sci, 12,* 381–396.

Van Horn, D. H., & Bux, D. A. (2001). A pilot test of motivational interviewing groups for dually diagnosed inpatients. *J Subst Abuse Treat, 20,* 191–195.

Vannicelli, M. (1982). Group psychotherapy with alcoholics: Special techniques. *J Stud Alcohol, 43,* 17–37.

Vannicelli, M., Canning, D., & Griefen, M. (1984). Group therapy with alcoholics: A group case study. *Int J Group Psychother, 34,* 127–147.

Vischi, T. R., Jones, K. R., Shank, E. L., & Lima, L. H. (1980). *The alcohol, drug abuse and mental health national data book* (DHHS Publication No. 80-983). Washington, DC: U.S. Government Printing Office.

Wells, B. (1987). Narcotics Anonymous (NA): The phenomenal growth of an important resource [Editorial]. *Br J Addict, 82,* 581–582.

Yalom, I. D., Bloch, S., & Bond, G. (1978). Alcoholics in interactional group therapy. *Arch Gen Psych, 35,* 419–425.

Zweben, J. E. (1987). Can the patient on medication be sent to 12-step programs? *J Psychoactive Drugs, 19,* 299–300.

CHAPTER 24

Family-Based Treatment
Stages and Outcomes

M. DUNCAN STANTON
ANTHONY W. HEATH

The importance of the family in the genesis, maintenance, and alleviation of substance abuse has been well established. Although it is widely acknowledged that genetic and/or other biological components are important in the etiology of many alcohol and drug abuse cases, addiction generally develops within a family context, frequently reflects other family difficulties, and is usually maintained and exacerbated by family interaction. Other factors can also be critical (e.g., environmental, economic, cultural), but family variables hold a position of salience in addiction.

Not surprisingly, treatment focused on changing family dynamics has a firm footing in the substance abuse treatment field. Family-based therapy is commonly part of most successful substance abuse treatment programs and is usually considered an essential element in relapse prevention. As Craig (1993) has noted in an overview of the field, "The need to address family issues in a comprehensive treatment program is now widely recognized in drug abuse treatment" (p. 185). More specifically, a national survey by Fals-Stewart and Birchler (2001) of 398 randomly selected adult outpatient alcohol and/or drug treatment programs found that 82% offered family- or couples-based counseling. Regarding younger patients, a review of treatments for adolescent substance abusers by Williams and Chang (2000) concluded that "outpatient family therapy appears superior to other forms of outpatient treatment" (p. 138), and that it should be a component of any treatment program for such youth. It is therefore no accident that, of 10 adolescent substance abuse treatment programs identified as exemplary models by the U.S. Department of Health and Human Services (three of which were modified therapeutic communities), all include family members, particularly parents: seven apply family therapy, two incorporate multifamily therapy, and one has groups for parents (Stevens & Morral, 2003).

Over two dozen books have been written about family therapy for adult and/or adolescent substance abusers. These books, plus hundreds of chapters, journal articles, and papers, have described many different modalities of family therapy, including couple therapy, parents' group therapy, concurrent parent and index patient therapy, therapy with individual families (both inpatient and outpatient), sibling-oriented therapy, multifamily therapy, social network therapy, and family therapy with one person. However, rather than reviewing this vast literature, the intent in the present chapter is, first, to set forth some of the fundamental methods, or principles, of family/couples assessment and treatment with substance abusers and their families, and, second, to summarize the documented effectiveness of family- and couples-based therapies for this patient population. Readers interested in further pursuit of this subject matter are referred to overviews by O'Farrell and Fals-Stewart (2002, 2003) and Rowe and Liddle (2003), plus other literature cited later, for a more detailed understanding of the full range of theoretical and clinical approaches within the overall family/couples therapy approach to substance abuse. In addition, a brief synopsis of family systems concepts and theory is given in Stanton (1985), while a clinically oriented presentation of the foundations and key elements in family therapy, per se, may be found in Hanna and Brown (1999).

FAMILY PATTERNS OF ADDICTION

Addicted people are commonly in close contact with their families of origin or the people who raised them (Bekir, McLellan, Childress, & Gariti, 1993; Cervantes, Sorenson, Wermuth, Fernandez, & Menicucci, 1988; Douglas, 1987/1988; Stanton, 1982). Either they live with one or both parents (at five times the national rates for same-age adults) or are in touch on a daily or weekly basis. This pattern extends to adult alcoholics (Stanton & Heath, 2004). Overall, 30 of 32 reports, across seven countries, attest to such living arrangements or regularity of contact (Stanton, 2004; Stanton & Heath, 2004). These data indicate that addicted people's families are important to them, and that they are important to their families.

Stanton, Todd, and Associates (1982) summarized a number of other characteristics that distinguish drug-abusing families from other seriously dysfunctional families. The distinguishing qualities include the following:

1. A higher frequency of multigenerational chemical dependency, particularly alcohol, plus a propensity for other addictive behaviors, such as gambling. Such practices model behavior for children and can develop into family "traditions."
2. More primitive and direct expressions of conflict in addictive families.
3. More overt alliances (e.g., between addict and overinvolved parent).
4. "Conspicuously unschizophrenic" parental behavior.
5. A drug-oriented peer group to which the addict retreats following family conflict, thus gaining an illusion of independence.
6. "Symbiotic" child-rearing practices on the part of addicts' mothers, lasting longer into the addicts' adulthood.
7. A preponderance of death themes and premature, unexpected, and untimely deaths in the addict's family.
8. "Pseudoindividuation" of the addict across several levels, from the individual pharmacological level to that of the drug subculture.
9. More frequent acculturation problems and parent–child cultural disparity within families of addicts.

This list should be considered no more than a sketch of the addictive family. Readers are referred to Stanton, Todd, and colleagues (1982) for references to the original studies on which the outline is based, plus an update by Lawson and Lawson (2004). For thorough summaries of family dynamics in alcoholism, see Steinglass, Bennett, Wolin, and Reiss (1987), as well as Lawson and Lawson (1998).

INDICATIONS FOR THE USE OF FAMILY THERAPY IN ADDICTION

Families suffer when one or more members abuse drugs and/or alcohol. Parents worry about whether their abusing children will come home alive. They rage at their lack of control, suffer the guilt of the damned, and grasp at any suggestion of hope. Spouses shamefully hide advancing drinking/drugging problems from their neighbors and employers, struggle to maintain their illusions that drinking/drugging is temporary, and wonder what they have done wrong. Children of alcoholics/addicts also wonder what they did wrong and assume the burdens of maturity at startlingly young ages. They beg their parents to come home without stopping at the tavern or meeting the dealer. Grown children of alcoholics/addicts are haunted by their pasts, despairing in relationships that inflict substantial pain. Substance abuse affects every member of the family for decades and for generations.

Family therapy offers family members an opportunity to resolve the problems that plague them. Family therapists believe that family treatment is indicated when any man, woman, or child has a complaint concerning alcohol or drug abuse, whether the individual is the abuser or the "abused." Because they figuratively cast such a large net, family therapists encounter and serve many clients who initiate therapy for other reasons but later present concerns about substance abuse in their families. These concerns include issues of abuse, addiction, and recovery for adult and adolescent substance abusers, as well as corresponding issues for "codependents," children of alcoholics, and adult children of alcoholics for several generations (Elkin, 1984; Treadway, 1989).

Substance abusers themselves rarely seek the services of therapists. In fact, the most characteristic feature of substance abuse may be the abuser's denial that the use of the substance is a problem at all. Similarly, it is almost universally accepted that family members often overlook substance abuse; some families unintentionally encourage it. Recognizing this fact, family therapists offer their services to *anyone* who wants to discuss substance abuse and often inquire about the individual's use of alcohol and drugs. As in Al-Anon and related self-help programs, family therapists generally believe that every family member can be helped to "recover" from the abuse, whether the substance abuser stops drinking/drugging or not.

Family therapy begins when a family member, a therapist, a treatment program, or a social institution, such as a court, initially identifies the problem. Family treatment is indicated (a) when the family is mustering its forces to convince the abuser of the extent of the problem and the need for change, (b) during residential treatment for the substance abuse (when it is used), and (c) during recovery, when the family learns new ways to go on in life without chemicals. We offer guidelines for each of these stages of treatment later in this chapter.

An absence of family-oriented services in substance abuse treatment can have calamitous consequences. Without concurrent treatment for nonabusing members, families have been known to attempt sabotage of treatment efforts when those efforts begin to succeed (Brown & Lewis, 1999; Stanton, Todd, et al., 1982). Examples of sabotage are commonly cited in the literature. The examples range from the spouse who gives a holiday bottle of liquor to a recovering alcoholic, to the parents who refuse to work together in maintaining rules for their substance-abusing adolescent. On the other hand, Steinglass and colleagues (1987) asserted, at least regarding alcohol treatment, that the evidence is compelling that "involvement of a nonalcoholic spouse in a treatment program significantly improves the likelihood that the alcoholic individual will participate in treatment as well" (pp. 331–332).

Problems also occur after residential treatment, if families are left out of the treatment process. Sobriety for an individual often has difficult consequences for other family members, who may gain sudden awareness of their own problems or of other family problems. Divorce is not uncommon when adult substance abusers "dry out" or "clean up" (Stanton, 1985). The family is crucial in determining whether or not someone remains addicted, and the social context of the abuser must be changed for treatment to "take hold."

Families can prove to be a highly positive influence in recovery as well. Eldred and Washington (1976) found that heroin addicts rated their families of origin or their in-laws as most likely to be helpful to them in their attempts to give up drugs; the addicts' second choice was their partner. Similarly, Levy (1972) found, in a 5-year follow-up of narcotics addicts, that patients who successfully overcame drug abuse most often had family support, while Simpson and Sells (1990) got 75% crediting family as a major reason for their entering treatment. In short, family therapists enlist the inherent leverage of family members.

Like other treatment professionals who have worked with substance-abusing families, family therapists know the difficulty involved in treating substance abuse. Only by working *together* with extended families, specialists in the field of chemical dependence, physicians monitoring pharmacotherapy, and self-help programs, can substance abuse and its related problems be ameliorated.

Finally, professionals must talk to each other, if therapy is to succeed. For example, outpatient family therapists must visit local treatment centers and get to know the treatment teams. This investment facilitates referrals to residential treatment and subsequent referral for continued therapy upon release.

STAGES OF FAMILY THERAPY

Our purpose here is to present a model of the stages of family therapy that synthesizes much of the literature on family/couple therapy with (1) alcoholic adults (e.g., Berenson, 1976a, 1986, 1992; Davis, 1987; O'Farrell, 1993; O'Farrell & Fals-Stewart, 2000, 2001, 2002; Steinglass et al., 1987), (2) drug-abusing adults (e.g., Fals-Stewart, O'Farrell, Birchler, Cordova, & Kelley, 2005; Kosten, Jalali, & Kleber, 1982–1983; Stanton & Todd, 1992; Stanton, Todd, et al., 1982), and (3) substance-abusing adolescents (e.g., Alexander & Parsons, 1982; Fishman, Stanton, & Rosman, 1982; Henggeler & Borduin, 1990; Landau & Garrett, 1998; Liddle & Hogue, 2001; Piercy & Frankel, 1989; Stanton & Landau-Stanton, 1990; Szapocznik & Kurtines, 1989; Todd & Selekman, 1991; Waldron, Slesnick, Brody, Turner, & Peterson, 2001). One reason we can do this is because there is already a relatively high degree of consensus among many of these authors. Although detailed descriptions of the techniques of family therapy are, again, beyond the scope of this chapter, the literature cited herein comprises a veritable treasure chest of useful family therapy methods.

This presentation will, however, additionally incorporate a more recent, integrative model, developed in great part from working with substance abusers, called *transitional family therapy*, or TFT (Horwitz, 1997; Landau & Stanton, 2000; Landau-Stanton, Clements, & Stanton, 1993; Landau-Stanton, Griffiths, & Mason, 1982; Seaburn, Landau-Stanton, & Horwitz, 1995; Stanton, 1981a, 1984; Watson & McDaniel, 1998). Based both on structural-strategic (Stanton, 1981a; Stanton & Todd, 1992) and intergenerational (e.g., Guerin & Pendagast, 1976) methods, it integrates (1) the management of the substance abuse problem, (2) the larger psychosocial environment (ecosystem and network)—in line with Henggeler and Borduin (1990), Liddle and Hogue (2001), and Speck and Attneave (1973; Speck, 2003)—and (3) exploration and interventions pertaining to how the problem originated in the family's history. TFT's "geodynamic balance" theory of change (Stanton, 1984) posits that all therapeutic interventions can be subsumed within a complementary dichotomy of "compression" and "diversion" techniques. Compression (e.g., strategic, paradoxical) methods push a family interaction sequence further in the way it normally unfolds, that is, exaggerating it so as to get a counteraction—and thus a new sequence—among family members. Diversion (e.g., structural, behavioral) methods introduce competing behaviors that block the family's typical sequence and induce it to experience, and then to practice, a different and more functional pattern.

Stage 1: Problem Definition and Contracting

The first stage of family therapy begins when someone contacts a therapist and requests help from the full range of service settings and treatment providers. Family therapists also work in therapeutic communities, where families once were excluded. By making family therapy available, such therapeutic communities bring the "real world" into the center and help each family prepare for its reunion.

The therapist's first step is to convene enough of the family to gain adequate leverage to initiate change in family interaction regarding the substance abuse. As previously discussed, this may involve 1, 2, or 30 family members, and may include other members of the substance abuser's community. Family therapists generally start by working with the most motivated family member or members, convening other family members as necessary (Berenson, cited in Stanton, 1981b).

Next, family therapists attempt to understand and define the problem. When substance abuse is suspected, many therapists ask simple questions, such as "Who drinks?" or "What medications are used in your family?" We ironically refer to these as loaded questions and ask them of all our clients.

To assess the degree of substance abuse, particularly with adult clients, Davis (1987) suggests the use of a standardized questionnaire, such as the Michigan Alcoholism Screening Test (Selzer, 1971). History of the abuse, degree of physiological addiction, organic consequences of long-term addiction, prior treatment contacts, family perception of the abuse and its consequences, codependence, and coping behaviors are also topics that deserve careful assessment by qualified practitioners (Steinglass et al., 1987). If the therapist is not medically trained, clients are commonly referred to a physician for diagnosis and medical treatment when substance abuse has been chronic and/or when there is any indication of organic impairment due to substance abuse or disease. Family therapists often suggest that another family member accompany the substance abuser to the physician, to offer support and to inform the physician of the history of the abuse. Efforts must be made to get the consent of the patient to involve and to communicate with family to satisfy Federal and other privacy statutes and regulations.

The therapist can use the information gathered during the assessment to conclude and to state with confidence that—by some objective standards—the family has a serious drug or alcohol problem. Such confidence is necessary to overcome denial that a substance abuse problem exists, a common reaction in such families (Bepko & Krestan, 1985).

Once the problem is defined, the therapist and family identify and prioritize their goals for treatment, starting with the primary goal of helping the substance abuser become "clean and sober," and directly relating each subsequent goal to this primary one. When families bring up additional issues, the therapist may ask family members to justify them as relevant to the main goal of sobriety (Stanton & Todd, 1992). Considered together, these goals form the basis for determining whether an acceptable treatment contract can be agreed on with the family (Steinglass et al., 1987).

If the decision is made to work with an adult couple, the behavioral couple therapy approach works toward implementing, within the first two sessions, a daily Sobriety Contract (O'Farrell, 1993; O'Farrell & Fals-Stewart, 2000, 2002)—a method that has accreted empirical support in 11 of 12 studies where it was examined (O'Farrell & Fals-Stewart, 2003). When applicable, the contract may also incorporate daily Antabuse (disulfiram) ingestion. The procedure, applied on a day-to-day basis, involves the substance-abusing patient's agreeing not to use alcohol or drugs during that day (in line with the "one day at a time" tradition), while the spouse/partner expresses support for the patient's efforts to stay abstinent. The spouse/partner then records the patient's performance on a daily calendar. The partners also agree to reserve for therapy sessions, and not to discuss at home, either past substance abuse or fears about future alcohol/drug abuse, since such conflictual conversations can precipitate relapse. At each therapy session the couple both reviews the contract calendar with the therapist, and actually *practices* the behaviors included in the contract. In other words, they engage in what Minuchin and Fishman (1981) termed "enactment" of the new interactional pattern, thus expanding both their repertoire and their options as to how they deal with one another.

From the beginning, family therapists work to establish alliances with the senior sober family members. If the abuser is an adolescent or young adult, the therapist tries to engage both parents in these alliances whenever possible. Parents are kept working *together* and are steered away from discussing their marital difficulties, which could divide them and deter them from the primary objective of therapy (Stanton & Todd, 1992). This alliance forms the basis for establishing appropriate parental influence in families with substance-abusing adolescents (Alexander & Parsons, 1982; Fishman et al., 1982; Henggeler & Borduin, 1990; Landau & Garrett, 1998; Liddle & Hogue, 2001; Piercy & Frankel, 1989; Stanton & Landau-Stanton, 1990; Szapocznik & Kurtines, 1989; Todd & Selekman, 1991).

Family therapists' alliances with sober family members and parents of substance abusers help them motivate their clients. Family members are the most effective motivators known. Even the most evangelistic therapist cannot do as well. Thus, by forming alliances and encouraging sober family members to step up the pressure, family therapists help motivate substance abusers to pursue and maintain sobriety. Similarly, other professional helpers (e.g., school counselors, teachers, police officers, and probation officers) can be enlisted to exert benevolent influence. Here, the family therapist serves as coach, promoting the effective use of every reasonable threat, promise, and consequence to encourage abstinence. Later, therapists encourage families to serve as recovering addicts' sponsors to help prevent relapse. For an interesting example of the motivating influence of a family member, we recommend Heard's (1982) rich description of how a deathbed wish of a deceased grandfather was used to promote recovery in a 23-year-old heroin addict.

Family therapists consider it extremely important during this stage to assume a *nonblaming stance* (Alexander, Waldron, Barton, & Mas, 1989; Stanton & Todd, 1992) toward the entire family. We find that the confronting techniques used in group therapy with substance abusers tend to fan the fires of resistance and to inspire counterattack. Challenges can still be offered to families, but they must be expressed in nonpejorative ways. Many family therapists use positive interpretation when they comment on family members' behavior. Stanton and Todd (1992) have referred to this as "ascribing noble intentions" or "noble ascriptions" (see also, Stanton, Todd, et al., 1982). Examples include statements such as "He's defending the family like any good son would" and "You're trying your best to be a good mother." Such statements tune into both the caring and frustration that most family members experience, and seem to lessen client resistance and promote compliance.

Steinglass and colleagues (1987) emphasized that it is essential to label the substance abuse as a *family* problem and to convince the family members that they are all essential players in the recovery process. Writing about alcoholism, these authors stated that whenever alcoholism is identified as a problem, the therapist must, in the same session, "get across to the family that there is no issue more important at this stage of the work than the cessation of drinking, and that the family and the therapist must mobilize all resources toward that goal and that goal alone" (p. 354). Family therapists characteristically invite family members to become part of the solution to problems.

A powerful, ecosystemic expansion of the above notion is to apply the methods of psychiatrist Ross V. Speck (2003; Speck & Attneave, 1973) and involve the family's social network in the treatment endeavor. This can include extended family, friends, work associates, and, commonly, other professionals involved with the case. Callan, Garrison, and Zerger (1975) described such an approach with adults who are addicted to drugs, while van der Velden, Ruhf, and Kaminsky (1991) have applied it with adolescents who abuse substances. It is also regularly used in TFT (Landau & Garrett, 1998; Landau & Stanton, 2000; Seaburn et al., 1995; Stanton & Landau-Stanton, 1990), in which a major thrust of the first session or two is to attain consensus across the network on what the primary goals of treatment are, and how change in each can be objectively defined. Thus all members are working in accord, and (often unintentional) competing agendas among subsystems are minimized: Everybody agrees both on what needs to be done and on how to know when that has occurred.

By the second session, TFT also begins to build three graphic constructions with the family, all of them printed with a marker on a large newsprint flip chart mounted on an easel. These are: (1) a list of the goals of treatment; (2) a list of the tasks to be performed toward meeting those goals, including who is to do them and, if applicable, by when; and (3) a three-generational genogram (Guerin & Pendagast, 1976; McGoldrick, Gerson, & Shellenberger, 1999) that includes all members, living and deceased. These graphics are brought to each session and hung on the walls (e.g., with masking tape) so as to be readily available for reference. Such techniques help to clarify, make more concrete, and provide perspective on the problem(s)—both as to how they developed and the ways the family has devised to contend with them.

The therapist should also be aggregating information for a fourth graphic, the family "time line" (Stanton, 1992). This method clearly spreads out facts as to, for instance, when the substance abuse problem, and the latest relapse, began and what changes (e.g., illnesses, unemployment, relocation, immigration), losses (e.g., deaths, divorces, breakups of relationships), or other family stressors were occurring around those times. However, it may be too early at this stage in therapy to construct the time line publicly with the family. Therefore, the technique is discussed at greater length below.

Many families—in attempting to answer the question, "Why did this happen to me?"—accept that genetics and/or a disease process is responsible for substance abuse, particularly when the problem is alcoholism (see below). At best, these theoretical explanations can reduce guilt, blame, and shame in families, facilitate participation in therapy, and promote recovery. Genetic or disease explanations are almost always more useful than moralistic explanations. At worst, though, these explanations (1) provoke fear and enable discouraged, wallowing inaction and irresponsible behavior in the family; and (2) engender inaction in a therapist who can only envision a medical pathway for change.

Incidentally, it is wise for family therapists not to allow themselves or their clients to become discouraged by the disease explanation of the cause of drug and alcohol addiction. They cannot afford to wait for a pill or a tissue implant to cure the disease. Instead, they help families to understand that by working together, they can overcome the disease's symptoms, reverse the ostensible destiny, and lead happy, chemical-free lives.

Of course, there are—and probably always will be—people who reject genetic and disease explanations for addiction. Regarding the former, they may be at least partly justified, since the majority of people who develop drinking or drug problems do not demonstrate a genetic predisposition. Only 15–36% of children of alcoholics develop drinking problems (Stabenau, 1988). A high proportion of the people who become problem drinkers—including at least half of those who are actually hospitalized for alcoholism—have no obvious genetic loading (Goodwin & Warnock, 1991; Searles, 1991). Furthermore, most of the genetic effects that have been identified for alcoholism in males tend to be somewhat weaker, or less clear, both for females and for other substances of abuse (Anthenelli & Schuckit, 1997; Cadoret, Yates, Troughton, Woodworth, & Stewart, 1995; van den Bree, Svikis, & Pickens, 1998). But in any case, people who do develop addiction problems can learn to live responsibly and avoid blame and shame. They can work together with their loved ones to overcome their problems.

Stage 2: Establishing the Context for a Chemical-Free Life

When substance abuse is identified as a problem, and a therapeutic contract is negotiated, family therapy enters a second stage in which a context for sobriety is established. Berenson (1976b) stated that this stage involves "management of an ongoing, serious drinking problem and setting up a context so that the alcoholic will stop drinking" (p. 33).

Family therapists generally accept cessation of substance abuse as a prerequisite for further treatment (e.g., Bepko & Krestan, 1985). Furthermore, many believe that therapists must consistently demonstrate conviction of the importance of abstinence over the course of therapy (e.g., Davis, 1987). In the words of Steinglass and colleagues (1987):

> Meaningful therapy with an Alcoholic Family cannot proceed if the therapist adopts a laissez-faire attitude about drinking behavior and acquiesces in a decision to allow the identified alcoholic to continue drinking. The therapist must take a

firm stand on this issue at the start of therapy, while at the same time acknowledging that it may not be an easy task and that there may be a number of slips before abstinence is achieved. (p. 343)

On the other hand, Berenson, whose innovative work was described by Stanton (1981a), believes that therapists should concern themselves with achieving substantial changes in drunken behavior instead of abstinence from drinking. Berenson considers it tactically unwise to take a resolute stand in favor of total abstinence, even though abstinence is usually the ultimate goal. This position on abstinence runs counter to the beliefs of several others, including Davis (1987) and Bepko and Krestan (1985). It is consistent, however, with the problem-solving models that have been applied to drug problems by Haley (1997), Stanton and Todd (1992), and others (e.g., Heath & Ayers, 1991), who often prefer to leave the decision about the importance of total abstinence to parents or others. These authors believe that therapists who assume a less adamant, less certain position on the necessity of abstinence enjoy more maneuverability in therapy. For example, a therapist who states that he or she is not sure whether abstinence will prove necessary may be able to stay out of a couple's argument over the issue long enough to help them try out several new solutions to the problems brought on by the substance abuse (e.g., Berg & Miller, 1992).

Independent of the issue of abstinence, Berenson believes that the therapist must exert a major effort to get the family system calmed down, ergo reducing the emotionality and increasing the psychological distance between family members. Families at this stage of therapy are often overwrought and involved in intense battles and patterns of over- and underresponsibility that lock members together. (See Bepko & Krestan, 1985, for a thorough discussion of the therapeutic process of assessing and interrupting overresponsible and underresponsible behaviors.)

On another tack, behavioral couple therapy for substance abuse is directed toward increasing positive behaviors as a means for countering the kind of negativity—particularly surrounding drinking or drug-taking—which usually creeps into, and may even predominate, the partners' relationship. Early on in therapy each partner is encouraged to acknowledge pleasing behaviors in the other, such as through homework assignments to, each day, "catch your partner doing something nice" and record it on a special sheet provided by the therapist (O'Farrell, 1993; O'Farrell & Fals-Stewart, 2000, 2002). This exercise is eventually guided toward the implementation of "love days" (Weiss, Hops, & Patterson, 1973) or "caring days" (Stuart, 1980), in which each person plans ahead to surprise their partner during the week "with a day when they do some special things to show their caring" (O'Farrell & Fals-Stewart, 2000, p. 52). As examples, Paolino and McCrady (1977) note the set of special behaviors "might include such minor actions as saying hello when the husband comes home at night, clearing the table, rinsing out a glass after having a drink of milk rather than leaving the glass on the counter, asking how the other's day was, giving a back rub, and so on" (p. 161). These various pleasure-inducing actions help to increase "the overall rewardingness of the relationship, which would enable the couple to more willingly work on problematic aspects of the relationship, while making the overall relationship more fun" (p. 161). In a sense, the newer, positive experiences compete with and crowd out the older, "nastier" ones.

Regarding self-help groups, family therapists often refer family members to Al-Anon, Nar-Anon, Alateen, Alatot, and related programs at this stage, encouraging clients to shop around until they find groups that are "socially compatible and geographically accessible" (Davis, 1987, p. 56). According to Bepko and Krestan (1985), the goal of this involvement is to help the family members "shift their role behavior significantly both in the interest of their greatest well-being and with the expectation that a change in their part of the family interaction will eventually lead to the drinker's sobriety" (p. 104). Davis (1987) suggests that therapists must consistently assign visits to self-help groups, because participation in groups enhances family therapy in several ways. Participation in self-help groups encourages detachment from substance-abusing behavior, provides validating experiences and 24-hour crisis support through sponsors, and emphasizes personal responsibility (Davis, 1987).

Many family therapists supplement the work of self-help groups by helping the spouses of substance abusers to achieve a greater degree of emotional detachment. Berenson begins by getting spouses of alcoholics into support groups, usually Al-Anon or other spouses' groups (Stanton, 1981b). Next, he prepares spouses for the impending period of pain and depression, perhaps even noting that they may have suicidal thoughts as a part of "hitting bottom." Finally, Berenson helps spouses gain distance from their alcoholic partners, often by suggesting brief separations (e.g., a week away from home) in order to promote differentiation. Berenson warns spouses that their alcoholic partners may try to get them back by intensifying the symptom, usually by increased drinking.

At this point Berenson may involve the alcoholics more in therapy, empathizing with how isolated and alone they may feel. Concomitantly, he helps spouses stick to the plan, so that the drunks have a chance to get sober. He tells spouses that they should not expect the alcoholic to improve but suggests that when they realize that the alcoholics cannot be controlled, the alcoholics may be able to make a change for the better. Berenson does not support hostile moves against the alcoholic but only supports moves the spouses make for themselves.

Berenson has suggested several helpful rules for therapists working through this stage of family therapy (Stanton, 1981b). First, therapists must have no expectations that change will occur; rather than "hoping," they must be "hopeless." Second, therapists should want family members to feel both helpless and hopeless—that is, to "hit bottom," if they have not done so already. Third, therapists must not look for a single strategic intervention to reverse the multitude of problems in these families but should work patiently in a simple, straightforward manner.

It is also during this stage that the TFT therapist considers publicly constructing a time line with the family (Stanton, 1992). By now, enough information about both the nuclear and the extended family should have been collected to provide a clear picture of how family life events have contributed to the onset of the family's problems. Stanton (1992) gives as an example a 17-year-old male, "Pat," who initiated substance abuse when an aunt with whom he was very close went through a divorce, and whose abuse became heavy when his close, 19-year-old cousin (the aunt's son) died suddenly in a traffic accident. The family finally entered therapy when his paternal grandmother and her live-in boyfriend of many years broke up, and she tried to induce Pat to leave his nuclear family and move 1,000 miles away to live with her.

Finally, many family therapists work to get the substance abuser to AA, Narcotics Anonymous (NA), or Cocaine Anonymous (CA) as the final step in the second stage of therapy. Bepko and Krestan (1985) suggest that it is not advisable for therapists to argue with clients about the value of AA, but they should describe AA and its purpose "in a way that is palatable to the particular client" (p. 103). Most family therapists emphasize that AA is one of the most effective treatments for addiction. We help each substance abuser find a group with which he or she feels comfortable, then encourage attendance for a while before making a decision whether to continue. For the individuals who feel uncomfortable with AA's use of the "Higher Power," we recommend secular sobriety groups (Christopher, 1988).

Stage 3: Halting Substance Abuse

In family therapy, there always comes a moment of truth. As a result of the changes in their family members' behavior and the firm position of the therapist, substance abusers suddenly become aware that they are going to have to choose between their families and their drugs. Substance abusers, when consistently confronted (or abandoned) by parents, spouses, children, friends, employers, and perhaps even recovering people in self-help groups and/or a therapist, often "hit bottom" and turn to the therapist for help in changing their ways.

At this juncture, Steinglass and colleagues (1987) suggest that there are basically three ways for therapists to proceed. First, when physical dependence on alcohol or drugs is identified, the therapist should arrange safe detoxification for the addicted person and refuse to continue therapy unless this option is completed. Without medical intervention, the addict's independent withdrawal is unlikely and possibly dangerous. Second, the therapist can agree to let the family attempt detoxification on an outpatient basis, on the condition that if there has been no meaningful progress made toward detoxification in 2 weeks (maximum), medical treatment will be pursued. Third, except in cases where the dependence is on sedative hypnotics (e.g., alcohol, barbiturates), and given proper medical backup, the therapist can work with the family as the "treatment team" and conduct the detoxification in the home environment (Scott & Van Deusen, 1982; Stanton, Todd, et al., 1982). In fact, home detoxification appears to be a cost-effective option in many cases, with savings of 70–85% of the cost of hospitalization (Stanton & Shadish, 1997; Stanton, Steier, Cook, & Todd, 1997).

Whichever of these courses of action is selected, family therapists try to keep family members involved in the change process. One benefit is that the members will be able to realize some responsibility for the success of the treatment (Stanton & Todd, 1992). When treatment is left to the "professionals," families often fail to realize their responsibility for change. And later, should the recovery process go awry, they blame the setback on the treatment program.

Finally, a parallel activity engaged in during this stage by transitional family therapists is to begin to expand the family genogram to include four, five, or more generations. The idea is to engage the family in an examination of its pedigree toward answering certain key questions (which were developed by psychiatrist Judith Landau) about the etiology of the problem, that is: When did the substance abuse start? With which generation? What was happening across the extended family at that time? In other words, when, in this family's history, was the family so stressed that it had to change its relational patterns or organization and develop a drinking or drug problem (Landau & Stanton, 2000)?

Stage 4: Managing the Crisis and Stabilizing the Family

When the substance abuser becomes "clean and sober," the family therapist should be prepared for a new set of problems (Brown & Lewis, 1999). Family members, stunned by the unfamiliar behavior of the sober or clean family member, and often frightened, have been known to make seemingly irrational statements, such as "I liked you better when you were drinking." One woman we know gave a bottle of bourbon to her recently sober husband for his birthday. No wonder the rate of relapse is high in this stage.

In discussing alcoholic families, Steinglass and colleagues (1987) identified an analogous stage, "the emotional desert." In their rich qualitative description, families that have been organized around alcohol for many years experience a profound sense of emptiness when the drinking stops. Steinglass and colleagues explain that these families "have the sensation of having been cut adrift, loosened from their familiar moorings, lost in a desert without any landmarks upon which to focus to regain their bearings" (p. 344). Instead of experiencing joy over the newfound sobriety, the family members feel empty and depressed. It is not surprising that members of newly sober families tend to interact in the same way they did while one of their own was abusing alcohol and/or drugs.

Couples often experience a feeling of "walking on eggshells" at home and drift into a kind of emotional divorce. Both partners want to preserve sobriety and peace, so they interact sparingly and hesitantly, unwittingly reestablishing the same patterns of closeness and distance that they enacted previously. For example, a recently sober alcoholic, wanting to talk with his wife about his feelings, approached her late at night, waking her from a sound sleep, just as he did when he was drunk. She, in turn, rebuffed his awkward attempt at communication, leaving him to go sulk alone, just as once he went off to drink alone. Thus, when recovering couples get to know each other anew, they often find themselves bored, irrationally angry, and unable to resolve problems that were once avoided with the help of intoxicants (e.g., O'Farrell, 1993).

In the case of addicted young people, a family crisis can be anticipated 3 or 4 weeks into this part of treatment (Stanton & Todd, 1992). Commonly, the crisis occurs in the marital relationship of the parents, who take steps toward separation. Many addicts have become "dirty" again to reunite their families.

Siblings and children of recovering substance abusers also can exert unintentional pressure to revert to old ways. Gradually, families begin to notice other problems, long hidden from attention by the magnitude of substance abuse. As the blur of intoxication clears, children who were once considered helpful are suddenly seen as withdrawn and depressed; children who were once seen to be doing fine in school may be seen as just getting by, and the teenager's marijuana smoking may be noticed for the first time.

Family therapists disagree about how quickly family problems should be resolved in this stage. Berenson suggested that it is advisable to begin this stage with a hiatus from therapy while things calm down; thus, he does not schedule regular appointments but tells clients, "Get back to me in a month or so" (Stanton, 1981b). Meanwhile, he encourages his clients to continue their self-help group activities, with the understanding that if their distress continues beyond 6–12 months, family therapy will resume on a more regular basis. Then, after a period of sobriety, Berenson returns to a more orthodox therapy schedule. Others (e.g., Bepko & Krestan, 1985; Steinglass et al., 1987) believe that regularly scheduled family therapy sessions can be very helpful at these times, especially if they focus on solving the series of problems that hound these families and wear them down.

Therapy in this stage should be focused on keeping family members as calm as possible (Bepko & Krestan, 1985), while they establish a newfound stability that is not based on substance abuse (Steinglass et al., 1987). Toward this end, therapists work to minimize stress and deescalate conflict, congratulate individuals for their contributions to family recovery, encourage individuals to focus on their own issues, predict and address common difficulties in recovery and fears about relapse, and facilitate minor structural changes in the family to allow adequate parenting (Bepko & Krestan, 1985). Changes in parenting practices are especially vital when the recovering substance abuser is an adolescent (Alexander & Parsons, 1982; Fishman et al., 1982; Henggeler & Borduin, 1990; Landau & Garrett, 1998; Liddle & Hogue, 2001; Piercy & Frankel, 1989; Stanton & Landau-Stanton, 1990; Szapocznik & Kurtines, 1989; Todd & Selekman, 1991; Waldron et al., 2001).

Whenever a relapse into drinking or drug taking occurs, the question of responsibility arises. Who is responsible for the relapse? Although conventional drug treatment programs and many individual therapists either thrust the responsibility on the substance abuser or accept it themselves, family therapists tend to assign the responsibility to the abuser's family. As Stanton and Todd (1992) suggested, "It should be remembered that the addicted individual was raised by, and in most cases is still being maintained by, his family of origin. It is thus with the family that responsibility rests, and the therapist should help the family either to accept it or to *effectively* disengage from the addict so that the addict must accept it on his or her own" (p. 55, original emphasis).

Similarly, the therapist must assign credit to the entire family when credit is due (Stanton, 1981c). Each member, particularly the often-neglected spouse, is praised for his or her contribution to the growing "health" of the family. By identifying and rewarding individual contributions, family therapists spread the glory that is usually bestowed on recovering abusers and promote long-lasting changes in family interaction.

Stage 5: Family Reorganization and Recovery

Whereas families in Stage 4 remained organized around substance abuse and therapy was focused on resolving difficulties with substance abuse, Stage 5 is concerned with helping families move away from interaction focused on substance abuse issues and toward fundamentally better relationships. Here, the substance abuser is stabilized and "clean and sober." Therapy now focuses on developing a better marriage, establishing more satisfactory parent–child relationships, and perhaps confronting long-standing family-of-origin and codependence issues.

Steinglass and colleagues (1987) called this process "family reorganization" (p. 344). Although some families restabilize before reaching this phase and remain organized around alcohol issues ("dry alcoholic" families), we have observed that for others, the previous stages of therapy culminate in a serious family crisis. This crisis then leads to disorganization and ultimately to a fundamentally different organizational pattern that is encouraged in this stage of therapy.

Bepko and Krestan (1985) enumerated four goals for their analogue of this stage, which they have termed "rebalancing" (p. 135):

1. Shift extremes of behavior from rigid complementarity to greater symmetry or more overt complementarity (improved complementarity for the specific relationship).
2. Help the couple/family to resolve issues of power and control.
3. Directly address the pride structures of both partners, so that new forms of role behavior are permitted without the need for alcohol.
4. Help the couple to achieve whatever level of closeness and intimacy is desirable for them. (pp. 135–136)

See Bepko and Krestan (1985), O'Farrell (1993), Fals-Stewart and colleagues (2005), and O'Farrell and Fals-Stewart (2000, 2002) for detailed discussions of therapeutic methods used to implement these and related goals.

Davis (1987) also emphasized that therapists must help family members to reconsider and redefine the substance abuser's role in the family at this stage of therapy. Old expectations and behavioral patterns, based on living with addiction, must be replaced by new adaptive ones. For example, a family that has grown used to an alcoholic husband/father may continue to withdraw every time he shows a hint of anger, leave him out of family decisions, and disregard his parenting efforts. In this stage of therapy, the father must learn to deal with his anger, to participate in making responsible decisions, and to function as a father, *and* the family members must let him change.

In the treatment of a family with a young addict during this stage, the therapy evolves beyond Stage 4 crisis management and toward other issues, such as finding the recovering addict gainful employment and a place to live away from home (Stanton & Todd, 1992). Family therapists work to involve parents in these "launchings," so they will share the addict's eventual success. Over time, it becomes increasingly possible to shift the parents' attention to other siblings, grandchildren, or retirement planning, thereby allowing both the parents and the recovering addict to let go. Should marital issues surface, as they often do, family therapists try to keep young addicts out of their parents' marriage issues.

Berenson focuses his work in this stage on the couple's relationship, with the aim of increasing emotional closeness within the couple, without a return either to drinking or to discussions centered on alcohol (Stanton, 1981b). In conjoint sessions with couples and/or multiple-couple groups, Berenson and other family therapists often focus on the severe sexual problems that are common in such marriages (Stanton, 1981b) and teach new skills for dealing with stress and conflict (Bepko & Krestan, 1985; Fals-Stewart et al., 2005; O'Farrell & Fals-Stewart, 2000, 2002). Therapy sessions with the extended family are scheduled when relatives or in-laws are disruptive (Speck, 2003; Stanton & Landau-Stanton, 1990).

Finally, it is also during this stage that a number of family therapists (e.g., Bowser, Word, Stanton, & Coleman, 2003; Coleman, Kaplan, & Downing, 1986; Horwitz, 1997; Reilly, 1975, 1984; Rosenbaum & Richman, 1972) deal with the often unexpected and unresolved losses and deaths that so many chemically dependent families have experienced. These issues may not need to be covered to effect abstinence initially, but unresolved grief can "eat away" at progress unless it is brought to terms.

More particular to this issue, it is important to recognize that most substance abusers have been fulfilling a script prescribed by family history. Similar to Walsh's (1978) finding that, in comparison with "normals," people who become schizophrenic are more likely to have been born close to the time when a grandparent died, Reilly (1975) has noted that addicted people are frequently dealt with as replacements, or "revenants," of other family members who were lost, often unexpectedly. Reilly also observed a tendency for adolescents who abuse substances to be named after a relative who was an alcoholic. His observation is supported by a national survey of adults in the United States by Stanton, Adams, Landau, and Black (1998) in which it was found that drug- or alcohol-dependent people were three times more likely to be named after a relative with a substance abuse problem than were people named after relatives with no such problem. An example is the case of the young man, "Pat," mentioned earlier: He was named after, and viewed as very similar to, his paternal grandfather who manufactured illegal alcohol during the Prohibition period. Pat was later pressured by his paternal grandmother—who called Pat her "pride and joy"—to fill in as a replacement for the longtime boyfriend who had left her (Stanton, 1992; Stanton & Landau-Stanton, 1990).

Transitional family therapy specifically deals with the kinds of loss and scripting dynamics mentioned above. The material revealed in the genogram as to when the problem began in the family's history, and the loss and grief that likely attended that onset, are dealt with in a direct manner. The family is taken back to the point of loss and symbolically "goes through" it again from a present-day vantage point. This joins the poles of past, present, and future—spanning the family's generations. The process also depathologizes those members from the past who had problems, and reinstates them, instead, as people who may have been pained and besieged. By granting the forebears their honorable place, honor is also bestowed on the living, their descendants. Such uncovering and rebuilding gives the family members the kind of information that can free them up to make a choice: Whether to keep, revise, or replace the intergenerational instructions (scripts) that have been carried down. In other words, it helps the family come to grips with the question of whether, and how, to move on in life. In experience with several thousand cases, as well as more systematic qualitative study with over 200 clinical and nonclinical families, TFT has shown great promise in bringing about long-term change in the intergenerational family addiction pattern (Landau & Stanton, 2000).

Stage 6: Ending Therapy

In the ideal course of therapy with substance-abusing families, treatment comes to an end when the clients and therapist agree to stop meeting regularly. Family therapists tend to agree to stop when they believe that the serious structural and functional problems that have maintained substance abuse have been replaced with new family rules, roles, and interactional patterns. Optimally, substance abuse has not been replaced with other addictive behaviors. Family therapists tend to tolerate socially acceptable "addictions" (e.g., "workaholism") as long as family members tolerate them.

In TFT, as the therapist hands over control to the family, a renewed commitment for support is requested from the network. Strategic predictions are made, helping the family to understand the likelihood that the substance abuser may once again test their commitment to his or her abstinence. Plans are made for dealing with this possibility. Finally, a formal, end-of-treatment ritual is designed and orchestrated by the family (Landau & Stanton, 2000).

The length of therapy and the specific definition of successful treatment vary widely among models of therapy and among individual families. Stanton and Todd (1992), in describing their brief therapy model for treating drug addicts, have broadly stated that therapy is appropriately concluded when "adequate change has occurred and been maintained long enough for the family to feel a sense of real accomplishment" (p. 56). Adherents of other models would not even attempt to reorganize family structure in the ways prescribed in our fifth stage. Instead, they conclude treatment when family members feel satisfied that the problems originally presented have been resolved (e.g., Heath & Ayers, 1991).

Once all parties agree to cease regularly scheduled sessions, occasional inoculatory follow-up sessions ("checkups") may be scheduled, one at a time, at intervals of 2–6 months. Therapists make it clear that clients are welcome to schedule future appointments at any time and to cancel sessions that seem unnecessary. Therapy clients, like medical patients, are not necessarily made permanently "healthy," even after a course of treatment. The door to the therapist's office, like that of the family physician, remains open (Heath, 1985).

Family therapy sometimes ends unexpectedly and prematurely, at least as seen by the therapist. No matter how skilled the therapist, and no matter what the stage of treatment, families generally stop coming to therapy when they want. In such circumstances, responsible therapists make every reasonable effort to determine whether client families are satisfied or dissatisfied with services rendered and to respond accordingly. They offer additional services or referrals for any family member, as well as professional opinions about remaining problems and caveats, when appropriate.

In conclusion, the six-stage model presented here is intentionally inclusive. We have made no effort to spell out or resolve differences among models of family therapy, or to examine the differences between treating drug addicts and alcoholics. Instead, we have broadly sketched a viable course of treatment for families with substance-abusing members. Clinicians may wish to emphasize some stages of therapy more than others.

SPECIAL CONSIDERATIONS IN FAMILY THERAPY

A number of special clinical considerations concern family therapists when they work with substance abusers and their families. The most salient of these considerations are discussed next. Interested readers will find insightful discussions of many of the day-to-day issues that face family therapists in the various texts referenced previously.

Engaging the Substance Abuser in Treatment or Self-Help

It is well known within the substance abuse field that, at least in the United States and Canada, in any given year the vast majority (90–95%) of people who are actively abusing drugs or alcohol do not obtain help for their problems (e.g., Kessler et al., 1994; Sobell, Cunningham, & Sobell, 1996). Consequently, recent years have seen considerable attention devoted to the means for getting reluctant substance abusers either to enroll in treatment, or to begin attending a self-help group such as Alcoholics Anonymous or Narcotics Anonymous. At least 11 different approaches have been developed that involve family members and/or significant others toward this end. Ten of the approaches have been examined in 19 outcome studies (nine of which included Hispanic cases) across three countries. Reviews of this literature (e.g., O'Farrell & Fals-Stewart, 2003; Rowe & Liddle, 2003; Stanton, 1997, 2004) indicate that significant progress is being made in terms of certain of these approaches both becoming more effective, and explicating their methods so others may apply them.

Regarding the results from the aforementioned 19 engagement outcome studies, Stanton (2004) has both summarized the various methods themselves and compared them as to results. His review applied an "intent-to-treat" criterion, that is, that a method's effectiveness should be gauged on the proportion of cases that become engaged of those to whom it is offered. Otherwise, if only 10 of 100 cases agree to attempt an approach, and nine of those succeed, the approach may claim "90% success" for what is actually 9% success.

Some rather surprising findings emerged from this synopsis. For instance, the well-known Johnson Institute "Intervention" actually succeeds in engaging in treatment/self-help only 0–36% of cases (average across studies = 20%). These low rates seem to be due to the fact that many of the people, such as family members, who are trying to get help for a substance abuser believe that the confrontive and secretive Intervention process is too stressful and damaging to relationships. Thus, many families have refused to proceed with Intervention.

Some other findings from this review of outcome studies are as follows:

1. Later (1995 on) studies generally attained higher engagement success rates than earlier studies (69 vs. 52%).
2. Adult drug users appear to be easier to engage than adult alcoholics (78

vs. 49%), although this may be confounded by age, because the alcoholic samples tended to be older.

3. The overall engagement success rates for adolescent and adult drug abusers do not differ significantly.

4. When a parent is the primary, or only, person mounting the engagement effort (vs. a spouse/partner, other relative, or friend), the likelihood of success is increased. This holds for both adolescent and adult cases.

5. Engagement is also more likely, and requiring of less effort on the part of the engagement professional, when more people (family, friends, work associates, etc.) are actively involved in the effort. In particular, Landau and colleagues (2004) found a high, and statistically significant, correlation between (a) the number of people involved and (b) scores on an engagement success/efficiency index ($r = .69, p < .0001$).

Stanton's (2004) review also singles out the approaches that appear to be the "best options" with particular kinds of cases (e.g., adult drug abusers, adult alcohol abusers, adolescent substance abusers) in terms of both success rate and cost-effectiveness. Regarding cost-effectiveness, specifically—that is, having the highest success rate for the least amount of professional effort—two approaches stand out, both of which are nonsecretive (in other words, the substance abuser is informed of the effort from the very beginning). Both involve an average of only 1.5–2 hours of staff time to get most substance abusers into treatment/self-help, and they generally accomplish this within 1–2 weeks. These approaches are: (1) for adolescents, the behaviorally based "intensive parent and youth attendance intervention" by Donahue and colleagues (1998), which attained an 89% success rate through the use of a standardized telephone program orientation with the parent to set up an appointment, plus motivational telephone reminder calls to both the parent *and* the youth 2–3 days before the scheduled intake session; and (2) for adults, a TFT-based approach called "A Relational Intervention Sequence for Engagement" (ARISE; Garrett, Landau-Stanton, Stanton, Stellato-Kabat, & Stellato-Kabat, 1997), which had engagement rates of 87% for drug abusers and 77% for alcohol abusers (Landau et al., 2004). ARISE uses a manual-guided, rapid-response, stepped approach in handling the first call from someone who is concerned about a substance abuser, as well as quickly expanding the system involved to both increase leverage with the substance abuser and provide additional support to the person who originally called (Garrett et al., 1998, 1999; Landau et al., 2000).

Convening Difficulties

One of the problems identified by therapists working with substance abusers and their families is the difficulty in convening the whole family for therapy

(Stanton & Todd, 1981; Stanton, Todd, et al., 1982). The families of addicts are particularly difficult to engage in such an endeavor. Fathers, in particular, often appear threatened by treatment and defensive about their contribution to the problem. Because many have drinking problems themselves, they may also fear being blamed.

Experienced family therapists, recognizing this hesitancy to participate in therapy, work hard to recruit families into therapy. They do not rely on other family members to do the recruiting, because this approach often fails. Instead, they work energetically and enthusiastically to extend personal invitations to the reluctant. With emotionally healthier families, one telephone call may enable a therapist to reassure family members that their contributions are important to the solution of the substance abuse. With less healthy families, it may be necessary to meet on "neutral turf" (e.g., a restaurant), to write multiple letters, or even (Stanton, Steier, & Todd, 1982) to pay family members for participation in treatment. Wermuth and Scheidt (1986) and Stanton and associates (Stanton & Todd, 1981; Stanton, Todd, et al., 1982) have described engagement procedures in considerable detail, the latter group also presenting 21 principles for getting reluctant families into therapy.

Control of the Case

To shift the responsibility for dealing with the substance abuser's problems to the family, a family therapist needs to have command of the case. The family therapist must be allowed (e.g., by other elements in the treatment system) to direct the overall case management, including the treatment plan, the use of medication and drug tests (see below), and decisions about hospitalization. When one therapist is in charge, substance abusers are less likely to manipulate relationships among treatment professionals.

Stanton, Todd, and colleagues (1982) estimated that approximately half the effectiveness of treatment of drug addicts and their families depends on the efficiency and cohesiveness of the treatment system. If family members receive varied advice, they often end up arguing about the therapy rather than working toward recovery. Cohesion in the treatment system of substance abusers necessarily includes the self-help programs used by their families. Again, it is vital for therapists to know the local self-help groups and to collaborate with them for the sake of their clients.

Medication and Management

Family therapists who work with substance abusers and their families must have at least a basic knowledge of pharmacology. This information aids them during the detoxification process and reduces the overcaution in the use of medications that sometimes occurs among less informed therapists.

With regard to the use of pharmacotherapy, it is vital that physicians, family therapists, and drug counselors work as a treatment team. Cooperation and open lines of communication help to counteract the manipulative behaviors of many substance abusers. Within that team, the family therapist and physician have to work together to encourage family or spouse/partner compliance with prescribed medications, as well as to share information on patient and family functioning (Fals-Stewart et al., 2005; Woody, Carr, Stanton, & Hargrove, 1982).

Family therapists must have influence over the use of methadone. Families tend to believe that their recovering members are inherently helpless, fragile, handicapped people; thus, families forgive the most outrageous behavior. For family therapists to argue effectively that addicts can be competent and function adequately without drugs, they must assert that they are primarily concerned with the addicts' detoxifying and getting off all drugs, including methadone. To encourage the cessation of methadone use, family therapists and the families themselves must have significant input into how it is dispensed (Stanton, Todd, et al., 1982; Woody et al., 1982).

Epidemiologists have taught us that 30–60% of substance abusers have concurrent mental health comorbidities that include major depression, major anxiety, and personality disorders (Leshner, 1999). Since effective treatment for mental health comorbidities typically involves pharmacotherapy, many questions occur about how to use medications in substance-abusing populations. Suffice it to say that family therapists must work closely with clients, psychiatrists, substance abuse treatment specialists, and family physicians to determine the optimal treatment approach for every patient.

Involving Parents in Decisions

When a substance abuser is an adolescent or a young adult, family therapists believe that parents must be involved in all decisions about the treatment of their children. Parents should be included in decisions about hospitalization, medication, and drug tests. Family therapists make parents part of the treatment team, because it helps to get couples working together, and the responsibility for the resolution of the problem is rightly theirs. When the parents of the young person are divorced or unmarried, the same holds true. Furthermore, given the evidence that the majority of *all* adult substance abusers are in close contact with one or both of their parents, it makes sense to include the parents.

OUTCOMES WITH FAMILY/COUPLE THERAPY

Consistent with the greater emphasis given to evidence-based treatments in the behavioral health industry (mental health and addiction treatment), family/couples treatment outcomes for substance abuse have received increased attention in recent years. As we have documented elsewhere (Stanton & Heath, 2004), since 1997, at least 16 reviews have been published incorporating 65 randomized clinical trials of the effectiveness of family/couples treatment for alcohol and/or other drug problems. The clinical trials are about equally distributed between alcohol and other drug abuse samples. About two-thirds of the alcohol treatment studies evaluate couples approaches, and two-thirds of the drug abuse treatment studies—many of which are with adolescents—examine conjoint family approaches.

O'Farrell and Fals-Stewart (2001) have updated the Edwards and Steinglass (1995) meta-analysis of the outcomes of family treatment for alcohol use disorders. The authors obtained a highly significant effect size in favor of family-involved treatment relative to individually based treatment or wait-list control conditions (median effect size = .30, p < .00001). The authors found further support for these conclusions in a subsequent review that included more clinical trials (O'Farrell & Fals-Stewart, 2003), and noted that the evidence for couples approaches was somewhat stronger than for conjoint family approaches.

Additional confirmations emerged from an evaluation of the efficacy of family/couples approaches to alcohol abuse by Miller, Johnson, Sandberg, Stringer-Seibold, and Gfeller-Strouts (2000). These authors determined that for adults, effectiveness is now (1) "established" for behavioral couples treatment, and (2) "probable" for psychodynamic/eclectic conjoint couples groups.

Stanton and Shadish (1997) reviewed and meta-analyzed the randomized clinical trials for family therapy with drug abuse and concluded the following:

1. Studies that compared family/couples treatment for drug abuse with nonfamily treatment (e.g., individual, group, or psychoeducational treatment) found better results for family therapy. Family therapy was found to be more effective, less expensive, or both, than the other treatment types.
2. Family therapy works equally well for adolescent and adult drug abusers.
3. Comparisons between different "schools" of family therapy were not conclusive.
4. Family therapy has shown higher rates of engagement and retention in treatment than nonfamily approaches.

Since the Stanton and Shadish (1997) meta-analysis, the number of family/couples clinical trials for drug abuse has more than doubled, with an increase, in particular, in couples treatment studies. Sixteen of the 17 newer trials supported the conclusions of the 1997 review. Furthermore, in conjunction with and expanding upon the Miller and colleagues (2000) review of the effectiveness of specific approaches, Stanton and Heath (2004) have concluded that effectiveness is now "established" for three family approaches and one couples approach, and "probable" for a fourth family approach. In summary, these, and the other reviews cited by Stanton and Heath make the case that involving families/partners in treatment of substance abuse can both reduce treatment dropout and improve outcomes.

The family has also been found to be an essential factor in evidence-based substance abuse *prevention* programs. Using 20 years of social science research as a foundation, the U.S. National Institute on Drug Abuse has identified risk and protective factors that predict substance abuse in adolescence and early adulthood (Cire, 2002). Today, an increasing number of prevention programs relate to family form and function in both their content and their activities. For example, family risk factors for substance abuse include chaotic home environments, ineffective parenting, and lack of parent–child attachments. Protective factors include strong and positive family bonds, parental monitoring of children's activities, clear rules of conduct that are consistently enforced, and involvement of parents in the lives of their children (Risk and Protective Factors, 2002).

Research has shown that the same family risk factors apply to the prevention of other social problems, including youth violence, delinquency, school dropout, risky sexual behaviors, and teen pregnancy. There is also evidence of the economic value of evidence-based prevention. One dollar spent in prevention saves four dollars in the cost of substance abuse treatment (Pentz, 1998).

CONCLUSION

Substance abuse affects everyone in the family. Family therapy is an ecological and inclusive intervention that can benefit all those involved and change the multigenerational dynamics of substance abuse. Research now supports family/couple therapy as an effective and efficient approach to both treatment *and* prevention. Given society's overt concerns about substance abuse and its incredible cost to our country, family/couple therapy appears to be making a significant contribution to the well-being of our people.

REFERENCES

Alexander, J. F., & Parsons, B. V. (1982). *Functional family therapy.* Monterey, CA: Brooks/Cole.

Alexander, J. F., Waldron, H. B., Barton, C., & Mas, C. H. (1989). Minimizing blaming attributions and behaviors in delinquent families. *J Consult Clin Psychol, 57,* 19–24.

Anthenelli, R. M., & Schuckit, M. A. (1997). Genetics. In J. H. Lowinson, P. Ruiz, R. B. Millman, & J. G. Langrod (Eds.), *Substance abuse: A comprehensive textbook* (3rd ed., pp. 41–51). Baltimore: Williams & Wilkins.

Bekir, P., McLellan, T., Childress, A. R., & Gariti, P. (1993). Role reversals in families of substance misusers: A transgenerational phenomenon. *Int J Addict, 28,* 613–630.

Bepko, C., & Krestan, J. (1985). *The responsibility trap*. New York: Free Press.

Berenson, D. (1976a). Alcohol and the family system. In P. J. Guerin, Jr. (Ed.), *Family therapy: Theory and practice* (pp. 284–297). New York: Gardner Press.

Berenson, D. (1976b). A family approach to alcoholism. *Psychiatr Opin, 13*, 33–38.

Berenson, D. (1986). The family treatment of alcoholism. *Fam Ther Today, 1*, 1–2, 6–7.

Berenson, D. (1992). The therapist's relationship with couples with an alcoholic member. In E. Kaufman & P. Kaufmann (Eds.), *The family therapy of drug and alcohol abuse* (2nd ed., pp. 224–235). Needham Heights, MA: Allyn & Bacon.

Berg, I. K., & Miller, S. D. (1992). *Working with the problem drinker: A solution-focused approach*. New York: Norton.

Bowser, B. P., Word, C. O., Stanton, M. D., & Coleman, S. B. (2003). Death in the family and HIV risk-taking among intravenous drug users. *Fam Process, 42*, 291–304.

Brown, S., & Lewis, V. (1999). *The alcoholic family in recovery: A developmental model*. New York: Guilford Press.

Cadoret, R. J., Yates, W. R., Troughton, E., Woodworth, G., & Stewart, M. A. (1995). Adoption study demonstrating two genetic pathways to drug abuse. *Arch Gen Psychiatry, 52*, 42–52.

Callan, D., Garrison, J., & Zerger, F. (1975). Working with the families and social networks of drug abusers. *J Psychedelic Drugs, 7*, 19–25.

Cervantes, O. F., Sorenson, J. L., Wermuth, L., Fernandez, L., & Menicucci, L. (1988). Family ties of drug abusers. *Psychol Addict Behav, 2*, 34–39.

Christopher, J. (1988). *How to stay sober: Recovery without religion*. Buffalo, NY: Prometheus Books.

Cire, B. (2002, February). NIDA conference reviews advances in prevention science, announces new national research initiative, *NIDA Notes, 16*(6), 1, 5–7. *www.drugabuse.gov/nida_notes/nnindex.html*

Coleman, S., Kaplan, J., & Downing, R. (1986). Life cycle and loss: The spiritual vacuum of heroin addiction. *Fam Process, 25*, 5–23.

Craig, R. J. (1993). Contemporary trends in substance abuse. *Prof Psychol, 24*, 182–189.

Davis, D. (1987). *Alcoholism treatment: An integrative family and individual approach*. New York: Gardner Press.

Douglas, L. J. (1987/1988). *Perceived family dynamics of cocaine abusers, as compared to opiate abusers and non-drug abusers* [Doctoral dissertation, University of Florida, Gainesville]. *Dissert Abstr Int, 49*(04A), 730.

Donahue, B., Azrin, N. H., Lawson, H., Friedlander, J., Teicher, G., & Rindsberg, J. (1998). Improving initial session attendance of substance abusing and conduct disordered adolescents: A controlled study. *J Child Adol Subst Abuse, 8*, 1–13.

Edwards, M., & Steinglass, P. (1995). Family therapy treatment outcomes for alcoholism. *J Marital Fam Ther, 21*, 475–509.

Eldred, C., & Washington, M. (1976). Interpersonal relationships in heroin use by men and women and their role in treatment outcome. *Int J Addict, 11*, 117–130.

Elkin, M. (1984). *Families under the influence: Changing alcoholic patterns*. New York: Norton.

Fals-Stewart, W., & Birchler, G. R. (2001). A national survey of the use of couples therapy in substance abuse treatment. *J Subst Abuse Treat, 20*, 277–283.

Fals-Stewart, W, O'Farrell, T., Birchler, G. R., Cordova, J., & Kelley, M. L. (2005).

Behavioral couples therapy for alcoholism and drug abuse: Where we've been, where we are, and where we're going. *J Cog Psychotherapy, 19*(2).

Fishman, H. C., Stanton, M. D., & Rosman, B. (1982). Treating families of adolescent drug abusers. In M. D. Stanton, T. C. Todd, & Associates, *The family therapy of drug abuse and addiction* (pp. 335–357). New York: Guilford Press.

Garrett, J., Landau, J., Shea, R., Stanton, M. D., Baciewicz G., & Brinkman-Sull, D. (1998). The ARISE Intervention: Using family and networks links to engage addicted persons in treatment. *J Subst Abuse Treat, 15,* 333–343.

Garrett, J., Landau-Stanton, J., Stanton, M. D., Stellato-Kabat, J., & Stellato-Kabat, D. (1997). ARISE: A method for engaging reluctant alcohol- and drug-dependent individuals in treatment. *J Subst Abuse Treat, 14,* 235–248.

Garrett, J., Stanton, M. D., Landau, J., Baciewicz, G., Brinkman-Sull, D., & Shea, R. R. (1999). The "Concerned Other" call: Using family links and networks to overcome resistance to addiction treatment. *Subst Use Misuse, 34,* 363–382.

Goodwin, D. W., & Warnock, J. K. (1991). Alcoholism: A family disease. In R. J. Frances & S. I. Miller (Eds.), *Clinical textbook of addictive disorders* (pp. 485–500). New York: Guilford Press.

Guerin, P. J., Jr., & Pendagast, E. G. (1976). Evaluation of family system and genogram. In P. J. Guerin, Jr. (Ed.), *Family therapy: Theory and practice* (pp. 450–464). New York: Gardner Press.

Haley, J. (1997). *Leaving home: The therapy of disturbed young people* (2nd ed.). New York: McGraw-Hill.

Hanna, S. M., & Brown, J. H. (1999). *The practice of family therapy: Key elements across models* (2nd ed.). Belmont, CA: Brooks/Cole-Wadsworth.

Heard, D. (1982). Death as a motivator: Using crisis induction to break through the denial system. In M. D. Stanton, T. C. Todd, & Associates, *The family therapy of drug abuse and addiction* (pp. 203–234). New York: Guilford Press.

Heath, A. (1985). Some new directions in ending family therapy. In D. Breunlin (Ed.), *Stages: Patterns of change over time* (pp. 33–40). Rockville, MD: Aspen.

Heath, A., & Ayers, T. (1991). MRI brief therapy with adolescent substance abusers. In T. C. Todd & M. Seleckman (Eds.), *Family therapy approaches with adolescent substance abusers* (pp. 49–69). Boston: Allyn & Bacon.

Henggeler, S. W., & Borduin, C. M. (1990). *Family therapy and beyond: A multisystemic approach to treating the behavior problems of children and adolescents.* Pacific Grove, CA: Brooks/Cole.

Horwitz, S. H. (1997). Treating families with traumatic loss: Transitional family therapy. In C. R. Figley, B. E. Bride, & N. Mazza (Eds.), *Death and trauma: The traumatology of grieving* (pp. 211–230). Washington, DC: Taylor & Francis.

Kessler, R. C., McGonagle, K. A., Zhao, S., Nelson, C. B., Hughes, M., Eshleman, S., et al. (1994). Lifetime and 12-month prevalence of DSM-III-R psychiatric disorders in the United States: Results from the National Comorbidity Survey. *Arch Gen Psychiatry, 51,* 8–19.

Kosten, T., Jalali, B., & Kleber, H. (1982–1983). Complementary marital roles of male heroin addicts: Evolution and intervention tactics. *Am J Drug Alcohol Abuse, 9,* 155–169.

Landau, J., & Garrett, J. (1998). *Transitional family therapy treatment manual for use with adolescent alcohol abuse and dependence.* Albany, NY: Linking Human Systems, LLC.

Landau, J., Garrett, J., Shea, R. R., Stanton, M. D., Brinkman-Sull, D., & Baciewicz G. (2000). Strength in numbers: The ARISE method for mobilizing family and network to engage substance abusers in treatment. *Am J Drug Alcohol Abuse, 26,* 379–398.

Landau, J., & Stanton, M. D. (2000, March). *Transitional Family Therapy for adolescent substance abuse: An integration of structural–strategic and multigenerational approaches.* Paper presented at the meeting of the Kentucky Association for Marriage and Family Therapy, Louisville, KY.

Landau, J., Stanton, M. D., Brinkman-Sull, D., Ikle, D., McCormick, D., Garrett, J., et al. (2004). Outcomes with the ARISE approach to engaging reluctant drug- and alcohol-dependent individuals in treatment. *Am J Drug Alcohol Abuse, 30,* 711–748.

Landau-Stanton, J., Clements, C., & Stanton, M. D. (1993). Psychotherapeutic intervention: From individual through group to extended network. In J. Landau-Stanton, C. Clements, & Associates, *AIDS, health and mental health: A primary sourcebook* (pp. 212–266). New York: Brunner/Mazel.

Landau-Stanton, J., Griffiths, J. A., & Mason, J. (1982). The extended family in transition: Clinical implications. In F. Kaslow (Ed.), *The international book of family therapy* (pp. 360–369). New York: Brunner/Mazel.

Lawson, A. W., & Lawson, G. W. (2004). Families and drugs. In R. H. Coombs (Ed.), *Addiction counseling review* (pp. 175–202). Mahwah, NJ: Erlbaum.

Lawson, G. W., & Lawson, A. W. (1998). *Alcoholism and the family: A guide to treatment and prevention* (2nd ed.). Gaithersburg, MD: Aspen.

Leshner, A. I. (1999, November). Drug abuse and mental disorders: Comorbidity is reality. *NIDA Notes, 14*(4), 3–4.

Levy, B. (1972). Five years later: A follow-up of 50 narcotic addicts. *Am J Psychiatry, 7,* 102–106.

Liddle, H. A., & Hogue, A. (2001). Multidimensional family therapy for adolescent substance abuse. In E. F. Wagner & H. B. Waldron (Eds.), *Innovations in adolescent substance abuse interventions* (pp. 229–261). New York: Pergamon/Elsevier Science.

McGoldrick, M., Gerson, R., & Shellenberger, S. (1999). *Genograms: Assessment and intervention* (2nd ed.). New York: Norton.

Miller, R. B., Johnson, L. N., Sandberg, J. G., Stringer-Seibold, T. A., & Gfeller-Strouts, L. (2000). An addendum to the 1997 outcome research chart. *Am J Fam Ther, 28,* 347–354.

Minuchin, S., & Fishman, H. C. (1981). *Family therapy techniques.* Cambridge, MA: Harvard University Press.

O'Farrell, T. J. (1993). A behavioral marital therapy couples group program for alcoholics and their spouses. In T. J. O'Farrell (Ed.), *Treating alcohol problems: Marital and family interventions* (pp. 170–209). New York: Guilford Press.

O'Farrell, T. J., & Fals-Stewart, W. (2000). Behavioral couples treatment for alcoholism and drug abuse. *J Subst Abuse Treat, 18,* 51–54.

O'Farrell, T. J., & Fals-Stewart, W. (2001). Family-involved alcoholism treatment: An update. In M. Galanter (Ed.), *Recent developments in alcoholism: Vol. 15. Services research in the era of managed care* (pp. 329–356). New York: Plenum Press.

O'Farrell, T. J., & Fals-Stewart, W. (2002). Marital and family therapy. In R. Hester & W. R. Miller (Eds.), *Handbook of alcoholism treatment approaches* (3rd ed., pp. 188–212). Boston: Allyn & Bacon.

O'Farrell, T. J., & Fals-Stewart, W. (2003). Alcohol abuse. *J Marital Fam Ther*, 29(1), 121–146.

Paolino, T. J., & McCrady, B. S. (1977). *The alcoholic marriage: Alternative perspectives*. New York: Grune & Stratton.

Pentz, M. A. (1998). Costs, benefits, and cost effectiveness of comprehensive drug abuse prevention. In W. J. Bukoski & R. I. Evans (Eds.), *Cost effectiveness and cost benefit research of drug abuse prevention: Implications for programming and policy* (NIDA Research Monograph, No. 176, NIH Pub. No. 98-4021, pp. 111–129). Rockville, MD: National Institute on Drug Abuse.

Piercy, F., & Frankel, B. (1989). The evolution of an integrative family therapy for substance-abusing adolescents: Toward the mutual enhancement of research and practice. *J Fam Psychol*, 3, 149–171.

Reilly, D. (1975). Family factors in the etiology and treatment of youthful drug abuse. *Fam Ther*, 2, 149–171.

Reilly, D. M. (1984). Family therapy with adolescent drug abusers and their families: Defying gravity and achieving escape velocity. *J Drug Issues*, 2, 381–391.

Risk and protective factors. (2002, February) *NIDA Notes*, 16(6), 5.

Rosenbaum, M., & Richman, J. (1972). Family dynamics and drug overdoses. *Suicide Life Threat Behav*, 2, 19–25.

Rowe, C. L., & Liddle, H. A. (2003). Substance abuse. *J Marital Fam Ther*, 29(1), 97–120.

Scott, S., & Van Deusen, J. (1982). Detoxification at home: A family approach. In M. D. Stanton, T. C. Todd, & Associates, *The family therapy of drug abuse and addiction* (pp. 310–334). New York: Guilford Press.

Seaburn, D., Landau-Stanton, J., & Horwitz, S. (1995). Core techniques in family therapy. In R. H. Mikesell, D.-D. Lusterman, & S. H. McDaniel (Eds.), *Integrating family therapy: Handbook of family psychology and systems theory* (pp. 5–26). Washington, DC: American Psychological Association.

Searles, J. S. (1991). The genetics of alcoholism: Impact on family and sociological models of addiction. *Fam Dyn Addiction Qrtly*, 1, 8–21.

Selzer, M. (1971). The Michigan Alcoholism Screening Test (MAST): The quest for a diagnostic instrument. *Am J Psychiatry*, 127, 89–94.

Simpson, D. D., & Sells, S. B. (Eds.). (1990). *Opioid addiction and treatment: A 12-year follow-up*. Malabar, FL: Krieger.

Sobel, L. C., Cunningham, J. A., & Sobel, M. B. (1996). Recovery from alcohol problems with and without treatment: Prevalence in two population surveys. *Am J Public Health*, 86, 966–972.

Speck, R. V. (2003). Social network intervention. In G. P. Sholevar & L. D. Schwoeri (Eds.), *Textbook of family and couples therapy: Clinical applications* (pp. 193–201). Washington, DC: American Psychiatric Association.

Speck, R. V., & Attneave, C. L. (1973). *Family networks: Retribalization and healing*. New York: Pantheon Books.

Stabenau, J. R. (1988). Family pedigree studies of biological vulnerability to drug dependence. In R. W. Pickens & D. S. Svikis (Eds.), *Biological vulnerability to drug abuse* (NIDA Research Monograph No. 89, DHHS Pub. No. [ADM] 88-1590, pp. 25–40). Rockville, MD: National Institute on Drug Abuse.

Stanton, M. D. (1981a). An integrated structural/strategic approach to family therapy. *J Marital Fam Ther*, 7, 427–439.

Stanton, M. D. (1981b). Strategic approaches to family therapy. In A. Gurman & D. Kniskern (Eds.), *Handbook of family therapy* (pp. 361–402). New York: Brunner/ Mazel.

Stanton, M. D. (1981c). Who should get credit for change which occurs in therapy? In A. S. Gurman (Ed.), *Questions and answers in the practice of family therapy* (pp. 519– 522). New York: Brunner/Mazel.

Stanton, M. D. (1982). Appendix A: Review of reports on drug abusers' family living arrangements and frequency of family contact. In M. D. Stanton, T. C. Todd, & Associates, *The family therapy of drug abuse and addiction* (pp. 427–431). New York: Guilford Press.

Stanton, M. D. (1984). Fusion, compression, diversion and the workings of paradox: A theory of therapeutic/systemic change. *Fam Process, 23,* 135–167.

Stanton, M. D. (1985). The family and drug abuse. In T. Bratter & G. Forrest (Eds.), *Alcoholism and substance abuse: Strategies for clinical intervention* (pp. 398–430). New York: Free Press.

Stanton, M. D. (1992). The time line and the "Why now?" question: A technique and rationale for therapy, training, organizational consultation and research. *J Marital Fam Ther, 18,* 331–343.

Stanton, M. D. (1997). The role of family and significant others in the engagement and retention of drug dependent individuals. In L. Onken, J. D. Blaine, & J. J. Boren (Eds.), *Beyond the therapeutic alliance: Keeping the drug dependent individual in treatment* (NIDA Research Monograph No. 165, NIH Publication No. 97-4142, pp. 157–180). Rockville, MD: National Institute on Drug Abuse.

Stanton M. D. (2004). Getting reluctant substance abusers to engage in treatment/self-help: A review of outcomes and clinical options. *J Marital Fam Ther, 30,* 165–182.

Stanton, M. D., Adams, E., Landau, J., & Black, G. S. (1998). *Names as "scripts" in the family transmission of drug and alcohol abuse patterns: Results from a national survey.* Unpublished manuscript, University of Rochester and the Gordon S. Black Corporation.

Stanton, M. D., & Heath, A. W. (2004). Family/couples approaches to treatment engagement and therapy. In J. H. Lowinson, P. Ruiz, R. B. Millman, & J. G. Langrod (Eds.), *Substance abuse: A comprehensive textbook* (4th ed., pp. 680–690). Baltimore: Lippincott Williams & Wilkins.

Stanton, M. D., & Landau-Stanton, J. (1990). Therapy with families of adolescent substance abusers. In H. Milkman & L. Sederer (Eds.), *Treatment choices in substance abuse* (pp. 329–339). Lexington, MA: Lexington Books.

Stanton, M. D., & Shadish, W. R. (1997). Outcome, attrition, and family/couples treatment for drug abuse: A meta-analysis and review of the controlled, comparative studies. *Psychol Bull, 122,* 170–191.

Stanton, M. D., Steier, F., Cook, L., & Todd, T. C. (1997). *Narcotic detoxification in a family and home context: Updated summary of Final Report results—1997* (Grant No. R01 DA 03097). Rockville, MD: National Institute on Drug Abuse, Treatment Research Branch.

Stanton, M. D., Steier, F., & Todd, T. C. (1982). Paying families for attending sessions: Counteracting the dropout problem. *J Marital Fam Ther, 8,* 371–373.

Stanton, M. D., & Todd, T. C. (1981). Engaging resistant families in treatment: II. Principles and techniques in recruitment. *Fam Process, 20*(3), 261–280.

Stanton, M. D., & Todd, T. C. (1992). Structural-strategic family therapy with drug addicts. In E. Kaufman & P. Kaufmann (Eds.), *Family therapy of drug and alcohol abuse* (2nd ed., pp. 46–62). Needham Heights, MA: Allyn & Bacon.

Stanton, M. D., Todd, T. C., & Associates. (1982). *The family therapy of drug abuse and addiction*. New York: Guilford Press.

Steinglass, P., Bennett, L., Wolin, S., & Reiss, D. (1987). *The alcoholic family*. New York: Basic Books.

Stevens, S. J., & Morral, A. R. (Eds.). (2003). *Adolescent substance abuse treatment in the United States: Exemplary models from a national evaluation study*. New York: Haworth Press.

Stuart, R. B. (1980). *Helping couples change: A social learning approach to marital therapy*. New York: Guilford Press.

Szapocznik J., & Kurtines, W. M. (1989). *Breakthroughs in family therapy with drug abusing and problem youth*. New York: Springer.

Todd, T. C., & Selekman, M. D. (Eds.). (1991). *Family therapy approaches with adolescent substance abusers*. Needham Heights, MA: Allyn & Bacon.

Treadway, D. (1989). *Before it's too late: Working with substance abuse in the family*. New York: Norton.

van den Bree, M. B., Svikis, D. S., & Pickens, R. W. (1998). Genetic influences in antisocial personality and drug use disorders. *Drug Alcohol Depend, 49*, 177–187.

van der Velden, E. H., Ruhf, L. L., & Kaminsky, K. (1991). Network therapy: A case study. In T. C. Todd & M. D. Selekman (Eds.), *Family therapy approaches with adolescent substance abusers* (pp. 209–225). Needham Heights, MA: Allyn & Bacon.

Waldron, H. B., Slesnick, N., Brody, J. L., Turner, C. W., & Peterson, T. R. (2001). Treatment outcomes for adolescent substance abuse at 4- and 7-month assessments. *J Consult Clin Psychol, 69*, 802–813.

Walsh, F. (1978). Concurrent grandparent death and birth of schizophrenic offspring: An intriguing finding. *Fam Process, 17*, 457–463.

Watson, W. H., & McDaniel, S. H. (1998). Assessment in transitional family therapy: The importance of context. In J. W. Barron (Ed.), *Making diagnosis meaningful: Enhancing evaluation and treatment of psychological disorders* (pp. 161–195). Washington, DC: American Psychological Association.

Weiss, R. L., Hops, H., & Patterson, G. R. (1973). A framework for conceptualizing marital conflict, a technology for altering it, some data for evaluating it. In L. A. Hamerlynck, L. C. Handy, & E. J. Mash (Eds.), *Behavior change: Methodology, concepts and practice* (pp. 309–342). Champaign, IL: Research Press.

Wermuth, L., & Scheidt, T. (1986). Enlisting family support in drug treatment. *Fam Process, 25*, 25–34.

Williams, R. J., & Chang, S. Y. (2000). A comprehensive and comparative review of adolescent substance abuse treatment outcome. *Clin Psychol, 7*, 138–166.

Woody, G., Carr, E., Stanton, M. D., & Hargrove, H. (1982). Program flexibility and support. In M. D. Stanton, T. C. Todd, & Associates, *The family therapy of drug abuse and addiction* (pp. 393–402). New York: Guilford Press.

CHAPTER 25

Treating Adolescent Substance Abuse

YIFRAH KAMINER
OSCAR G. BUKSTEIN

The consequences of substance use, as well as substance use disorders (SUDs), continue to present a major public health concern. Level of substance use is associated with leading causes of adolescent morbidity and mortality in the United States, including motor vehicle accidents, suicidal behavior, violence, delinquency, drowning, and unprotected sexual behavior. Adolescent SUDs, which include substance abuse and substance dependence as defined in the fourth edition of the *Diagnostic and Statistical Manual of Mental* Disorders (DSM-IV-TR; American Psychiatric Association, 2000), are also associated with drug-related chronic problems in several life domains, including psychiatric comorbidity, school or employment performance, family function, peer social relationships, legal status, and recreational activities.

Regional studies reveal that between 7 and 10% of adolescents are in need of treatment (Harrison, Fulkerson, & Beebe, 1998; Lewinsohn, Hops, Roberts, & Seeley, 1993; Reinharz, Giaconia, Lefkowitz, Pakiz, & Frost, 1993; Ungemack, Hartwell, & Babor, 1997). However, due to limited resources, only a small segment of the adolescent subpopulation with alcohol and other substance use disorders (AOSUDs), in particular, those with high severity of AOSUDs, comorbid psychiatric disorders, and legal problems, usually end up in treatment (Kaminer, 2001).

Our objectives in this chapter are to review the trends in adolescent substance use, nosology, etiology of substance use and its transition to adolescent SUDs, psychiatric comorbidity, prevention, assessment, and the treatment–aftercare continuum. As a point of clarification, the generic term "substance use" refers here to nonpathological use of any licit drug (tobacco, alcohol, and inhalants) or illicit drug (controlled substances, both those that are essentially proscribed for everyone and those that are available by prescription). The term "substance abuse" is used generically to indicate pathological use. Terms such as "substance abuse," "substance dependence," and "SUDs" are specifically mentioned as part of a formal classification system (e.g., DSM-IV-TR).

EPIDEMIOLOGY

Substance use among American youth in the 1980s and early 1990s dropped to a low point, then rose continuously between 1992 and 1997; since then, the use of several specific drugs has leveled off or has declined. The main consistent source of information on adolescent substance use has been the Monitoring the Future (MTF) surveys, which in 2002 covered nationally representative samples of 43,000 8th, 10th, and 12th graders in 394 schools (National Institute on Drug Abuse, 2002). Although the prevalence rates derived from the survey fail to reflect adequately the magnitude of high-risk behaviors, clinical significance, and adolescent health problems, they may serve at best as a periodic "snapshot" of adolescent substance use.

In the 2002 MTF, specific decreases were noted in the use of marijuana, cigarettes, alcohol, inhalants, D-lysergic acid diethylamide (LSD), amphetamines, and Ecstasy. Abuse of anabolic steroids, methylphenidate, and heroin remained stable. The only significant increase in drug use in 2002 was past year crack use by 10th graders and sedative use by 12th graders. Attitudes and beliefs about drugs, which may play a critical role in deterring use, began to change in all three grades, because perceived risk of harm, personal disapproval, and perceived availability are associated with the level of drug use.

There are surprisingly few community epidemiological studies on the prevalence of SUDs in adolescents. In community studies, lifetime diagnosis of alcohol abuse ranged from 0.4% in the Great Smoky Mountain Study (Costello et al., 1996) to 8.2 and 9.6% in the Pittsburgh Adolescent Alcohol Research Center (Martin, Kaczynski, Maisto, Bukstein, & Moss, 1995) and the National Cormorbidity Study (Kendler, 1994), respectively. Lifetime diagnoses of alcohol dependence ranged from 0.6% (Costello et al., 1996) to 4.3% in the Oregon Adolescent Depression Project (Lewinsohn, Hops, Roberts, & Seeley, 1993; Lewinsohn, Rohde, & Seeley, 1996). The lifetime prevalence of drug abuse or dependence has ranged from 3.3% in 15-year-olds to 9.8% in 17- to 19-year-olds (Kashani et al., 1987; Reinherz et al., 1993).

Age of Initiation

Based on retrospective reports of grade level of first use, the data provided by eighth graders indicated that three substances were initiated by more than 50%

of users in sixth grade or earlier. These "gateway drugs" were alcohol, tobacco, and inhalants (O'Malley, Johnston, & Bachman, 1995).

Gender and Ethnic Group

In general, male students use more substances of all kinds than female students; however, the differences are consistently getting smaller (Wallace et al., 2003). O'Malley and colleagues (1995) suggested that "closing the gap" by adolescent females may have to do with slightly earlier female maturation and with their tendency to associate with older male students. Excluding Native American youth, Hispanic students score highest among all other ethnic subpopulations at 8th grade for all illicit drug classes. At 12th grade, they are the highest for cocaine, heroin, and steroids. Hispanic males and females manifest the highest levels of marijuana use and binge drinking similar to white youth (in excess of 40% for 10th graders). Asian American students manifest the lowest rates of use.

NOSOLOGY

Substance use and abuse occurs on a continuum, and the cutoff point for making a diagnosis of abuse/dependence is somewhat arbitrary, particularly in adolescents (Rohde, Lewinsohn, & Seeley, 1996). Clinical psychiatry has traditionally followed the dichotomous paradigm of the DSM nosology regardless of its limitation providing information in terms of pathogenesis and treatment response (Bukstein & Kaminer, 1994). In addition, the serious negative impact of drugs on adolescents or adults who experience subdiagnostic levels of problematic substance use has been recognized but has not been addressed by the DSM system (Lewinsohn et al., 1996).

The same DSM-IV-TR diagnostic criteria are utilized for both adolescents and adults in the diagnosis of substance abuse and dependence. Empirical data generally support the utility of DSM-IV-TR criteria for alcohol dependence among adolescents (Martin et al., 1995). Lewinsohn and colleagues (1996) reported on the strong similarity between adolescents and adults in the frequency of 8 of the 11 symptoms in DSM-IV-TR criteria for abuse and dependence. Among adolescents with a diagnosis, the most frequently reported symptoms were reduced activities, tolerance, consuming more than intended, and desire to cut down (Lewinsohn et al., 1996; Stewart & Brown, 1995).

Abuse and dependence are distinctly separate (Hasin, Grant, & Endicott, 1990). A majority of adults diagnosed as abusers never progress to dependence. Abuse is not necessarily a prodrome, and it may be developmentally limited in many adolescents. "Diagnostic orphans" are those youth who have subthreshold symptomatology of alcohol dependence (i.e., one or two symptoms only) but no abuse symptoms (Pollock & Martin, 1999). A 3-year follow-up study demonstrated that this entity has a unique trajectory that is not dissimilar to either abuse or dependence.

ETIOLOGY AND PATHOGENESIS

Genetic and biological factors, as well as environmental variables, have been extensively researched to address questions regarding the etiology of SUDs. Most researchers acknowledge a multifactorial consensus, as presented in the biopsychosocial paradigm for the etiology and pathogenesis of these disorders.

Genetic and Biological Factors

Most of the data regarding the genetic and biological contribution to the development of substance abuse are derived from alcoholism research. It has been suggested that individuals may enter life with a certain level of genetic predisposition toward AOSUDs. Convergent evidence from twin, adoption, and biological response studies suggests that genetic factors may indeed play a role in the etiology of alcoholism (Bohman, Sigvardsson, & Cloninger, 1981; Cloninger, Bohman, & Sigvardsson, 1981). Investigations of neuropsychological and physiological precursors or markers of alcoholism, conducted with sons of alcoholics and nonalcoholics, suggest some possible biological differences that may increase vulnerability to alcoholism. For example, children of alcoholics may be deficient in serotonin or may have an increased level of serotonin in the presence of alcohol (Goodwin, 1985). The "addictive cycle"—a pattern in which a person initially drinks to feel good and then later has to resume drinking after an abstinence period to stop feeling bad—may result from such a problem with serotonin. Children of alcoholics are also suspected to have increased tolerance to alcohol.

There are indications that adolescent substance abuse may be part of a broader genetic constellation. Some theorists suggest that polydrug abuse (abuse of a wide variety of substances) constitutes evidence against a genetic interpretation of addiction. Cadoret, Troughton, O'Gorman, and Heywood (1986) suggest instead that some underlying biochemical route may be involved both in substance abuse and in problem or deviant behavior, especially delinquency, and that at least one genetic pathway occurs through antisocial behavior.

Temperament deviations are associated with an increased risk for psychopathology and substance abuse (Reich, Earls, Frankel, & Shayka, 1993). For example, children with a "difficult temperament" more commonly manifest externalizing and internalizing behavior problems by middle childhood (Earls & Jung, 1987) and in adolescence (Maziade, Caron, Cote, Boutin, & Thivierge, 1990) compared to children whose temperament is normative.

Increased behavioral activity level is noted in both youth at high risk for substance abuse and those having an SUD (Tarter, Laird, Mostefa, Bukstein, & Kaminer, 1990). Other temperamental trait deviations found in high-risk youth include reduced attention span persistence (Schaeffer, Parson, & Yohman, 1984), increased impulsivity (Noll, Zucker, Fitzgerald, & Curtis, 1992; Shedler & Block, 1990), and negative affect states such as irritability (Brook, Whiteman, Gordon, & Brook, 1990) and emotional reactivity (Blackson, 1994). Tarter, Kirisci, Hegedeus, Mezzich, and Yanyukov (1994) developed a difficult temperament index to classify adolescent alcoholics. Those adolescents with a difficult temperament displayed a high conditional probability to develop psychiatric disorders such as conduct disorder, attention-deficit/hyperactivity disorder, anxiety disorders, and mood disorders (Tarter et al., 1994).

Environmental Theories

The evidence supporting genetic and, presumably, biological factors in alcoholism and substance abuse is paralleled by evidence supporting the role of psychosocial, familial, peer, and other environmental and interactional variables.

Problem behavior theory, formulated by Jessor and associates, explains substance use as a component of a "deviance syndrome" or "proneness" to problem behavior (Jessor, 1987). Together, the personality system, the perceived environment system, and the behavior system generate a dynamic state called "proneness," which specifies the likelihood of occurrence of normative development or problem behavior that departs from the social and legal norms.

Also, longitudinal studies have documented that personality characteristics such as aggressiveness and rebelliousness are predictive factors that precede the use of substances and can be identified in preschoolers. Kandel (1982) made two pivotal contributions. She formulated four broad classes of predictors: (1) parental influences, (2) peer influences, (3) adolescent beliefs and values, and (4) adolescent involvement in various shared activities. Kandel also conceptualized the "gateway" theory to adolescent substance use and abuse. According to Kandel (1982, 2003), alcohol and marijuana are pivotal "gateway" substances, and she formulated several distinct developmental stages in the initiation and progression of substance use by adolescents, including (1) beer or wine, (2) cigarettes or hard liquor, (3) marijuana, and (4) other illicit substances. Participation in each stage is a necessary but not a sufficient condition for progression into a latter stage. Problem drinking may take place between marijuana and other illicit drug use; therefore, it represents an additional stage in the transition of substance use (Donovan & Jessor, 1983). Morral, McCaffrey, and Paddock (2002) argued that a marijuana gateway effect to hard drugs might exist, particularly among specific ethnic groups such as African Americans, although a common factor model may suffice to explain this association.

Parental Influences

Three different types of parental characteristics predict initiation of adolescent substance use: parental substance use/abuse behaviors, parental attitudes toward substances, and parent–child interactions, which include quality of parent–child communication and parental supervision and monitoring. Studies suggest that a caretaker who exposes a child (particularly a young child) to substance abuse behavior, and to the nonfulfillment of parental responsibilities that follows, affects the child by providing models and by reinforcement of related behaviors. In a study of environmental influences, the number of household users of substances and the degree of children's involvement were found to be the best predictors of both expectations of use and actual abuse of alcohol, as well as a strong predictor of children's cigarette and marijuana use (Ahmed, Bush, Davidson, & Iannotti, 1984). Among the environmental characteristics of these families, the following factors were noted to predict adolescent substance use: high stress, poor and inconsistent family management skills, increased separation, divorce, death, parental prison terms, and decreased family activities.

Families with addicted members are often socially isolated from the community, partly because of their need for secrecy and partly because of community rejection. Parents in substance-abusing families have fewer friends and are less involved in recreational, social, religious, and cultural activities (Kumpfer & Demarsh, 1986). Because of such families' social isolation, the children have fewer opportunities to interact with other children, have fewer friends, and the children express a desire to have more friends but doubt their abilities to make friends. Emotional neglect is frequently reported; substance-abusing parents have only a limited ability to involve themselves meaningfully and emotionally with their children and also have been found to spend less time in planned and structured activities with their children (Kumpfer & Demarsh, 1986). In addition, more psychopathology and significantly more depression have been detected in substance-abusing parents. The emotional impact on children from these families results in the children's difficulty with identifying and expressing positive feelings. Substance-abusing parents are also characterized by difficulty in coping with everyday realities and responsibilities, the presence of comorbid psychiatric disorders, decreased ability to supervise and monitor their children's activities or appreciate that their children may be participating in deviant activities such as substance use, and lack of energy for better parenting, because of the drain on the family's time, finances, and emotional–social resources created by the substance abuse (Kumpfer & Demarsh, 1986).

Resentment, embarrassment, anger, fear, loneliness, depression, and insecurity are often identified or reported among these children. Intense fear of separation and abandonment is very common. Because psychopathology and emotional disturbances often precede substance abuse, these children are at high risk for the development of substance abuse and dependence.

Peer Influences

Peer influences play a crucial role in the process of involvement in the use and abuse of all substances—tobacco, alcohol, and illicit substances (especially marijuana). Because only a small fraction of adolescent substance users may progress to substance abuse, it is of a significant clinical importance to differentiate between the causes for substance use and substance abuse. Most substance use occurs due to social influences and can be attributed to the adolescent's immediate subculture and lifestyle. Substance abuse is more strongly tied to a developmental process involving biobehavioral factors (Glantz & Pickens, 1992), and it occurs as a part of a cluster of behaviors that form a syndrome of problem behavior (Jessor & Jessor, 1977) or general deviance (Newcomb, 1995).

Peer relationships have a significant effect on the initiation, development, and maintenance of substance abuse. The most consistent and reproducible finding in substance abuse research is the strong relationship between an individual's substance use behavior and the concurrent substance use of his or her friends (Jessor & Jessor, 1977). Such an association may result from socialization, as well as from a process of interpersonal selection (assortative pairing), in which adolescents with similar values and behaviors seek each other out as friends (Kandel, 1982). Susceptibility to peer influence is related to earlier involvement in peer-related activities and to a greater degree of attachment and reliance on peers rather than parents (Kandel, 1978).

Regarding values and attitudes in adolescent substance abusers, substance abuse is correlated negatively with conventional behaviors and beliefs, such as church attendance, good scholastic performance, value of academic achievement, and beliefs in the generalized expectations, norms, and values of society (Jessor, 1987). Substance abuse is correlated positively with risk-taking behavior, sensation-seeking behavior, early sexual activity, higher value of independence, and greater involvement in delinquent behavior (Jessor, 1987).

Delinquent peer groups may engage in many shared deviant behaviors, such as using the same drugs of choice, Satanism and related rituals, drug trafficking, and violence. Such activities are deeply rooted in the identity-creating process of these groups and are inseparable components of their code of values.

PSYCHIATRIC COMORBIDITY

The presence of one or more comorbid psychiatric disorders, both internalizing and/or externalizing types, is often noted in populations of adolescents with SUDs (Bukstein, Glancy, & Kaminer, 1992; Riggs, Baker, Mikulich, Young, & Crowley, 1995). Psychiatric disorders in childhood, featured by disruptive behavior disorders, as well as mood or anxiety disorders, confer an increased risk for the development of SUDs in a majority of the cases in adolescence (Bukstein, Brent, & Kaminer, 1989; Christie et al., 1988; Loeber, 1988). The etiological mechanisms have not been systematically researched. However, a number of possible relationships exist between SUD and psychopathology. Psychopathology may precede SUD, may develop as a consequence of a preexisting SUD, may influence the severity of an SUD, may not be related, or may originate from a common vulnerability (Hovens, Cantwell, & Kiriakos, 1994).

African American and Hispanic youth may both present with high-above-threshold symptom rates of co-occurring disorders, while Hispanic youths may have higher rates of externalizing symptoms than African American youths (Robbins et al., 2002). Among youth with SUDs, males have higher rates of disruptive disorders, while females have higher rates of depression (Latimer, Stone, Voight, Winters, & August, 2002).

A number of psychiatric disorders are commonly associated with SUDs in youth (Bukstein et al., 1989). Conduct disorder and constituent criteria, such as aggression, usually precede, predict, and accompany adolescent SUDs (Ferdinand, Blum, & Verhulst, 2001; Loeber, 1988). Clinical populations of adolescents with SUDs show rates of conduct disorder regularly ranging from 50% to almost 80%. Conduct disorder is a poor prognostic sign for treatment (Hser et al., 2003; Kaminer, Tarter, Bukstein, & Kabene, 1992). Although attention-deficit/hyperactivity disorder (ADHD) is commonly noted in substance-using and -abusing youth, the observed association is likely due to the high level of comorbidity between conduct disorder and ADHD (Barkley, Fischer, Edelbrock, & Smallish, 1990; Kaminer, 1992a; Levin & Kleber, 1995; Wilens, Biederman, Spencer, & Frances, 1994). An earlier onset of conduct problems and aggressive behavior, in addition to the presence of ADHD, may increase the risk for later substance abuse (Loeber, 1988). Adolescents with and without ADHD may have a similar risk for SUDs mediated by conduct and bipolar disorders (Biederman et al., 1997).

Aggressive behaviors are present in many adolescents who have SUDs. Consumption of substances such as alcohol, amphetamines, and phencyclidine may increase the likelihood of subsequent aggressive behavior (Moss & Tarter, 1993). The direct pharmacological effects resulting in aggression may be further exacerbated by the presence of preexisting psychopathology, the use of multiple agents simultaneously, and the frequent relative inexperience of the adolescent substance user. Other compulsive deviant behaviors such as gambling and pathological gambling are common among adolescents with SUDs (Griffiths, 1995).

Mood disorders, especially depression, frequently have onsets both preceding and consequent to the onset of substance use and SUD in adolescents (Bukstein et al., 1992; Deykin, Buka, & Zeena, 1992; Deykin, Levy, & Wells, 1987; Hovens et al., 1994). The prevalence of depressive disorders in these studies ranged from 24% to more than 50%.

The literature supports SUDs among adolescents as a risk factor for suicidal behavior, including ideation, attempts, and completed suicide (Bukstein et al.,

1993; Crumley, 1990; Kaminer, 1996). Possible mechanisms for this relation-ships include acute and chronic effects of psychoactive substances. Adolescent suicide victims are frequently using alcohol or other drugs at the time of suicide (Brent, Perper, & Allman, 1987). The acute substance use may produce tran-sient but intense dysphoric states, disinhibition, impaired judgment, and in-creased level of impulsivity or may exacerbate preexisting psychopathology, including depression or anxiety disorders.

A number of studies of clinical populations show high rates of anxiety dis-orders among youth with SUDs (Clark et al., 1995; Clark & Sayette, 1993). In clinical populations of adolescents with SUDs, the prevalence of anxiety disor-der ranged from 7% to over 40% (Clark et al., 1995; DeMilio, 1989; Stowell, 1991). The order of appearance of comorbid anxiety and SUD appears to be variable, depending on the specific anxiety disorder. Social phobia usually pre-cedes abuse, whereas panic and generalized anxiety disorder more often follow the onset of a SUD (Kushner, Sher, & Beitman, 1990). Adolescents with SUDs often have a history of posttraumatic stress disorder (PTSD) following acute or chronic physical and sexual abuse (Clark et al., 1995; Van Hasselt, Null, Kemp-ton, & Bukstein, 1993). Bulimia nervosa is also commonly associated with ado-lescents having substance use disorders (Bulik, 2002). SUDs are very common among individuals diagnosed with schizophrenia (Kutcher, Kachur, & Marton, 1992; Regier et al., 1990). Personality disorders (Cluster B in particular) among adolescents with SUDs are highly prevalent (Grilo et al., 1995). Finally, as sug-gested by studies showing language deficits in youth affected by or at high risk for SUDs, learning disabilities or disorders may also show an increased inci-dence of comorbidity (Moss, Kirisci, Gordon, & Tarter, 1994). Patients with comorbid psychiatric disorders continue to be a challenge for clinicians and researchers in the assessment and treatment domains.

PREVENTION

Efforts to curtail substance abuse concentrate on activities designed for supply-and-demand reduction. It has been reported that the use of alcohol by youths declines when either the price of alcoholic beverages or the legal drinking age increases (Coate & Grossman, 1987). Similarly, a reduction in car accidents among youth resulted from the increase of the minimum drinking age to 21 (O'Malley & Wagenaar, 1991).

The goal of primary prevention among children and adolescents is to defer or preclude initiation of gateway substances such as cigarettes, alcohol, and marijuana. The traditional education program is a prevention strategy used to increase knowledge of the consequences of drug use. Investigators (Schinke, Botvin, & Orlani, 1991) found the assumption that increased knowledge decreases drug use to be invalid. Affective education, which increases self-esteem and enhances responsible decision making, and alternative activities programs for adolescents were found to be ineffective in the prevention of drug use based on meta-analysis of the literature (Bangert-Drowns, 1988; Tobler, 1986). Furthermore, all the prevention strategies noted previously were reported to increase interest in drugs among some of the participants (Schinke et al., 1991). A more advanced prevention strategy is based on a psychosocial approach. These prevention programs are aimed at enhancing self-esteem (Schaps, Moskowitz, & Malvin, 1986), social skills, and assertive skills for resisting substance use (Botvin, Baker, Filazola, & Botvin, 1990). However, these techniques failed to be successful in enhancing secondary prevention (Pentz, Dwyer, & MacKinnon, 1989).

A study by Botvin, Baker, Dusenbury, Botvin, and Diaz (1995) implemented a curriculum covering life skills training (LST) and skills for resisting social influences to use drugs. This curriculum included booster sessions during the 2 years after completion of the intervention. The investigators reported a significant and durable reduction in drug use 6 years later. The generalizability of the LST prevention approach for African American and Hispanic youth has been supported (Botvin & Griffin, 2001). Most middle schools however, use proven prevention programs that combine effective content and delivery. Universal prevention programs may delay onset of drinking among low-risk baseline abstainers; however, there is little evidence supporting their utility for at-risk adolescents (Masterman & Kelly, 2003). Brief interventions such as motivational interviewing within a harm reduction framework may be well suited to for many adolescents.

The challenge for health care providers is to identify individuals at high risk before or shortly after initiation of substance use and to intervene to reduce transitional risk. One of the largest subpopulations of children at risk are those with at least one biological parent diagnosed with alcohol or substance dependence. These individuals are at greater risk of developing the same disorder, fourfold and 10-fold, respectively (Goodwin, 1985; Tarter, 1992). Children of opioid-dependent parents were reported to have high rates of psychopathology and significant dysfunction in the academic, family, and legal life domains (Kolar, Brown, Haertzen, & Michaelson, 1994; Wilens, Biederman, Kiely, Bredin, & Spencer, 1995). Contrary to public perception, there is a need for a more balanced view regarding the natural history of children of alcoholics (COAs) primarily because (1) regardless of popular models of dysfunctional COAs, the majority of offspring raised with a dysfunctional alcoholic parent do not develop alcoholism (Wilson & Crowe, 1991) and (2) the negative labeling of adolescent COAs regardless of their current behavior was reported to be robust and potentially harmful (Burk & Sher, 1990). Resilence and protective factors are also important to consider (Wolin & Wolin, 1996).

The heterogeneity of adolescent subpopulations needs to be recognized to better understand substance use and its transition to substance abuse and dependence. This recognition is followed by determining the level of interven-tion required, whether primary, secondary, or tertiary prevention. The preven-tion effort must also address adolescent needs in all domains of life, including attitudes, expectations, and interactions with the community.

Implications for policy-related initiatives have to do with supply reduc-tion. Effective prevention programs are cost-effective. For every $1 spent on drug use prevention, communities can save $4–5 in costs for drug abuse treat-ment and counseling. The National Institute on Drug Abuse (NIDA; 2001) has established a set of prevention principles, based on research of effective model programs. These principles state that prevention programs should (1) enhance "protective factors" and reverse or reduce known "risk factors"; (2) target all forms of drug abuse, including the use of tobacco, alcohol, marijuana, and inhalants; (3) teach skills to resist drugs when offered, strengthen personal commitments against drug use, and increase social competence (e.g., in com-munications, peer relationships, self-efficacy, and assertiveness), in conjunction with reinforcement of attitudes against drug use; (4) use interactive methods, such as peer discussion groups, rather than didactic teaching techniques alone; (5) include a parent or caregiver component that reinforces what the children are learning and opens opportunities for family discussions about use of legal and illegal substances, and family policies about their use; (6) last long term over the school career, with repeat interventions to reinforce the original pre-vention goals; (7) use family-focused prevention efforts that have a greater impact than strategies that focus on parents only or children only; (8) use com-munity programs that include media campaigns and policy changes, such as new regulations that restrict access to alcohol, tobacco, or other drugs; (9) use community programs to strengthen norms against drug use in all drug abuse pre-vention settings, including the family, the school, and the community; (10) offer school-based opportunities to reach all populations and also serve as important settings for specific subpopulations at risk for drug abuse, such as children with behavior problems or learning disabilities and those who are potential dropouts; (11) be adapted to address the specific nature of the drug abuse problem in the local community; (12) be more intensive for high-risk tar-get populations, and the earlier age it must begin; and (13) be age-specific, developmentally appropriate, and culturally sensitive.

ASSESSMENT

A significant step toward addressing the need for better therapeutic interventions for adolescents with SUDs has been the recognition of the assessment and treat-ment of SUDs as potentially a multistep task. The expert committee of the Insti-tute of Medicine report (1990) of the adolescent assessment/referral system devel-oped by the NIDA (Rahdert, 1991; Tarter, 1990) recommend a three-phase process. An initial screening phase involves identification of health disorders, psychiatric problems, and psychosocial maladjustment. Based on the screening phase, a minority of adolescents are required to go through the second extensive assessment phase. This assessment provides a diagnostic summary that identifies the adolescent's treatment needs within specific life domains, such as substance use, psychiatric status, physical health status, school adjustment, vocational status, family function, peer relationship, leisure and recreation activity, and legal situation. The third phase involves the preparation and implementation of an integrated, problem-focused, and comprehensive treatment plan.

Substance use and SUDs are multidimensional behaviors that demand a thorough assessment of several dimensions of substance use behavior in addition to quantity and frequency of use. Within the domain of substance use behavior, important dimensions include the pattern of use (quantity, frequency, onset, and types of agents used), negative consequences (school–vocational, social–peer–family, emotional–behavioral, legal and physical), context of use (time–place, peer use–attitudes, mood antecedents, consequences, expectancies, and overall social milieu), and control of use (view of use as a problem, attempts to stop or limit use, other DSM-IV-TR dependence criteria).

Clinicians frequently question whether any self-report by an adolescent about substance use is accurate. Self-reports may, however, provide reliable and valid information, particularly when no legal contingencies for drug use are pending (Barnea, Rahav, & Teichman, 1987; Winters, 1992). The clinician may attempt to substantiate suspected use by reports from third parties or through the use of urine or blood toxicology. Parents, however, tend to underreport their child's level of drug involvement and resulting problems (Burleson & Kaminer, in press; Winters, Stinchfield, & Opland, 2000).

A variety of instruments are available and others are being developed to assist in the screening and detailed assessment of substance use, and related behaviors and problems. Although readers are referred elsewhere for a more detailed discussion of individual instruments (Leccese & Waldron, 1994; Winters, Latimer, & Stinchfield, 2001), we provide several examples of types of instruments.

Screening instruments are used to identify the potential presence of SUD as a preliminary step toward a more detailed, comprehensive assessment, although many substance use/abuse screening instruments are designed to measure the substance use domain only, such as the CAGE (cut down, annoyed, guilty, eye opener) developed by Ewing (1984). The CRAFFT (car, relax, alone, forget, friends, trouble), a longer, modified version of the CAGE, has shown superior psychometric properties (Knight, Sherritt, Shrier, Harris, & Chang, 2002). Other instruments screen other domains for psychosocial functioning; Problem-Oriented Screening Instrument for Teenagers (POSIT; Rahdert, 1991); Drug Use Screening Inventory (DUSI; Tarter, 1990); Personal Experience Screening Questionnaire (PESQ; Winters, 1992); and Substance

Abuse Subtle Screening Inventory—Adolescent Version (SASSI-A; Miller, 1990). Comprehensive assessment instruments usually provide more detailed information about substance use behavior, as well as other domains of functioning. The formats for comprehensive instruments vary, with some being self-report questionnaires (e.g., Personal Experience Inventory [PEI]; Winters & Henly, 1988), others being structured interviews (e.g., Adolescent Drug Abuse Diagnosis [ADAD]; Friedman & Utada, 1989), and still others being semistructured interviews (e.g., Adolescent Problem Severity Index [APSI]; Metzger, Kushner, & McLellan, 1991; Teen Addiction Severity Index [T-ASI]; Kaminer, Bukstein, & Tarter, 1991; Kaminer, Wagner, Plummer, & Seifer, 1993); and the Global Appraisal of Individual Needs [GAIN]; Dennis, Titus, White, Unsicker, & Hodgkins, 2003).

Toxicology of bodily fluids, usually urine, but also blood and hair samples, can be used as a screen to detect the presence of specific substances for both initial assessment and as an ongoing check for substance use. The optimal use of urine screens requires proper collection techniques, including visual proof of sample authenticity, evaluation of positive results, and a specific plan of action should the specimen be positive for the presence of substance(s) (Casavant, 2002; Cole, 1997). Clinicians should establish rules regarding the confidentiality of the results prior to testing.

LEVEL OF CARE

Placement of adolescents with SUDs at a particular level of care is based on several factors. Dispositional options (triage) involve a variety of possibilities, which may also depend on service availability. Despite certain inherent advantages of residential programs in terms of intensity and control, the generalization of improvement made during these programs is uncertain. More emphasis should be given to community-based programs that may guide the adolescent and his or her family through their real-life problems and experiences.

Appropriate referrals to an inpatient unit or residential program may include (1) adolescents with SUDs who have either failed or do not qualify for outpatient treatment; (2) dually diagnosed adolescents with moderate or severe psychiatric disorders; (3) adolescents who display a potentially morbid or mortal behavior toward themselves or others (e.g., suicidal and self-injurious behavior); (4) adolescents who are intravenous drug abusers, drug dependent, or need to be detoxified; (5) patients with accompanying moderate-to-severe medical problems; (6) adolescents who need to be isolated from their community to ensure treatment without interruptions; and (7) pregnant adolescents who manifest SUDs that endanger the fetus (Kaminer, 1994).

Enrollment criteria in a drug-free outpatient or partial hospitalization setting include (1) SUDs and other psychiatric disorders that do not require inpatient treatment (i.e., psychiatric disorder severity less than moderate); (2) previous successful outpatient treatment follow-up after completion of inpatient treatment; and (3) agreement to a contingency contract that will delineate frequency of visits, compliance with curriculum, including random urine screening, consequences of noncompliance and relapse, and participation in the community network, including self-help groups. Similar placement criteria for adolescents with SUDs, such as the American Society for Addiction Medicine (ASAM) criteria tailored from the Cleveland Criteria (Hoffmann, Halikas, & Mee-Lee, 1987), have some level of face validity; however, no research regarding their reliability or predictive validity supports them. The ASAM Placement Criteria (2001), specify five broad levels of care for each group: Level 0.5, Early Intervention; Level I, Outpatient Treatment; Level II, Intensive Outpatient/ Partial Hospitalization; Level III, Residential/Inpatient Treatment; and Level IV, Medically Managed Intensive Inpatient Treatment. Within these broad levels of service is a range of specific levels of care. Admission criteria for these levels of care are based on severity scores for the following six dimensions: acute intoxication/withdrawal potential; biomedical conditions and complications; emotional, behavioral, or cognitive conditions and complications; readiness to change; relapse, continued use, or continued problem potential; and recovery environment.

TREATMENT

Although there are over 1,000 studies on drug and alcohol treatment in adults (Kranzler, Amin, Modesto-Lowe, & Onken, 1999), there are a relatively small number of adolescent treatment outcome studies. The limited literature on efficacy studies is characterized, however, by significant methodological limitations (Kaminer, 2000), including small sample size, lack of placebo-controlled condition, different selection criteria, inadequate measurement of psychosocial and comorbid psychiatric conditions, failure to indicate compliance and attrition rates, little description of actual treatment involved or measures to maintain treatment fidelity by counselors, unmanualized interventions (making replication difficult), therapist variability, lack of or deficiency in objective measurement, such as drug urinalysis for treatment outcome, and inadequate follow-up of both treatment completers and noncompleters.

Catalano and associates' (1990–1991) review of adolescent treatment outcome in 16 studies concluded that treatment is better than no treatment. Pretreatment factors associated with outcome were race, seriousness of substance use, criminality, and educational status. The in-treatment factors predictive of outcome were time in residential treatment, involvement of family, use of practical problem solving, and provision of comprehensive services, such as housing, academic assistance, and recreation. Posttreatment variables, which were thought to be the most important determinants of outcome, included association with nonusing peers, involvement in leisure time activities, work, and school.

In more recent reviews of the literature (Deas & Thomas, 2001; Williams & Chang, 2000; Winters, 1999), similar variables were reported to be most consistently related to successful outcome: treatment completion, low pretreatment use, peer and parent social support, and nonuse of substances. These more recent reviews also found evidence that treatment was superior to no treatment. Although insufficient evidence was found to compare the effectiveness of treatment modalities, early reports indicated that outpatient family therapy appeared to be superior to other forms of outpatient treatment. These findings however, have not been supported by most recent studies.

The Drug Abuse Treatment Study for Adolescents (DATOS-A) is a multisite, prospective treatment outcome study of 1,732 adolescent admissions to 23 programs in four U.S. cities (Grella, Hser, Joshi, & Rounds-Bryant, 2001; Hser et al., 2001). In the year following treatment, patients reported decreased heavy drinking, marijuana and other illicit drug use, and decreased criminal involvement, as well as improved psychological adjustment and school performance. Although the length of time in treatment was generally short, longer treatment stays were associated with several favorable outcomes. Nearly two-thirds (63%) of the sample reported at least one comorbid DSM-IV-TR disorder. At baseline, when compared with noncomorbid youth with SUDs, these youth with comorbid disorders were more likely to be alcohol- or other-drug-dependent and to have more problems with family, school, and criminal involvement. Although comorbid youth reduced their drug use and problem behaviors after treatment, they were more likely to use marijuana and halluci-nogens, and to engage in delinquent behavior in the 12 months after treatment when compared with noncomorbid adolescents (Grella et al., 2001).

Data indicate that most adolescents return to some level of alcohol or other drug abuse following treatment (Brown, Vik, & Creamer, 1989; Brown et al., 1990). Adolescents in substance abuse treatment begin substance use at an earlier age and progress rapidly to the use of multiple drugs, followed by the development of SUDs (Brown et al., 1989; Myers & Brown, 1990). Other clinical features of adolescents entering treatment include high levels of coexisting psychopathology or early personality difficulties; deviant behavior; school difficulties, including high levels of truancy; and family disruption and substance abuse (Bukstein et al., 1992; Doyle, Delaney, & Trobin, 1994). Several pretreatment characteristics predict completion of treatment by adolescents, including greater severity of alcohol problems; greater use of drugs other than alcohol, marijuana, and tobacco; a higher level of internalizing problems; and lower self-esteem (Blood & Cornwall, 1994; Doyle et al., 1994, Kaminer, 1992a). Premorbid psychopathology (e.g., conduct disorder) is negatively correlated with treatment completion and with future abstinence (Kaminer, Burleson, & Goldberger, 2002; Myers, Brown, & Mott, 1995). Although factors such as severity of substance use may predict short-term treatment outcomes, most longer term outcomes may depend on social–environmental factors. This is consistent with studies of relapse among adolescent populations, which suggest that relapse in adolescents is more often associated with social pressures to use rather than situations involving negative affect, as is usually found in adult relapse (Brown, Myers, Mott, & Vik, 1994; Vik, Grisel, & Brown, 1992). Adolescents' attendance at self-support or aftercare groups is associated with higher rates of abstinence and other measure of improved outcome when compared with those adolescents who did not attend such groups (Harrison & Hoffmann, 1989).

Despite a higher level of return to substance use among adolescents after treatment, abstinent teens may expect decreased interpersonal conflict, improved academic functioning, and increased involvement in social and occupational activities (Brown et al., 1994). Patterns of substance abuse among adolescents appear to become more stable between 6 and 12 months after treatment (Brown et al., 1994). An extensive review of treatment outcome studies conducted in the 1970s and 1980s concluded that treatment can be effective and is better than no treatment (Catalano et al., 1990–1991). However, an unequivocal superiority of specific treatment modalities or components has not been demonstrated (Winters, 1999).

Psychosocial treatment strategies that have shown promise in reducing SUDs among adolescents include family therapies such as multisystemic therapy (Henggeler, Pickrel, & Brondino, 1996), functional family therapy (Waldron, Slesnick, Brody, Turner, & Peterson, 2001), and multidimensional family therapy (Liddle, Dakov, & Diamond, 2001), as well as behavioral therapy (Azrin, Donohue, & Besalel, 1994), cognitive-behavioral therapy (Kaminer, Blitz, Burleson, Sussman, & Rounsaville, 1998; Kaminer, Burleson, & Goldberger, 2002), Motivational Interviewing (Monti, 1999), contingency management reinforcement (Corby, Roll, & Ledgerwood, 2000), the Minnesota 12-step model (Winters et al., 2000), and integrative models of treatment (Dennis et al., 2004; Kaminer, 2001). A common recommendation for youth is to attend 12-step groups. It is noteworthy, however, that little is known regarding the effects of this approach on adolescents. Kelly, Myers, and Brown (2000) reported modest beneficial effects of 12-step attendance, which were mediated by motivation but not by coping or self-efficacy.

PHARMACOTHERAPY OF DUAL DIAGNOSES

Pharmacotherapy or medication treatment potentially targets several areas, including treatment of withdrawal, use to counteract or decrease the subjective reinforcing effects of illicit substance use, and treatment of comorbid psychopathology. Unfortunately, no systematic research evaluates the efficacy and safety of any psychotropic medication in the treatment of adolescents with SUDs (Kaminer, 1995). Although clinically significant withdrawal symptoms appear to

be rare in adolescents (Martin et al., 1995), there is little rationale for using different detoxification protocols than those used for adults. The use of agents to block
the reinforcing effects of various substances, as aversive agents (e.g., disulfiram) or
to relieve craving during and after acute withdrawal, has been studied in adults
but has received scant attention in adolescents. Kaminer (1992b) described the
use of desipramine in an adolescent with cocaine dependence. Aversive pharmacological treatment with agents such as disulfiram is rare in adolescents. In two
case studies, Myers, Donaue, and Goldstein (1994) expressed caution in using
disulfiram in adolescents. The opiate antagonist naltrexone, used safely and effectively in adults to reduce cravings for alcohol, may hold promise for the treatment
of adolescents with alcohol use disorder according to a case study reported by
Wold and Kaminer (1997).

The high prevalence of coexisting psychiatric disorders in adolescents with
SUD presents additional targets for pharmacological agents (Bukstein &
Kithas, 2003; Bukstein et al., 1989). Potential targets for pharmacological treatment include depression and other mood problems, ADHD, severe levels of
aggressive behavior, and anxiety disorders. Unfortunately, few data in the literature demonstrate the efficacy of pharmacological agents prescribed for adolescents with a SUD and comorbid psychiatric disorders. Preliminary data suggest
that selective serotonergic reuptake inhibitors may reduce problem drinking in
adult drinkers (Naranjo, Kadlec, Sanheuza, Woodley-Remus, & Sellars, 1990),
and both depression and drinking behavior in depressed adult alcoholics
(Cornelius et al., 1993). However, a recent study indicates that these agents
have a limited clinical utility (Kranzler et al., 1995). In general, clinicians
should use the same caution in considering pharmacological treatment for adolescents with a comorbid SUD and psychiatric disorders, as they do in youth
with psychiatric symptoms alone.

Only more recently has there been research evaluating the efficacy and
safety of any psychotropic medication in the treatment of adolescents with
SUDs (Bukstein & Kithas, 2003; Kaminer, 2001). Open trials with pemoline
and bupropion for ADHD, and fluoxetine for depression, in a population of
drug-dependent delinquents have shown promise (Riggs, Milkovich, Coffman,
& Crowley, 1997; Riggs, Leon, Mikulich, & Pottle, 1998). More recently, a
double-blind, placebo-controlled trial of a stimulant medication demonstrated
the efficacy of medication improving ADHD symptoms in adolescents with
comorbid ADHD and an SUD. This study also demonstrated that medication treatment of ADHD alone, without specific SUD or other psychosocial
treatment, did not decrease substance use (Riggs, Hall, Mikulich-Gilbertson,
Lohman, & Kayser, 2004). Lithium, in a randomized controlled trial (Geller et
al., 1998), and serotonergic reuptake inhibitors, in open trials (Cornelius et al.,
2001; Riggs et al., 1997), have produced significant improvements in adolescents with an SUD and comorbid mood disorders.

An SUD may increase the potential for intentional or unintentional overdose. Some pharmacological agents may have inherent abuse potential. Critical

issues in the use of pharmacotherapy include avoiding the precipitation or exacerbation of psychiatric symptoms by the abused substances and the need to achieve some level of abstinence or control of substance use before a more optimal assessment of symptoms and starting pharmacological treatment, the potential of acute drug effects resulting in intentional or unintentional overdose, and the potential abuse of the pharmacotherapeutic agents themselves. The treatment of ADHD among populations with SUDs remains problematic due to the abuse potential of central nervous system stimulants by the patient, family, and peers (Coetzee, Kaminer, & Morales, 2002; Kaminer, 1995). The use of therapeutic stimulants by patients correctly diagnosed with ADHD does not lead to initiation of an SUD (Wilens, Faraone, Biederman, & Guanawardene, 2003). In addition to close supervision of medication compliance, clinicians should consider the use of effective agents with much lower abuse potential, such as tricyclic antidepressants, bupropion, and pemoline. Longer acting stimulants, while not immune from being abused, may have a lower abuse potential than shorter acting stimulants.

Although pharmacotherapy of adolescents with SUDs offers a strong potential adjunct for treatment, the use of medications does not alleviate the need for psychosocial treatment that directly addresses substance use and related behaviors.

Although not specifically studied, the multiple areas of possible dysfunction in adolescents with SUDs and the many available treatment modalities suggest a multimodal approach. Treatment matching, or matching adolescents with specific characteristics with appropriate levels of care and types of treatment modalities, is a concept that has received much attention in the adult literature. Psychiatric severity may be the best identified guide to matching (McLellan, Luborsky, Woody, O'Brien, & Druley, 1983). Despite two decades of specific treatment for adolescents with SUDs, we know little about the "dose" of treatment necessary for successful outcomes, nor do we know much about the specific effects of characteristics such as gender, race, and comorbid psychopathology on outcome. Research into adolescent treatment lags considerably behind adult treatment research. As the focus of treatment for adolescents with SUDs shifts from inpatient and residential settings to outpatient, partial hospitalization, and home/family-based treatments, the need for research into treatment effectiveness is critical.

DISCHARGE AND AFTERCARE

Maintenance of treatment gains in the months after treatment ends has been problematic in youth with AOSUDs. An approximately 60% relapse rate was reported during the first 3 months after treatment completion, and an additional 20% relapsed during the rest of the first year (Brown et al., 1989). About 60% of adolescents continued either to vacillate in and out of recovery after discharge from the Cannabis Youth Treatment study (Dennis et al., 2004) or to manifest at least some form of substance abuse (Kaminer, Burleson, et al., 2002). Lack of continuity of care or aftercare programs for adolescents with AOSUDs is the rule rather than the exception.

Partially overlapping terms such as "aftercare," "continued care," or "transition of care" have been used in the literature interchangeably to describe interventions used in the postacute treatment period. The Continuity of Care Guidelines for Addiction Services developed by the American Academy of Addiction Psychiatry (AAAP) defined "continuity" as follows: "Transitions should incorporate relevant elements of any preexisting treatment plan. Treatment plans should be relevant to the entire course of an episode of illness/disability so that they can provide a degree of continuity in the context of change" (Sowers, 2003, p. 2).

The timing and level of therapeutic services in important. The more ancillary community therapeutic services received during treatment, the better the short-term outcome (Burleson & Kaminer, in press). The more therapeutic services received posttreatment, however, the poorer the short-term outcome.

Godley, Godley, and Dennis (2002) reported that adolescents referred from residential treatment to continuing care services were significantly more likely to initiate and receive more continuing care services, to be abstinent from marijuana 3 months postdischarge, and to reduce their 3-month postdischarge days of alcohol use when assigned to an assertive continuing care protocol involving case management and the adolescent community reinforcement approach as compared to usual continuing care. Because of the stated importance of aftercare, we need continued exploration of how to improve engagement and retention in aftercare. One of the most prominent aftercare options is school-based interventions. Most patients return to school; therefore, school-based tertiary prevention in the form of counseling, peer-led groups, and support group for "recovered" adolescents is warranted (Wagner, Kortlander, & Morris, 2001). Adolescents enrolled in these programs may also be instrumental as role models in school-based primary and secondary prevention groups for high-risk youth. Also, continued participation in self-help groups, follow-up with an outpatient clinic, and rigorous maintenance of a contingency discharge contract are helpful for relapse prevention.

Parents/caretakers should be encouraged to support the recovery process and to maintain a risk-free lifestyle for the adolescent (e.g., be aware of ominous signs of relapse, keep curfew hours, and avoid enabling behavior).

CONCLUSION

Despite the progress achieved in the understanding of different aspects of SUDs in adolescents, more research is needed to advance the field. Among the priority areas for further research are interventions including prevention, and effectiveness studies in general, and for dually diagnosed youth in particular. Finally, advancement of aftercare/continued care is necessary in order to reduce the high rates of relapse among youth. An incorporation of a developmental psychopathology perspective in subtyping adolescents with SUDs and related problems includes describing the phenomenology of these problems and developing an age-appropriate nosology. Based on this research and a developmental perspective, clinicians should develop comprehensive intervention programs that include the family, peers, and the community.

REFERENCES

Ahmed, S. W., Bush, P. J., Davidson, F. R., & Iannotti, R. J. (1984). *Predicting children's use and intentions to use abusable substances.* Paper presented at the annual meeting of the American Public Health Association, Anaheim, CA.

American Psychiatric Association. (2000). *Diagnostic and statistical manual of mental disorders* (4th ed., text rev.). Washington, DC: Author.

American Society of Addiction Medicine. (2001). ASAM *placement criteria for the treatment of substance-related disorders* Chevy Chase, MD: Author.

Azrin, N. H., Donohue, B., & Besalel, V. A. (1994). Youth drug abuse treatment: A controlled outcome study. *J Child Adolesc Subst Abuse, 3,* 1–16.

Bangert-Drowns, R. L. (1988). The effects of school-based substance abuse education: A meta-analysis. *J Drug Educ, 18,* 243–264.

Barkley, R. A., Fischer, M., Edelbrock, C. S., & Smallish, L. (1990). The adolescent outcome of hyperactive children diagnosed by research criteria: I. An 8-year prospective follow-up study. *J Am Acad Child Adolesc Psychiatry, 29,* 546–557.

Barnea, A., Rahav, G., & Teichman, M. (1987). The reliability and consistency of self-reports of substance use in longitudinal study. *Br J Addict, 82,* 891–898.

Biederman, J., Wilens, T., Mick, E., Farone, S., Weber, W., Curtis, S., et al. (1997). Is ADHD a risk factor for psychoactive substance use disorders?: Findings from a four-year prospective follow-up study. *J Am Acad Child Adolesc Psychiatry, 36,* 21–29.

Blackson, T. C. (1994). Temperament: A salient correlate of risk factors for alcohol and drug abuse. *Drug Alcohol Depend, 36,* 205–214.

Blood, L., & Cornwall, A. (1994). Pretreatment variables that predict completion of an adolescent substance abuse treatment program. *J Nerv Ment Dis, 182,* 14–19.

Bohman, M., Sigvardsson, S., & Cloninger, C. R. (1981). Maternal inheritance of alcohol abuse. *Arch Gen Psychiatry, 38,* 965–969.

Botvin, G. J., Baker, E., Dusenbury, L., Botvin, E. M., & Diaz, T. (1995). Long-term follow-up results of a randomized drug abuse prevention trial in a white middle class population. *JAMA, 273,* 1106–1112.

Botvin, G. J., Baker, E., Filazzola, A., & Botvin, E. M. (1990). A cognitive behavioral approach to substance abuse prevention: One year follow-up. *Addict Behav, 15,* 47–63.

Botvin, G. J., & Griffin, K. W. (2001). Life skills training: Theory, methods, and effectiveness of a drug abuse prevention approach. In E. F. Wagner & H. B. Waldron

(Eds.), *Innovations in adolescent substance abuse interventions* (pp. 31–50). Amsterdam: Pergamon.

Brent, D. A., Perper, J. A., & Allman, C. (1987). Alcohol, firearms and suicide among youth: Temporal trends in Allegheny County, Pennsylvania, 1960 to 1983. *JAMA, 257,* 3369–3372.

Brook, J. S., Whiteman, M., Gordon, A. S., & Brook, D. W. (1990). The psychosocial etiology of adolescent drug use: A family interactional approach. *Genet, Soc Gen Psychol Mon, 116,* 2.

Brown, S. A., Myers, M. G., Mott, M. A., & Vik, P. W. (1994). Correlates of success following treatment for adolescent substance abuse. *Appl Prevent Psychol, 3,* 61–73.

Brown, S. A., Vik, P. N., & Creamer, V. (1989). Characteristics of relapse following adolescent substance abuse treatment. *Addict Behav, 14,* 291–300.

Brown, S. A., Vik, P. W., McQuaid, J. R., Patterson, T., Irwin, M. R., & Grant, I. (1990). Severity of psychosocial stress and outcome of alcoholism treatment. *J Abnorm Psychol, 99,* 344–348.

Bukstein, O. G., Brent, D. A., & Kaminer, Y. (1989). Comorbidity of substance abuse and other psychiatric disorders in adolescents. *Am J Psychiatry, 146,* 1131–1141.

Bukstein, O. G., Brent, D. B., Perper, J. A., Mortiz, G., Schweers, J., Roth, C., & Balach, L. (1993). Risk factors for completed suicide among adolescents with a lifetime history of substance abuse: A case control study. *Acta Psychiatr Scand, 88,* 403–408.

Bukstein, O. G., Glancy, L. J., & Kaminer, Y. (1992). Patterns of affective comorbidity in a clinical population of dually-diagnosed substance abusers. *J Am Acad Child Adolesc Psychiatry, 31,* 1041–1045.

Bukstein, O. G., & Kaminer, Y. (1994). The nosology of adolescent substance abuse. *Am J Addict, 3,* 1–13.

Bukstein, O. G., & Kithas, J. (2002). Adolescent substance use disorders. In D. Rosenberg, P. A. Davanzo, & S. Gershon (Eds.), *Child-adolescent psychopharmacology* (pp. pp. 675–710). New York: Marcel Dekker.

Bulik, C. M. (1987). Eating disorders in adolescents and young adults. *Child Adolesc Psychiat Clin NA, 11,* 201–218.

Burk, J. P., & Sher, K. J. (1990). Labeling the child of an alcoholic: Negative stereotyping by mental health professionals and peers. *J Stud Alcohol, 51,* 156–163.

Burleson, J., & Kaminer, Y. (in press). Correlation between youth parent report and objective measurement of substance abuse and related problems. *J Child Adolesc Subst Abuse.*

Cadoret, R. J., Troughton, E., O'Gorman, T. W., & Heywood, E. (1986). An adoption study of genetic and environmental factor in drug abuse. *Arch Gen Psychiatry, 43,* 1131–1136.

Casavant, M. J. (2002). Urine drug screening in adolescents. *Pediatr Clin North Am, 49,* 317–327.

Catalano, R. F., Hawkins, D., Kreuz, C., Gillmore, M., Morrison, D., Wells, E., & Abbott, R. (1993). Using research to guide culturally appropriate drug abuse prevention. *J Consult Clin Psychol, 61,* 804–811.

Catalano, R. F., Hawkins, J. D., Wells, E. A., Miller, J., & Brewer, D. (1990–1991). Evaluation of the effectiveness of adolescent drug abuse treatment, assessment of risks for relapse, and promising approaches for relapse prevention. *Int J Addict, 25*, 1085–1140.

Christie, K. A., Burke, J. D., Regier, D. A., Rae, D. S., Boyd, J. H., & Locke, B. Z. (1988). Epidemiologic evidence for early onset of mental disorders and higher risk of drug abuse in young adults. *Am J Psychiatry, 145*, 971–975.

Clark, D. B., Bukstein, O. G., Smith, M. G., Kaczynski, N. A., Mezzich, A. C., & Donovan, J. E. (1995). Identifying anxiety disorders in adolescents hospitalized for alcohol abuse or dependence. *Psychiatr Serv, 46*, 618–620.

Clark, D. B., & Sayette, M. A. (1993). Anxiety and the development of alcoholism. *Am J Addict, 2*, 56–76.

Cloninger, C. R., Bohman, M., & Sigvardsson, S. (1981). Inheritance of alcohol abuse. *Arch Gen Psychiatry, 38*, 861–871.

Coate, D., & Grossman, N. (1987, Fall). Change in alcoholic beverage prices and legal drinking age. *Alcohol Health Res World*, pp. 22–25.

Coetzee, M., Kaminer, Y., & Morales, A. (2002). Megadose intranasal methylphenidate (Ritalin) abuse in adult with attention deficit hyperactivity disorder. *Subst Abuse, 23*, 165–169.

Cole, E. J. (1997). New developments in biological measures of drug prevalence. In L. Harrison & A. Hughes (Eds.), *Validity of self-reported drug use: Improving the accuracy of survey estimates* (NIDA Research Monograph 167, pp. 108–130). Rockville, MD: National Institute on Drug Abuse.

Corby, E. A., Roll, J. M., & Ledgerwood, D. M. (2000). Contingency management interventions for treating the substance abuse of adolescents: A feasibility study. *Exp Clin Psychopharmacol, 8*, 371–376.

Cornelius, J. R., Bukstein, O. G., Birmaher, B., Salloum, I. M., Lynch, K., Pollock, N. K., et al. (2001). Fluoxetine in adolescents with major depression and an alcohol use disorder: An open label trial. *Addict Behav, 26*, 735–739.

Cornelius, J. R., Salloum, I. M., Cornelius, M. D., Perel, J. M., Thase, M. E., Ehler, J. G., & Marm, J. (1993). Fluoxetine trial in suicidal depressed alcoholics. *Psychopharmacol Bull, 29*, 195–199.

Costello, J. E., Angold, A., Burns, B. J., Stangl, D. K., Tweed, D. L., Erkanli, A., & Wotrthman, C. M. (1996). The Smoky Mountains study of youth: Goals, design, methods, and the prevalence of DSM-II-R disorders. *Arch Gen Psychiatry, 53*, 1129–1136.

Crumley, F. E. (1990). Substance abuse and adolescent suicidal behavior. *JAMA, 263*, 3051–3056.

Deas, D., & Thomas, S. E. (2001). An overview of controlled studies of adolescent substance abuse treatment. *Am J Addict, 10*, 178–189.

DeMilio, L. (1989). Psychiatric syndromes in adolescent substance abusers. *Am J Psychiatry, 146*, 1212–1214.

Dennis, M. L., Godley, S. H., Diamond, G., Tims, F., Babor, T., Donaldson, J., et al. (2004). Main findings of the Cannabis Youth Treatment randomized field experiment. *J Subst Abuse Treat, 27*, 197–213.

Dennis, M. L., Titus, J. C., White, M., Unsicker, J., & Hodgkins, D. (2003). *Global Appraisal of Individual Needs (GAIN): Administration guide for the GAIN and related measures* (5th ed.). Bloomington, IL: Chestnut Health Systems.

Deykin, E. Y., Buka, S. L., & Zeena, T. H. (1992). Depressive illness among chemically dependent adolescents. *Am J Psychiatry, 149,* 1341–1347.

Deykin, E. Y., Levy, J. C., & Wells, V. (1987). Adolescent depression, alcohol, and drug abuse. *Am J Public Health, 77,* 178–182.

Donovan, J. E., & Jessor, R. (1983). Problem drinking and the dimension of involvement with drugs: A Guttman scalogram analysis of adolescent drug use. *Am J Public Health, 73,* 5433–5452.

Doyle, H., Delaney, W., & Trobin, J. (1994). Follow-up study of young attendees at an alcohol unit. *Addiction, 89,* 183–189.

Earls, F., & Jung, K. (1987). Temperament and home environment characteristics in the early development of child psychopathology. *J Am Acad Child Psychiatry, 26,* 491–498.

Ewing, J. A. (1984). Detecting alcoholism: The CAGE questionnaire. *JAMA, 252,* 1905–1907.

Ferdinand, R. F., Blum, M., & Verhulst, F. C. (2001). Psychopathology in adolescence predicts substance use in young adulthood. *Addiction, 96,* 861–870.

Friedman, A. S., & Utada, A. (1989). A method for diagnosing and planning the treatment of adolescent drug abusers (the Adolescent Drug Abuse Diagnosis [ADAD] instrument). *J Drug Educ, 19,* 285–312.

Geller, B., Cooper, T. B., Sun, K., Zimermann, B., Frazier, J., Williams, M., & Heath, J. (1998). Double-blind and placebo-controlled study of lithium for adolescent bipolar disorders with secondary substance dependency. *J Am Acad Child Adolesc Psychiatry, 37,* 171–178.

Glantz, M., & Pickens, R., (Eds.). (1992). *Vulnerability to drug abuse.* Washington, DC: American Psychological Association.

Godley, M. D., Godley, S. H., & Dennis, M. L. (2002). Preliminary outcomes from the assertive continuing care experiment for adolescents discharged from residential treatment. *J Subst Abuse Treat, 23,* 21–32.

Goodwin, D. W. (1985). Alcoholism and genetics: The sins of the fathers. *Arch Gen Psychiatry, 42,* 171–174.

Grella, C. E., Hser, Y., Joshi, V., & Rounds-Bryant, J. (2001). Drug treatment outcomes for adolescents with comorbid mental and substance use disorders. *J Nerv Ment Dis, 189,* 384–392.

Griffiths, M. (1995). *Adolescent gambling.* London, Routledge.

Grilo, C. M., Becker, D. F., Walker, M. L., Levy, K. N., Edell, W. S., & McGlashan, T. H. (1995). Psychiatric comorbidity in adolescent inpatients with substance use disorders. *J Am Acad Child Adolesc Psychiatry, 34,* 1085–1091.

Harrison, P. A., Fulkerson, J. A., & Beebe, T. J. (1998). DSM-IV substance use disorder criteria for adolescents: A critical examination based on a statewide school survey. *Am J Psychiatry, 155,* 486–492.

Harrison, P. A., & Hoffmann, N. (1989). *CATOR report: Adolescent treatment completers one year later.* St. Paul, MN: Chemical Abuse/Addiction Treatment Outcome Registry.

Hasin, D. S., Grant, B., & Endicott, J. (1990). The natural history of alcohol abuse implications for definitions of alcohol use disorders. *Am J Psychiatry, 147,* 337–341.

Henggeler, S. W., Pickrel, S. G., & Brondino, M. J., (1996). Eliminating treatment dropout of substance abusing or dependent delinquents through home-based multisystemic therapy. *Am J Psychiatry, 153*, 427–428.

Hoffman, N. G., Halikas, J. A., & Mee-Lee, D. (1987). *The Cleveland admission, discharge, and transfer criteria: Model for chemical dependency treatment programs.* Cleveland, OH: Chemical Dependency Directors Association.

Hovens, J., Cantwell, D. P., & Kiriakos, R. (1994). Psychiatric comorbidity in hospitalized adolescent substance abusers. *J Am Acad Child Adolesc Psychiatry, 33*, 476–483.

Hser, Y., Grella, C. E., Collins, C., & Teruya, C. (2003). Drug-use initiation and conduct disorder among adolescents in treatment. *J Adolesc, 26*, 331–345.

Hser, Y., Grella, C. E., Hubbard, R. L., Hsieh, S., Fletcher, B. W., Brown, B. S., & Anglin, M. (2001). An evaluation of drug treatments for adolescents in 4 U.S. cities. *Arch Gen Psychiatry, 58*, 689–695.

Institute of Medicine. (1990). *Broadening the base of treatment for alcohol problems.* Washington, DC: National Academy Press.

Jessor, R. (1987). Problem-behavior theory, psychosocial development and adolescent problem drinking. *Br J Addict, 82*, 331–342.

Jessor, R., & Jessor, S. L. (1977). *Problem behavior and psychosocial development: A longitudinal study of youth.* New York: Academic Press.

Kaminer, Y. (1992a). Clinical implications of the relationship between attention-deficit/hyperactivity disorder and psychoactive substance use disorders. *Am J Addict, 1*, 257–264.

Kaminer, Y. (1992b). Desipramine facilitation of cocaine abstinence in an adolescent. *J Am Acad Child Adolesc Psychiatry, 31*, 312–317.

Kaminer, Y. (1994). *Adolescent substance abuse: A comprehensive guide to theory and practice.* New York: Plenum Medical.

Kaminer, Y. (1995). Issues in the pharmacological treatment of adolescent substance abuse. *J Child Adolesc Psychopharmacol, 5*, 93–106.

Kaminer, Y. (1996). Adolescent substance abuse and suicidal behavior. In S. L. Jaffe (Ed.), Adolescent substance abuse and dual disorders [Special issue]. *Child Adolescent Psychiatry Clin North Am, 5*, 59–72.

Kaminer, Y. (2000). Contingency management (CM) reinforcement procedures for adolescent substance abuse. *J Am Acad Child Adolesc Psychiatry, 39*, 1324–1326.

Kaminer, Y. (2001). Adolescent substance abuse treatment: Where do we go from here? *Psychiatr Serv, 52*, 147–149.

Kaminer, Y., Blitz, C., Burleson, J., Sussman, J., & Rounsaville, B. J. (1998). Psychotherapies for adolescent substance abusers: Treatment outcome. *J Nerv Ment Dis, 186*, 684–690.

Kaminer, Y., Bukstein, O. G., & Tarter, R. E. (1991). The Teen-Addiction Severity Index: Rationale and reliability. *Int J Addict, 26*, 219–226.

Kaminer, Y., Burleson, J., & Goldberger, R. (2002). Psychotherapies for adolescent substance abusers: Short-and long-term outcomes. *J Nerv Ment Dis, 190*, 737–745.

Kaminer, Y., Burleson, J., & Jadamec, A. (2002). Gambling behavior in adolescent substance abusers. *Subst Abuse, 23*, 191–198.

Kaminer, Y., Tarter, R, E., Bukstein, O., & Kabene, M. (1992). Comparison between treatment completers and noncompleters among dually diagnosed substance abusing adolescents. *J Am Acad Child Adolesc Psychiatry, 31,* 1046–1049.

Kaminer, Y., Wagner, E., Plummer, B., & Seifer, R. (1993). Validation of the Teen-Addiction Severity Index (T-ASI). *Am J Addict, 2,* 250–254.

Kandel, D. B. (1978). *Longitudinal research on drug use: Empirical findings and methodological issues.* New York: Hemisphere/Wiley.

Kandel, D. B. (1982). Epidemiological and psychosocial perspective on adolescent drug use. *J Am Acad Child Psychiatry, 20,* 328–347.

Kandel, D. B. (2003). Does marijuana use cause the use of other drugs? *JAMA, 289,* 482–483.

Kashani, J. H., Beck, N. C., Hoeper, E. W., Fallahi, C., Corcoran, C. M., McAllister, J. A., et al. (1987). Psychiatric disorders in a community sample of adolescents. *Am J Psychiatry, 144,* 584–589.

Kelly, J. F., Myers, M. G., & Brown, S. A. (2000). A multivariate process model of adolescent 12-step attendance and substance use outcome following inpatient treatment. *Psychol Addict Behav, 14,* 376–389.

Kendler, K. S. (1994). Lifetime and 12-month prevalence of DSM-III-R psychiatric disorders in the United States: Results from the National Comorbidity survey. *Arch Gen Psychiatry, 51,* 8–19.

Knight, J. R., Sherritt, L., Shrier, L. A., Harris, S. K., & Chang, G. (2002). Validity of the CRAFFT substance abuse screening test among adolescent clinic patients. *Arch Pediatr Adolesc Med, 156,* 607–614.

Kolar, A. F., Brown, B. S., Haertzen, C. A., & Michaelson, B. S. (1994). Children of substance abusers: The life experiences of children of opiate addicts in methadone maintenance. *Am J Drug Alcohol Abuse, 20,* 159–171.

Kranzler, H. R., Amin, H., Modesto-Lowe, V., & Oncken, C. (1999). Pharmacologic treatments for drug and alcohol dependence. *Psychiatr Clin North Am, 22,* 401–423.

Kranzler, H. R., Burleson, J. A., Korner, P., Del Boca, F. K., Bohn, M. J., & Brown, J. (1995). Fluoxetine differentially alters alcohol intake and other consummatory behavior in problem drinkers. *Clin Pharmacol Ther, 47,* 490–498.

Kumpfer, K. L., & Demarsh, J. (1986). Future issues and promising directions in the prevention of substance abuse among youth. *J Child Contemp Soc, 18,* 49–91.

Kushner, M. G., Sher, K. J., & Beitman, B. D. (1990). The relation between alcohol problems and anxiety disorders. *Am J Psychiatry, 147,* 685–695.

Kutcher, S., Kachur, E., & Marton, P. (1992). Substance use among adolescents with chronic mental illnesses: A pilot study of descriptive and differentiating features. *Can J Psychiatry, 37,* 428–431.

Latimer, W. W., Stone, A. L., Voight, A., Winters, K. C., & August, G. J. (2002). Gender differences in psychiatric comorbidity among adolescents with substance use disorder. *Exp Clin Psychopharmacol, 10,* 310–315.

Leccese, M., & Waldron, H. B. (1994). Assessing adolescent substance use: A critique of current measurement instruments. *J Subst Abuse Treat, 11,* 553–563.

Levin, F. R., & Kleber, H. D. (1995). Attention-deficit/hyperactivity disorder and substance abuse: Relationships and implications for treatment. *Harv Rev Psychiatry, 2,* 246–258.

Lewinsohn, P. M., Hops, H., Roberts, R. E., & Seeley, J. R. (1993). Adolescent psychopathology: I. Prevalence and incidence of depression and other DSM-III-R disorders in high school students. *J Abnorm Psychol, 102,* 133–144.

Lewinsohn, P. M., Rohde, P., & Seeley, J. R. (1993). Adolescent psychopathology: III. The clinical consequences of comorbidity. *J Am Acad Child Adolesc Psychiatry, 34,* 510–519.

Lewinsohn, P. M., Rohde, P., & Seeley, J. R. (1996). Alcohol consumption in high school adolescents: Frequency of use and dimensional structure of associated problems. *Addiction, 91,* 375–390.

Liddle, H. A., Dakof, G. A., & Diamond, G. (2001). Multidimensional family therapy for adolescent substance abuse: Results of a randomized clinical trial. *Am J Drug Alcohol Abuse, 27,* 651–687.

Loeber, R. (1988). Natural histories of conduct problems, delinquency and associated substance use. In B. B. Lahey & A. E. Kazdin (Eds.), *Advances in clinical child psychology* (Vol. 11, pp. 73–124). New York: Plenum Press.

Martin, C. S., Kaczynski, N. A., Maisto, S. A., Bukstein, O. G., & Moss, H. B. (1995). Patterns of DSM-IV alcohol abuse and dependence symptoms in adolescent drinkers. *J Stud Alcohol, 56,* 672–680.

Masterman, P. W., & Kelly, A. B. (2003). Reaching adolescents who drink harmfully: Fitting intervention to developmental reality. *J Subst Abuse Treat, 24,* 347–355.

Maziade, M., Caron, C., Cote, P., Boutin, P., & Thivierge, J. (1990). Extreme temperament and diagnosis: A study in a psychiatric sample of consecutive children. *Arch Gen Psychiatry, 47,* 477–484.

McLellan, A. T., Luborsky, L., Woody, G. E., O'Brien, C. P., & Druley, K. A. (1983). Predicting response to alcohol and drug abuse treatment: Role of psychiatric severity. *Arch Gen Psychiatry, 40,* 620–628.

Metzger, D. S., Kushner, H., & McLellan, A. T. (1991). *Adolescent Problem Severity Index: Administration manual.* Philadelphia: Biomedical Computer Research Institute.

Miller, G. (1990). *Substance abuse Subtle Screening Inventory—Adolescent (SASSI-A).* Bloomington, IN:SASSI Institute.

Monti, P. M. (1999). Innovations in adolescent substance abuse intervention. In E. F. Wagner (Ed.), *Alcoholism* [Special issue]. *Clin Exp Res, 23,* 236–249.

Morral, A. R., McCaffrey, D. F., & Paddock, S. M. (2002). Reassessing the marijuana gateway effect. *Addiction, 97,* 1493–1504.

Moss, H. B., Kirisci, L., Gordon, H. W., & Tarter, R. E. (1994). A neuropsychological profile of adolescent alcoholics. *Alcohol: Clin Exp Res, 18,* 159–163.

Moss, H. B., & Tarter, R. E. (1993). Substance abuse, aggression and violence: What are the connections? *Am J Addict, 2,* 149–160.

Myers, M. G., & Brown, S. A. (1990). Coping responses and relapse among adolescent substance abusers. *J Subst Abuse, 2,* 177–190.

Myers, M. G., Brown, S. A., & Mott, M. A. (1995). Preadolescent conduct disorder behaviors predict relapse and progression of addiction for adolescent alcohol and drug abusers. *Alcohol: Clin Exp Res, 19,* 1528–1536.

Myers, W. C., Donaue, J. E., & Goldstein, M. R. (1994). Disulfiram for alcohol use disorders in adolescents. *J Am Acad Child Adolesc Psychiatry, 33,* 484–489.

Naranjo, C. A., Kadlec, K. E., Sanheuza, P., Woodley-Remus, D., & Sellars, E. M.

(1990). Fluoxetine differentially alters alcohol intake and other consummatory behavior in problem drinkers. *Clin Pharmacol Ther, 47*, 490–498.

National Institute on Drug Abuse. (2001). *Preventing drug use among children and adolescents: A research-based guide.* Rockville, MD: Author.

National Institute on Drug Abuse. (2002). *NIDA Info Facts.* Retrieved from *www.nda.nh.gov/drugpages/mtf.html*

Newcomb, M. D. (1995). Identifying high-risk youth: Prevalence and patterns of adolescent drug abuse. In E. Rahdert & D. Czechowicz (Eds.), *Adolescent drug abuse: Clinical assessment and therapeutic interventions* (NIH Publication No. 95-3908, pp. 7–38). Rockville, MD: National Institute on Drug Abuse.

Noll, R. B., Zucker, R. A., Fitzgerald, H. E., & Curtis, W. J. (1992). Cognitive and motoric functioning of sons of alcoholic fathers and controls: The early childhood years. *Dev Psychol, 28*, 665–675.

O'Malley, P. M., Johnston, L. D., & Bachman, J. G. (1995). Adolescent substance use: Epidemiology and implications for public policy. In P. D. Rogers & M. J. Werner (Eds.), Substance abuse [Special issue]. *Pediatr Clin North Am, 42*, 241–260.

O'Malley, P. M., & Wagenaar, A. C. (1991). Effects of minimum drinking age laws on alcohol use, related behaviors and traffic crash involvement among American youth: 1976–1987. *J Stud Alcohol, 52*, 478–491.

Pentz, M. A., Dwyer, J. H., & MacKinnon, D. P. (1989). A multicommunity trial for primary prevention of adolescent drug abuse. *JAMA, 261*, 3259–3266.

Pollock, N. K., & Martin, C. S. (1999). Diagnostic orphans: Adolescent with alcohol symptoms who do not qualify for DSM-IV abuse or dependence diagnoses. *Am J Psychiatry, 156*, 897–901.

Rahdert, E. (Ed.). (1991). *The adolescent assessment and referral system manual* (DHHS Publication No. ADM 91-1735). Rockville, MD: National Institute on Drug Abuse.

Regier, D. A., Farmer, M. E., Rae, D. S., Locke, B. Z., Keith, S. J., Judd, L. L., & Goodwin, F. R. (1990). Comorbidity of mental disorders with alcohol and other drug abuse. *JAMA, 264*, 2511–2518.

Reich, W., Earls, F., Frankel, O., & Shayka, J. (1993). Psychopathology in children of alcoholics. *J Am Acad Child Adolesc Psychiatry, 32*, 995–1002.

Reinherz, H. Z., Giaconia, R. M., Lefkowitz, E. S., Pakiz, B., & Frost, A. K. (1993). Prevalence of psychiatric disorders in a community population of older adolescents. *J Am Acad Child Adolesc Psychiatry, 32*, 369–377.

Riggs, P. D., Baker S., Mikulich, S. K., Young, S. E., & Crowley, T. J. (1995). Depression in substance-dependent delinquents. *J Am Acad Child Adolesc Psychiatry, 34*, 764–771.

Riggs, P. D., Hall, S., Mikulich-Gilbertson, S., Lohman, M., & Kayser, A. (2004). A randomized controlled trial of pemoline for attention deficit hyperactivity disorder in substance abusing adolescents. *J Am Acad Child Adolesc Psychiatry, 43*, 420–429.

Riggs, P. D., Leon, S. L., Mikulich, S. K., & Pottle, L. C. (1998). An open trial of bupropion for ADHD in adolescents with substance use disorders and conduct disorder. *J Am Acad Child Adolesc Psychiatry, 37*, 1271–1278.

Riggs, P. D., Mikovich, S. K., Coffman, L. M., & Crowley, T. J. (1997). Fluoxetine in drug-dependent delinquents with major depression: An open trial. *J Child Adolesc Subst Abuse Psychopharmacol, 7*, 87–95

Robbins, M. S., Kumar, S., Walker-Barnes, C., Feaster, D. J., Briones, E., & Szapocznik, J. (2002). Ethnic differences in comorbidity among substance abusing adolescents referred to outpatient therapy. *J Am Acad Child Adolesc Psychiatry, 41,* 394–401.

Rohde, P., Lewinsohn, P. M., & Seeley, J. R. (1996). Psychiatric comorbidity with problematic alcohol use in high school students. *J Am Acad Child Adolesc Psychiatry, 35,* 101–109.

Schaeffer, K., Parson, O., & Yohman, J. (1984). Neuropsychological differences between male familial alcoholics and nonalcoholics. *Alcohol: Clin Exp Res, 8,* 347–351.

Schaps, E., Moskowitz, J., & Malvin, J. (1986). Evaluation of seven school based prevention programs: A final report of the Napa report. *Int J Addict, 21,* 1081–1112.

Schinke, S. P., Botvin, G. J., & Orlani, M. A. (1991). *Substance abuse in children and adolescents: Evaluation and intervention.* Newbury Park, CA: Sage.

Shedler, J., & Block, J. (1990). Adolescent drug use and psychological health: A longitudinal inquiry. *Am Psychol, 45,* 612–630.

Sowers, W. (2003, Winter). Continuity of care and transition planning in addiction services [News insert]. *Am Acad Addict Psychiatry,* pp. 1–4.

Stewart, D. G., & Brown, S. A. (1995). Withdrawal and dependency symptoms among adolescent alcohol and drug abusers. *Addiction, 90,* 627–635.

Stowell, R. J. (1991). Dual diagnosis issues. *Psychiat Ann, 21,* 98–104.

Tarter, R. E. (1990). Evaluation and treatment of adolescent substance abuse: A decision tree method. *Am J Drug Alcohol Abuse, 16,* 1–46.

Tarter, R. E. (1992). Prevention of drug abuse: Theory and application. *Am J Addict, 1,* 2–20.

Tarter, R. E., Kirisci, L., Hegedus, A., Mezich, A., & Yanyukov, M. (1994). Heterogeneity of adolescent alcoholism. In T. F. Babor, V. Hesselbrock, R. E. Meyer, & W. Shoemaker (Eds.), Types of alcoholics: Evidence from clinical, experimental and genetic research [Special issue]. *Ann NY Acad Sc, 708,* 172–180.

Tarter, R. E., Laird, S. B., Mostefa, K., Bukstein, O. G., & Kaminer, Y. (1990). Drug abuse severity in adolescents is associated with magnitude of deviation in temperamental traits. *Br J Addict, 85,* 1501–1504.

Tobler, N. S. (1986). Meta-analysis of 143 adolescent drug prevention programs: Quantitative outcome results of program participants compared to a control or comparison group. *J Drug Issues, 16,* 537–567.

Ungemack, J. A., Hartwell, S. W., & Babor, T. F. (1997). Alcohol and drug abuse among Connecticut youth: Implications for adolescent medicine and public health. *Conn Med, 9,* 577–585.

Van Hasselt, V. B., Null, J. A., Kempton, T., & Bukstein, O. G. (1993). Social skills and depression in adolescent substance abusers. *Addict Behav, 18,* 9–18.

Vik, P. W., Grisel, K., & Brown, S. A. (1992). Social resource characteristics and adolescent substance abuse relapse. *J Adolesc Chem Depend, 2,* 59–74.

Wagner, E. F., Kortlander, S. E., & Morris, S. (2001). The teen intervention project. In E. F. Wagner & H. B. Waldron (Eds.), *Innovations in adolescent substance abuse interventions* (pp. 21, 89–203). Amsterdam: Pergamon/Elsevier Science.

Waldron, H. B., Slesnick, N., Brody, J. L., Turner, C. W., & Peterson, T. R. (2001). Treatment outcomes for adolescent substance abuse at 4- and 7-month assessments. *J Consult Clin Psychol, 69,* 802–813.

Wallace, J. M., Bachman, J. G., O'Malley, P. M., Schulenberg, J. E., Cooper, S. M., & Johnston, L. D. (2003). Gender and ethnic differences in smoking, drinking and illicit drug use among American 8th, 10th, and 12th grade students, 1976–2000. *Addiction, 98,* 225–234.

Wilens, T. E., Biederman, J., Kiely, K., Bredin, E., & Spencer, T. J. (1995). Pilot study of behavioral and emotional disturbances in the high-risk children of parents with opioid dependence. *J Am Acad Child Adolesc Psychiatry, 34,* 779–785.

Wilens, T. E., Biederman, J., Spencer, T. J., & Frances, R. J. (1994). Comorbidity of attention-deficit disorder and psychoactive substance use disorders. *Hosp Community Psychiatry, 45,* 421–435.

Wilens, T, E., Faraone, S, V., Biederman, J., & Guanawardene, J. (2003). Stimulant therapy of ADHD beget later substance abuse: A meta-analytic review of the literature. *Pediatrics, 111,* 179–185.

Williams, R. J., & Chang, S. Y. (2000). A comprehensive and comparative review of adolescent substance abuse treatment outcome. *Clin Psychol: Sci Pract, 7,* 138–166.

Wilson, J. R., & Crowe, L. (1991). Genetics of alcoholism: Can and should youth at risk be identified? *Alcohol Health World Rep, 15,* 11–17.

Winters, K. C. (1992). Development of an adolescent alcohol and drug abuse screening scale: Personal Experience Screening Questionnaire. *Addict Behav, 17,* 479–490.

Winters, K. C. (1999). Treating adolescents with substance use disorders: An overview of practice issues and treatment outcome. *Subst Abuse, 20,* 203–225.

Winters, K. C., & Henly, G. (1988). *Personal Experience Inventory (PEI).* Los Angeles: Western Psychological Services.

Winters, K. C., Latimer, W. W., & Stinchfield, R. (2001). Assessing adolescent substance use. In E. F. Wagner & H. B. Waldron (Eds.), *Innovations in adolescent substance abuse interventions* (pp. 1–29). Amsterdam: Pergamon.

Winters, K. C., Stinchfield, R. D., & Opland, E. (2000). The effectiveness of the Minnesota Model approach in the treatment of adolescent drug abusers. *Addiction, 95,* 601–612.

Wold, M., & Kaminer, Y. (1997). Naltrexone for adolescent alcohol use disorders. *J Am Acad Child Adolesc Psychiatry, 36,* 6–7.

Wolin, S., & Wolin, S. J. (1996). The challenge model: Working with strengths in children of substance-abusing parents. In S. L. Jaffe (Ed.), Adolescent substance abuse and dual disorders [Special issue]. *Child Adolesc Psychiatry Clin North Am, 5,* 243–255.

CHAPTER 26

Psychopharmacological Treatments

ELINORE F. McCANCE-KATZ
THOMAS R. KOSTEN

This chapter reviews pharmacotherapies for abuse of nicotine, alcohol, benzo-diazepines, opioids, and cocaine. Pharmacotherapies for substance use disorders (SUDs) have been developed to address two broad treatment categories: (1) acute withdrawal or the initial attainment of abstinence and (2) chronic maintenance or the prevention of relapse. Agents for acute withdrawal are most relevant to dependence on opioids and alcohol.

Maintenance agents might directly benefit any protracted withdrawal syndrome, but the general rationale for maintenance pharmacotherapies is that they are either blocking or substitution agents. For example, the competitive opioid antagonist naltrexone completely blocks the effects of heroin, including the subjective euphoria and the production of physiological dependence from repeated heroin use. Before administering blocking agents, detoxification is required to prevent withdrawal from the abused drug. In contrast, substitution agents maintain the dependent state and will not cause withdrawal when given to dependent patients. Substitution agents prevent illicit drug use by both reducing drug hunger and withdrawal and producing cross-tolerance. "Cross-tolerance" means that tolerance, which is the diminished intensity of a drug's effects after repeated and sustained dosing, will develop not only to the precise drug that is being taken repeatedly but also to other drugs from the same pharmacological class (e.g., methadone and heroin, which are both opioids). Examples of substitution agents that produce cross-tolerance to heroin and have been shown to be effective in reducing illicit opioid use are methadone, levo-alpha-acetyl methadol (LAAM), and buprenorphine.

Blocking and substitution are not necessarily incompatible, and partial agonists provide a pharmacological tool to combine both approaches in treating drug dependence. At low doses partial agonists such as buprenorphine, suppress withdrawal symptoms in dependent patients and produce some subjective reinforcing properties, whereas at higher dosages, these same medications block the reinforcement from full agonists. Thus, buprenorphine at low doses suppresses heroin withdrawal and at high doses blocks the euphoric Finally, any of these pharmacotherapies should be administered in the context of psychosocial interventions developed to encourage adherence to medications to facilitate the rehabilitation that is a necessary component to any successful treatment.

In the following sections, we review a variety of standard treatments for SUDs, as well as several new agents. The goal is to provide an overview of current pharmacological treatments for nicotine, alcohol, sedative/hypnotic, opioid, and cocaine use disorders.

NICOTINE PHARMACOTHERAPIES

A variety of pharmacotherapies are available for the treatment of nicotine dependence. Pharmacotherapies for nicotine dependence, which have been shown to have some efficacy for smoking cessation and the relief of acute withdrawal symptoms, include nicotine replacement therapy, several antidepressants, and clonidine. A nicotine antagonist is also available.

Acute Withdrawal Medications

Nicotine polacrilex gum contains 2 or 4 mg of nicotine; 50–90% of the nicotine is released, depending on the rate of chewing, and is absorbed through the buccal mucosa, with peak nicotine concentrations reached in 15–30 minutes (Lee & D'Alonzo, 1993). Scheduled dosing (i.e., 1 piece of gum per hour) is more effective than using the gum as needed for craving (Hughes, 1996). Absorption of nicotine is decreased in an acidic environment, and patients should be instructed not to consume acidic beverages such as coffee, juices, and soda immediately before, during, or after use of the gum (Henningfield, Stapleton, Benowitz, Grayson, & London, 1993). Nicotine polacrilex has been shown to reduce withdrawal symptoms of anger, irritability, anxiety, depression, and decreased concentration, although craving for cigarettes is unaffected (Lee & D'Alonzo, 1993). The average length of treatment is 4–6 weeks (Hatsukami, Huber, Callies, & Skoog, 1993). One-year follow-up studies show that quit rates for nicotine polacrilex gum range from 8 to 10% when given with physician advice and minimal support. This increases to 29% when combined with behavioral treatment (Hall, Hall, & Ginsberg, 1990). The 4 mg dose of nicotine polacrilex gum is more effective than the 2 mg nicotine dose in the treatment of highly dependent smokers who smoke in excess of 25 cigarettes daily (Hughes, Goldstein, Hurt, & Schiffman, 1999).

Transdermal nicotine administration is another variation of the nicotine replacement approach to smoking cessation. These systems are available in regimens that deliver nicotine over a 16- or 24-hour duration (delivering 15 mg and 21–22 mg, respectively) (Palmer, Buckley, & Faulds, 1992). Nicotine is slowly absorbed, with peak levels reached 6–10 hours after application, and nicotine levels are about half those obtained through smoking. It is recommended that those smoking more than 10 cigarettes daily use the highest dose nicotine patch, while those smoking fewer than 10 cigarettes per day can use the lower dose patches. Patch use is generally recommended for 8 weeks, with 4 weeks at the highest dose, followed by 2 weeks each at the lower doses prior to discontinuation. No advantage has been shown by use of the nicotine patch after 8 weeks (Fiore et al., 2000). Abrupt cessation of patch use has not been associated with significant withdrawal; therefore, tapering may not be necessary (Fiore, Smith, Jorenby, & Baker, 1994). Transdermal nicotine systems have been generally well tolerated, with minor side effects of local irritation at the application site, mild gastric disturbances, and sleep disturbances, and their use has been reported to be associated with delayed weight gain. Nicotine patches produce end-of-treatment smoking cessation rates from 18 to 77% (about twice that of placebo-treated subjects), and 6-month abstinence rates range from 22 to 42% (compared to 5–28% for placebo-treated subjects) with some fluctuation depending on counseling (Fiore, Jorenby, Baker, & Kenford, 1992). For those who fail with either gum or patch alone, the two may be combined. In these cases, the highest dose of the nicotine patch available should be used with the 2 mg nicotine gum. Other nicotine delivery systems used less frequently in clinical practice include a nasal spray and an inhaler.

The observed relationship between nicotine dependence and mood disorders led to research examining the potential for antidepressant medications as effective pharmacotherapies for cigarette smoking cessation (Glassman, 1997), including tricyclic, monoamine oxidase (MAO) inhibiting, serotonin reuptake–inhibiting, and other forms of antidepressants. Two large, multicenter clinical trials demonstrated the efficacy of bupropion for the treatment of nicotine dependence, and it is recommended as a first-line treatment for smoking cessation (Fiore et al., 2000). Disadvantages of bupropion include more frequent adverse events of tremor, rash, headache, urticaria, insomnia, and dry mouth, resulting in an 8–12% discontinuation rate in clinical trials. Bupropion also lowers seizure threshold and should not be used in those at risk for seizures (American Psychiatric Association, 1996). The antidepressant dose is the same as that for the treatment of depression, allowing for the pharmacological treatment of both disorders simultaneously.

Two positive clinical trials (Hall et al., 1998; Prochaska et al., 1998) have led to the recommendation of nortriptyline as a second-line choice for smoking cessation (Fiore et al., 2000). The target dose of this drug for treatment of nicotine dependence is 75–100 mg daily, but it should be used with caution in those with cardiovascular disease given its possible effects on cardiac function. Like bupropion, nortriptyline is an antidepressant and may be useful in the treatment of depressed cigarette smokers. Another antidepressant related medication, selegiline, an MAO inhibitor, has shown some recent efficacy in reducing smoking (George et al., 2003).

Finally, clonidine, a noradrenergic alpha$_2$ agonist that decreases central sympathetic activity, may be an effective treatment for those who do not want nicotine replacement therapy or who have failed other smoking cessation methods.

ALCOHOL PHARMACOTHERAPIES

Acute Withdrawal Medications

Acute withdrawal from alcohol is a serious medical condition that can precipitate adrenergic activation, seizures, or delirium tremens, a condition with up to 15% mortality when untreated (Kosten & O'Connor, 2003). The current standard approach to alcohol detoxification uses tapering dosages of benzodiazepines, such as chlordiazepoxide or clonazepam, which are effective in relieving the autonomic hyperactivity of withdrawal and will prevent seizures. Benzodiazepines are initially made available on an as-needed basis, with parameters for dosing based on appearance of withdrawal symptoms including agitation, diaphoresis, tremor, hypertension, and tachycardia. Withdrawal symptoms can be assessed over the course of the detoxification using the Clinical Institute Withdrawal Assessment of Alcohol Scale, revised (CIWA-Ar; Sullivan, Sykora, Schneiderman, Naranjo, & Sellers, 1989). This extensively studied scale has been shown to have good reliability, reproducibility, and validity. The scale measures 10 symptoms associated with withdrawal, each of which can be scored in increasing severity on a scale of 0–7 (with the exception of orientation and clouding of sensorium, which are scored on a scale of 0–4. Scores above 10 indicate a need for medication to treat withdrawal symptoms. Furthermore, the CIWA predicts that those with a score of greater than 15 are at increased risk for severe alcohol withdrawal, with higher scores conveying higher risk. Although detoxification schedules must be individualized, a benzodiazepine taper can usually be accomplished in 3–4 days. Patients with hepatic disease should be detoxified with lorazepam or oxazepam, shorter-acting drugs that, unlike the other benzodiazepines, have no active metabolites requiring hepatic clearance. Lorazepam is also a good choice for detoxification of the patient with severe vomiting, because it is well absorbed by the intramuscular route of administration.

Anticonvulsants have been shown to be equal in effectiveness to benzodiazepines in the treatment of alcohol withdrawal (Malcolm, Myrick, Brady, & Ballenger, 2001). Multiple studies support the efficacy of sodium valproate

(1,000 mg daily in divided doses) in reducing the symptoms associated with alcohol withdrawal. Further double-blind studies are needed before routine use of this drug can be recommended in alcohol detoxification. Several studies reported on the use of valproate, which appears to show good success when used alone for alcohol detoxification (Hillbom et al., 1989; Roy-Byrne, Ward, & Donnelly, 1989). Sodium valproate should not be used in those with preexisting hepatic or hematological abnormalities. The extended release formulation of valproate now available may be superior for detoxification in order to have once daily dosing, less variation in blood levels, reduction in toxicity (peak levels), and reduced symptom breakthrough during dosing (trough levels).

Carbamazepine, an anticonvulsant that has been widely used in alcohol withdrawal, has been shown to be superior to placebo in the rapidity with which it relieves alcohol withdrawal symptoms, including tremor, sweating, palpitations, sleep disturbances, depression, anxiety, and anorexia (Bjorkquist et al., 1976). In outpatient randomized clinical trials comparing carbamazepine to tapering dosages of benzodiazepines, the patients receiving carbamazepine had higher success rates and fewer withdrawal symptoms during alcohol detoxification (Agricola, 1982; Malcolm, Ballenger, Sturgis, & Anton, 1989). In a study comparing carbamazepine to lorazepam for treatment of alcohol withdrawal, participants were treated over 5 days with a fixed-dose taper of carbamazepine 800 mg versus lorazepam 8 mg on day 1. Follow-up showed that both drugs effectively suppress withdrawal symptoms, but carbamazepine-treated individuals showed less posttreatment drinking behavior, and those who reported drinking stated that they drank less following carbamazepine treatment (Malcolm et al., 2002). This finding has yet to be replicated in additional studies. Carbamazepine has common side effects of dizziness, nausea, and vomiting. It may induce the metabolism of drugs that are substrates of hepatic cytochrome P450-3A4 and should not be used in persons with severe hepatic or hematological disease(s). Its efficacy has also not been established in severe alcohol withdrawal. However, carbamazepine can be effective alone as a withdrawal medication in mild to moderate alcohol withdrawal syndromes.

The combination of anticonvulsants and moderate doses of benzodiazepines can facilitate successful alcohol detoxification in those with a history of previous alcohol withdrawal seizures or head trauma (Kasser, Geller, Howell, & Wartenberg, 1997). In these cases, the anticonvulsant should be administered concomitantly with benzodiazepines in dosages that will provide therapeutic anticonvulsant blood levels. The anticonvulsant should be tapered within a week of completion of the benzodiazepine taper. There is no indication for continuation of anticonvulsant therapy in individuals who have experienced generalized, nonfocal seizures secondary to alcohol withdrawal. It is, however, important to assess such patients carefully, because any focal neurological signs may be indicative of an underlying neurological disorder requiring treatment.

Two newer anticonvulsants, vigabatrin and gabapentin, have been examined as adjunctive therapies for the treatment of alcohol withdrawal (Myrick, Brady, & Malcolm, 2001; Myrick, Malcolm, & Brady, 1998), but further controlled studies are needed. Two older medicines, phenytoin and phenobarbital are not recommended for routine use.

Protracted withdrawal consisting of subtle symptoms such as sleep dysregulation, anxiety, irritability, and mood instability lasting weeks to months are reported by some alcohol-dependent patients. Patients experiencing such symptoms are more vulnerable to relapse.

Maintenance Medications

A variety of agents have been used for reducing relapse to alcohol use, including disulfiram and naltrexone. Other medications include agents such as serotonin reuptake inhibitors (SRIs), ondansetron, topiramate, buspirone, and acamprosate.

Disulfiram is a relatively nonspecific, irreversible inhibitor of sulfhydryl-containing enzymes (Wright & Moore, 1990). The target enzyme for the pharmacological effect of disulfiram in the treatment of alcohol addiction is aldehyde dehydrogenase, which converts acetaldehyde to acetate in alcohol metabolism. When ethyl alcohol is present in the liver, disulfiram causes acetaldehyde to accumulate, leading to the disulfiram–alcohol reaction: flushing, weakness, nausea, tachycardia, and, in some instances, hypotension (Wright & Moore, 1990). Disulfiram has not been shown to be effective in achieving abstinence or delaying relapse (Fuller & Roth, 1979). However, in motivated patients who are intelligent, not impulsive, and have no comorbid major psychiatric disorder, and in combination with psychosocial treatments, disulfiram may be effective (Fuller et al., 1986). Treatment of the disulfiram reaction is primarily supportive and includes fluid hydration, oxygen, and Trendelenburg posture (Elenbaas, 1977). Disulfiram must not be initiated until alcohol is completely eliminated (usually 24 hours after the last drink). Standard daily dose is 250 mg orally (range, 125–500 mg daily). The time to onset of aldehyde dehydrogenase inhibition sufficient to result in a reaction on alcohol consumption is 12 hours, and aldehyde dehydrogenase recovery is complete within 6 days of the last disulfiram dose (Helander & Carlsson, 1990). Patients taking disulfiram must be warned to avoid alcohol-containing products and foods. Disulfiram may also produce a variety of adverse effects, which are rare, but the most severe are hepatotoxicity and neuropathies. This medication should be avoided in patients with moderate to severe hepatic dysfunction, peripheral neuropathies, pregnancy, renal failure, or cardiac disease.

Opioid antagonists can be used in the treatment of alcohol dependence. Volpicelli, Alterman, O'Brien, and Hayashida (1992) conducted a double-blind, controlled study in which 35 male veterans were randomized to naltrexone (50 mg daily) and 35 to placebo. Naltrexone was found to significantly reduce alcohol craving, days of drinking per week, and the rate of relapse among those who drank. The second study (O'Malley et al., 1992) involved 97 subjects and used a 2 × 2 design in which two of the groups received naltrexone, 50 mg daily, and two of the groups received placebo combined with either coping skills therapy or a supportive therapy. During this 12-week trial, the rate of relapse in those patients treated with naltrexone was 45%, whereas patients on placebo had a 90% relapse rate. Naltrexone was well tolerated and appeared to reduce alcohol consumption and relapse rates. The psychotherapy also had an interesting interaction with naltrexone treatment. Although the patients in the coping skills group were more likely to initiate drinking, they were less likely to relapse than were patients treated with supportive therapy. For those subjects who drank during the study, the most success in avoiding relapse was attained by the naltrexone and coping skills group, which had a relapse rate of less than 35%. The worst outcome was in the placebo and supportive therapy group, where 90% relapsed, and for this placebo group, most of the relapses occurred within 30 days of initiating the study. Thus, the second study showed promise for not only this pharmacotherapy but also its combination with a specific psychotherapeutic intervention.

A 6-month follow-up study reported on the persistence of naltrexone and psychotherapy effects following discontinuation after 12 weeks of treatment for alcohol dependence (O'Malley et al., 1996). Subjects who received naltrexone were less likely to drink heavily (defined as more than 5 drinks/day in men, and more than 4 drinks/day in women) or meet criteria for alcohol abuse or dependence than those who received placebo, but only through the first month of follow-up, suggesting that some patients may benefit from a period of naltrexone treatment exceeding 12 weeks. Others have also demonstrated a modest but consistent effect of naltrexone treatment on drinking outcomes (Anton et al., 1999).

Other drugs and administration forms include long-acting, depot formulations of naltrexone being developed as an alternative to daily or thrice weekly oral dosing of the drug. (Volpicelli, Rhines, & Rhines, 1997). The opiate antagonist, nalmefene, is also being examined as a treatment for alcohol dependence. It may have advantages over naltrexone in that it is active not only at mu opioid receptors but also at kappa and delta opioid receptors. It may have fewer gastrointestinal side effects, better bioavailability, and less liver toxicity associated with its use (Mason, Salvato, & Williams, 1999).

Serotonergic agents, including buspirone (5-HT$_{1A}$ agonist) (Kranzler et al., 1994), SRIs, and ondansetron (5-HT$_3$ antagonist) (Sellers, Higgins, Tompkins, & Romach, 1992), have been studied as treatments for alcohol dependence but results have been limited. The possible matching of medications to patient type or comorbid condition may be an effective approach to treatment of alcohol dependence, but this remains to be demonstrated in clinical trials (Myrick et al., 2001). Studies showed that ondansetron reduced alcohol craving in early-onset (but not late-onset) alcoholics, and reduced drinking in these individuals (Johnson et al., 2000), but these results need to be replicated in larger controlled trials.

Not yet available in the United States, acamprosate (calcium acetylhomotaurinate), an analogue of homocysteic acid, has a structure similar to gamma-aminobutyric acid (GABA) and, as such, has been reported to stimulate inhibitory GABA transmission and to antagonize excitatory amino acids (Zeise, Kasparov, Capogna, & Zieglgansberger, 1993). These properties have been postulated to be important to reduction in alcohol craving (Littleton, 1995). Acamprosate has no abuse potential, hypnotic muscle relaxant, or anxiolytic properties. Furthermore, it is not hepatically metabolized and is, instead, excreted as unchanged drug by the kidneys, allowing its safe use in those with liver impairment, although it should not be administered to those with renal insufficiency (Wilde & Wagstaff, 1997). A review of acamprosate studies showed that in 14 of 16 controlled clinical trials, those treated with acamprosate had higher rates of treatment completion for alcohol dependence, longer abstinence period to first drink, and higher overall abstinence rates than those treated with placebo (Mason, 2001; Mason & Ownby, 2000). Acamprosate treatment in several studies also was associated with decreases in laboratory indices of alcohol consumption, including gamma-glutamyltransferase and carbohydrate-deficient transferrin (Graham, Wodak, & Whelan, 2002). The drug was found to be well tolerated and acceptable to patients.

Several studies have compared naltrexone and acamprosate treatment for alcohol dependence. In a 1-year follow-up study, no differences were observed in time to first drink, but time to first relapse was shorter in acamprosate-treated patients, while those treated with naltrexone were found to have a greater cumulative number of days of abstinence, to consume fewer drinks at one time, and to have less craving for alcohol (Rubio, Jimenez-Arriero, Ponce, & Palomo, 2001). In a study comparing naltrexone, acamprosate, naltrexone and acamprosate in combination, and placebo, both active drugs and the combination were associated with significantly longer time to first drink and relapse to alcohol use relative to placebo. Additionally, there was a trend toward more positive outcomes in the naltrexone-treated group relative to the acamprosate-treated group. The combination was more effective than placebo or acamprosate but not naltrexone (Kiefer et al., 2003).

BENZODIAZEPINE PHARMACOTHERAPIES

The benzodiazepines are some of the most frequently prescribed medications in the United States due to their efficacy as anxiolytics and muscle relaxants, rapid onset of action, and relatively low risk of toxicity relative to other medications with similar indications. However, benzodiazepines, similar to alcohol, have abuse liability, and produce physiological and psychological dependence. Physiological dependence occurs with longer term (greater than 30 days) use, requiring tapering of the drug, and tolerance that develops with prolonged use can lead to escalating dosages. Interestingly, severity of the withdrawal syndrome does not correlate significantly with difficulty in benzodiazepine taper (Rickels, De Martinis, Rynn, & Mandos, 1999). Personality psychopathology appears to contribute to withdrawal severity and lack of successful taper. Furthermore, a study examining benzodiazepine taper in a sample of sedative/hypnotic-dependent patients reported that those with personality pathology were more likely to drop out of the taper in the early stage prior to significant dose reductions (Rickels, Schweizer, Case, & Garcia-Espana, 1988). In a 3-year follow-up study of outcomes, it was determined that those who participated in a taper leading to a 50% reduction in daily benzodiazepine use had a 39% rate of being benzodiazepine-free. Eighty-six percent of those who refused a taper continued benzodiazepine use at 3 years, and those who successfully ended benzodiazepine use reported significantly lower levels of anxiety compared to patients who continued to use benzodiazepines (Rickels, Case, Schweizer, Garcia-Espana, & Fridman, 1991).

Benzodiazepine taper can be undertaken rapidly in an inpatient setting or slowly on an outpatient basis. The taper of a benzodiazepine is usually undertaken with the substitution of another benzodiazepine, particularly if the patient is dependent on a drug with a short half-life. These drugs can be tapered by converting the daily reported use of a benzodiazepine reduced by 50% to the equivalent dose of chlordiazepoxide, clonazepam, or, in cases where there is concern for hepatic disease and a decreased ability to metabolize the benzodiazepine and its active metabolites, or concern about inability of the patient to take oral medications, lorazepam. The total daily dose required to stabilize the patient on the first day of the taper can be reduced by up to 10–20% daily, leading to detoxification over several days.

OPIOID PHARMACOTHERAPIES

Treatment of Overdose

Opioid overdose is a medical emergency and can be life threatening when complications of coma and/or respiratory arrest occur. Naloxone is an injectable drug that rapidly reverses effects of opioid overdose by displacing the opioid from receptors in the brain. Naloxone may be administered intravenously or, in those without venous access, by subcutaneous injection. A dosage of 0.4–0.8 mg should reverse most opioid overdoses. In dependent patients, lower doses (0.1–0.2 mg) may be sufficient; furthermore, it is not advisable to precipitate withdrawal in these patients. Therefore, in these cases, treatment should begin with lower naloxone doses, with the dosage increased as clinically indicated.

Once the symptoms of overdose have abated, it is important to continue to monitor level of consciousness and respiratory status, because long-acting opioids may require prolonged naloxone treatment that can be administered by intravenous infusion. Patients with opioid overdose should react within minutes to this treatment. Failure to do so should call into question the working diagnosis and prompt additional evaluation.

Treatment of Acute Withdrawal

Clonidine reduces the severity of acute opioid withdrawal. Using the opioid antagonists naloxone or naltrexone to precipitate withdrawal, while simultaneously treating the patient with relatively high doses of clonidine, has enabled opioid-dependent patients to become drug free within as little as 3 days, while minimizing the antagonist-precipitated symptoms (Charney et al., 1982; Kleber, Topazian, Gaspari, Riordan, & Kosten, 1987; Vining, Kosten, & Kleber, 1988). The duration of withdrawal using this approach was equivalent for methadone- or heroin-dependent patients; ordinarily withdrawal symptoms last nearly twice as long after abruptly stopping methadone, just as they do after stopping heroin (Kleber, 1981).

Administering an antagonist such as naltrexone precipitates withdrawal within minutes for both types of patients, and this process of precipitation appears to equalize the duration of subsequent withdrawal symptoms. The amount of clonidine needed to ameliorate these symptoms was also lessened by larger initial doses of naltrexone. Detoxification with a starting dose of 12.5 mg of naltrexone required clonidine for only 4 days, with a total dose of 1.7 mg and a peak dose of 0.6 mg on day 1 (Vining et al., 1988). Thus, a more rapid and comfortable procedure has evolved for acute detoxification relative to the use of clonidine alone. Another study showed that clonidine, and clonidine and naltrexone in combination, are both efficacious regimens for the ambulatory treatment of opioid withdrawal, with 70% of subjects completing detoxification (O'Connor et al., 1995).

Tapering doses of methadone are often used in ambulatory detoxification, but the protracted withdrawal syndrome associated with methadone cessation contributes to a high rate of relapse to opioid use (Senay, Dorus, Goldberg, & Thornton, 1977). Methadone can be administered in starting doses of 10–20 mg to patients showing evidence of opioid withdrawal. Failure to suppress withdrawal symptoms in 30–60 minutes can be followed with an additional dose of 5–10 mg. A dose similar to the initial dose may be given 12 hours later, if necessary, although this is not usually practical in ambulatory detoxification settings. On day 2, the total dose administered on day 1 can be administered in a single dose. The methadone dose can then be decreased by 5 mg daily, or by 5 mg daily until a dose of 10 mg daily is reached, at which time the dose continues to be tapered by 2 mg daily (for an additional 5 days).

Khan, Mumford, Rogers, and Beckford (1997) reported that lofexidine, an alpha$_2$ adrenergic agonist that produces less hypotension than clonidine, can be a useful adjunctive medication during methadone detoxification. Lofexidine was equal to clonidine in reducing symptoms of opioid withdrawal, and side effects of hypotension and lethargy were reported by substantially fewer patients in the lofexidine group. Clonidine can also be used as an adjunctive medication to assist with emerging withdrawal symptoms during detoxification, but medical complications related to hypotension and sedation can limit tolerance for this drug. Methadone detoxification should be completed within 3 weeks (Van den Brink, Goppel, & van Ree, 2003). Detoxification protocols are summarized in Figure 26.1.

Opioid detoxification can also be undertaken with buprenorphine, an opioid partial agonist (Kosten & Kleber, 1988; Lewis, 1985). In one study, heroin addicts and methadone-maintained patients were converted to buprenorphine for a month of stabilization at once-daily doses ranging from 2 to 8 mg sublingually. Following this period, buprenorphine was abruptly stopped, and the patient was given a high dose of intravenous naloxone (35 mg) to precipitate withdrawal from the buprenorphine (Kosten et al., 1989). This withdrawal syndrome was relatively mild and treated with clonidine, if needed. Following precipitated withdrawal, it was possible for the patient to be started on naltrexone the same day. Additional studies in which the sublingual formulations of buprenorphine are used for detoxification are ongoing at this time. Buprenorphine can also be combined with clonidine and naltrexone for a highly successful rapid detoxification that is medically safe and preferred by patients to the alternative of clonidine alone or clonidine plus naltrexone in heroin- or methadone-stabilized patients. The details for such a buprenorphine protocol are also provided in Figure 26.1.

Another method of opiate detoxification has been termed "rapid" or "ultrarapid" detoxification in which withdrawal is precipitated by administration of either naloxone or naltrexone, with heavy sedation or anesthesia to ease withdrawal symptoms. This procedure produces more severe withdrawal than standard opioid detoxification procedures, but the hypothesis is that the use of an opioid antagonist to induce withdrawal will curtail the duration of the withdrawal syndrome. This procedure has been associated with severe adverse events, including complications of anesthesia, severe withdrawal symptoms lasting for several days following the procedure, and, rarely, death (Badenoch, 2002; Cucchia, Monat, Spagnoli, Ferrero, & Gertschy, 1998; O'Connor & Kosten, 1998; Rabinowitz, Cohen, & Atias, 2002; Scherbaum et al., 1998). Furthermore, this procedure has not been associated with better long-term outcomes in terms of relapse to opiate dependence, calling into question the expense and risk of the procedure relative to other procedures for opioid withdrawal (Cucchia et al., 1998; Lawental, 2000; Rabinowitz et al., 2002; Scherbaum et al., 1998).

Clonidine detoxification (9-day protocol)

	1	Detoxification day 2 3 4	5 6 7	8 9
Clonidine[a,b]	0.1–0.2 mg (oral) Max. dose: 1 mg on day 1	Every 4 hours as needed Max. dose: 1.2 mg on days 2–4	Taper to 0 on days 5–8	
Naltrexone[b]				25 mg 50 mg

Clonidine with naltrexone induction (5-day protocol)

Clonidine[b]	Preload: 0.2–0.4 mg Max. dose: 1.2 mg on days 1–2		Taper to 0 on days 3–5		
Oxazepam[b]	Preload: 30–60 mg				
Naltrexone[b]	12.5 mg	25 mg	50 mg	50 mg 50 mg	

Note. As needed: oxazepam 30–60 mg every 6 hours for cramps, insomnia; ibuprofen 600 mg every 6 hours for cramps; prochlorperazine 5 mg i.m. every 6 hours for vomiting.
[a] Hold for systolic blood pressure < 90 mm Hg or diastolic blood pressure < 60.
[b] Oral dosing.

Methadone detoxification	Detoxification day 1	2	3
Methadone	10–20 mg; may give additional 5–10 mg 12 hours later if symptoms reemerge	Give entire day 1 methadone amount as one dose	Decrease by 5 mg daily or decrease by 5 mg daily until 10 mg/day; then decrease by 2 mg daily to complete taper

Buprenorphine detoxification	Day 1	Day 2	Day 3	Day 4	Days 5–7
Buprenorphine at dose of 8–20 mg daily tapered to 4 mg daily for ≥ 2 days	Discontinue buprenorphine for 24–96 hours				
Clonidine		0.1 mg × 3 (9, 10, and 11 A.M.); each dose spaced by 1 hour as tolerated (check blood pressure and hold if orthostatic); continue every 6 hours as tolerated; give one additional dose before leaving clinic	0.1–0.3 mg at 9 A.M.; then every 6 hours	0.1–0.3 mg at 9 A.M.; begin clonidine taper by 25% daily	Continue taper by 25% daily
Naltrexone		12.5 mg at noon	25 mg at 11 A.M.	50 mg at 11 A.M.	50 mg daily

FIGURE 26.1. Ambulatory opioid detoxification medication protocols.

Success rates for detoxification treatments have generally assessed only short-term outcomes of becoming either opioid-free or opioid-free with concomitant naltrexone treatment, which is not a widely used treatment. Consideration should be given to maintaining such patients on an opioid antagonist medication such as naltrexone, because relapse to illicit opioid use following medical withdrawal is frequent ($\geq$ 90%) over a 6- to 12-month period without sustained outpatient treatment (Kleber, 1981; Kosten & Kleber, 1984). In a study of methadone maintenance versus a 180-day methadone detoxification program with enhanced psychosocial treatment services, methadone maintenance therapy resulted in greater treatment retention and lower heroin use than did the enhanced detoxification treatment (Sees et al., 2000). This observation underscores the difficulty of successfully undertaking opiate detoxification in heroin-addicted patients and speaks to the need to increase the availability of opiate therapy programs that can provide long-term opiate pharmacotherapy to this population (Rounsaville & Kosten, 2000).

Maintenance Medications

There are currently four drugs approved for the maintenance treatment of opioid dependence: naltrexone, methadone, LAAM, and the opioid partial agonist buprenorphine. These medication treatments are summarized below.

Naltrexone, an opioid antagonist that is administered orally, can be used in those patients who do not want to be maintained on opioids. Naltrexone should not be initiated until the patient is completely detoxified from opioids to avoid precipitating withdrawal (with the exception of the use of the clonidine–naltrexone detoxification procedure described earlier). An abstinence period of 7–10 days from short-acting opioids (e.g., heroin) and 10 days of abstinence from long-acting opioids (e.g., methadone) is usually required. If doubt exists as to the opioid history, a "naloxone challenge" may be given: Lack of withdrawal symptoms indicates the absence of current physiological opioid dependence, and naltrexone can then be administered. To perform a naloxone challenge, 2 ml of naloxone (0.4 mg/ml) solution is prepared, and an initial dose of 0.5 ml of this solution (0.2 mg of naloxone) is administered intravenously. Symptoms of opioid withdrawal (mydriasis, dysphoria, diaphoresis, and gastrointestinal discomfort) in approximately 30 seconds indicate that the patient remains dependent. If no withdrawal is observed, the remaining naloxone solution is administered and observation is continued. If intravenous access is not available, 2 ml of the naloxone solution may be administered subcutaneously, with an observation period of 45 minutes (Galloway & Hayner, 1993).

The standard dose of naltrexone is 50 mg daily, although this drug can also be administered less frequently at larger doses (100 mg every 2 days, or 150 mg every third day). Naltrexone will attenuate/block effects of opioid agonists and assist in relapse prevention. Naltrexone should be administered for at least 6 months, and discontinuation should be carefully planned. Naltrexone side effects are few, but hepatotoxicity has been reported, and hepatic function should be monitored before and during administration. The biggest problem with naltrexone has been a lack of patient and clinician acceptance of the treatment.

For patients who chronically relapse to opioid dependence, the treatment of choice is maintenance with a long-acting opioid agonist. The goal of treatment with any long-acting opioid is to achieve a stable dose that reduces or, ideally, eliminates illicit opioid craving and use, and facilitates the engagement of the patient in a comprehensive program that promotes substance abuse rehabilitation. Because treatment with long-acting opioids results in dependence, it is important to select patients who have a history of prolonged dependence (greater than 1 year) and demonstrate physiological dependence (positive urine toxicology screen for opioids and evidence of opiate withdrawal prior to initiation of treatment).

Methadone, the most widely used of these long-acting opioids, is effective in decreasing psychosocial consequences and medical morbidity associated with opioid dependence. It is also an important tool in decreasing the spread of human immunodeficiency virus infection in and by injection drug users. The efficacy of methadone spans a wide range of doses, and each patient's dose must be individually titrated. Methadone, 40–60 mg daily, will block opioid withdrawal symptoms, but doses of 70–80 mg daily are more often needed to curb craving. Generally, doses greater than 60 mg daily are associated with better retention in treatment and less illicit opioid use (Ball & Ross, 1991).

LAAM, a methadone congener that is longer acting and was thought to have had potential advantages over methadone, has been associated with cardiac electrophysiological complications in some patients, resulting in revised labeling that includes a black box warning recommending that an electrocardiogram (EKG) be performed prior to treatment, 12–14 days after initiation of LAAM, and then periodically thereafter to rule out any alterations in the QT interval (Orlaam Package Insert, 2001). The finding that LAAM and its metabolites, norLAAM and dinorLAAM exert negative chronotropic effects and negative ionotropic responses in cardiac tissue, and the association of LAAM with several lethal cardiac dysrhythmias (including torsades de dointes) has resulted in its no longer being a first-line treatment for opioid dependence in the United States (Expert Panel Consensus Guidelines, 2002). LAAM has been removed from the market in the European Union.

Buprenorphine, an opioid partial agonist, was approved for use as a treatment for opioid dependence in October 2002. Buprenorphine, formulated as a sublingual tablet, is available as a single agent or as a combination tablet containing buprenorphine and naloxone in a ratio of 4:1. The latter combination product was designed to prevent the drug from being diverted to injection drug use. The injection of this drug in those addicted to full mu agonist drugs (e.g., heroin, methadone, LAAM) would produce opiate withdrawal symptoms. Buprenorphine has been shown to be a safer drug than methadone in that a plateau was observed for dose effects in terms of subjective responses and respiratory depression (Walsh, Preston, Stitzer, Cone, & Bigelow, 1994). Several clinical trials have been reported in which buprenorphine showed comparable efficacy to other opiate therapies. Johnson and colleagues (2000) reported that in a 17-week randomized study, compared to low-dose methadone maintenance (20 mg daily), high-dose methadone maintenance (60–100 mg daily), LAAM (75–100 mg daily), and buprenorphine (16–32 mg daily) substantially reduced the use of illicit opioids. The recommended daily dose of buprenorphine is 16 mg, although a range of 12–24 mg daily is possible, and dosage should be individualized for each patient.

Induction with buprenorphine is a straightforward clinical procedure in which the patient is instructed to present for induction not having used opioids for at least 4 hours and in mild withdrawal. An initial dose of 4 mg is administered and may be followed 2 hours later by another dose of 4 mg (not to exceed 8 mg on day 1). On the second day, a dose of 12–16 mg may be administered. Once a dose of 16 mg is reached, the patient should be followed for several days to determine whether the dose is one that suppresses withdrawal and reduces drug craving. Adjustments up or down should be based on clinical examination. Another potential advantage to buprenorphine is that it can be dosed three times per week or daily (Schottenfeld et al., 2000). A study of outcomes after 1 year of buprenorphine treatment (16 mg daily) or placebo given with psychosocial interventions showed a highly significant positive treatment effect of buprenorphine both in terms of retention in treatment and reduction in the use of illicit drugs (opiates, stimulants, cannabinoids, and benzodiazepines) (Kakko, Svanborg, Kreek, & Heilig, 2003).

The significant advantage to buprenorphine is that it is the first opioid therapy for the treatment of opioid dependence that can be obtained by prescription from the patient's primary care physician or psychiatrist. Physicians who wish to prescribe buprenorphine must have special training to comply with governmental regulations.

Drug–Drug Interactions

Individuals with SUDs often suffer with comorbid medical or mental disorders that themselves require pharmacotherapy. The prescribing of multiple medications to the same patient can result in adverse interactions between medications, leading to adverse events and, in many cases, nonadherence to medication regimens, increased use of illicit drugs, drug toxicities, and lack of therapeutic benefit of treatment regimens. These interactions can be especially difficult in the opioid-dependent patient who is maintained on an opiate therapy. These patients are at risk for opiate withdrawal syndromes when prescribed medications that induce the metabolism of opioids (e.g., inducers of cytochrome P450-3A4) and for opiate toxicity should a coadministered medication inhibit opioid metabolism. Similarly, if an opioid delays absorption of a medication or inhibits the metabolism of the drug; toxicity from the drug may occur. Table 26.1 summarizes drug interactions that have been shown to occur in opioid-maintained patients treated with medications for comorbid medical or psychiatric disorders.

COCAINE PHARMACOTHERAPIES

Cocaine affects multiple neurotransmitters, including release and reuptake blockade of dopamine, norepinephrine, and serotonin (Koe, 1976). Many medications, including antidepressants, anticonvulsants, and dopaminergic agents, have been studied as potential treatments for cocaine dependence. However, none has been proven an effective pharmacotherapy in randomized, controlled clinical trials, and none have been approved by the U.S. Food and Drug Administration (FDA) for this indication (Boyarsky & McCance-Katz, 2000; Jin & McCance-Katz, 2003; McCance-Katz, 1997; Silva de Lima et al., 2002).

One outpatient, randomized clinical trial in which disulfiram, 250 mg daily, was administered in combination with psychotherapies in cocaine-dependent, alcohol-abusing patients showed that disulfiram significantly reduced cocaine and alcohol use. Few adverse events were observed in this study (Carroll, Nich, Ball, McCance, & Rounsaville, 1998). A 1-year follow-up evaluation with 96 of the participants in this study showed that the effects of disulfiram in reducing cocaine and alcohol use were sustained (Carroll et al., 2000). Subsequently, Petrakis and colleagues (2000) showed, in a double-blind, randomized, controlled study, that disulfiram treatment decreased cocaine and alcohol use in methadone-maintained patients who were also cocaine dependent. George and colleagues (2000) showed similar findings in buprenorphine-maintained, opioid-addicted patients who were also cocaine dependent.

Naltrexone, an opioid antagonist approved for the treatment of opioid and alcohol dependence, is also being examined as a treatment for cocaine dependence. Although results of earlier studies in patients with comorbid cocaine and alcohol dependence were not encouraging, Oslin and colleagues (1999) reported that dosing of naltrexone, 150 mg daily, in cocaine- and alcohol-dependent individuals was associated with decreased cocaine and alcohol use. Naltrexone, 50 mg daily, was found to be associated with significantly less cocaine use when administered in combination with relapse prevention therapy (Schmitz, Stotts, Rhoades, & Grabowski, 2001). The results from these studies suggest that the effectiveness of naltrexone may depend on multiple factors, including other substance comorbidity, dose of naltrexone, length of treatment,

TABLE 26.1. Drug Interactions between Methadone or LAAM and Medications Used to Treat Other Common Conditions in Opioid-Dependent Patients

	Indication	Interaction with methadone or LAAM
Psychotropic medications		
Fluvoxamine	Depression	↑ Methadone levels with potential toxicity (Eap et al., 1997)
Desipramine	Depression	↑ Desipramine levels (Gourevitch & Friedland, 2000)
Sertraline	Depression	↑ Methadone levels without reported toxicity (Hamilton et al., 2000)
Valproic acid	Seizure disorder, bipolar affective disorder	None reported (Saxon et al., 1989)
Carbamazepine	Seizure disorder, bipolar affective disorder	↓ Methadone levels (Eap et al., 2002)
Other medications		
Phenytoin	Seizure disorder	↓ Methadone levels (Eap et al., 2002)
Phenobarbital	Seizure disorder	↓ Methadone levels (Eap et al., 2002)
Rifampin	Tuberculosis	↓ Methadone levels (Raistrick et al., 1996)
Rifabutin	Tuberculosis	No change in methadone levels (Brown et al., 1996)
Fluconazole	Fungal infection	↑ Methadone levels by ≈ 35%; clinical significance unknown (Cobb et al., 1998)
Ciprofloxacin	Bacterial infection	↑ Methadone levels with toxicity reported (Herrlin et al., 2000)
Zidovudine (AZT)	HIV	↑ Methadone associated with increase in AZT levels (McCance-Katz et al., 2002)
Didanosine (ddI)	HIV	↓ ddI levels by 63% (Rainey et al., 2000)
Lamivudine	HIV	None
Lamivudine/ zidovudine	HIV	None (Rainey et al., 2002)
Stavudine (d4T)	HIV	None (Rainey et al., 2000)
Abacavir	HIV	↑ Methadone clearance (Sellers et al., 1999)

(*continued*)

TABLE 26.1. (continued)

	Indication	Interaction with methadone or LAAM
Other medications (cont.)		
Nevirapine	HIV	↓ Methadone levels, withdrawal symptoms (Altice et al., 1999)
Delavirdine	HIV	No significant effect on methadone; ↑ LAAM levels (McCance-Katz et al., 2003)
Efavirenz	HIV	↓ Methadone levels associated with withdrawal (Clarke et al., 2000; McCance-Katz et al., 2002)
Nelfinavir	HIV	↓ Methadone levels, but no withdrawal symptoms observed (Hsyu et al., 2000); case report of methadone withdrawal (McCance-Katz et al., 2000)
		↑ norLAAM and ↓ dinerLAAM (McCance-Katz et al., 2003)
Ritonavir	HIV	No significant effect on methadone (McCance-Katz et al., 2003)
Lopinavir	HIV	↓ Methadone levels, withdrawal symptoms (McCance-Katz et al., 2003)

Note. Data from McCance-Katz, Cropsey, and Gourevitch.

and type of psychotherapeutic intervention. Naltrexone will need to be examined in larger, controlled clinical trials to determine its efficacy as a cocaine pharmacotherapy.

Future Directions for Cocaine Pharmacotherapy

Medications development continues for the treatment of cocaine addiction. Preclinical research focusing on medications that bind the dopamine D_1, D_2, and D_3 receptors is ongoing, although no studies have yet been conducted in humans. A cocaine vaccine is also in clinical trials. Anticocaine antibodies have been developed and have been shown in animal studies to inhibit self-administration. The presence of antibody has also been shown to reduce brain cocaine levels following intravenous or intranasal cocaine administration (Fox, Kantak, & Edwards, 1996). The vaccine is structurally similar to cocaine, but is coupled to a carrier protein that prevents rapid metabolism, thus making it possible to mount an immune response to cocaine (Fox, 1997). The results of clinical trials for efficacy in humans have shown excellent safety, adequate antibody development, and reductions in cocaine abuse (Kosten et al., 2002; Kosten & O'Connor, 2003).

INTERFACE OF PSYCHIATRIC COMORBIDITY AND SUBSTANCE USE DISORDERS

Psychotropic medication treatment of dually diagnosed patients is similar to that of psychiatric patients without SUDs, with several caveats. Patients with psychotic disorders treated with medications that block dopamine receptors may develop postsynaptic dopaminergic supersensitivity, which has been demonstrated in animal studies (Kosten, 1997). This supersensitivity may enhance euphoria from a wide range of abused drugs. Furthermore, patients with chronic psychotic disorders often experience negative symptoms of schizophrenia and dysphoria that may be exacerbated by conventional neuroleptics. These patients will benefit from selection of an atypical neuroleptic that lacks strong dopaminergic antagonism (Kosten & Ziedonis, 1997). Patients with psychotic disorders who are also alcoholic should be carefully evaluated before being treated with disulfiram, a dopamine beta-hydroxylase inhibitor that could exacerbate psychosis in such patients.

Attention-deficit/hyperactivity disorder (ADHD) can occur as a comorbid condition in cocaine abusers who may self-medicate with this stimulant. Cocaine use in this population is often described as ingestion of small amounts of cocaine taken intermittently throughout the day rather than the classic binge pattern characterized by use of multiple doses of cocaine in rapid succession described by those with primary cocaine dependence. Treatment with standard agents used for ADHD, including stimulant medications, may result in cessation of cocaine use.

Depressive disorders are common in those with cocaine and alcohol use disorders. SRIs may be a good choice for these patients because they are less likely to have significant cardiovascular interactions with cocaine and to be lethal in overdose. Monoamine oxidase inhibitors (MAOIs) should never be used in cocaine abusers, because of the risk of hypertensive crisis. Benzodiazepines should be used with caution in those with cormorbid psychiatric and SUDs, and particularly in alcoholic patients, because of cross-tolerance with alcohol and additive effects if combined with alcohol. Benzodiazepines may be required initially to stabilize patients with exacerbation of psychosis or severe agitation but should be tapered as antipsychotics and/or mood stabilizers become therapeutic. Alcoholic patients with anxiety disorders can usually be effectively treated with serotonergic agents (SRIs or partial agonists) or, in some cases, tricyclic antidepressants.

NEUROLOGICAL AND COGNITIVE EFFECTS OF DRUG ABUSE

The neurocognitive effects of drug abuse, while not yet fully elucidated, are likely to have several negative sequelae in drug abusers. Cognitive impairment observed clinically may be associated with perfusion deficits identified in neuroimaging studies. Drug abusers with these deficits may have more difficulty grasping concepts imparted in drug abuse psychotherapy important for initiating and maintaining abstinence. Drug users may be less able to utilize skills taught in psychotherapy interventions aimed at drug and alcohol abuse. These deficits may underlie the observation that some patients with SUDs have high relapse rates despite participation in substance abuse treatment. Finally, these deficits may place drug users at higher risk for medical complications of drug and alcohol use due to both a primary effect of perfusion deficits and secondary effect of cognitive impairment that may contribute to high-risk behaviors leading to medical morbidity. These findings indicate a need to address the issue of cognitive impairment in the drug abuser and point to a new direction in the development of pharmacotherapies for SUDs in the future.

SUMMARY

Substantial progress has been made in the development of pharmacotherapies for the treatment of SUDs. FDA-approved medication therapies are now available for the treatment of nicotine, alcohol, and opiate use disorders. These treatments, utilized in conjunction with a program addressing the psychosocial needs of the patient, represent the most effective regimens available to treat addictive disorders. Research is ongoing to continue to broaden the number of pharmacotherapies available for these disorders. The search for effective medication treatments for other SUDs, such as stimulant use disorders, continues.

ACKNOWLEDGMENTS

This work was supported by Grant Nos. K02-DA00478 (to Elinore F. McCance-Katz) and K05-DA00454 (to Thomas R. Kosten) from the National Institute on Drug Abuse.

REFERENCES

Agricola, R. (1982). Treatment of acute alcohol withdrawal syndrome with carbamazepine: A double-blind comparison with tiapride. *J Int Med Res*, 10, 160–165.

Altice, F. L., Friedland, G. H., & Cooney, E. L. (1999). Nevirapine induced opiate withdrawal among injection drug users with HIV infection receiving methadone. *AIDS*, *13*, 957–962.

Anton, R. F., Moak, D. H., Waid, L. R., Latham, P. K., Malcolm, R. J., & Dias, J. K. (1999). Naltrexone and cognitive behavioral therapy for the treatment of outpatient alcoholics: Results of a placebo-controlled trial. *Am J Psychiatry*, *156*, 1758–1764.

Badenoch, J. (2002). A death following ultra-rapid opiate detoxification: The General Medical Council adjudicates on a commercialized detoxification. *Addiction*, *97*, 475–477.

Ball, J., & Ross, A. (Eds.). (1991). *The effectiveness of methadone maintenance treatment*. New York: Springer-Verlag.

Bjorkquist, S. E., Isohanni, M., Makela, R., & Malinen, L. (1976). Ambulant treatment of alcohol withdrawal symptoms with carbamazepine: A formal multicentre, double-blind comparison with placebo. *Acta Psychiatr Scand*, *53*, 333–342.

Boyarsky, B. K., & McCance-Katz, E. F. (2000). Improving the quality of substance abuse dependency treatment with pharmacotherapy. *Subst Use Misuse*, *35*, 2095–2125.

Brown, L. S., Sawyer, R. C., Li, R., Cobb, M. N., Colborn, D. C., & Narang, P. K. (1996). Lack of a pharmacologic interaction between rifabutin and methadone in HIV-infected former injecting drug users. *Drug Alcohol Depend*, *43*, 71–77.

Carroll, K. M., Nich, C., Ball, S. A., McCance, E., Frankforter, T. L., & Rounsaville, B. J. (2000). One-year follow-up of disulfiram and psychotherapy for cocaine-alcohol users: Sustained effects of treatment. *Addiction*, *95*, 1335–1349.

Carroll, K. M., Nich, C., Ball, S. A., McCance, E., & Rounsaville, B. J. (1998). Treatment of cocaine and alcohol dependence with psychotherapy and disulfiram. *Addiction*, *93*, 713–728.

Charney, D. S., Riordan, C. E., Kleber, H. D., Murburg, M., Braverman, P., Sternberg, D. E., et al. (1982). Clonidine and naltrexone: A safe, effective and rapid treatment of abrupt withdrawal from methadone therapy. *Arch Gen Psychiatry*, *39*, 1327–1332.

Clarke, S., Mulcahy, D., Back, S., Gibbons, S., Tija, J., & Barry, M. (2000). *Managing methadone and non-nucleoside reverse transcriptase inhibitors: Guidelines for clinical practice*. Paper presented at the 7th Conference on Retroviruses and Opportunistic Infections, San Francisco.

Cobb, M. N., Desai, J., Brown, L. S., Zannikos, P. N., & Rainey, P. M. (1998). The effect of fluconazole on the clinical pharmacokinetics of methadone. *Clin Pharmacol Ther*, *63*, 655–662.

Cucchia, A. T., Monnat, M., Spagnoli, J., Ferrero, F., & Gertschy, G. (1998). Ultra-rapid opiate detoxification using deep sedation with oral midazolam: Short and long-term results. *Drug Alcohol Depend*, *52*, 243–250.

Eap, C.B., Bertschy, G., Powell, K., & Baumann, P. (1997). Fluvoxamine and fluoxetine do not interact in the same way with the metabolism of the enantiomers of methadone. *J Clin Psychopharmacol*, *17*, 113–117.

Eap, C. B., Buclin, T., & Baumann, P. (2002). Interindividual variability of the clinical pharmacokinetics of methadone: Implications for the treatment of opioid dependence. *Clin Pharmacokinet*, *41*, 1153–1193.

Elenbaas, R. M. (1977). Drug therapy reviews: Management of the disulfiram–alcohol reaction. *Am J Hosp Pharm, 34*, 827–831.

Expert Panel Clinical Guidelines. (2002). *LAAM in opioid agonist therapy* (Technical Assistance Publication [TAP] Series). Rockville, MD: U.S. Dept. of Health and Human Services, Center for Substance Abuse Treatment.

Fiore, M. C., Bailey, W. C., Cohen, S. J., Dorfman, S. F., Goldstein, M. G., Gritz, E. R., et al. (2000). *Treating tobacco use and dependence: Clinical practice guideline.* Rockville, MD: U.S. Department of Health and Human Services, Public Health Service.

Fiore, M. C., Jorenby, D. E., Baker, T. B., & Kenford, S. L. (1992). Tobacco dependence and the nicotine patch: Clinical guidelines for effective use. *JAMA, 268*, 2687–2694.

Fiore, M. C., Smith, S. S., Jorenby, D. E., & Baker, T. B. (1994). The effectiveness of the nicotine patch for smoking cessation: A meta analysis. *JAMA, 271*, 1940–1946.

Fox, B. S. (1997). Development of a therapeutic vaccine for the treatment of cocaine addiction. *Drug Alcohol Depend , 48*, 153–158.

Fox, B. S., Kantak, K. M., & Edwards, M. A. (1996). Efficacy of a therapeutic cocaine vaccine in rodent models. *Nat Med, 2*, 1129–1132.

Fuller, R. F., Branchey, L., Brightwell, D. R., Derman, R. M., Emrick, C. D., Iber, F. L., et al. (1986). Disulfiram treatment of alcoholism: A Veteran's Administration cooperative study. *JAMA, 256*, 1449–1455.

Fuller, R. F., & Roth, H. P. (1979). Disulfiram for the treatment of alcoholism: An evaluation in 128 men. *Ann Intern Med, 90*, 901–904.

Galloway, G., & Hayner, G. (1993). Haight-Ashbury Free Clinics' drug detoxification protocols: Part 2: Opioid blockade. *J Psychoactive Drugs, 25*, 251–252.

George, T. P., Chawarski, M. C., Pakes, J., Carroll, K. M., Kosten, T. R., & Schottenfeld, R. S. (2000). Disulfiram versus placebo for cocaine dependence in buprenorphine-maintained subjects: A preliminary trial. *Biol Psychiatry, 47*, 1080–1086.

George, T. P., Vessicchio, J. C., Termine, A., Jatlow, P. I., Kosten, T. R., & O'Malley, S. S. (2003). A preliminary placebo-controlled trial of selegiline hydrochloride for smoking cessation. *Biol Psychiatry, 53*, 136–143.

Glassman, A. H. (1997). Cigarette smoking and its comorbidity (NIDA Research Monograph No. 172, p. 52–60). Washington, DC: U.S. Government Printing Office.

Gourevitch, M. N., & Friedland, G. H. (2000). Interactions between methadone and medications used to treat HIV infection: A review. *Mt Sinai J Med, 67*, 429–436.

Graham, R., Wodak, A. D., & Whelan, G. (2002). New pharmacotherapies for alcohol dependence. *Med J Aust, 177*, 103–107.

Hall, S. M., Hall, R. G., & Ginsberg, D. (1990). Pharmacology and behavioral treatment for cigarette smoking. In M. Hersen, R. M. Eisler, & P. M. Miller (Eds.), *Progress in behavior modification* (pp. 86–118). Newbury Park, CA: Sage.

Hall, S. M., Reus, V. I., Munoz, R. F., Sees, K. L., Humfleet, G., Hartz, D. T., et al. (1998). Nortriptylene and cognitive-behavioral therapy in the treatment of cigarette smoking. *Arch Gen Psychiatry, 55*, 683–690.

Hamilton, S. P., Nunes, E. V., Janal, M., & Weber, L. (2000). The effect of sertraline on methadone plasma levels in methadone-maintenance patients. *Am J Addict, 9*, 63–69.

Hatsukami, D. K., Huber, M., Callies, A., & Skoog, K. (1993). Physical dependence on nicotine gum: Effect of duration of use. *Psychopharmacology, 111*, 449–456.

Helander, A., & Carlsson, S. (1990). Use of leukocyte aldehyde dehydrogenase activity to monitor inhibitory effect of disulfiram treatment in alcoholism. *Alcohol Clin Exp Res, 14*, 48–52.

Henningfield, J. E., Stapleton, J. M., Benowitz, N. L., Grayson, R. F., & London, E. D. (1993). Higher levels of nicotine in arterial than in venous blood after cigarette smoking. *Drug Alcohol Depend, 33*, 23–29.

Herrlin, K., Segerdahl, M., Gustafsson, L. L., & Kalso, E. (2000). Methadone, ciprofloxacin, and adverse reactions. *Lancet, 356*, 2069–2070.

Hillbom, M., Tokola, R., Kuusela, V., Karkkainen, P., Kalli-Lemma, L., Pilke, A., & Kaste, M. (1989). Prevention of alcohol withdrawal seizures with carbamazepine and valproic acid. *Alcohol, 6*, 223–226.

Hsyu, P. H., Lillibridge, J. H., Maroldo, L., Weiss, W. R., & Kerr, B. M. (2000). *Pharmacokinetic (PK) and pharmacodynamic (PD) interactions between nelfinavir and methadone.* Paper presented at the 7th Conference on Retroviruses and Opportunistic Infections, San Francisco.

Hughes, J. R. (1996). Treatment of nicotine dependence. In C. R. Schuster, S. W. Gust, & M. J. Kuhar (Eds.), *Pharmacological aspects of drug dependence: Toward an integrative neurobehavioral approach* (pp. 599–618). New York: Springer-Verlag.

Hughes, J. R., Goldstein, M. G., Hurt, R. D., & Schiffman, S. (1999). Recent advances in the pharmacotherapy of smoking cessation. *JAMA, 281*, 72–76.

Jin, C., & McCance-Katz, E. F. (2003). Cocaine use disorders. In A. Tasman, J. Kay, & J. A. Lieberman (Eds.), *Psychiatry* (2nd ed., pp. 807–826). Philadelphia: Saunders.

Johnson, R. E., Chutaupe, M. A., Strain, E. C., Walsh, S. L., Stitzer, M. L., & Bigelow, G. E. (2000). A comparision of levomethadyl acetate, buprenorphine, and methadone for opioid dependence. *N Engl J Med, 343*, 1290–1297.

Kakko, J., Svanborg, K. D., Kreek, M. J., & Heilig, M. (2003). One-year retention and social function after buprenorphine assisted relapse prevention treatment for heroin dependence in Sweden: A randomized, placebo-controlled trial. *Lancet, 361*, 662–668.

Kasser, C., Geller, A., Howell, E., & Wartenberg, A. (1997). Detoxification: Principles and protocols. In B. B. Wilford (Ed.), *Topics in addiction medicine* (pp. 1–51). Chevy Chase, MD: American Society of Addiction Medicine.

Keifer, F., Holger, J., Timo, T., Hauke, H., Briken, P., Holzbach, R., et al. (2003). Comparing and combining naltrexone and acamprosate in relapse prevention of alcoholism. *Arch Gen Psychiatry, 60*, 92–99.

Khan, A., Mumford, J. P., Rogers, G. A., & Beckford, H. (1997). Double-blind study of lofexidine and clonidine in the detoxification of opiate addicts in hospital. *Drug Alcohol Depend, 44*, 57–61.

Kleber, H. D. (1981). Detoxification from narcotics. In J. H. Lowinson & P. Ruiz (Eds.), *Substance abuse: Clinical problems and perspectives* (pp. 317–338). Baltimore: William & Wilkins.

Kleber, H. D., Topazian, M., Gaspari, J., Riordan, C. E., & Kosten, T. (1987).

Clonidine and naltrexone in the outpatient treatment of heroin withdrawal. *Am J Drug Alcohol Abuse, 13*, 1–17.

Koe, B. K. (1976). Molecular geometry of inhibitors of the uptake of catecholamines and serotonin in synaptosomal preparations of rat brain. *J Pharmacol Exp Ther, 199*, 649–661.

Kosten, T. A. (1997). Enhanced neurobehavioral effects of cocaine with chronic neuroleptic exposure in rats. *Schizophr Bull, 23*, 203–213.

Kosten, T. R., & Kleber, H. D. (1984). Strategies to improve compliance with narcotic antagonists. *Am J Drug Alcohol Abuse, 10*, 249–266.

Kosten, T. R., & Kleber, H. D. (1988). Buprenorphine detoxification from opioid dependence: A pilot study. *Life Sci, 42*, 635–641.

Kosten, T. R., Krystal, J. H., Charney, D. S., Price, L. H., Morgan, C. H., & Kleber, H. D. (1989). Rapid detoxication from opioid dependence. *Am J Psychiatry, 146*, 1349.

Kosten, T. R., & O'Connor, P. G. (2003). Current concepts—management of drug withdrawal. *N Engl J Med, 348*, 1786–1795.

Kosten, T. R., Rosen, M., Bond, J., Settles, M., St. Clair Roberts, J., Shields, J., et al. (2002). Human therapeutic cocaine vaccine: Safety and immunogenicity. *Vaccine, 20*, 1196–1204.

Kosten, T. R., & Ziedonis, D. M. (1997). Substance abuse and schizophrenia. *Schizophr Bull, 23*, 181–186.

Kranzler, H. R., Burleson, J. A., Del Boca, F. K., Babor, T. F., Korner, P., Brown, J., & Bohn, M. (1994). Bupsirone treatment of anxious alcoholics. *Arch Gen Psychiatry, 51*, 720–731.

Lawental, E. (2000). Ultra rapid opiate detoxification as compared to 30-day inpatient detoxification program—a retrospective follow-up study. *J Subst Abuse, 11*, 173–181.

Lee, E. W., & D'Alonzo, G. E. (1993). Cigarette smoking, nicotine addiction, and its pharmacologic treatment. *Arch Intern Med, 153*, 34–48.

Lewis, J. W. (1985). Buprenorphine. *Drug Alcohol Depend, 14*, 363–372.

Littleton, J. (1995). Acamprosate in alcohol dependence: How does it work? *Addiction, 90*, 1179–1188.

Malcolm, R., Ballenger, J. C., Sturgis, E. T., & Anton, R. (1989). Double-blind controlled trial comparing carbamazepine to oxazepam treatment of alcohol withdrawal. *Am J Psychiatry, 146*, 617–621.

Malcolm, R., Myrick, H., Brady, K. T., & Ballenger, J. C. (2001). Update on anticonvulsants for the treatment of alcohol withdrawal. *Am J Addict, 10*(Suppl), 16–23.

Malcolm, R., Myrick, H., Roberts, J., Wang, W., Anton, R. F., & Ballenger, J. C. (2002). The effects of carbamazepine and lorazepam on single versus multiple previous alcohol withdrawals in an outpatient randomized trial. *J Gen Intern Med, 17*, 349–355.

Mason, B. (2001). Treatment of alcohol-dependent outpatients with acamprosate: A clinical review. *J Clin Psychiatry, 62*(Suppl), 42–48.

Mason, B., & Ownby, R. (2000). Acamprosate for the treatment of alcohol dependence: A review of double-blind, placebo-controlled trials. *CNS Spectrum, 5*, 58–69.

Mason, B., Salvato, F., & Williams, L. (1999). A double-blind, placebo-controlled study of oral nalmefene for alcohol dependence. *Arch Gen Psychiatry, 56,* 719–724.

McCance-Katz, E. F. (1997). *Pharmacotherapies for cocaine dependence an overview and new directions* (NIDA Research Monograph No. 175, pp. 36–72). Washington, DC: U.S. Government Printing Office.

McCance-Katz, E. F., Cropsey, K., & Gourevitch, M. (in press). *Responding to intravenous drug use (IDU) among people living with HIV/AIDS: An international review.* Unpublished paper, World Health Organization.

McCance-Katz, E. F., Leal, J., & Schottenfeld, R. S. (1995). Attention deficit hyperactivity disorder and cocaine abuse. *Am J Addict, 4,* 88–91.

McCance-Katz, E. F., Rainey, P., Friedland, G., & Jatlow, P. (2003). The protease inhibitor, Kaletra (Lopinavir/Ritonavir) may produce opiate withdrawal in methadone-maintained patients. *Clin Infect Dis, 37,* 476–482.

McCance-Katz, E. F., Rainey, P. M., Friedland, G., Kosten, T. R., & Jatlow, P. (2002). Effect of opioid dependence pharmacotherapies on zidovudine disposition. *Am J Addict, 10*(4), 296–307.

McCance-Katz, E. F., Rainey, P., Smith, P., Morse, G., Friedland, G., Gourevitch, M., & Jatlow, P. (2003). Drug interactions between opioid and antiretroviral medications: Interaction between methadone, LAAM, and nelfinavir. *Am J Addict.*

McCance-Katz, E. F., Selwyn, P., Farber, S., & O'Connor, A. H. (2000). The protease inhibitor nelfinavir decreases methadone levels. *Am J Psychiatry, 157,* 481.

Myrick, H., Brady, K. T., & Malcolm, R. (2001). New developments in the pharmacotherapy of alcohol dependence. *Am J Addict, 10*(Suppl), 3–15.

Myrick, H., Malcolm, R., & Brady, K. T. (1998). Gabapentin treatment of alcohol withdrawal. *Am J Psychiatry, 155,* 1632.

O'Connor, P. G., & Kosten, T. R. (1998). Rapid and ultrarapid opioid detoxification techniques. *JAMA, 279*(3), 229–234.

O'Connor, P. G., Waugh, M. E., Carroll, K. M., Rounsaville, B. J., Diakogiannis, I. A., & Schottenfeld, R. S. (1995). Primary care-based ambulatory opioid detoxification: The results of a clinical trial. *J Gen Intern Med, 10,* 255–260.

O'Malley, S. S., Jaffe, A. J., Chang, G., Rode, S., Schottenfeld, R. S., Meyer, R. E., & Rounsaville, B. J. (1996). Six-month follow-up of naltrexone and psychotherapy for alcohol dependence. *Arch Gen Psychiatry, 53,* 217–224.

O'Malley, S. S., Jaffe, A. J., Chang, G., Schottenfeld, R. S., Meyer, R. E., & Rounsaville, B. J. (1992). Naltrexone and coping skills therapy for alcohol dependence: A controlled study. *Arch Gen Psychiatry, 49,* 881–887.

Orlaam Package Insert (Revised May 2001). Columbus, OH: Roxane Laboratories, Inc.

Oslin, D. W., Pettinati, H. M., Volpicelli, J. R., Wolf, A. L., Kampman, K. M., & O'Brien, C. P. (1999). The effects of naltrexone on alcohol and cocaine use in dually addicted patients. *J Subst Abuse Treat, 16,* 163–167.

Palmer, K. J., Buckley, M. M., & Faulds, D. (1992). Transdermal nicotine: A review of its pharmacodynamic and pharmacokinetic properties, and therapeutic efficacy as an aid to smoking cessation. *Drugs, 44,* 498–529.

Petrakis, I. L., Carroll, K. M., Nich, C., Gordon, L. T., McCance-Katz, E. F., Frankforter, T., & Rounsaville, B. J. (2000). Disulfiram treatment for cocaine dependence in methadone-maintained opioid addicts. *Addiction, 95,* 219–228.

Prochaska, A. V., Weaver, M. J., Keller, R. T., Fryer, G. E., Licari, P. A., & Lofaso, D.

(1998). A randomized trial of nortriptylene for smoking cessation. *Arch Intern Med*, *158*, 2035–2039.

Rabinowitz, J., Cohen, H., & Atias, S. (2002). Outcomes of naltrexone maintenance following ultra rapid opiate detoxification versus intensive inpatient detoxification. *Am J Addict*, *11*, 52–56.

Rainey, P. M., Friedland, G., McCance-Katz, E. F., Andrews, L., Mitchell, S. M., Charles, C., & Jatlow, P. (2000). Interaction of methadone with didanosine (ddI) and stavudine (d4T). *J Acquir Immune Defic Syndr*, *24*, 241–248.

Rainey, P. M., Friedland, G. H., Snidow, J. W., McCance-Katz, E. F., Mitchell, S. M., Andrews, L., et al. (2002).The pharmacokinetics of methadone following co-administration with a lamivudine/zidovudine combination tablet in opiate dependent subjects (NZTA4003). *Am J Addict*, *11*, 66–74.

Raistrick, D., Hay, A., & Woldd, K. (1996). Methadone maintenance and tuberculosis treatment. *Br Med J*, *313*(7062), 925–926.

Rickels, K., Case, W. G., Schweizer, E., Garcia-Espana, F., & Fridman, R. (1991). Long-term benzodiazepine users 3 years after participation in a discontinuation program. *Am J Psychiatry*, *148*, 757–761.

Rickels, K., De Martinis, N., Rynn, M., & Mandos, L. (1999). Pharmacologic strategies for discontinuing benzodiazepine treatment. *J Clin Psychopharmacol*, *19*, 12S–16S.

Rickels, K., Schweizer, E., Case, W. G., & Garcia-Espana, F. (1988). Benzodiazepine dependence, withdrawal severity, and clinical outcome: Effects of personality. *Psychopharmacol Bull*, *24*, 415–420.

Rounsaville, B. J., & Kosten, T. R. (2000). Treatment for opioid dependence: Quality and access. *JAMA*, *283*, 1337–1339.

Roy-Byrne, P. P., Ward, N. G., & Donnelly, P. J. (1989). Valproate in anxiety and withdrawal syndromes. *J Clin Psychiatry*, *50*(Suppl), 44–48.

Rubio, G., Jimenez-Arriero, M. A., Ponce, G., & Palomo, T. (2001). Naltrexone vs. acamprosate: One year follow-up of alcohol dependence treatment. *Alcohol Alcohol*, *36*, 419–425.

Saxon, A. J., Whittaker, S., & Hawker, C. S. (1989). Valproic acid, unlike other anticonvulsants, has no effect on methadone metabolism: Two cases. *J Clin Psychiatry*, *50*, 228–229.

Scherbaum, N., Klein, S., Kaube, H., Kienbaum, P., Peters, J., & Gastpar, M. (1998). Alternative strategies of opiate detoxification: Evaluation of the so-called ultra-rapid detoxification. *Pharmacopsychiatry*, *31*, 205–209.

Schmitz, J. M., Stotts, A. L., Rhoades, H. M., & Grabowski, J. (2001). Naltrexone and relapse prevention treatment for cocaine-dependent patients. *Addict Behav*, *26*, 167–180.

Schottenfeld, R. S., Pakes, J., O'Connor, P., Chawarski, M., Oliveto, A., & Kosten, T. R. (2000). Thrice weekly versus daily buprenorphine maintenance. *Biol Psychiatry*, *47*, 1072–1079.

Sees, K. L., Delucci, K. L., Masson, C., Rosen, A., Clark, H. W., Robillard, H., et al. (2000). Methadone maintenance vs. 180-day psychosocially enriched detoxification for treatment of opioid dependence. *JAMA*, *283*, 1303–1310.

Sellers, E., Higgins, G., Tompkins, D., & Romach, M. (1992). Serotonin and alcohol drinking. *NIDA Res Monogr*, *119*, 141–145.

Senay, E. C., Dorus, W., Goldberg, F., & Thornton, W. (1977). Withdrawal from methadone maintenance: Rate of withdrawal and expectation. *Arch Gen Psychiatry, 34,* 361–367.

Silva de Lima, M., Garcia de Olivereiro Soares, B., Alves Pereira Reisser, A., & Farrell, M. (2002). Pharmacological treatment of cocaine dependence: A systematic review. *Addiction, 97,* 931–949.

Sullivan, J. T., Sykora, K., Schneiderman, J., Naranjo, C. A., & Sellers, E. M. (1989). Assessment of alcohol withdrawal: The revised Clinical Institute Withdrawal Instrument for Alcohol Scale (CIWA-Ar). *Br J Addict, 84,* 1353–1357.

Van den Brink, W., Goppel, M., & van Ree, J. M. (2003). Management of opioid dependence. *Curr Opin in Psychiatry, 16,* 297–304.

Vining, E., Kosten, T. R., & Kleber, H. D. (1988). Clinical utility of rapid clonidine naltrexone detoxification for opioid abusers. *Br J Addict, 83,* 567–575.

Volpicelli, J., Alterman, A. I., O'Brien, C. P., & Hayashida, M. (1992). Naltrexone in the treatment of alcohol dependence. *Arch Gen Psychiatry, 49,* 867–880.

Volpicelli, J., Rhines, K., & Rhines, J. (1997). Naltrexone and alcohol dependence: Role of subject compliance. *Arch Gen Psychiatry, 54,* 737–742.

Walsh, S. L., Preston, K. L., Stitzer, M. L., Cone, E. J., & Bigelow, G. E. (1994). Clinical pharmacology of buprenorphine: Ceiling effects at high doses. *Clin Pharmacol Ther, 55,* 569–580.

Wilde, M. I., & Wagstaff, A. J. (1997). Acamprosate: A review of its pharmacology and clinical potential in the management of alcohol dependence after detoxification. *Drugs, 53,* 1038–1053.

Wright, C., & Moore, R. D. (1990). Disulfiram treatment of alcoholism. *Am J Med, 88,* 647–655.

Zeise, M. L., Kasparov, S., Capogna, M., & Zieglgansberger, W. (1993). Acamprosate (calciumacetylhomotaurinate) decreases postsynaptic potentials in the rat neocortex: Possible involvement of excitatory amino acid receptors. *Eur J Pharmacol, 231,* 47–52.

CHAPTER 27

Dialectical Behavior Therapy for Individuals with Borderline Personality Disorder and Substance Use Disorders

M. ZACHARY ROSENTHAL
THOMAS R. LYNCH
MARSHA M. LINEHAN

Dialectical behavior therapy for substance use disorders (DBT-SUD) is a comprehensive psychosocial treatment for substance users with borderline personality disorder (BPD). DBT-SUD is an extension of standard dialectical behavior therapy (DBT; Linehan, 1993a, 1993b), a treatment for BPD that has been investigated to the extent that the treatment can be considered "well-established" according to criteria outlined by Chambless and Hollon (1998). It is the subject of several well-controlled randomized clinical trials (RCTs) for the treatment of BPD, and efficacy has been demonstrated across independent research teams (Koons et al., 2001; Linehan, Armstrong, Suarez, Allmon, & Heard, 1991; Linehan et al., 1999; Linehan, Dimeff, et al., 2002; Verheul et al., 2003). Across studies, the evidence suggests that DBT is an efficacious treatment for reducing a variety of problems associated with BPD, including self-injurious behavior, suicide attempts, suicidal ideation, hopelessness, depression, bulimia, and substance use.

This chapter provides an overview of the modifications of standard DBT that comprise DBT-SUD. The philosophy and theory behind DBT-SUD, the biosocial model of BPD, as well as treatment modes and functions, skill modules, and treatment strategies in DBT-SUD are outlined. For a comprehensive description of this treatment approach, interested readers are referred to the DBT treatment manual and group skills training manual (Linehan, 1993a, 1993b) and the DBT-SUD treatment manual (Linehan, Dimeff, & Sayrs, 2004).

WHY IS A TREATMENT FOR SUBSTANCE USERS WITH BORDERLINE PERSONALITY DISORDER NEEDED?

Separately, SUDs and BPD are serious public health problems associated with significant psychosocial impairment. Together, however, the combination of BPD and SUD is associated with greater problems than substance abuse alone (Links, Heslegrave, Mitton, van Reekum, & Patrick, 1995). For example, substance users with personality disorders are at risk for poor treatment outcome (Moos, Moos, & Finney, 2001). The presence of BPD specifically may lead to a number of impediments in standard substance abuse treatments. In one study, a diagnosis of BPD among opiate addicts treated with methadone predicted greater psychiatric problems and alcoholism following treatment (Kosten, Kosten, & Rousaville, 1989). Between 5 and 32% of individuals with SUD meet criteria for BPD (Brooner, King, Kidorf, Schmidt, & Bigelow, 1997; Weiss et al., 1993), and the two disorders often share core features (e.g., impulsivity; Trull, Sher, Minks-Brown, Durbin, & Burr, 2001). The extension of DBT from clients with BPD to those with BPD and SUD can be attributed, in part, to the high severity and comorbidity of the two separate disorders, along with the evidence that standard DBT is efficacious for individuals with BPD.

TARGET POPULATION FOR DBT-SUD

DBT-SUD was originally developed and tested with female clients meeting full diagnostic criteria for BPD and polysubstance abuse disorder or SUDs for opiates, cocaine, amphetamines, sedative/hypnotics, hallucinogens, or anxiolytics. Individuals with mental retardation, schizophrenia, schizoaffective disorder, bipolar affective disorder, and psychosis disorder not otherwise specified (NOS) have been excluded from studies evaluating the efficacy of DBT-SUD. As a result, DBT-SUD has been tested in a relatively specific population. Although it may be impossible to limit the use of DBT-SUD to such a specific population in clinical practice, it is recommended that DBT-SUD be used with clients similar to the population from DBT-SUD clinical trials, until future outcome studies support the efficacy of DBT-SUD in different populations.

EMPIRICAL SUPPORT

Two randomized trials examining DBT-SUD have been conducted. Linehan and colleagues (1999) compared DBT-SUD to treatment as usual (TAU) in the community in a sample of 28 women diagnosed with BPD and either SUD or polysubstance use disorder. Subjects received 1 year of treatment, and were assessed at 4, 8, 12, and 16 months after treatment, and were matched at pretreatment on age, severity of drug dependence, readiness to change, and global adjustment. Subjects in the DBT-SUD condition attended significantly more individual psychotherapy sessions during treatment, dropped out of treatment less, and, importantly, evidenced significantly less drug use, as determined by urinary analyses. At 16-month follow-up, subjects in the DBT-SUD condition had higher scores on measures of global adjustment and social adjustment compared to subjects in the TAU condition.

In a second study, 23 subjects with BPD and heroin dependence were randomly assigned to receive 1 year of DBT-SUD or comprehensive validation therapy, a treatment consisting of therapist validation coupled with 12-step methods (Linehan, Dimeff, et al., 2002). Subjects also received ORLAAM concurrently as an opiate replacement medication, and were matched at pretreatment on age, cocaine dependence, antisocial personality disorder, and global functioning. Although subjects in both conditions had a small proportion of positive urinary analyses at follow-up, in the last 4 months of treatment, those in the DBT-SUD condition maintained treatment gains, whereas those in the comprehensive validation condition had a significant increase in opiate use during this period. In addition, subjects in both conditions reported greater social adjustment and general adjustment following treatment. Taken together, these studies suggest that DBT-SUD is an efficacious treatment for substance users with BPD.

PHILOSOPHY AND THEORY

Philosophers such as Hegel and Kant discussed dialectics as a means of understanding or synthesizing apparent contradictions. Dialectics includes both a worldview and a process of change in DBT-SUD. From a dialectical worldview, behavior is conceptualized as interrelated, contextually determined, and systemic. The dialectical process of change is guided by the fundamental notions that (1) for every point an opposite position can be held, and (2) natural tensions can be resolved and adaptive change can occur when workable syntheses emerge from the consideration of contradicting polarities or opposing ideas. For example, clients might insist that substance use helps them feel less bored, whereas the therapist might insist that substance use is the problem. Using a dialectical perspective, the therapist and client could jointly create a synthesis by discussing how substance use is *both* understandable as a means of reducing bordeom *and* simultaneously a cause of much long-term suffering. Working together, the therapist and client would look for ways to feel better temporarily without creating long-term suffering.

There are many dialectical tensions in DBT-SUD. However, the central dialectic is that of *acceptance and change.* For the therapist, this entails balancing an acceptance of clients as they are in the present moment with an explicit, long-term goal of meaningful change. For clients, changing behaviors must be balanced by accepting unpleasant thoughts, emotions, or the reality that unpleasant events have occurred. As an example in DBT-SUD, clients are encouraged to accept the reality that painful emotions will occur, while concurrently working to prevent unnecessary emotional suffering caused by dysfunctional behavior. A compromise between acceptance and change is not necessarily the goal. Instead, a synthesis of polarities may be more acceptance-based in one moment and more change-focused in another, depending on the context and what is likely to be effective. This is similar to how a golfer might hit the ball toward one side of the fairway or the other, depending on the direction and strength of the wind in the present moment, the shape of the fairway, and the obstacles that lie to the side. The target is to hit the ball as close to the putting green or cup as possible, without the ball going out of play, not to hit the ball down the exact middle of the fairway.

BIOSOCIAL MODEL

Linehan (1993a, 1993b) suggests that BPD is fundamentally a disorder of the emotion regulation system and results from a reciprocal transaction between an emotional vulnerability, an invalidating environment, and emotional dysregulation (see Figure 27.1). Emotional vulnerability is considered to be the key

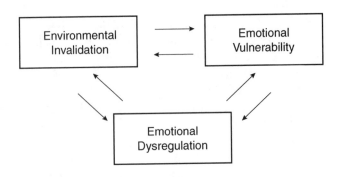

FIGURE 27.1. Components of the biosocial theory of borderline personality disorder.

diathesis, environmental invalidation is the primary socially mediated process, and emotional dysregulation is the multidimensional construct thought to underlie BPD criterion behaviors.

Emotional Vulnerability

According to Linehan (1993a), BPD is characterized by emotional vulnerability, a biologically mediated predisposition for affective instability involving genetic, intrauterine, and temperamental factors that is defined by heightened emotional sensitivity, heightened emotional reactivity, and a slow return to baseline level of emotional arousal; that is, individuals with BPD respond quickly to stimuli, respond with a high magnitude of arousal, and take a long time before arousal decreases to baseline. Similar to the intense physical pain felt when someone with a serious lower back injury tries to walk, emotionally vulnerable individuals often feel acute emotional pain in response to what appear to others to be ordinary events.

The Invalidating Environment

Broadly put, the invalidating environment is described by Linehan (1993a) as an environment characterized by pervasive criticizing, minimizing, trivializing, punishing, or erratically reinforcing communication of internal experiences (e.g., thoughts and emotions), and oversimplifying the ease of problem solving. For example, a parent may pervasively communicate, "You're not hurt, you just think you are" or "This is easy, just deal with it!" In addition, verbal communication is indiscriminately rejected, and the individual is chronically pathologized as having undesirable personality traits (e.g., too sensitive, paranoid, lazy, or unmotivated). Because appropriate emotional expression is chronically punished and extreme emotional displays are intermittently reinforced, escalation of emotional expressions (e.g., suicidal behavior) may occur. In addition to emotional invalidation, prototypical examples of invalidation are childhood sexual or physical abuse (Wagner & Linehan, 1997).

Emotional Dysregulation

In the context of environmental invalidation and emotional vulnerability, the biosocial model suggests that emotional dysregulation occurs, leading to problems with behavioral–motoric, physiological, and cognitive–experiential emotional systems. Such problems with emotion are hypothesized by Linehan (1993a) to underlie BPD criterion behaviors, and, as shown in Table 27.1, can be organized across domains of functioning (emotional, behavioral, cognitive, and interpersonal). Linehan suggests that emotional dysregulation in BPD is characterized by problems with up–down regulation of physiological arousal,

**TABLE 27.1. DSM-IV Criteria
for Borderline Personality Disorder**

- Emotion dysregulation
    Affective instability
    Problems with anger
- Behavioral dysregulation
    Impulsive behavior
    Self-injurious behavior
- Cognitive dysregulation
    Dissociation
    Paranoia
- Interpersonal dysregulation
    Chaotic relationships
    Fears of abandonment
- Self-dysregulation
    Identity disturbances
    Chronic feelings of emptiness

inhibiting mood-dependent behavior, excessive reliance on avoidant coping strategies, attentional control, processing emotional information, self-soothing, and self-validation. For example, an inability to decrease intense physiological arousal may precede the behavioral dyscontrol that is a hallmark of BPD, such as self-injury or impulsive substance use. Although substance use may occur in response to dysregulated emotional systems, in DBT-SUD, substance use also can be conceptualized as a means of emotion regulation; that is, substance use can function as an attempt to regulate emotions or as the outcome of emotional dysregulation.

TREATMENT

DBT-SUD is a principle-driven, flexible, and comprehensive treatment. As a behavioral therapy, it is change-focused. As an acceptance-based therapy, DBT-SUD incorporates strategies to use when changing behavior may not be possible or effective. Treatment begins by orienting clients to the therapeutic assumptions, agreements, levels and modes of treatment, and includes obtaining a commitment to treatment.

Assumptions and Agreements

In DBT-SUD, assumptions and agreements are openly delineated with clients in the first few "pretreatment" sessions (see Tables 27.2 and 27.3). During these sessions, the therapist discusses the requirement that clients commit to treat-

TABLE 27.2. Patient and Therapy Assumptions in Dialectical Behavior Therapy

Patients

1. Patients are doing the best they can.
2. Patients want to improve.
3. Patients need to do better, try harder, and be more motivated to change.
4. Patients must solve their current problems, regardless of who caused these problems.
5. Patients are living lives that are unbearable as they are currently being lived.
6. Patients must learn new behaviors in all relevant contexts.

Therapy

1. Patients can not fail in DBT, but the therapy or therapist can fail the patient.
2. Helping patients work toward their ultimate goals in life is the most caring thing a therapist can do.
3. DBT therapists need support.
4. The therapeutic relationship is a relationship of two equals.
5. Principles of behavior are universal, affecting both patients and therapists alike.

TABLE 27.3. Patient and Therapist Agreements in Dialectical Behavior Therapy

Patient agreements

1. Stay in therapy for a specified period of time, usually 1 year.
2. Attend all therapy sessions.
3. Therapy will be discontinued if four consecutive sessions are missed.
4. Work toward terminating self-injurious behavior and other therapeutic targets.
5. Participate in skills training.
6. Abide by relevant research conditions of therapy.
7. Pay agreed upon fees for service.

Therapy agreements

1. Maintain competence and effort.
2. Provide ethical and professional treatment.
3. Be available for weekly sessions and phone consultation.
4. Treat patients humanely, with respect and integrity.
5. Maintain confidentiality.
6. Seek appropriate consultation.

ment. Although standard DBT often uses a variety of commitment strategies during pretreatment sessions, in DBT-SUD, clients must, at a minimum, agree to work toward abstinence from all drugs. Because commitment to treatment often ebbs and flows, it is necessary to monitor ongoing changes in committed behavior throughout treatment.

Treatment Targets

Clients with BPD often present for treatment with severe behavioral dyscontrol (e.g., self-injurious behavior), treatment-interfering behaviors (e.g., not showing up to treatment), and problems affecting physical (e.g., sleep problems), emotional (e.g., excessive emotionality), and cognitive (e.g., hopelessness) functioning. To treat this range of therapeutic targets consistently, a hierarchy for problem behaviors is used in DBT-SUD: (1) Reduce acute life-threatening and intentional self-injurious behaviors; (2) reduce treatment-interfering behaviors; and (3) reduce quality-of-life interfering behaviors, beginning with drug use, and including such problems as eating disorders, anxiety, depression, and physical health problems. The complete and total cessation of all drug use is the primary target in the quality-of-life interfering behaviors.

Within this larger treatment hierarchy, DBT-SUD outlines the "path to clear mind" in order to provide specific treatment targets addressing substance use. The overarching, and, accordingly, first SUD-specific target is the reduction of all substance abuse, including illicit and licit drug abuse. In accomplishing this, the next target in the path to clear mind is to maintain an adequate dose of drug replacement medications, when relevant, and more generally to decrease the physical discomfort associated with abstinence. Physical pain and psychological distress are targeted for change when possible. However, acceptance skills are used to tolerate pain that cannot be reduced directly.

Clients also learn how to monitor cravings, to evaluate the intensity of cravings, to identify when cravings are particularly likely to increase drug use, to reduce cravings, and to avoid using drugs once cravings occur. On the one hand, clients learn that cravings should be expected to occur; on the other hand, they learn how to actively problem-solve ways to cope with cravings without using. Unlike standard DBT, in which clients are frequently encouraged to turn their attention toward the experience of aversive emotions, DBT-SUD clients are encouraged to use skills to turn their attention *away from* cravings and urges to use. As coping skills are acquired and generalized, DBT-SUD emphasizes community reinforcement of "nonaddict wise-mind" behaviors; that is, clients increase activities associated with a decreased likelihood for drug use, such as Alcoholics Anonymous (AA) and Narcotics Anonymous (NA) meetings, gaining steady and legitimate employment, and socializing whenever possible with nonaddicts in mainstream settings.

Next, "apparently unimportant behaviors" are targeted. Patterned after Marlatt's work on apparently irrelevant decisions (Marlatt & Gordon, 1985), in DBT-SUD, behaviors (both observable events and privately experienced events, such as thoughts) that are links on the chain toward drug use are targeted. Examples range from obvious (e.g., selling drugs) to less obvious (e.g., going into an environment with many cues associated with drug use). Finally, on the path to clear mind, DBT-SUD targets closing options to use drugs, including, for example, ending contacts and throwing away contact information with those who sell and use drugs, getting rid of all drug paraphernalia, and not lying about drug use.

Dialectical Abstinence

The goal of DBT-SUD is to stop using drugs, with the ideal outcome of treatment being complete and indefinite abstinence. However, the cold reality suggested by clinical observation and supported by treatment outcome studies is that even in the best treatments for substance use, abstinence may not last indefinitely. Harm reduction approaches take into account the likelihood of lapse following treatment (e.g., Marlatt & Gordon, 1985), aiming to reduce the impact of substance use rather than focus exclusively on abstinence. In DBT-SUD, abstinence is the goal, not harm reduction. However, the synthesis between complete abstinence and a harm reduction approach is struck. The resulting perspective, called "dialectical abstinence," refers to the position of targeting complete abstinence on the one hand, while being prepared for and responding effectively to drug lapse on the other hand; that is, dialectical abstinence is achieved through the therapist targeting 100% abstinence with the client, while also planning for the possibility of relapse by developing a relapse management plan.

Attachment Strategies

Although similar to BPD clients without substance use problems, those with co-occurring BPD–SUD disorders appear to have important differences. Linehan (1993a) characterizes individuals with BPD as either "attached" or as "butterflies." Whereas attached BPD clients communicate often with therapists, rarely miss appointments, and appear closely affiliated to their therapists, butterfly clients do the opposite. Substance-abusing BPD clients are often butterflies, possibly because their drug use has become more reinforcing than social interactions, and this clinical observation has led to the addition of a set of attachment strategies in DBT-SUD. For example, to develop rapport, the first several sessions include a large amount of therapist validation, with less emphasis on immediate change and/or interpersonal aversive contingencies than in standard DBT. In addition, because these clients tend to come into and go out of therapy, therapists may become easily demoralized. Thus, a strong emphasis is made on remoralizing and motivating therapists during consultation team meetings. Other attachment strategies include orienting the client to this problem, increasing contact with clients toward the beginning of treatment, frequent contacts with clients via voice mail, *in vivo* therapy sessions, decreasing or increasing session length as needed, family and friends network meetings, and calling clients when they are avoiding them when they repeatedly do not show up for appointments or respond to telephone calls.

Modes and Functions of Treatment

DBT-SUD includes methods for learning adaptive coping skills, generalizing such skills into relevant contexts, enhancing commitment to treatment, and preventing demoralization of both the therapist and client. There are four primary modes of treatment: group skill training, individual therapy, phone consultation, and consultation team. Because of the need for replacement medication and the frequent comorbidity of Axis I disorders, DBT-SUD also can incorporate a pharmacotherapy mode. Next, the function, process, and structure of treatment modes are briefly reviewed.

Skills Training

Weekly 2-hour skills training classes occurs in a group format. The primary function of skills training classes is the acquisition of new behavioral and cognitive skills. Skills training classes are co-led by two skills trainers, and include both homework review of previously learned skills and didactic presentation of new skills from the skills training manual (Linehan, 1993b). Specifically, there are separate skill modules for mindfulness, distress tolerance, emotion regulation, and interpersonal effectiveness.

Mindfulness

Derived from Eastern meditative and Christian contemplative traditions, mindfulness is the practice of paying attention in a particular way: on purpose, in the present moment, and without judgment. In this module, clients learn that their behavior is a function of current emotions (emotion mind) or logical analysis (reasonable mind). "Wise mind" knowing and behavior is emphasized as a synthesis of emotion and reasonable minds, such that decisions and actions are both effective and remain within personal values. For example, in order to change a client's identity as an addict, wise mind is emphasized as behaviors that are inconsistent with identity as an addict.

Mindfulness skills specifically include the ability to observe, describe, and participate fully in one's actions and experiences in a nonjudgmental, one-mindful, and effective manner. Observing refers to noticing experiences without becoming attached, allowing thoughts or other internal experiences to flow freely with full awareness. Describing follows observing and involves labeling or putting words on experiences. Participating is somewhat different and involves behaving effectively, without observing and describing internal experiences (e.g., an athlete at peak performance). Being nonjudgmental, including being aware of judgments and letting go of their literal truth, is a central skill repeatedly practiced by DBT clients and therapists. Being one-mindful entails a sharpening of attentional focus on one thing or activity at a time. This skill involves staying in the present moment and not becoming distracted by thoughts about the past or future. Finally, the focus on effectiveness is a key aspect of mindfulness. Effectiveness refers to behaving in a flexible manner across contexts in a way that is consistent with one's values and long-term goals. The emphasis on effectiveness as a DBT skill illustrates how mindfulness is a behavioral, psychological, and spiritual practice, extending beyond formal meditation practice.

Additional mindfulness skills specific to DBT-SUD include "urge surfing" and "alternative rebellion." Urge surfing stems from Marlatt's treatment for alcohol abuse (Marlatt & Gordon, 1985) and involves awareness of urges to use, coupled with the use of imagery of a wave as the urge is "surfed." As is always the case with waves, urges eventually cease. For many, use of this skill helps considerably in preventing substance use following cravings to use. Alternative rebellion refers to identifying ways to rebel against society, parents, or others in a skillful way that does not involve drug use. This skill is relevant for those drug users whose identity as an addict functions as a way to be different and unique. As a mindfulness skill, alternative rebellion is linked to being effective and could include dyeing one's hair, getting a tattoo, or wearing unusual clothes.

Distress Tolerance

The distress tolerance module is designed to teach clients how to tolerate aversive emotional experiences without behaving maladaptively. A list of crisis management skills is taught, including strategies for effective temporary distraction, such as activities eliciting opposite emotions, and squeezing ice or a rubber ball. Self-soothing skills are introduced, whereby clients learn to soothe themselves intentionally during periods of crisis, with calming visual stimuli, sounds, smells, tastes, and objects to touch. In addition, other skills, such as imaginal and relaxation exercises, are taught to improve the current moment, in order to avert crises. Other distress tolerance skills include awareness, breathing, and half-smile exercises, as well as radical acceptance of reality as it is in the present moment. Overall, distress tolerance skills are intended to interrupt and change habitual, problematic, and often context-insensitive responses to emotional distress, allowing the opportunity for new responses to aversive stimulation that cannot be directly changed and the emergence of a broader repertoire of skillful behavior.

Two new skills added to the distress tolerance module are "adaptive denial" and "burning your bridges." Adaptive denial is a skill that draws on what is often considered an inherent problem among many substance users, denial. As a skill, adaptive denial includes identifying a craving to use drugs and relabeling it as a craving for something that is not harmful and to which one has access; that is, the idea is to reattribute a drug craving as a craving for something else. For example, clients may be taught to recognize their craving to use drugs and to practice telling themselves that it is really a craving for a flavored toothpick. Of course, in this example, it would be necessary for the client to carry around flavored toothpicks, putting one in the mouth each time as adaptive denial of the drug craving.

"Burning your bridges" is a skill derived from the notion of willingness. In order to help tolerate distress associated with no longer using drugs, burning your bridges involves radical acceptance that drugs will no longer be used. However, the key component of this skill is that such acceptance is accompanied completely by a willingness, as evidenced by behavior, to cut off all previous links to drug use and the identity of being a drug user. This skill is compatible with the target on the path to clear mind described as eliminating options to use drugs (e.g., telling the truth).

Emotion Regulation

The emotion regulation skills module is designed to help clients better understand their emotions, reduce emotional vulnerability, and decrease emotional suffering. Specific skills taught include an increased awareness of emotions, identifying and challenging distorted ways of thinking about emotions, learning how emotions are related to problem behaviors, accurately labeling emotions, understanding the functions of emotions, reducing emotional vulnerability, increasing pleasant emotions, and *acting opposite* to behavioral urges associated with emotions. Although all of these skills are useful, the opposite action skill is particularly helpful, because it can be applied in many contexts to change a variety of problem behaviors.

The opposite action skill uses an algorithm for knowing when to change emotion. This includes first determining whether the emotion is justified, based on the current situation. Next, it is important to know the action urge of the emotion being experienced. Each emotion has its own urging component (e.g., anger—attack, fear—run, sadness—withdraw, guilt—repair, shame—hide). When the client is experiencing an unjustified emotion that he or she wishes to change, the skill is to go opposite to the action urge of the emotion.

For example, if a client is feeling guilty for disagreeing with a friend, the opposite action skill would be to teach the client to ask him- or herself first whether the behavior was egregious according to his or her own values. If the disagreement was done in a manner inconsistent with the client's values (e.g., disrespectfully and judgmentally disagreeing), then a repair (e.g., apology) would be suggested as a way to lower justified guilt. However, if the disagreement did not violate the client's values and guilt was unjustified (i.e., respectfully and nonjudgmentally disagreeing), then the client would be instructed not to repair but to repeat the behavior (i.e., effective opinion giving) multiple times. As the client learns that giving opinions does not always result in negative outcomes, over time, the unjustified guilt response to disagreeing effectively would extinguish.

Interpersonal Effectiveness

Because chaotic interpersonal relationships are a key characteristic of BPD, the development of interpersonal skills is crucial. This skill module teaches clients how to identify factors interfering with interpersonal effectiveness, challenge common cognitive distortions associated with interpersonal situations, and determine the appropriate level of intensity for making requests or saying "no" a given situation. Specific guidelines for being taken seriously, attending to relationships, and preserving self-respect are taught, and clients are instructed to practice developing new interpersonal skills based on these guidelines in a wide variety of situations, including frequent rehearsal and role playing during group and individual sessions. When teaching interpersonal effectiveness in DBT-SUD, the specific skills taught are designed to avoid drug-using contexts (e.g., drug refusal interpersonal skills) and to respond effectively when such contexts cannot be avoided (e.g., craving tolerance skills).

Individual Therapy

Individual therapy sessions with a DBT-SUD therapist are typically 50–60 minutes once per week. The individual therapist provides psychoeducational information to the client early in treatment, including handouts that describe the pros and cons of participating in DBT-SUD compared to other treatments and facts about drug addiction. However, a primary function of individual therapy is to develop and maintain client motivation to overcome obstacles to change. A validating environment is created, whereby clients are treated with compassion and acceptance in the context of targeting behavioral change. Factors interfering with progress in treatment are discussed, preventing problems that might interfere with the development of new skills and helping clients remain in treatment despite urges to dropout. Episodes of emotional dysregulation from the previous week are discussed in light of skills that could have been used. In

addition, skills are practiced during session and are woven into plans in anticipation of upcoming events.

Diary Cards

In order to monitor a variety of targets, a daily diary card is used. For example,
clients may rate their mood, monitor the frequency of self-injurious behavior
and drug use urges, and track other relevant targets. The diary card is reviewed
at the beginning of each session, and the therapy session is organized around
targets evident on the diary card. Given the plethora of treatment targets and
the possibility that clients will not remember salient events from the previous
week, the diary card is instrumental in directing therapy sessions toward highly
relevant targets.

Behavioral Analysis

To change dysfunctional behaviors, DBT-SUD uses a number of problem-
solving strategies. Behavioral analysis is used to identify problem behaviors and
to understand the relevant contexts in which these behaviors generally occur.
Behavioral analysis involves an active, directive effort by the therapist to identify specific antecedents and consequences associated with the problem behavior. A thorough elaboration of events before, during, and after problem behaviors facilitates the selection of appropriate treatment interventions. Based on a
functional-analytic approach to behavioral assessment, the goal of behavioral
analysis is prediction and control of functional classes of problem behavior
rather than traditional diagnostic assessment of disease entities (Hayes &
Follette, 1992; Kanfer & Saslow, 1969). In other words, in DBT-SUD, borderline symptoms and substance use are conceptualized as problem *behaviors*. These
may be external, publicly observable behaviors, such as self-mutilation or
impulsive aggression, or internal, publicly unobservable experiences, such as
self-judgmental thoughts or urges to use substances.

Because behavioral analysis in DBT-SUD involves explicating the links in
a specific chain of events, it is often referred to as a "chain analysis." During a
chain analysis, the topography, intensity, and duration of the target problem is
discussed. As links in the chain of events (including internal experiences and
external events) before and after the target behavior are explored, the therapist
considers the role of classical and instrumental conditioning. Classically conditioned (respondent) behaviors are under the control of an antecedent stimulus,
and instrumentally conditioned (operant) behaviors are under the control of
consequent events. For example, strong urges to use substances may be classically conditioned to occur after interpersonal conflicts. On the other hand, substance use may be instrumentally conditioned by the consequences that follow,
such as less hostility or increased attention from others. A chain analysis is a

detailed assessment of one instance of a problem behavior. As chain analyses are conducted repeatedly across sessions, an understanding of the relevant controlling variables (i.e., antecedent or consequence) of a problem behavior is determined, informing the choice of interventions. Strategies for changing antecedents include behavioral exposure (e.g., rehearsing saying "no" to a drug dealer) and stimulus control (e.g., avoiding drug dealers). In addition, other behavioral principals used during chain analyses are positive and negative reinforcement, punishment, extinction, and shaping.

Dysfunctional links uncovered in a chain analysis are examined and replaced with more adaptive responses during a *solution analysis*. Typically, this is guided by three questions:

1. Can the client change the circumstance (e.g., flush the drugs down the toilet, quit the job)?
2. Can the client change an emotional reaction (e.g., go opposite to the emotion action urge)?
3. Can the client better tolerate the pain associated with the problem (e.g., radically accept the problem)?

Together, client and therapist collaboratively develop strategies to replace problematic links and then commit to using new solutions the next time the problem behavior emerges. The solution analysis does not stop there, however. Once the client has committed to using new behavior in future chains of events that could lead to problem behaviors, it is important to continue searching for possible links in the solution chain that could lead the client back to the problem behavior. This can be challenging, because many therapists may be satisfied with their chain analysis and the client's commitment to skillful solutions targeting reduced substance use or other problems. From a dialectical perspective, however, the identification and commitment to a specific solution does not mean that solution is the best choice of solutions, nor does it mean that the solution will actually work at all. If solutions were easy to implement, then most substance-abusing clients with BPD might not have such severe and enduring problems. Accordingly, solutions are analyzed for apparent problems, and newly improved solutions emerge. The process is akin to predicting where the leaks might be when preparing to fix the plumbing under the sink. Although a reasonable plan may exist, the skillful plumber considers where the plan may fail, making adjustments as necessary, before implementing the plan.

Skills Enhancement

A primary goal of individual therapy is to enhance skills learned during group. One way to do this is to ask clients to rehearse behavior in session. Behavioral rehearsal may occur in the form of covert rehearsing of challenges to distorted cognitions or by role-playing interpersonal scenarios. Therapists provide reinforcement and coaching during rehearsals and role plays, with an emphasis on skills use. Whenever skillful behavior occurs in session, the therapist reinforces such behavior. Ineffective behavior during the session, on the other hand, is often extinguished. When repeated attempts to extinguish ineffective behavior in session fail to work, the therapist may use mildly aversive responses to such behavior. However, the standard stance of the therapist is to be warm, nurturing, and validating, using aversive contingencies infrequently and only as needed to evoke skillful behavior.

Another method of facilitating skills use is behavioral exposure and response prevention in session. Clients will often become angry, ashamed, or fearful in session, and a range of behaviors may be evoked in response to these emotions. BPD clients who feel angry may lash out, while those who feel ashamed may look down or dissociate, and clients who feel fearful may suddenly leave a session. Behavioral exposure and response prevention applied to these emotions in session target paying attention to these emotions nonjudgmentally, observing urges to behave ineffectively, and blocking these urges by helping clients not to lash out, to keep eye contact, or to remain in the therapy room.

Validation

Verification of what the client does effectively and disconfirmation of what is ineffective is a commonality across many psychotherapies. Although validation of clients may be defined in various ways, in DBT-SUD, validation is a core strategy operationalized on several levels (see Table 27.4). Validation may be explicitly verbal, or it may occur more implicitly and functionally, such as when the therapist offers a tissue when an emotionally inhibited client appears on the verge of tears. Validation may be used as pure acceptance, with no directed effort toward change. In DBT-SUD, there is an explicit emphasis on the thera-

---

TABLE 27.4. Levels of Validation in Dialectical Behavior Therapy

1. Listening and observing
2. Accurate reflection of patient experiences
3. Helping patients articulate unverbalized emotions, thoughts, and patterns of behavior
4. Communicating an understanding of behavior as valid given past learning history or biological vulnerability
5. Communicating an understanding of behavior as valid given a current context or what is deemed normative
6. Therapist providing radical genuineness, treating the individual as an equal and not as a sick and fragile patient

---

pist providing a warm, genuine, and compassionate interpersonal style. In many cases, these clients were raised in invalidating family environments (e.g., physical, sexual, or emotional abuse), continue to be surrounded by invalidating people associated with drug using, and describe their previous mental health treatments as invalidating. The DBT-SUD therapist attempts to create a relationship that is different from past relationships. The deep pain and suffering experienced by these clients is attended to and validated in an authentic and compassionate way.

Importantly, however, therapist validation of client behavior is targeted specifically to that which makes sense, is legitimate, or is effective. DBT-SUD therapists attempt to validate what is valid, and, at times, invalidate what is invalid. This requires the DBT therapist to discern carefully what is valid, and to apply validation in accordance with the conceptualization of each client's problem behaviors. For example, after a relapse, the therapist might warmly and compassionately validate how and why it makes sense that the client used drugs to reduce short-term misery, but would not validate drug use as an effective, long-term solution to reducing pain. In DBT-SUD, validation is essential, because clients often come and go from treatment, and may not be as attached to therapists compared to standard DBT clients with BPD and no substance use problems. Consequently, aversive interpersonal contingencies are held to a minimum, unless, of course, such contingencies assist in reducing problem behaviors.

Dialectical Strategies

In DBT, dialectical strategies are fundamentally based around acceptance (e.g., validation) and change (e.g., problem solving). Dialectical reasoning is pursued with the client, whereby the therapist helps the client move from a polarized position of "either–or" to a dialectical synthesis of "both–and." Any therapist strategy that challenges the client's position (thesis), and instead involves actively searching for what might be missing (antithesis), can be considered a dialectical strategy if the tension between the thesis and antithesis produces a synthesis, or solution, that is ultimately useful for therapeutic change. There is no assumption that a single synthesis is the "correct" solution to a problem. Instead, the therapeutic process is one that continually works dialectically, yielding a number of possible solutions to a given problem; that is, the underlying principle of dialectical strategies is a focus on the process of change within a fluid context. Specifically, however, there are a number of dialectical strategies used with clients (see Table 27.5; for descriptions, see Linehan, 1993b). In order to be effective, these strategies must be used in a manner that is genuine, and not as simple mechanical techniques. In addition, from a dialectical perspective, the therapist must be willing to let go of the truth or rightness of any dialectical strategy, and instead continually search for ways to help clients

TABLE 27.5. Dialectical Strategies Used in Dialectical Behavior Therapy

1. Acceptance and change-focused interventions
2. Nurturing the patient and demanding that patients help themselves
3. Being stable and persistent, as well as flexible
4. Highlighting patient's strengths and deficits
5. Structuring session with an agenda, and responding to in-session patient behaviors as they occur
6. Highlighting both ends of continua, and making synthesizing statements
7. Pointing out paradoxes when present (e.g., patient's behavior, therapeutic process)
8. Using metaphors
9. Playing the devil's advocate
10. Extending the seriousness or implications of patient's communication
11. Helping patient activate "wise mind"
12. Helping make lemonade out of lemons
13. Allowing natural changes in therapy

Note. Adapted from Linehan (1993a, p. 206). Copyright 1993 by The Guilford Press. Adapted by permission.

change problem behaviors. This approach probably helps reduce therapist burnout, and also helps ensure a validating and warm therapeutic environment. In addition, dialectical strategies are used in a manner that is often unpredictable to the client, and when any specific strategy does not help bring about new client behavior, another strategy is used.

Telephone Consultation

Clients with BPD and substance abuse problems experience a profound sense of suffering. Between treatment sessions, there often are times when emotional pain (e.g., shame) and dysregulation occur, or events transpire that historically have prompted drug use. To reduce the effects of emotional dysregulation in the client's natural environment, to prevent substance abuse, and, more broadly, to enhance generalization of skills, clients are encouraged to contact their individual therapists on an ad hoc basis for brief telephone consultation between sessions. On the one hand, because these individuals may experience unrelenting crises, therapists observe personal limits associated with telephone consultation. Clients call for help in implementing skills in necessary situations, ideally before crises occur. On the other hand, many DBT-SUD clients, particularly those who are less attached to their therapists, will infrequently use the telephone for skills coaching. As a result, some clients not only are encouraged to call but also will be asked to practice calling their therapist between sessions. In all consultation calls, therapists assess for immediate danger and provide appropriate assistance if the client is deemed to be in imminent danger of harming him- or herself or others.

TABLE 27.6. Consultation Team Agreements in Dialectical Behavior Therapy

1. Meet weekly for 1–2 hours.
2. Discuss cases according to the treatment hierarchy (i.e., self-injurious/life-threatening behavior, treatment-interfering behavior, and quality-of-life interfering behavior).
3. Accept a dialectical philosophy.
4. Consult with the patient on how to interact with other therapists, and do not tell other therapists how to interact with the patient.
5. Consistency of therapists with one another (even across the same patient) is not expected.
6. All therapists observe their own limits without fear of judgmental reactions from other consultation group members.
7. Search for nonpejorative empathic interpretation of patient's behavior.
8. All therapists are fallible.

Consultation Team

As mentioned earlier, the consultation team is a necessary mode of treatment. Team members commit to weekly meetings and agree to a team structure and process (see Table 27.6). In important ways, team members treat each other by providing validation, support, and motivation. This support is invaluable and can help DBT-SUD therapists have a more balanced approach toward their clients. A consultation team also provides opportunities for fresh perspectives and new solutions, helping therapists get unstuck and remain hopeful. It is not uncommon for DBT-SUD therapists periodically to become rigid in their thinking and behavior with a client. The consultation team offers problem solving and validation for the therapist, and team members actively use a dialectical process to help find effective syntheses between polarized positions. For example, the team can help remind the therapist to continue managing contingencies in session appropriately (e.g., not being warm in response to client hostility). If possible, it is extremely helpful to videotape and watch important segments of the therapy session during the consultation team meeting, because this engenders a full appreciation for the difficulty a therapist may be having, and allows the team to ensure that all members are indeed adhering to the treatment.

Pharmacotherapy

Five principles organize the management of psychotropic medications in DBT-SUD. First, and most importantly, safe and nonlethal medications must be prescribed and used in a safe manner. This principle is considered in light of each individual. For those with a history of medication abuse, the DBT-SUD pharmacotherapist would observe the medication being ingested and provide the client with a small supply of take-home medications. Second, simple medication regimens are used in order to mitigate problems with side effects and drug interactions, both of which can interfere with treatment. Third, specific symptoms are targeted first, rather than general problems such as affective instability. Fourth, choice of medications is guided by controlled efficacy studies. Finally, speed of clinical improvement is imperative, with, for example, opiate replacement rapidly adjusted to the desirable therapeutic maintenance dose.

DBT-SUD Case Management

Because substance users with BPD often encounter problems obtaining and maintaining adequate food, housing, and employment, case management can be added to DBT-SUD. Unlike standard case management approaches that intervene directly in the environment (e.g., making a phone call on behalf of a client), however, DBT-SUD case management emphasizes actively coaching the client to intervene on his or her own behalf. The DBT-SUD case manager does not manage clients' resources; instead, clients manage their resources with skills coaching from the case manager or individual therapist. The case manager is utilized by the individual therapist on an ad hoc basis in one of the following ways: (1) as a resource to the therapist for referrals or advice, (2) to provide information or referrals directly to the client, or (3) to provide *in vivo* skills coaching in the client's natural environment.

FUTURE DIRECTIONS

To date, the efficacy of DBT-SUD has been demonstrated in two small clinical trials. As described earlier, these studies suggest that DBT-SUD is a promising, manual-based treatment for substance users with BPD. The next step in the development and evaluation of DBT-SUD is a Stage II efficacy trial. Such work is currently underway on a two-site study at the University of Washington (Linehan) and Duke University (Lynch). In this National Institute of Drug Abuse–sponsored project, 172 individuals with BPD and opioid dependence will be randomly assigned to receive DBT-SUD or *Individual Drug Counseling with Group Drug Counseling* (Mercer & Woody, 1999). Both treatment conditions will receive Suboxone, an opiate replacement medication that consists of an opiate partial agonist (buprenorphine) and antagonist (naloxone). This will be the largest study ever to evaluate the efficacy of DBT-SUD.

SUMMARY

DBT-SUD is a comprehensive psychosocial treatment designed to treat substance users with BPD. The philosophy, theory, structure, skills modules, treatment modes and functions, and treatment strategies are equivalent to those of standard DBT. However, notable additions to DBT-SUD include (1) treatment targets that aim to reduce drug-related behaviors, (2) new coping skills for managing drug cravings and withdrawal, (3) new "wise mind" skills, (4) attachment strategies, (5) increased use of validation and less aversive interpersonal contingencies, (6) increased use of case management to assist in housing and other crises via direct environmental intervention, and (7) a pharmacotherapy mode. Overall, DBT-SUD is a promising new treatment that is grounded in philosophy and theory, supported by preliminary empirical findings, and, importantly, offers hope for substance users with BPD.

REFERENCES

Brooner, R. K., King, V. L., Kidorf, M., Schmidt, C. W., & Bigelow, G. E. (1997). Psychiatric and substance use comorbidity among treatment-seeking opioid abusers. *Arch Gen Psychiatry, 54,* 71–80.

Chambless, D. L., & Hollon, S. D. (1998). Defining empirically supported therapies. *J Consult Clin Psychol, 66,* 7–18.

Hayes, S. C., & Follette, W. C. (1992). Can functional analysis provide a substitute for syndromal classification? *Behav Assess, 14,* 345–365.

Kanfer, F. H., & Saslow, G. (1969). Behavioral diagnosis. In C. M. Franks (Ed.), *Behavior therapy: Appraisal and status.* New York: McGraw-Hill.

Koons, C. R., Robins, C. J., Tweed, J. L., Lynch, T. R., Gonzalez, A. M., Morse, J. Q., et al. (2001). Efficacy of dialectical behavior therapy in women veterans with borderline personality disorder. *Behav Ther, 32,* 371–390.

Kosten, R. A., Kosten, T. R., & Rousaville, B. J. (1989). Personality disorders in opiate addicts show prognostic specificity. *J Subst Abuse Treat, 6,* 163–168.

Linehan, M. M. (1993a). *Cognitive-behavioral treatment of borderline personality disorder.* New York: Guilford Press.

Linehan, M. M. (1993b). *Skills training manual for treating borderline personality disorder.* New York: Guilford Press.

Linehan, M. M., Armstrong, H. E., Suarez, A., Allmon, D., & Heard, H. L. (1991). Cognitive-behavioral treatment of chronically parasuicidal borderline patients. *Arch Gen Psychiatry, 48,* 1060–1064.

Linehan, M. M., Dimeff, L. A., Reynolds, S. K., Comtois, K. A., Welch, S. S., Heagerty, P., & Kivlahan, D. R. (2002). Dialectical behavior therapy versus comprehensive validation therapy plus 12-step for the treatment of opioid dependent women meeting criteria for borderline personality disorder. *Drug Alcohol Depend, 67,* 13–26.

Linehan, M. M., Dimeff, L. A., & Sayrs, J. H. R. (2004). *Dialectical behavior therapy for substance abusers with borderline personality disorder: An extension of standard DBT.* Unpublished manuscript.

Linehan, M. M., Schmidt, H., III, Dimeff, L. A., Craft, J. C., Kanter, J., & Comtois, K. A. (1999). Dialectical behavior therapy for patients with borderline personality disorder and drug-dependence. *Am J Addict, 8,* 279–292.

Links, P. S., Heslegrave, R. J., Mitton, J. E., van Reekum, R., & Patrick, J. (1995). Borderline personality disorder and substance use: Consequences of comorbidity. *Can J Psychiatry, 40,* 9–14.

Marlatt, G. A., & Gordon, J. R. (1985). *Relapse prevention: Maintenance strategies in the treatment of addictive behaviors.* New York: Guilford Press.

Mercer, D., & Woody, G. (1999). *Individual drug counseling.* Rockville, MD: National Institute on Drug Abuse.

Moos, R. H., Moos, B. S., & Finney, J. W. (2001). Predictors of deterioration among patients with substance-use disorders. *J Clin Psychol, 57,* 1403–1419.

Trull, T. J., Sher, K. J., Minks-Brown, C., Durbin, J., & Burr, R. (2001). Borderline personality disorder and substance use disorders: A review and integration. *Clin Psychol Rev, 20,* 235–253.

Verheul, R., van den Bosch, L. M. C., Koeter, M. W. J, de Ridder, M. A. J, Stijnen, T., & van den Brink, W. (2003). Dialectical behaviour therapy for women with borderline personality disorder: 12-month, randomised clinical trial in the Netherlands. *Br J Psychiatry, 182,* 135–140.

Wagner, A. W., & Linehan, M. M. (1997). Biosocial perspective on the relationship of childhood sexual abuse, suicidal behavior, and borderline personality disorder. In M. Zanarini (Ed.), *Role of sexual abuse in the etiology of borderline personality disorder.* Washington, DC: American Psychiatric Press.

Weiss, R. D., Mirin, S. M., Griffin, M. L., Gunderson, J. G., & Hufford, C. (1993). Personality disorders in cocaine dependence. *Compr Psychiatry, 34,* 145–149.

CHAPTER 28

Matching and Differential Therapies
Providing Substance Abusers
with Appropriate Treatment

KATHLEEN M. CARROLL

Broadly defined, matching individuals to treatment means providing the individual with the treatment approach that is likely to maximize outcome. The past 20 years have been marked by both tremendous progress and increasing methodological rigor in substance abuse research, and hence, the development of a much wider range of empirically supported pharmacotherapies and behavioral therapies. Availability of a broader range of therapies has likewise heightened interest in differential treatment research, whether it be matching individuals to specific treatment approaches, matching patients to different levels of services, or identifying predictors of response to specific therapies.

To date however, empirical evidence supporting specific, a priori matching strategies has been modest at best (Magura et al., 2003; McKay, Cacciola, McLellan, Alterman, & Wirtz, 1997; McLellan & McKay, 1998; Project MATCH Research Group, 1993, 1997), in part due to the complexity of treatment decisions for many patients, who typically present for treatment with a complex array of substance use, psychiatric, legal, medical, and social problems, as well as limits of the service delivery system in accommodating the needs of diverse patients (Gastfriend, Lu, & Sharon, 2000). The complexities and challenging methodological requirements of matching research have also hampered progress in this area (Moyer, Finney, Elworth, & Kraemer, 2001).

There is some more consistency in the literature, however, regarding patient prognostic variables that have emerged across patient populations.

Briefly, greater severity of substance dependence, presence and severity of comorbid psychiatric problems, lower levels of social support, and unemployment have consistently related to poorer outcome reviews (McLellan & McKay, 1998). Larger scale studies have also demonstrated with some consistency that addressing comorbid issues and problems in treatment is generally associated with improved outcome (McLellan, Arndt, Metzger, Woody, & O'Brien, 1993; McLellan, Grissom, Zanis, & Randall, 1997).

Thus, appropriate matching to treatment implies provision of an effective, empirically supported therapy, with adjunct therapies appropriate to the specific co-occurring problems, as dictated by careful, thorough, assessment of the patient functioning and status across a range of domains. This review summarizes empirically supported therapies across the most common substance use disorders (SUDs), with special emphasis on how pharmacological and behavioral therapies can be combined to enhance outcome. When available, data regarding the types of individuals who may respond particularly well or poorly to specific approaches are reviewed. First, however, it is important to understand the respective roles of pharmacotherapy and behavioral approaches in terms of how these may be tailored, or combined, to meet the needs of specific individuals.

ROLES OF PHARMACOTHERAPY IN THE TREATMENT OF SUBSTANCE USE DISORDERS

The target symptoms addressed and roles typically played by pharmacotherapy differ from those of behavioral treatments in their course of action, time to effect, target symptoms, and durability of benefits (Elkin, Pilkonis, Docherty, & Sotsky, 1988). In general, pharmacotherapies have a much more narrow application than do most behavioral treatments for SUDs; that is, most behavioral therapies are applicable across a range of treatment settings (e.g., inpatient, outpatient, residential), modalities (e.g., group, individual, family), and to a wide variety of populations. For example, disease-model, behavioral, or motivational approaches have been used, with only minor modifications, regardless of whether the patient is an opiate, alcohol, cocaine, or marijuana user. On the other hand, most available pharmacotherapies tend to be applicable only to a single class of substance use and exert their effects over a narrow band of symptoms or clinical settings. For example, methadone produces cross-tolerance for opioids but has little effect on concurrent cocaine abuse; disulfiram produces nausea after alcohol ingestion, but not after ingestion of illicit substances. A notable exception is naltrexone, which is used to treat both opioid and, more recently, alcohol dependence.

Common roles and indications for pharmacotherapy in the treatment of substance dependence disorders are presented (Carroll, 2001; Rounsaville & Carroll, 1997).

Detoxification

For those classes of substances that produce substantial physical withdrawal syndromes (e.g., alcohol, opioids, sedatives/hypnotics), medications are often needed to reduce or control the often-dangerous symptoms associated with withdrawal. Benzodiazepines are often used to manage symptoms of alcohol withdrawal. Agents such as methadone, clonidine, naltrexone, and buprenorphine are typically used for the management of opioid withdrawal. Typically, the role of behavioral treatments during detoxification is typically extremely limited due to the level of discomfort, agitation, and confusion the patient may experience. However, studies have suggested the effectiveness of behavioral strategies in increasing retention and abstinence in the course of longer term outpatient detoxification protocols (Bickel, Amass, Higgins, Badger, & Esch, 1997).

Stabilization and Maintenance

A widely-used example of the use of a medication for long-term stabilization of drug users is methadone maintenance for opioid dependence, a treatment strategy that involves the daily administration of a long-acting opioid (methadone) as a substitute for the illicit use of short-acting opioids (typically heroin). Methadone maintenance permits the patient to function normally, without experiencing withdrawal symptoms, craving, or side effects. The large body of research on methadone maintenance confirms its importance in fostering treatment retention, providing the opportunity to evaluate and treat other problems and disorders that often coexist with opioid dependence (e.g., medical, legal, and occupational problems), reducing the risk of HIV infection and other complications through reducing intravenous drug use, and providing a level of stabilization that permits the inception of psychotherapy and other aspects of treatment.

Antagonist and Other
Behaviorally Oriented Pharmacotherapies

A more recent pharmacological strategy is the use of antagonist treatment, that is, the use of medications that block the effects of specific drugs. An example of this approach is naltrexone, an effective, long-acting opioid antagonist. Naltrexone is nonaddicting, does not have the reinforcing properties of opioids, has few side effects and, most important, effectively blocks the effects of opioids. Therefore, naltrexone treatment represents a potent behavioral strategy: Because opioid ingestion is not reinforced while the patient is taking naltrexone, unreinforced opioid use allows extinction of relationships between conditioned drug cues and drug use. For example, a naltrexone-maintained patient, anticipating that opioid use will not result in desired drug effects, may be more likely to learn to live in a world full of drug cues and high-risk situations without resorting to drug use.

Treatment of Coexisting Disorders

An important role of pharmacotherapy in the treatment of SUDs is as treatment for coexisting psychiatric syndromes that may precede or play a role in the maintenance or complications of drug dependence. The frequent co-occurrence of psychiatric disorders, particularly affective and anxiety disorders, with SUDs is well documented in a variety of populations and settings (Kessler et al., 1997; Regier et al., 1990). Given that psychiatric disorders often precede development of SUDs, several researchers and clinicians have hypothesized that individuals with primary psychiatric disorders may be attempting to self-medicate their psychiatric symptoms with drugs and alcohol. Thus, effective pharmacological treatment of the underlying psychiatric disorder may improve not only the psychiatric disorder but also the perceived need for, and therefore the use of, illicit drugs (Nunes & Levin, 2004). Examples of this type of approach include the use of antidepressant treatment for depressed alcohol- (Mason, Salvato, Williams, Ritvo, & Cutler, 1999), opioid- (Nunes et al., 1998), and cocaine-dependent (Rounsaville, 2004) individuals.

BEHAVIORAL TREATMENTS

Most behavioral approaches for SUDs address several common issues and tasks, despite often vast differences in theory, technique, and strategies. Although different approaches vary in the degree to which emphasis is placed on these common tasks, some attention to these issues is likely to be involved in any successful treatment (Rounsaville & Carroll, 1997). Moreover, it should be noted that currently available pharmacotherapies for drug dependence would be expected to have little or no effect in these areas commonly addressed by behavioral therapies.

Setting the Resolve to Stop

Rare is the substance abuser who seeks treatment without some degree of ambivalence regarding cessation of drug use. Even at the time of treatment seeking, which usually occurs only after substance-related problems have become severe, substance abusers usually can identify many ways in which they want or feel the need for drugs and alcohol, and have difficulty developing a clear picture of what life without drugs might be like (Rounsaville & Carroll, 1997). Moreover, given the substantial external pressures that may precipitate application for treatment, many patients are highly ambivalent about treatment itself. Ambivalence must be addressed if the patient is to experience him- or herself as an active participant in treatment; if the patient perceives treatment as wholly imposed upon him or her by external forces and does not have a clear sense of personal goals for treatment; it is likely that any form of treatment will be of limited usefulness. Treatments based on principles of motivational psychology, such as motivational interviewing (Miller & Rollnick, 2002), concentrate almost exclusively on strategies intended to bolster the patient's own motivational resources. However, most behavioral treatments include some exploration of what the patient stands to lose or gain through continued substance use as a means to enhance motivation for treatment and abstinence.

Teaching Coping Skills

Social learning theory posits that substance abuse may represent a means of coping with difficult situations, positive and negative affects, invitations by peers to use substances, and so on. By the time substance use is severe enough for treatment, use of substances may represent the individual's single, overgeneralized means of coping with a variety of situations, settings, and states. If stable abstinence is to be achieved, treatment must help patients to recognize the high-risk situations in which they are most likely to use substances and to develop other, more effective means of coping with them. Although cognitive-behavioral approaches concentrate almost exclusively on skills training as a means of preventing relapse to substance use (Marlatt & Gordon, 1985; Monti et al., 1989), most treatment approaches touch on the relationship between high-risk situations and substance use to some extent.

Changing Reinforcement Contingencies

By the time treatment is sought, many substance abusers spend the preponderance of their time involved in acquiring, using, and recovering from substance use, to the exclusion of other endeavors and rewards. The abuser may be estranged from friends and family, and have few social contacts who do not use drugs. If the patient is still working, employment often becomes only a means of acquiring money to buy drugs, and the fulfilling or challenging aspects of work have faded. Few other activities, such as hobbies, athletics, and involvement with community or church groups, can stand up to the demands of substance dependence. Typically, rewards available in daily life are narrowed progressively to those derived from drug use, and other diversions may be neither available nor perceived as enjoyable. When drug use is stopped, its absence may leave the patient with the need to fill the time that had been spent using drugs and to find rewards that can substitute for those derived from drug use. Thus, most behavioral treatments encourage patients to identify and develop fulfilling alternatives to substance use, as exemplified by the community reinforcement approach (CRA; Azrin, 1976) or contingency management (Budney & Higgins, 1998), which stresses the development of alternate reinforcers for substance use.

Fostering Affect Management

Among the most commonly cited reasons for relapse are powerful negative affects, and several clinicians have suggested that failure of affect regulation is a critical dynamic underlying the development of compulsive drug use. Moreover, the difficulty many substance abusers have in recognizing and managing affect states has been noted in several populations. Thus, an important common task in substance abuse treatment is to help develop ways of coping with powerful dysphoric affects, and to learn to recognize and identify the probable cause of these feelings (Rounsaville & Carroll, 1997). Again, while psychodynamically oriented treatments such as supportive–expressive therapy (Luborsky, 1984) emphasize the role of affect in the treatment of cocaine abuse, virtually all forms of psychotherapy for substance abuse include a variety of techniques for coping with strong affects.

Improving Interpersonal Functioning and Enhancing Social Supports

A consistent finding in the literature on relapse to substance abuse and dependence is the protective influence of an adequate network of social supports (Longabaugh, Beattie, Noel, Stout, & Malloy, 1993). Typical issues presented by drug abusers are loss of or damage to valued relationships occurring when using drugs was the principal priority, failure to have achieved satisfactory relationships even prior to having initiated drug use, and inability to identify friends or intimates who are not themselves drug users (Rounsaville & Carroll, 1997). Many forms of treatment, including family/couple therapy (E. E. Epstein & McCrady, 1998; Fals-Stewart, O'Farrell, & Birchler, 1997), 12-step approaches (Nowinski, Baker, & Carroll, 1992), interpersonal therapy (Rounsaville, Gawin, & Kleber, 1985), and network therapy (Galanter, 1993), make building and maintaining a network of social supports for abstinence a central focus of treatment.

Fostering Compliance with Pharmacotherapy

The difficulties of fostering adequate levels of treatment compliance with substance users are well known, so much so that substance abusers are typically excluded from clinical trials of treatments for other disorders. Thus, when pharmacotherapies are used in the treatment of substance abuse, it is not surprising that high rates of noncompliance are seen. A major role that behavioral treatments play when pharmacotherapies are used in the treatment of substance use is in fostering compliance, because most strategies to improve compliance are inherently psychosocial. These include, for example, regular monitoring of medication compliance through pill counts and medication serum levels; encouragement of patient self-monitoring of compliance (e.g., through medication logs or diaries); clear communication between patient and staff about the medication, its expected effects, side effects, and benefits; repeatedly stressing the importance of adherence; contracting with the patients for adherence; directly reinforcing adherence through incentives or rewards; providing telephone or written reminders about appointments or taking medication; preparing and educating patients about the disorder and its treatment; and frequent contact and the provision of extensive support and encouragement to the patient and his or her family.

TREATMENT APPROACHES FOR SPECIFIC CATEGORIES OF SUBSTANCE USE

Before moving to a review of empirically supported treatments for specific categories of substance use, three general issues regarding the current state of substance abuse treatment are highlighted. First, nonpharmacological, behavioral treatments continue to constitute the bulk of substance abuse treatment in the United States. Numerous uncontrolled studies, as well as randomized trials, consistently point to the benefits of purely behavioral approaches for many SUDs (McLellan & McKay, 1998; Simpson, Joe, & Brown, 1997), and effective pharmacotherapies, even in cases where they exist, tend to be underutilized Second, for most types of illicit drug use, no effective pharmacotherapies exist. Classes of drug use for which no effective, approved pharmacotherapies have been developed include marijuana, hallucinogens, amphetamines, inhalants, phencyclidine, and sedative/hypnotic/anxiolytics. Although major advances have been made in identifying physiological mechanisms of action for many of these substances, and in a few cases (e.g., marijuana) specific receptors have been identified that should accelerate progress in identifying pharmacological treatments, behavioral therapies remain the sole available treatment for many classes of drug dependence. Third, there is general consensus that even for our most potent pharmacotherapies for drug use, purely pharmacological approaches are insufficient for most substance abusers and best outcomes are seen for combined treatments. As described earlier, most pharmacotherapies are comparatively specific and narrow in their actions, and may help to detoxify, stabilize, or treat coexisting disorders, but are rarely considered "complete treatments" in and of themselves. Furthermore, because few patients will persist or comply with a purely pharmacotherapeutic approach, pharmacotherapies delivered alone, without any supportive or compliance-enhancing elements, are usually not considered feasible. Even where pharmacotherapy is seen as the primary treatment approach (as in the case of methadone maintenance), some form of psychosocial treatment is used to provide at least a minimal supportive structure within which pharmacotherapeutic treatment can be conducted effectively. Furthermore, medication effects can be enhanced or diminished with respect to the context in which they are delivered; that is, a medication administered in the context of a supportive clinician–patient relationship, with clear expectations of possible medication benefits and side effects, close monitoring of compliance, and encouragement for abstinence, is more likely to have enhanced effectiveness than a medication delivered without such elements. Thus, even for primarily pharmacotherapeutic treatments, a psychotherapeutic component is almost always included to foster patients' retention in treatment and compliance with pharmacotherapy, and to address the numerous comorbid psychosocial problems that occur so frequently among individuals with SUDs (Carroll, 2001).

TREATMENT OF ALCOHOL DEPENDENCE

There is now a comparatively wide range of empirically supported behavioral therapies for alcohol use disorders, including brief intervention, social skills training, cognitive-behavioral therapies, family/couple and network therapies, and motivational interviewing (DeRubeis & Crits-Christoph, 1998; Miller & Wilbourne, 2002). The availability of a much broader array of effective treatment options led in part to Project MATCH, a large, multisite study of a priori treatment-matching hypotheses, in which 1,726 alcohol-abusing or -dependent patients were randomly assigned to either motivational enhancement therapy (Miller, Zweben, DiClemente, & Rychtarik, 1992), 12-step facilitation (Nowinski et al., 1992), or cognitive-behavioral therapy (Kadden et al., 1992), all delivered as individual treatments over 12 weeks. While the results of this landmark study indicated few strong indicators of matching or differential response to these treatments, a major finding of Project MATCH was that these three therapies were followed by marked and sustained reductions in alcohol consumption (Project MATCH Research Group, 1997, 1998). To illustrate, in all three conditions, patients, on average, entered treatment drinking more than 80% of days, rapidly reduced their consumption to less than 15% of days, and kept those levels down at follow-up visits over 3 years. Thus, one implication of these findings is that delivery of a high-quality individual behavioral therapy can be associated with meaningful change in individuals with a wide range of alcohol disorders and associated problems.

There have been a number of developments in the pharmacotherapy of alcohol use disorders as well. The most commonly used pharmacological adjunct for the treatment of alcohol dependence remains disulfiram (Antabuse). Disulfiram interferes with normal metabolism of alcohol, which results in an accumulation of acetaldhyde; hence, drinking following ingestion of disulfiram results in an intense physiological reaction, characterized by flushing, rapid or irregular heartbeat, dizziness, nausea, and headache (see Nace, Chapter 5, this volume). Thus, disulfiram treatment is intended to work as a deterrent to drinking. Despite the sustained popularity and widespread use of disulfiram, a landmark multicenter, randomized clinical trial found that disulfiram was no more effective than inactive doses of disulfiram or no medication in terms of rates of abstinence, time to first drink, unemployment, or social stability (Fuller et al., 1986). However, for subjects who did drink, disulfiram treatment was associated with significantly fewer total drinking days. Rates of compliance with disulfiram in the study were low (20% of all subjects), but abstinence rates were reasonably good (43%) among compliant subjects. This study highlights several important problems with the use of disulfiram: (1) Compliance is a major problem and must be monitored closely, and (2) many patients are unwilling to take disulfiram (62% of those eligible for the study refused to participate).

Thus, several investigators have evaluated the effectiveness of behavioral treatments to improve retention and compliance with disulfiram. One of the most effective strategies is disulfiram contracts, in which the patient's spouse or a significant other agrees to observe the patient take disulfiram each day and reward the patient for compliance with disulfiram treatment (O'Farrell, Cutter, Choquette, & Floyd, 1992). Azrin, Sisson, Meyers, and Godley (1982) reported positive and durable results from a randomized clinical trial comparing unmonitored disulfiram to disulfiram contracts, where disulfiram ingestion was monitored by the patient's spouse or administered as part of a multifaceted behavioral program, the CRA. A broad-spectrum approach developed by Hunt and Azrin (1973), CRA incorporates skills training, behavioral family therapy, and job-finding training, as well as a disulfiram component. CRA has been found to be significantly more effective than traditional group approaches in fostering abstinence. Combined disulfiram–behavioral treatment for alcohol dependence illustrates how a pharmacotherapy that may be marginally effective when used alone can be highly effective when used with in combination with treatments that foster compliance and target other aspects of substance abuse.

Another major development in the treatment of alcohol dependence was the recent Food and Drug Administration (FDA) approval of naltrexone. The application of naltrexone, an opioid antagonist, to the treatment of alcoholism derives from findings that naltrexone reduces alcohol craving and use in humans. In randomized clinical trials, naltrexone has been shown to be more effective than placebo in reducing alcohol use and craving (O'Malley et al., 1992; Volpicelli, Alterman, Hayashida, & O'Brien, 1992). As with disulfiram, best responses are seen among patients who are compliant with naltrexone

(Volpicelli et al., 1997), which *underscores the importance of delivering naltrexone in conjunction with an effective behavioral approach that addresses compliance.*

Thus, it is not surprising that naltrexone's effects have been found to differ somewhat depending on the nature of the behavioral treatment with which it is delivered. For example, in the O'Malley and colleagues (1992) study, highest rates of abstinence were found when the patient received naltrexone plus a supportive clinical management psychotherapy condition that encouraged complete abstinence from alcohol and other substances. However, for patients who drank, the combination of a cognitive-behavioral coping skills approach and naltrexone was superior in terms of rates of relapse and drinks per occasion. Evaluation of naltrexone's effectiveness in combination with acamprosate, another promising medication, and with brief versus more intensive behavioral treatment that should shed light on important data regarding the types of patients who respond to lower versus higher intensity behavioral approaches with naltrexone, is ongoing (COMBINE Study Research Group, 2003).

TREATMENT OF OPIOID DEPENDENCE

The inception of methadone maintenance treatment revolutionized the treatment of opioid addiction, because it displayed the previously unseen ability to keep addicts in treatment and to reduce their illicit opioid use, outcomes with which nonpharmacological treatments had fared comparatively poorly. Beyond its ability to retain opioid addicts in treatment and help control opioid use, methadone maintenance also reduces the risk of HIV infection and other medical complications through reducing intravenous drug use (Ball & Ross, 1991), and provides the opportunity to evaluate and treat concurrent disorders, including medical problems and family and psychiatric problems. The bulk of the large body of literature on the effectiveness of methadone maintenance points to its success in retaining opioid addicts in treatment and reducing their illicit opioid use and illegal activity (Ball & Ross, 1991). Methadone maintenance treatment, especially when provided at adequate doses and combined with drug counseling, substantially decreases illicit opioid use, injection drug use, criminal activity, and morbidity and mortality risk (O'Brien, 1997). However, there is a great deal of variability in the success across different methadone maintenance programs, which appears to be largely associated with both variability in delivery of adequate dosing of methadone and in provision and quality of psychosocial services (Ball & Ross, 1991).

There remain, however, several problems with methadone maintenance, including illicit diversion of take-home methadone doses, difficulties with detoxification from methadone maintenance to a drug-free state, and the concurrent use of other substances, particularly alcohol and cocaine, among methadone-maintained individuals. Thus, a range of psychosocial treatments have been evaluated for their ability to address these drawbacks of methadone maintenance, as well as to enhance and extend the benefits of methadone maintenance. Several types of behavioral approaches have been identified as effective in enhancing and extending the benefits of methadone maintenance treatment, and these are summarized below (Carroll, 2001).

Before describing specific approaches that have been demonstrated to be effective in enhancing the effectiveness of opioid maintenance therapies, the context for such approaches should be set by a brief review of a study that authoritatively established the importance of psychosocial treatments even in the context of a pharmacotherapy as potent as methadone. McLellan and colleagues (1993) randomly assigned 92 opiate-dependent individuals to (1) methadone maintenance alone, without psychosocial services; (2) methadone maintenance with standard services, which included regular meetings with a counselor; and (3) enhanced methadone maintenance, which included regular counseling plus on-site medical/psychiatric, employment, and family therapy, in a 24-week trial. Although some patients did reasonably well in the methadone-alone condition, 69% of this group had to be transferred out of this condition within 3 months of the study inception, because their substance use did not improve or even worsened, or because they experienced significant medical or psychiatric problems that required a more intensive level of care. In terms of drug use and psychosocial outcomes, the best outcomes were seen in the enhanced methadone maintenance condition, with intermediate outcomes for the standard methadone services condition, and the poorest outcomes for the methadone-alone condition. This study illustrates that although methadone maintenance treatment has powerful effects in terms of keeping addicts in treatment and making them available for psychosocial treatments, a purely pharmacological approach is not sufficient for the large majority of patients, and better outcomes are closely associated with higher levels of psychosocial treatments.

More recently, among the most exciting findings regarding how the benefits of agonist maintenance therapies can be enhanced for a range of individuals has been the use of contingency management to reduce the use of illicit drugs in addicts who are maintained on methadone. In these studies, a reinforcer is provided to patients who demonstrate specified target behaviors, such as providing drug-free urine specimens, accomplishing specific treatment goals, or attending treatment sessions. For example, using methadone take-home privileges as rewards contingent on reduced drug use is an approach that capitalizes on an inexpensive reinforcer that is potentially available in all methadone maintenance programs. Stitzer, Iguchi, Kidorf, and Bigelow (1993) have done extensive work in evaluating methadone take-home privileges as a reward for decreased illicit drug use. In a series of well-controlled trials, this group of researchers has demonstrated (1) the relative benefits of positive over negative contingencies; (2) the attractiveness of take-home privileges over other incentives available within methadone maintenance clinics; (3) the effectiveness of targeting and rewarding drug-free urines over other, more distal behaviors, such as group attendance; and (4) the benefits of using take-home privileges contingent on drug-free urines over noncontingent take-home privileges.

Silverman and colleagues (1996), drawing on the compelling work of Steve Higgins and his colleagues (e.g., Budney & Higgins, 1998), evaluated a voucher-based contingency management system to address concurrent illicit drug use (typically cocaine) among methadone-maintained opioid addicts. In this approach, urine specimens are required three times weekly in order to detect systematically all episodes of drug use. Abstinence is reinforced through a voucher system in which the rewards help patients develop alternative reinforcers to drug use (e.g., movie tickets or sporting goods, but never money). To encourage longer periods of consecutive abstinence, the value of the points earned by a patient increases with each successive clean urine specimen, and the value of the points is reset when the patient relapses. In a very elegant series of studies, Silverman and his colleagues have demonstrated the efficacy of this approach in reducing illicit opioid and cocaine use, and in producing a number of treatment benefits among this very difficult population.

Although contingency management procedures appear quite promising in modifying previously intractable problems in methadone maintenance programs, particularly continued illicit drug use among clients, they have rarely been implemented in clinical practice. A major obstacle to the implementation of contingency management voucher approaches in regular clinical settings is their cost (up to $1,200 over 12 weeks). However, lower cost variable ratio contingency management approaches, in which patients earn opportunities to draw prizes from a bowl contingent on specific behavioral targets, have also received impressive empirical support in a range of populations (Petry, 2000; Petry & Martin, 2002). Moreover, there are indications that the positive effects of contingency management procedures may diminish over time when the behavioral intervention is no longer in effect. Studies evaluating the change in strength or preference of reinforcers over time within methadone maintenance programs are needed. For example, for clients from the street who enter a methadone program, contingency payments or dose increases may be highly motivating, whereas for clients who have been stabilized and are working, and who may have less free time, other reinforcers, such as take-home doses or permission to omit counseling sessions, may be more attractive later in treatment. While contingency management procedures may prove effective only over short periods of time, they may still be valuable in that they may provide an interruption in illicit drug use (or other undesirable behaviors) that may serve as an opportunity for other interventions and services to take effect.

Other Psychotherapies

Other studies have evaluated other forms of psychotherapy as strategies to enhance outcome from opioid maintenance therapies. The landmark study in this area was done by Woody and colleagues (1983) and replicated in community settings (Woody, McLellan, Luborsky, & O'Brien, 1995). While the original study is now more than 20 years old, it is reviewed in some detail here, because it remains the most impressive demonstration of the benefits and role of psychotherapy in the context of methadone maintenance programs. Moreover, it has generated several substudies that have added greatly to our understanding of the types of patients who benefit from psychotherapy in the context of methadone maintenance programs.

In this landmark study, 110 opiate addicts entering a methadone maintenance program were randomly assigned to one of three treatments: drug counseling alone, drug counseling plus supportive–expressive psychotherapy (SE), or drug counseling plus cognitive psychotherapy (CT). After a 6-month course of treatment, although the SE and CT groups did not differ significantly from each other on most measures of outcome, subjects who received either form of professional psychotherapy evidenced greater improvement in more outcome domains than the subjects who received drug counseling alone (Woody et al., 1983). Furthermore, gains made by the subjects who received professional psychotherapy were sustained over a 12-month follow-up, while subjects receiving drug counseling alone evidenced some attrition of gains (Woody, McLellan, Luborsky, & O'Brien, 1987). This study also demonstrated differential response to psychotherapy as a function of patient characteristics, which may point to the best use of psychotherapy (relative to drug counseling) when resources are scarce: While methadone-maintained opiate addicts with lower levels of psychopathology tended to improve regardless of whether they received professional psychotherapy or drug counseling, those with higher levels of psychopathology tended to improve only if they received psychotherapy. In addition, this study provides indications of differential response to psychotherapy by concurrent psychiatric disorder. For example, depressed addicts improved with psychotherapy, while addicts with antisocial personality disorder tended to show little or no improvement, unless they are also had a depressive disorder (Woody et al., 1995).

New Maintenance Therapies

New maintenance therapies that have recently been developed for opioid dependence hold the promise of making effective maintenance therapies more broadly available. This is significant, because access to methadone treatment is quite limited; currently, fewer than one in five heroin users receives treatment for drug dependence (Rounsaville & Kosten, 2000). Barriers to access to methadone maintenance include both limited patient and community acceptance of methadone, and regulatory restrictions and the lack of availability in many areas of the country. Development of alternative maintenance agents, and especially agents that can be more readily administered with reduced clinic attendance and outside of traditional methadone maintenance settings, may address some of the problems associated with limited access to treatment.

Buprenorphine, a partial mu agonist and kappa antagonist, represents a promising alternative to methadone and was recently approved by the FDA. Because of its unique pharmacological properties, there may be a number of advantages to its use, compared to either methadone or levo-alpha-acetyl methadol (LAAM), as a maintenance agent for the treatment of opioid dependence settings. Ceiling effects at higher buprenorphine doses result in a lower risk of overdose compared with methadone, and buprenorphine may also have a reduced abuse liability in opiate-dependent individuals (thus, less likelihood for diversion), because its use may precipitate withdrawal symptoms (Strain, Preston, Liebson, & Bigelow, 1995; Walsh, Preston, Bigelow, & Stitzer, 1995). Withdrawal symptoms following abrupt discontinuation of buprenorphine are also usually relatively mild (Cowan & Lewis, 1995; Fudala, Jaffe, Dax, & Johnson, 1990). Results of random assignment, double-blind clinical trials generally support the safety and dose-dependent efficacy of buprenorphine maintenance (Fudala et al., 2003; Ling, Wesson, Charavastra, & Klett, 1996; Schottenfeld, Pakes, Oliveto, Ziedonis, & Kosten, 1997).

Because buprenorphine have been made available only recently, very few studies have been done to identify predictors of patient response to methadone versus buprenorphine, or the minimal and optimal intensity of behavioral treatment to be administered in conjunction with these maintenance agents. However, it is likely that the same principles as those found in the methadone literature regarding use of behavioral therapies to enhance outcome with these agents as will emerge over time.

Naltrexone–Agonist Treatment

Opioid antagonist treatment (naltrexone) offers many potential advantages over methadone maintenance: It is nonaddicting and can be prescribed without concerns about diversion, it has a benign side-effect profile, and it may be less costly, in terms of demands on professionals and patients' time, than the daily or near-daily clinic visits required for methadone maintenance (Rounsaville, 1995). Most important are behavioral aspects of the treatment, because unreinforced opiate use allows extinction of relationships between cues and drug use. While naltrexone treatment is likely to be attractive only to a minority of opioid addicts (Cornish et al., 1997), naltrexone's unique properties make it an important alternative to methadone maintenance.

However, despite its many advantages, naltrexone has not fulfilled its promise. Naltrexone treatment programs remain comparatively rare and underutilized with respect to methadone maintenance programs (Rounsaville, 1995). This is in large part due to problems with retention, particularly during the induction phase, where, on average, 40% of patients drop out during the first month of treatment, and 60% drop out by 3 months (Greenstein, Fudala, & O'Brien, 1997). Naltrexone treatment has other disadvantages compared with methadone, including (1) discomfort associated with detoxification and protracted withdrawal symptoms, (2) lack of negative consequences for abrupt discontinuation, and (3) no reinforcement for ingestion—all of which may lead to inconsistent compliance with naltrexone treatment and high rates of attrition.

Preliminary evaluations of behavioral interventions targeted to address naltrexone's weaknesses were encouraging. Several investigators (e.g., Grabowski et al., 1979; Meyer et al., 1976) reported success using contingency payments as reinforcements for naltrexone consumption. Family therapy and counseling have also been used to enhance retention in naltrexone programs. For example, in a nonrandomized study of multiple family therapy, Anton, Hogan, Jalali, Riordan, and Kleber (1981) reported that during the first month of naltrexone therapy, addicts in family therapy had a much significantly lower dropout rate compared to those not in family therapy (92 vs. 62%). More recently, some of the most promising data regarding strategies to enhance retention and outcome in naltrexone treatment have come from investigators evaluating contingency management approaches. Preston and colleagues (1999) found improved retention and naltrexone compliance for an approach that provided vouchers for naltrexone compliance versus one that provided noncontingent or no-vouchers. Again, however, it is not clear to what extent these procedures can be implemented outside of research settings, nor how durable they are after the termination of the incentive program.

TREATMENT OF COCAINE DEPENDENCE

In contrast to the treatment of opioid dependence, where behavioral therapies have been most effective when combined with pharmacotherapies (particularly agonist approaches such as methadone maintenance), the cocaine treatment literature is marked by strong evidence that points to the effectiveness of purely behavioral approaches. Despite many clinical trials evaluating diverse pharmacological agents, there is currently no effective pharmacotherapy for general populations of cocaine abusers. In contrast, several studies have demonstrated that comparatively brief, purely behavioral approaches can be both sufficient and effective for the majority of patients who receive them.

Voucher-Based Contingency Management

Perhaps the most exciting findings pertaining to the effectiveness of psycho-social treatments for cocaine dependence have been reports by Higgins and colleagues (Higgins et al., 1991, 1994; Higgins, Wong, Badger, Haug-Ogden, & Dantona, 2000) of the effectiveness of a program incorporating positive incentives for abstinence, reciprocal relationship counseling, and disulfiram into a community reinforcement approach (CRA; Azrin, 1976). The Higgins strategy has four organizing features, which are grounded in principles of behavioral pharmacology: (1) Drug use and abstinence must be swiftly and accurately detected; (2) abstinence is positively reinforced; (3) drug use results in loss of reinforcement; and (4) emphasis is on the development of competing reinforcers to drug use (Higgins, Budney, Bickel, & Hughes, 1993).

In this program, urine specimens are required three times weekly. Abstinence, assessed through drug-free urine screens, is reinforced through a voucher system in which patients receive points redeemable for items consistent with a drug-free lifestyle, such as movie tickets, sporting goods, and the like, but patients never receive money directly. To encourage longer periods of consecutive abstinence, the value of the points earned by the patients increases with each successive clean urine specimen, and the value of the points is reset back to its original level when the patient produces a drug-positive urine screen or does not provide a urine specimen.

In a series of well-controlled clinical trials, Higgins and colleagues have demonstrated (1) high acceptance, retention, and rates of abstinence for patients receiving this approach (i.e., 85% completing a 12-week course of treatment, and 65% achieving 6 or more weeks of abstinence) relative to standard substance abuse counseling; (2) rates of abstinence that do not decline substantially when less valuable incentives are substituted for the voucher system; (3) the value of the voucher system itself (as opposed to other program elements) in producing good outcomes by comparing the behavioral system with and without the vouchers; and (4) the durable effects of the voucher system (Higgins et al., 1993, 2000; Higgins & Silverman, 1999). Higgins's initial work with voucher-based contingency management has now been widely replicated in other settings and samples: homeless substance abusers (Milby et al., 2000), pregnant substance users (Svikis, Haug, & Stitzer, 1997), drug users in a therapeutic workplace (Silverman et al., 2002), alcohol-dependent individuals (Petry, Martin, Cooney, & Kranzler, 2000), and cocaine-dependent individuals within methadone maintenance treatment programs (Silverman et al., 1998). In regard to matching, there is some evidence that individuals with antisocial personality disorder may respond comparatively well to contingency management approaches (Messina, Farabee, & Rawson, 2003), and that raising the level of reinforcement may improve response among individuals who do not respond initially to lower levels of reinforcement (Silverman, 1999).

Cognitive-Behavioral Therapies

Another behavioral approach that has been shown to be effective in treating cocaine abusers is cognitive-behavioral therapy (CBT), which is based on social learning theories on the acquisition and maintenance of SUDs. The goal of CBT (also frequently called relapse prevention or coping skills therapy) is to foster abstinence through helping the patient to master an individualized set of coping strategies as effective alternatives to substance use. Typical skills taught include fostering resolution to stop both cocaine and other substance use through exploring positive and negative consequences of continued use; functional analysis of substance use (i.e., understanding substance use in relationship to its antecedents and consequences), development of strategies for coping with high-risk situations, including cocaine craving, preparation for emergencies, and coping with a relapse to substance use; and identifying and confronting thoughts about substance use.

A number of randomized clinical trials among several diverse, cocaine-dependent populations have demonstrated that compared with other commonly used psychotherapies for cocaine dependence, CBT appears to be particularly more effective with more severe cocaine users or those with comorbid psychiatric disorders, especially depression (Carroll, Rounsaville, Gordon, et al., 1994; Maude-Griffin et al., 1998; Rohsenow, Monti, Martin, Michalec, & Abrams, 2000). Moreover, CBT appears to be a particularly durable approach, with several studies suggesting that patients treated with this approach may continue to reduce their cocaine use even after they leave treatment (Carroll, Rounsaville, Nich, et al., 1994; D. E. Epstein, Hawkins, Covi, Umbricht, & Preston, 2003; Rawson et al., 2002). Recent evidence also suggests that individuals with cognitive impairment may not respond as well to cognitive-behavioral approaches (Aharonovich, Nunes, & Hasin, 2003).

Manualized Disease Model Approaches

Until very recently, treatment approaches based on disease models were widely practiced in the United States, but virtually no well-controlled, randomized clinical trials had been done to evaluate their efficacy alone or in comparison with other approaches. Thus, another important finding that has emerged from recent randomized clinical trials and has potential significance for the clinical community is the effectiveness of manualized disease model approaches. One such approach is 12-step facilitation (TSF), a manual-guided, individual approach that is intended to be similar to widely used approaches that emphasize principles associated with disease models of addiction. While this treatment has no official relationship with Alcoholics Anonymous (AA) or Cocaine Anonymous (CA), its content is intended to be consistent with the 12 steps of AA, with primary emphasis given to steps 1–5 and the concepts of acceptance (e.g., to help patients accept that they have the illness, or disease, of addiction) and surrender (e.g., to help patients acknowledge that there is hope for sobriety through accepting help from others and from a "Higher Power")(Nowinski et al., 1992). In addition to abstinence from all psychoactive substances, a major goal of the treatment is to foster active participation in self-help groups, and patients are actively encouraged to attend AA or CA meetings and become involved in traditional fellowship activities. In a comparison of TSF, CBT, and clinical management (a supportive approach in which patients receive comparable empathy, support and other "common elements" of psychotherapy but none of the unique "active ingredients" of TSF or CBT) for alcoholic cocaine-dependent individuals, TSF was significantly more effective than clinical management and was comparable to CBT in reducing cocaine use (Carroll, Nich, Ball, McCance-Katz, & Rounsaville, 1998).

The National Institute on Drug Abuse (NIDA) Collaborative Cocaine Treatment Study (CCTS), a multisite, randomized trial of psychotherapeutic treatments for cocaine dependence (Crits-Christoph et al., 1999), also offered strong evidence of the effectiveness of a similar approach, individual drug counseling (Mercer & Woody, 1999). In this study, 487 cocaine-dependent patients were randomized to one of four manual-guided treatment conditions: (1) cognitive therapy plus group drug counseling; (2) SE, a short-term psychodynamically oriented approach, plus group drug counseling; (3) individual drug counseling plus group drug counseling; or (4) group drug counseling alone. Outcomes on the whole were good, with all groups significantly reducing cocaine use from baseline; however, the best cocaine outcomes were seen for subjects who received individual drug counseling. Considered together with the recent findings of the Project MATCH Research Group (1997), where TSF was found to be comparable to CBT and motivational enhancement therapy in reducing alcohol use among 1,726 alcohol-dependent individuals, the findings from these studies offer compelling support for the efficacy of manual-guided disease model approaches. This has important clinical implications, because these approaches are similar to the dominant model applied in most community treatment programs and may thus be more easily mastered by "real-world" clinicians than approaches such as contingency management or CBT, treatments whose theoretical underpinnings may not be seen as highly compatible with disease model approaches.

TREATMENT OF MARIJUANA DEPENDENCE

Although marijuana is the most commonly used illicit drug in the United States, treatment of marijuana abuse and dependence is a comparatively understudied area to date, in part because comparatively few individuals present for treatment with a primary complaint of marijuana abuse or dependence. Currently, no effective pharmacotherapies for marijuana dependence exist, and only a few controlled trials of psychosocial approaches have been completed; thus, there is as yet little data on the types of individuals who respond particularly well or poorly to these approaches. Stephens, Roffman, and Curtin (2000) compared a delayed treatment control, a two-session motivational approach, and the more intensive (14 session) relapse prevention approach, and found better marijuana outcomes for the two active treatments compared with the delayed treatment control group, but no significant differences between the brief and the more intensive treatment. More recently, a replication and extension of that study, involving a multisite trial of 450 marijuana-dependent patients, compared three approaches: (1) a delayed treatment control, (2) a two-session motivational approach, and (3) a nine-session combined motivational–coping skills approach. Results suggested that both active treatments were associated with significantly greater reductions in marijuana use than the delayed treatment control through a 9-month follow-up (MTP Research Group, 2004). Moreover, the nine-session intervention was significantly more effective than the two-session intervention, and this effect was also sustained through the 9-month follow-up. Adding contingency management has also been shown to improve outcomes in these populations (Budney, Higgins, Radonovich, & Novy, 2000). Moreover, some early evidence suggests that individuals who submit drug-negative urines at treatment inception may have better response to treatment (Moore & Budney, 2002), a finding that is consistent with that of the general drug abuse treatment literature (Ehrman, Robbins, & Cornish, 2001).

CONCLUSIONS

Recent years have been marked by enormous progress in the identification of a wide range of empirically validated pharmacological and behavioral therapies for SUDs. Important new treatment options, such as naltrexone and acamprosate for alcohol use disorders, and buprenorphine for opioid dependence, were unavailable 20 years ago, as were behavioral therapies, including contingency management, behavioral marital counseling, motivational interviewing, and CBT—all of which have demonstrated efficacy across a range of SUDs and populations. Equally promising are the findings that combining pharmacotherapies with behavioral therapies can extend, strengthen, and make treatment effects more durable. Nevertheless, the rapid, recent progress in the identification of efficacious therapies has not been matched by identification of moderating variables or consistent patient predictors of response to specific treatment approaches that can guide researchers' and clinicians' efforts to match individuals to optimal treatment strategies. Identification of moderators of response to efficacious therapies, as well as identification of the specific mechanisms by which those treatments achieve their effects, should be a primary focus in the years that lie ahead.

ACKNOWLEDGMENTS

Support was provided by National Institute on Drug Abuse Grant Nos. K05-DA00457 and P50-DA09241, and by the U.S. Department of Veterans Affairs VISN 1 Mental Illness Research, Education, and Clinical Center.

REFERENCES

Aharonovich, E., Nunes, E. V., & Hasin, D. (2003). Cognitive impairment, retention and abstinence among cocaine abusers in cognitive-behavioral treatment. *Drug Alcohol Depend, 71,* 207–211.

Anton, R. F., Hogan, I., Jalali, B., Riordan, C. E., & Kleber, H. D. (1981). Multiple family therapy and naltrexone in the treatment of opioid dependence. *Drug Alcohol Depend, 8,* 157–168.

Azrin, N. H. (1976). Improvements in the community-reinforcement approach to alcoholism. *Behav Res Ther, 14,* 339–348.

Azrin, N. H., Sisson, R. W., Meyers, R., & Godley, M. (1982). Alcoholism treatment by disulfiram and community reinforcement therapy. *J Behav Therapy Exp Psych, 13,* 105–112.

Ball, J. C., & Ross, A. (1991). *The effectiveness of methadone maintenance treatment.* New York: Springer-Verlag.

Bickel, W. K., Amass, L., Higgins, S. T., Badger, G. J., & Esch, R. A. (1997). Effects of adding behavioral treatment to opioid detoxification with buprenorphine. *J Consult Clin Psychol, 65,* 803–810.

Budney, A. J., & Higgins, S. T. (1998). *A community reinforcement plus vouchers approach: Treating cocaine addiction.* Rockville, MD: National Institute on Drug Abuse.

Budney, A. J., Higgins, S. T., Radonovich, K. J., & Novy, P. L. (2000). Adding voucher-based incentives to coping skills and motivational enhancement improves outcomes during treatment for marijuana dependence. *J Consult Clin Psychol, 68,* 1051–1061.

Carroll, K. M. (2001). Combined treatments for substance dependence. In M. T. Sammons & N. B. Schmidt (Eds.), *Combined treatments for mental disorders: Pharmacological and psychotherapeutic strategies for intervention* (pp. 215–238). Washington, DC: American Psychological Association Press.

Carroll, K. M., Nich, C., Ball, S. A., McCance-Katz, E., & Rounsaville, B. J. (1998). Treatment of cocaine and alcohol dependence with psychotherapy and disulfiram. *Addiction, 93,* 713–728.

Carroll, K. M., Rounsaville, B. J., Gordon, L. T., Nich, C., Jatlow, P. M., Bisighini, R. M., et al. (1994). Psychotherapy and pharmacotherapy for ambulatory cocaine abusers. *Arch Gen Psychiatry, 51,* 177–197.

Carroll, K. M., Rounsaville, B. J., Nich, C., Gordon, L. T., Wirtz, P. W., & Gawin, F. H. (1994). One year follow-up of psychotherapy and pharmacotherapy for cocaine dependence: Delayed emergence of psychotherapy effects. *Arch Gen Psychiatry, 51,* 989–997.

COMBINE Study Research Group. (2003). Testing combined pharmacotherapies and behavioral therapies in alcohol dependence: Rationale and methods. *Alcohol Clin Exp Res, 27,* 1107–1122.

Cornish, J. W., Metzger, D., Woody, G. E., Wilson, D., McLellan, A. T., Vandergrift, B., et al. (1997). Naltrexone pharmacotherapy for opioid dependent federal probationers. *J Subst Abuse Treat, 14,* 529–534.

Cowan, A., & Lewis, J. W. (1995). *Buprenorphine: Combating drug abuse with a unique opioid.* New York: Wiley.

Crits-Christoph, P., Siqueland, L., Blaine, J. D., Frank, A., Luborsky, L., Onken, L. S., et al. (1999). Psychosocial treatments for cocaine dependence: Results of the National Institute on Drug Abuse Collaborative Cocaine Study. *Arch Gen Psychiatry, 56,* 495–502.

DeRubeis, R. J., & Crits-Christoph, P. (1998). Empirically supported individual and group psychological treatments for adult mental disorders. *J Consult Clin Psychol, 66,* 37–52.

Ehrman, R. N., Robbins, S. J., & Cornish, J. W. (2001). Results of a baseline urine test predict levels of cocaine use during treatment. *Drug Alcohol Depend, 62,* 1–7.

Elkin, I., Pilkonis, P. A., Docherty, J. P., & Sotsky, S. M. (1988). Conceptual and methodologic issues in compartive studies of psychotherapy and pharmacotherapy: I. Active ingredients and mechanisms of change. *Am J Psychiatry, 145,* 909–917.

Epstein, D. E., Hawkins, W. E., Covi, L., Umbricht, A., & Preston, K. L. (2003). Cognitive behavioral therapy plus contingency management for cocaine use: Findings during treatment and across 12-month follow-up. *Psychol Addict Behav, 17,* 73–82.

Epstein, E. E., & McCrady, B. S. (1998). Behavioral couples treatment of alcohol and drug use disorders: Current status and innovations. *Clin Psychol Rev, 18,* 689–711.

Fals-Stewart, W., O'Farrell, T. J., & Birchler, G. R. (1997). Behavioral couples therapy for male substance-abusing patients: A cost outcomes analysis. *J Consult Clin Psychol, 65,* 789–802.

Fudala, P. J., Bridge, T. P., Herbert, S., Williford, W. O., Chiange, C. N., Jones, K., et al. (2003). Office-based treatment of opiate addiction with a sublingual-tablet formulation of buprenorphine and naloxone. *N Engl J Med, 329*(10), 949–958.

Fudala, P. J., Jaffe, J. H., Dax, E. M., & Johnson, R. E. (1990). Use of buprenorphine in the treatment of opioid addiction: II. Physiologic and behavioral effects of daily and alternate-day administration and abrupt withdrawal. *J Pharmacol Exp Ther, 47,* 525–534.

Fuller, R. K., Branchey, L., Brightwell, D. R., Derman, R. M., Emrick, C. D., Iber, F. L., et al. (1986). Disulfiram treatment of alcoholism: A Veterans Administration cooperative study. *JAMA, 256,* 1449–1455.

Galanter, M. (1993). *Network therapy for alcohol and drug abuse: A new approach in practice.* New York: Basic Books.

Gastfriend, D. R., Lu, S. H., & Sharon, E. (2000). Placement matching: Challenges and technical progress. *Subst Use Misuse, 35,* 2191–2213.

Grabowski, J., O'Brien, C. P., Greenstein, R. A., Long, M., Steinberg-Donato, S., & Ternes, J. (1979). Effects of contingent payments on compliance with a naltrexone regimen. *Am J Drug Alcohol Abuse, 6,* 355–365.

Greenstein, R. A., Fudala, P. J., & O'Brien, C. P. (1997). Alternative pharmacotherapies for opiate addiction. In J. H. Lowinson, P. Ruiz, R. B. Millman, & J. G. Langrod (Eds.), *Comprehensive textbook of substance abuse* (3rd ed., pp. 415–425). New York: Williams & Wilkins.

Higgins, S. T., Budney, A. J., Bickel, W. K., Foerg, F. E., Donham, R., & Badger, G. J. (1994). Incentives improve outcome in outpatient behavioral treatment of cocaine dependence. *Arch Gen Psychiatry, 51,* 568–576.

Higgins, S. T., Budney, A. J., Bickel, W. K., & Hughes, J. R. (1993). Achieving cocaine abstinence with a behavioral approach. *Am J Psychiatry, 150,* 763–769.

Higgins, S. T., Delany, D. D., Budney, A. J., Bickel, W. K., Hughes, J. R., Foerg, F., et al. (1991). A behavioral approach to achieving initial cocaine abstinence. *Am J Psychiatry, 148,* 1218–1224.

Higgins, S. T., & Silverman, K. (1999). *Motivating behavior change among illicit-drug abusers.* Washington, DC: American Psychological Association.

Higgins, S. T., Wong, C. J., Badger, G. J., Haug-Ogden, D. E., & Dantona, R. L. (2000). Contingent reinforcement increases cocaine abstinence during outpatient treatment and one year follow-up. *J Consult Clin Psychol, 68,* 64–72.

Hunt, G. M., & Azrin, N. H. (1973). A community-reinforcement approach to alcoholism. *Behav Res Ther, 11,* 91–104.

Kadden, R., Carroll, K. M., Donovan, D., Cooney, J. L., Monti, P., Abrams, D., et al. (1992). *Cognitive-behavioral coping skills therapy manual: A clinical research guide for therapists treating individuals with alcohol abuse and dependence.* Rockville, MD: National Institute on alcohol Abuse and Alcoholism.

Kessler, R. C., Crum, R. M., Warner, L. A., Nelson, C. B., Schulenberg, J., & Anthony, J. C. (1997). Lifetime co-occurence of DSM-III-R alcohol abuse and dependence with other psychiatric disorders in the National Comorbidity Study. *Arch Gen Psychiatry, 54,* 313–321.

Ling, W., Wesson, D. R., Charavastra, C., & Klett, C. J. (1996). A controlled trial comparing buprenorphine and methadone maintenance in opioid dependence. *Arch Gen Psychiatry, 53,* 401–407.

Longabaugh, R., Beattie, M., Noel, R., Stout, R. L., & Malloy, P. (1993). The effect of social support on treatment outcome. *J Stud Alcohol, 54,* 465–478.

Luborsky, L. (1984). *Principles of psychoanalytic psychotherapy: A manual for supportive–expressive treatment.* New York: Basic Books.

Magura, S., Staines, G., Kosanke, N., Rosenblum, A., Foote, J., DeLuca, A., et al. (2003). Predictive validity of the ASAM Patient Placement Criteria for naturalistically matched vs. mismatched alcoholism patients. *Am J Addict, 12,* 386–397.

Marlatt, G. A., & Gordon, J. R. (1985). *Relapse prevention: Maintenance strategies in the treatment of addictive behaviors.* New York: Guilford Press.

Mason, B. J., Salvato, F. R., Williams, L. D., Ritvo, E. C., & Cutler, R. B. (1999). A double-blind, placebo controlled study of oral nalmefene for alcohol dependence. *Arch Gen Psychiatry, 56,* 719–724.

Maude-Griffin, P. M., Hohenstein, J. M., Humfleet, G. L., Reilly, P. M., Tusel, D. J., & Hall, S. M. (1998). Superior efficacy of cognitive-behavioral therapy for crack cocaine abusers: Main and matching effects. *J Consult Clin Psychol, 66,* 832–837.

McKay, J. R., Cacciola, J. S., McLellan, A. T., Alterman, A. I., & Wirtz, P. W. (1997). An initial evaluation of the psychosocial dimensions of the American Society of Addiction Medicine criteria for inpatient versus outpatient substance abuse rehabilitation. *J Consult Clin Psychol, 58,* 239–252.

McLellan, A. T., Arndt, I. O., Metzger, D., Woody, G. E., & O'Brien, C. P. (1993). The effects of psychosocial services in substance abuse treatment. *JAMA, 269,* 1953–1959.

McLellan, A. T., Grissom, G. R., Zanis, D., & Randall, M. (1997). Problem-service "matching" in addiction treatment: A prospective study in four programs. *Arch Gen Psychiatry, 54,* 730–735.

McLellan, A. T., & McKay, J. R. (1998). The treatment of addiction: What can research offer practice? In S. Lamb, M. R. Greenlick, & D. McCarty (Eds.), *Bridging the gap between practice and research: Forging partnerships with community based drug and alcohol treatment* (pp. 147–185). Washington, DC: National Academy Press.

Mercer, D. E., & Woody, G. E. (1999). *An individual drug counseling approach to treat cocaine addiction: The Collaborative Cocaine Treatment Study Model.* Rockville, MD: National Institute on Drug Abuse.

Messina, N., Farabee, D., & Rawson, R. A. (2003). Treatment responsivity of cocaine-dependent patients with antisocial personality disorder to cognitive-behavioral and contingency management interventions. *J Consult Clin Psychol, 71*(2), 320–329.

Meyer, R. E., Mirin, S. M., Altman, J. L., & McNamee, H. B. (1976). A behavioral paradigm for the evaluation of narcotic antagonists. *Arch Gen Psychiatry, 33,* 371–377.

Milby, J. B., Schumacher, J. E., McNamara, C., Wallace, D., Usdan, S., McGill, T., et al. (2000). Initiating abstinence in cocaine abusing dually diagnosed homeless persons. *Drug Alcohol Depend, 60,* 55–67.

Miller, W. R., & Rollnick, S. (2002). *Motivational interviewing: Preparing people for change* (2nd ed.). New York: Guilford Press.

Miller, W. R., & Wilbourne, P. L. (2002). Mesa Grande: A methodological analysis of clinical trials of treatments for alcohol use disorders. *Addiction, 97,* 265–277.

Miller, W. R., Zweben, A., DiClemente, C. C., & Rychtarik, R. G. (1992). *Motivational enhancement therapy manual: A clinical research guide for therapists treating individuals with alcohol abuse and dependence.* Rockville, MD: National Institute on Alcohol Abuse and Alcoholism.

Monti, P. M., Rohsenow, D. J., Abrams, D. B., Zwick, W. R., Binkoff, J. A., Munroe, S. M., et al. (1989). *Treating alcohol dependence: A coping skills training guide in the treatment of alcoholism.* New York: Guilford Press.

Moore, B. A., & Budney, A. J. (2002). Abstinence at intake for marijuana dependence treatment predicts response. *Drug Alcohol Depend, 249*–257.

Moyer, A., Finney, J. W., Elworth, J. T., & Kraemer, H. C. (2001). Can methodological features account for patient-treatment matching findings in the alcohol field? *J Stud Alcohol, 62,* 62–73.

MTP Research Group. (2004). Treating cannabis dependence: Findings from a multisite study. *J Consult Clin Psychol, 72,* 455–466.

Nowinski, J., Baker, S., & Carroll, K. M. (1992). *Twelve-step facilitation therapy manual: A clinical research guide for therapists treating individuals with alcohol abuse and dependence.* Rockville, MD: National Institute on Alcohol Abuse and Alcoholism.

Nunes, E. V., & Levin, F. R. (2004). Treatment of depression in patients with alcohol or other drug dependence: A meta-analysis. *JAMA, 291,* 1887–1896.

Nunes, E. V., Quitkin, F. M., Donovan, S. J., Deliyannides, D., Ocepek-Welikson, K., Koenig, T., et al. (1998). Imipramine treatment of opiate dependent patients with depressive disorders: A placebo-controlled trial. *Arch Gen Psychiatry, 55,* 153–160.

O'Brien, C. P. (1997). A range of research-based pharmacotherapies for addiction. *Science, 278,* 66–70.

O'Farrell, T. J., Cutter, H. S., Choquette, K. A., & Floyd, F. J. (1992). Behavioral marital therapy for male alcoholics: Marital and drinking adjustment during two years after treatment. *Behav Ther, 23,* 529–549.

O'Malley, S. S., Jaffe, A. J., Chang, G., Schottenfeld, R., Meyer, R. E., & Rounsaville, B. J. (1992). Naltrexone and coping skills therapy for alcohol dependence: A controlled study. *Arch Gen Psychiatry, 49,* 881–887.

Petry, N. M. (2000). A comprehensive guide to the application of contigency management procedures in clinical settings. *Drug Alcohol Depend, 58,* 9–25.

Petry, N. M., & Martin, B. (2002). Low-cost contingency management for treating cocaine- and opioid abusing methadone patients. *J Consult Clin Psychol, 70,* 398–405.

Petry, N. M., Martin, B., Cooney, J. L., & Kranzler, H. R. (2000). Give them prizes and they will come: Contingency management treatment of alcohol dependence. *J Consult Clin Psychol, 68,* 250–257.

Preston, K. L., Silverman, K., Umbricht, A., DeJesus, A., Montoya, I. D., & Schuster, C. R. (1999). Improvement in naltrexone treatment compliance with contingency management. *Drug Alcohol Depend, 54,* 127–135.

Project MATCH Research Group. (1993). Project MATCH: Rationale and methods for a multisite clinical trial matching alcoholism patients to treatment. *Alcohol Clin Exp Res, 17,* 1130–1145.

Project MATCH Research Group. (1997). Matching alcohol treatments to client heterogeneity: Project MATCH posttreatment drinking outcomes. *J Stud Alcohol, 58,* 7–29.

Project MATCH Research Group. (1998). Matching alcoholism treatments to client heterogeneity: Project MATCH three-year drinking outcomes. *Alcohol Clin Exp Res, 22,* 1300–1311.

Rawson, R. A., Huber, A., McCann, M. J., Shoptaw, S., Farabee, D., Reiber, C., et al. (2002). A comparison of contingency management and cognitive-behavioral approaches during methadone maintenance for cocaine dependence. *Arch Gen Psychiatry, 59,* 817–824.

Regier, D. A., Farmer, M. E., Rae, D. S., Locke, B. Z., Keith, S. J., Judd, L. L., et al. (1990). Comorbidity of mental disorders with alcohol and other drug abuse:

Results from the Epidemiologic Catchment Area (ECA) study. *JAMA, 264*, 2511–2518.

Rohsenow, D. J., Monti, P. M., Martin, R. A., Michalec, E., & Abrams, D. B. (2000). Brief coping skills treatment for cocaine abuse: 12-month substance use outcomes. *J Consult Clin Psychol, 68*, 515–520.

Rounsaville, B. J. (1995). Can psychotherapy rescue naltrexone treatment of opioid addiction? In L. S. Onken & J. D. Blaine (Eds.), *Potentiating the efficacy of medications: Integrating psychosocial therapies with pharmacotherapies in the treatment of drug dependence* (pp. 37–52). Rockville, MD: National Institute on Drug Abuse.

Rounsaville, B. J. (2004). Treatment of cocaine dependence and depression. *Biol Psych, 15*, 803–809.

Rounsaville, B. J., & Carroll, K. M. (1997). Individual psychotherapy for drug abusers. In J. H. Lowinsohn, P. Ruiz, & R. B. Miller (Eds.), *Comprehensive textbook of substance abuse* (3rd ed., pp. 430–439). New York: Williams & Wilkins.

Rounsaville, B. J., Gawin, F. H., & Kleber, H. D. (1985). Interpersonal psychotherapy adapted for ambulatory cocaine abusers. *Am J Drug Alcohol Abuse, 11*, 171–191.

Rounsaville, B. J., & Kosten, T. R. (2000). Treatment for opioid dependence: Quality and access. *JAMA, 283*(10), 1337–1339.

Schottenfeld, R. S., Pakes, J. R., Oliveto, A., Ziedonis, D., & Kosten, T. R. (1997). Buprenorphine vs. methadone maintenance treatment for concurrent opioid dependence and cocaine abuse. *Arch Gen Psychiatry, 54*, 713–720.

Silverman, K. (1999). Voucher-based reinforcement of cocaine abstinence in treatment-resistant methadone patients: Effects of reinforcer magnitude. *Psychopharmacology (Berl), 146*(2), 128–138.

Silverman, K., Higgins, S. T., Brooner, R. K., Montoya, I. D., Cone, E. J., Schuster, C. R., et al. (1996). Sustained cocaine abstinence in methadone maintenance patients through voucher-based reinforcement therapy. *Arch Gen Psychiatry, 53*, 409–415.

Silverman, K., Svikis, D. S., Wong, C. J., Hampton, J., Stitzer, M. L., & Bigelow, G. E. (2002). A reinforcement-based therapeutic workplace for the treatment of drug abuse: Three year abstinence outcomes. *Exp Clin Psychopharmacol, 10*, 228–240.

Silverman, K., Wong, C. J., Umbricht-Schneiter, A., Montoya, I. D., Schuster, C. R., & Preston, K. L. (1998). Broad beneficial effects of cocaine abstinence reinforcement among methadone patients. *J Consult Clin Psychol, 66*, 811–824.

Simpson, D. D., Joe, G. W., & Brown, B. S. (1997). Treatment retention and follow-up outcomes in the Drug Abuse Treatment Outcome Study (DATOS). *Psychol Addict Behav, 11*, 294–307.

Stephens, R., Roffman, R. A., & Curtin, L. (2000). Comparison of extended versus brief treatments for marijuana use. *J Consult Clin Psychol, 68*, 898–908.

Stitzer, M. L., Iguchi, M. Y., Kidorf, M., & Bigelow, G. E. (1993). Contingency management in methadone treatment: The case for positive incentives. In L. S. Onken, J. D. Blaine, & J. J. Boren (Eds.), *Behavioral treatments for drug abuse and dependence* (pp. 19–36). Rockville, MD: National Institute on Drug Abuse.

Strain, E. C., Preston, K. L., Liebson, I. A., & Bigelow, G. E. (1995). Buprenorphine effects in methadone-maintained volunteers: Effects at two hours after methadone. *J Pharmacol Exp Ther, 272*, 628–638.

Svikis, D. S., Haug, N. A., & Stitzer, M. L. (1997). Attendance incentives for outpatient treatment: Effects in methadone- and nonmethadone maintained pregnant drug dependent women. *Drug Alcohol Depend, 25,* 33–41.

Volpicelli, J. R., Alterman, A. I., Hayashida, M., & O'Brien, C. P. (1992). Naltrexone in the treatment of alcohol dependence. *Arch Gen Psychiatry, 49,* 876–880.

Volpicelli, J. R., Rhines, K. C., Rhines, J. S., Volpicelli, L. A., Alterman, A. I., & O'Brien, C. P. (1997). Naltrexone and alcohol dependence: Role of subject compliance. *Arch Gen Psychiatry, 54*(8), 737–742.

Walsh, S. L., Preston, K. L., Bigelow, G. E., & Stitzer, M. L. (1995). Acute administration of buprenorphine in humans: Partial agonist and blockade effects. *J Pharmacol Exp Ther, 55,* 361–372.

Woody, G. E., Luborsky, L., McLellan, A. T., O'Brien, C. P., Beck, A. T., Blaine, J. D., et al. (1983). Psychotherapy for opiate addicts: Does it help? *Arch Gen Psychiatry, 40,* 639–645.

Woody, G. E., McLellan, A. T., Luborsky, L., & O'Brien, C. P. (1987). Twelve-month follow-up of psychotherapy for opiate dependence. *Am J Psychiatry, 144,* 590–596.

Woody, G. E., McLellan, A. T., Luborsky, L., & O'Brien, C. P. (1995). Psychotherapy in community methadone programs: A validation study. *Am J Psychiatry, 152,* 1302–1308.

Index